Brinker, Piermattei, and Flo's
Handbook of
SMALL ANIMAL
ORTHOPEDICS *and*
FRACTURE REPAIR

847 548 5300
An ER+Tx Cat.

Brinker, Piermattei, and Flo's
Handbook of

SMALL ANIMAL ORTHOPEDICS *and* FRACTURE REPAIR

THIRD EDITION

DONALD L. PIERMATTEI, D.V.M., Ph.D.

Diplomate, American College of Veterinary Surgeons
Professor Emeritus
Department of Clinical Sciences
College of Veterinary Medicine and Biomedical Sciences
Colorado State University
Fort Collins, Colorado

GRETCHEN L. FLO, D.V.M., M.S.

Professor
Department of Small Animal Surgery and Medicine
Michigan State University
College of Veterinary Medicine
East Lansing, Michigan

Illustrations by F. Dennis Giddings, A.M.I., and Richard M. Fritzler, A.M.I.

W.B. SAUNDERS COMPANY

A Division of Harcourt Brace & Company

Philadelphia   London   Toronto   Montreal   Sydney   Tokyo

W.B. SAUNDERS COMPANY
A Division of Harcourt Brace & Company

The Curtis Center
Independence Square West
Philadelphia, Pennsylvania 19106

Library of Congress Cataloging-in-Publication Data

Piermattei, Donald L.
    Brinker, Piermattei, and Flo's Handbook of small animal orthopedics and fracture
repair / Donald L. Piermattei, Gretchen L. Flo ; illustrations by F. Dennis Giddings
and Richard M. Fritzler.—3rd ed.
      p. cm.
    Rev. ed. of: Handbook of small animal orthopedics & fracture
treatment / Wade O. Brinker, Donald L. Piermattei, Gretchen L. Flo.
2nd ed. 1990.
    Includes bibliographical references and index.
    ISBN 0-7216-5689-7
    1. Dogs—Surgery—Handbooks, manuals, etc. 2. Cats—Surgery—
Handbooks, manuals, etc. 3. Dogs—Fractures—Treatment—Handbooks,
manuals, etc. 4. Cats—Fractures—Treatment—Handbooks, manuals,
etc. 5. Veterinary orthopedics—Handbooks, manuals, etc.
6. Fractures in animals—Treatment—Handbooks, manuals, etc.
I. Flow, Gretchen L. II. Brinker, Wade O. Handbook of small animal
orthopedics & fracture treatment. III. Title.
SF991.P54   1997
636.089′67—dc21

                                                       96-39430

HANDBOOK OF SMALL ANIMAL ORTHOPEDICS
AND FRACTURE REPAIR   ISBN 0-7216-5689-7

Copyright © 1997, 1990, 1983 by W. B. Saunders Company

Printed in the United States of America.

Last digit is the print number: 9   8   7   6   5   4   3   2

PREFACE

From our viewpoint, the most notable aspect of this third edition is the retirement of our mentor and colleague Wade O. Brinker. Although he did not participate in this revision, his influence permeates everything we have written. He was responsible for both our orthopedic training and instilling in us the basic philosophy of surgical management of orthopedic disease. It has been a privilege to have shared in this friendship and collegiality with one of the pioneers of modern veterinary orthopedic surgery.

The aims of this edition remain constant with those of previous editions: to present this material in a straightforward, well illustrated, and readily understandable manner, usable by both the student and practicing surgeon, with the goal of rapid and complete return to function following treatment of locomotor impairment in our patients. The text is profusely illustrated for clarity and easy reference, and we are delighted to have F. Dennis Giddings back for the revisions and additional illustrations in this edition.

This handbook is not intended as an exhaustive reference, and rare and unusual conditions have again been omitted. Cited references have been kept to a minimum, with most over 10 years old having been dropped, excepting those we felt truly represented landmark publications. Extensive reorganization of the contents has taken place, aiming for a topographic regional coverage, by keeping coverage of both fractures and other conditions of an anatomic region in close physical proximity to each other.

The chapter on orthopedic examination has been expanded and also includes diagnostic tools such as nuclear medicine, computerized tomography, arthrography, and arthrocentesis procedures. The fracture classification scheme of the AO Vet has been incorporated as a basis for discussion of all long bone fractures, and as a part of the Fracture Patient Scoring System of Palmer, Hulse, and Aron, which allows the clinician to evaluate a specific fracture in a specific patient and decide on an appropriate method of fixation. We hope this approach to decisions on fixation methodology will eliminate the tendency to look for an illustration of a fracture that matches the radiograph and then to simply copy the fixation without considering all the clinical factors involved. Extensive consideration has been given to the emergence of the external fixator and the concept of biological fixation as principal factors in fracture treatment. Principles of fracture fixation, Chapter 2, has been expanded to give a detailed explanation of general principles of application of all forms of fixation, and special considerations for specific bones are covered in the appropriate chapter. Joint diseases and therapies has been reorganized and updated emphasizing techniques we find work best for us. The elbow chapter has been expanded to include treatment of congenital diseases.

Finally we recognize the fine folks at W.B. Saunders, Ray Kersey, David Kilmer, and all the production staff who have been patient, helpful, and understanding of the many diversions that always appear in our lives to slow the gestation of such a revision as this.

Donald L. Piermattei
Gretchen L. Flo

CONTENTS

NOTICE

Companion animal practice is an ever-changing field. Standard safety precautions must be followed, but as new research and clinical experience grow, changes in treatment and drug therapy become necessary or appropriate. The authors and editors of this work have carefully checked the generic and trade drug names and verified drug dosages to assure that dosage information is precise and in accord with standards accepted at the time of publication. Readers are advised, however, to check the product information currently provided by the manufacturer of each drug to be administered to be certain that changes have not been made in the recommended dose or in the contraindications for administration. This is of particular importance in regard to new or infrequently used drugs. Recommended dosages for animals are sometimes in regard to new or infrequently used drugs. Recommended dosages for animals are sometimes based on adjustments in the dosage that would be suitable for humans. Some of the drugs mentioned here have been given experimentally by the authors. Others have been used in dosages greater than those recommended by the manufacturer. It is the responsibility of those administering a drug, relying on their professional skill and experience, to determine the dosages, the best treatment for the patient, and whether the benefits of giving a drug justify the attendant risk. The editors cannot be responsible for misuse or misapplication of the material in this work.

PART I

GENERAL PRINCIPLES OF DIAGNOSIS AND TREATMENT OF FRACTURES, LAMENESS, AND JOINT DISEASE

1

Orthopedic Examination and Diagnostic Tools

GENERAL EXAMINATION

An orthopedic examination must begin with an adequate history and general physical examination. A systemic approach to the examination ensures that multiple problems are discovered. The animal's general health should be ascertained prior to focusing on the orthopedic complaint. The entire examination varies with the complexity of the case, a history of recent trauma, the intended use of the animal (e.g., breeding, showing, racing, hunting), and economics dictated by owners. Severely traumatized animals with hemorrhaging wounds and unstable fractures with danger of becoming open fractures obviously need different immediate steps and will not be discussed in this chapter. This chapter will focus on the examination for orthopedic problems (Table 1–1) and presentation of some of the diagnostic tools available.

History

Specific historical information is useful for categorizing rule outs. This includes breed, age, gender, occurrence of trauma, owner identification of limb(s) involved, chronological progression of the problem, efficacy of treatments tried, and variability with weather, exercise, and arising from recumbency. In addition, other features such as fever, inappetance, lethargy, weight loss, etc., may indicate some systemic problem such as inflammatory joint conditions, or a ruptured bladder following trauma.

Certain historical facts and deviation from the "normal" presentation of certain orthopedic conditions alert the clinician to investigate further than the obvious by asking appropriate questions or performing additional tests or procedures. For example, a 10-year-old dog that falls down two stairs and sustains a fractured radius and ulna should be carefully scrutinized for pathological fracture. Normally, chronic luxating patellas usually do not suddenly cause a carrying-leg lameness, and cruciate ligament rupture may have become the more recent problem. Chronic osteoarthritic conditions usually do not cause severe pain. In older animals with severe progressive pain, neoplasia must always be considered. With pelvic fractures, trauma to the chest, abdomen, or spine often occurs. Answers to specific questions help assess concurrent problems. For example, knowing whether the recumbent animal has been eating, voiding large pools of urine, or moving the legs spontaneously is helpful. A good appetite

TABLE 1–1. CAUSES OF LAMENESS IN THE DOG (EXCLUDING FRACTURES AND MINOR SOFT TISSUE INJURIES)

Pelvic Limb	Forelimb
GROWING DOG	GROWING DOG
1. hip dysplasia	1. OCD—shoulder
2. avascular necrosis (Legg-Calvé-Perthes)	2. luxation/subluxation shoulder—congenital
3. avulsion of long digital extensor	3. avulsion supraglenoid tubercle
4. OCD—stifle	4. OCD—elbow
5. OCD—hock	5. UAP
6. luxating patella complex	6. FCP
7. genu valgum	7. UME
8. panosteitis	8. elbow incongruity
Medium–large breeds = 1, 3–8	a. congenital
Toy–small breeds = 2, 6	b. physeal injury
Chondrodystrophied breeds = 1, 2, 6, 8	9. radius curvus
	10. retained cartilaginous cores (ulna)
ADULT DOG	11. panosteitis
A. arthritis (or continuum) 1–7	12. HOD
B. luxating patella complex	13. congenital shoulder luxation
C. panosteitis	Medium–large breeds = 1, 4–7, 8b, 9–12
D. cruciate/meniscal syndrome	Toy–small breeds = 2, 8, 9, 13
E. inflammatory joint disease	Chondrodystrophied breeds = 2?, 5, 8a, 8b, 9, 11, 13
F. neoplasia	
Medium–large breeds = A_1, A 3–7, B, F	ADULT DOG
Toy–small breeds = A_2, B, D–F	A. arthritis (or continuum) 1–6, 8, 9
Chondrodystrophied breeds = A_1, A_2, B, D–F	B. UME
	C. panosteitis
	D. bicipital tenosynovitis
	E. calcification of supraspinatus tendon
	F. contracture of infraspinatus or supraspinatus
	G. bone/soft tissue neoplasia
	H. luxation/subluxation—shoulder
	I. inflammatory joint disease
	J. HO
	K. SCM
	Medium–giant breeds = A, 7, 11, I, J, K
	Toy–small breeds = 2, G, H, I, J, K
	Chondrodystrophied breeds = 2?, A–5, A–8, A–9, C, H, I, J, K

OCD = osteochondritis dissecans; UAP = ununited anconeal process; FCP = fragmented coronoid process; UME = ununited medial epicondyle; HOD = hypertrophic osteodystrophy; HO = hypertrophic osteopathy; SCM = synovial chondrometaplasia.

probably does not occur with significant internal injuries. "Urinating" or dribbling small amounts of urine does *not* mean the bladder is intact, and voluntary leg movement usually means serious thoracolumbar spinal injury has not occurred.

Distant Observation

The animal should be observed for general thriftiness and relative weight status. Patient disposition and potential lack of cooperation by owner and animal should be noted. Sedation should not be used if possible or at least until the area of involvement is known because tranquilizers may mask detection of painful regions. The animal should be observed for body conformation, decreased weight bearing, trembling, asymmetrical joint or soft tissue swellings, muscle atrophy, and digit and joint alignment. Dogs with tarsocrural osteochondritis dissecans (OCD) tend to be very straight legged in the pelvic limb, while dogs with elbow problems tend to have curvature of the forelimbs (Fig. 1–1).

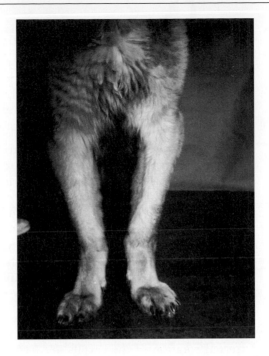

FIGURE 1–1. Typical forelimb curvature in a German shepherd affected with ununited anconeal process. Note varus angulation of the elbows and valgus of the carpi.

Gait

Observing the lameness is helpful prior to examining the limb. It helps confirm or contradict owner complaints. Often in an exam room environment, however, chronic lameness disappears. The gait is observed at a walk and if necessary a trot. Covert lameness may become apparent with tight circles or stair climbing. Abnormalities include a shortened stride, dragging of the toenails, "toeing-in" or "toeing-out," limb circumduction, hypermetria, stumbling, generalized weakness, ataxia, criss-crossing of the legs, abnormal sounds (e.g., clicks, snaps), and a head "bob," which is a bobbing motion of the head that occurs with foreleg lameness. The head elevates as the painful leg strikes the ground.

Standing Palpation

With the animal standing as symmetrically as possible, both hands examine the contralateral aspects of the limbs simultaneously observing for asymmetry produced by trauma, inflammation, neoplasia, degenerative joint changes, and congenital defects. Signs to palpate are swelling, heat, malaligned bony landmarks, crepitus, and muscle atrophy. Muscle atrophy may be palpated directly if the examiner can grasp around a muscle (e.g., gastrocnemius muscle), or indirectly by discerning a more prominent adjacent bone (e.g., acromion, trochanter major). With bilateral conditions, experience or radiography is used to distinguish abnormality.

Foreleg

Specific landmarks to observe in the foreleg are the acromion, spine and vertebral border of the scapula, greater tubercle of the humerus, humeral epicondyles, olecranon, and accessory carpal bone which is located at the level of the radiocarpal joint.

SCAPULOHUMERAL REGION ■ Trauma and neoplasia affect the scapula. The scapulohumeral region is affected with congenital OCD, developmental calcification of the supraspinatus, bicipital tendinitis, and joint luxation. The lateral aspect is palpated. The relative position and size of the greater tubercle of the humerus are noted, which are altered with shoulder luxation or tumors of the proximal humerus. Muscle atrophy from any chronic (over 3 to 4 weeks) foreleg lameness is often detected as a more prominent acromion.

ELBOW AND FOREARM ■ Traumatic and congenital elbow incongruities, congenitally unstable fragments, fracture, and luxation occur in the elbow. Elbow joint effusion is especially noted laterally between the lateral epicondyle of the humerus and the olecranon. Normally, only a thin anconeus muscle lies under the skin. With increased joint fluid, a bulge occurs between these two bony landmarks in the weight-bearing limb that often disappears with non–weight-bearing. Osteophytes are noted as an extra ridge lying between the epicondyle and the olecranon. The width of the condyles is compared to the opposite side and is increased with condylar fracture or elbow dislocation. The radius and ulnar regions are palpated for swelling and malalignment.

CARPUS AND PAW ■ The carpal and paw regions are affected with fracture, malalignment, joint swelling, and proliferative bony changes. Valgus and external rotation of the carpus are frequently seen with congenital elbow conditions (Fig. 1–1) and with growth plate injuries. The dorsal carpal and metacarpal regions are palpated for swelling. Further examination takes place in the recumbent animal.

NEUROLOGICAL EXAMINATION ■ Conscious proprioception of the foreleg is carried out at this point. With the animal standing with the forelegs parallel, the chest is supported while the paw is knuckled over on its dorsal aspect. This is repeated several times. The paw should quickly right itself. A normal animal will usually not even allow the dorsum of the paw to be placed on the floor, unlike the rear limb (Fig. 1–2). The neck is flexed and extended to elicit a painful response or stimulation of cervical muscle spasms. The dorsal spines of the thoracolumbar regions are pressed downward to elicit pain. In dogs with lumbosacral disease, this pressure may cause a sudden sitting position.

The thoracic and abdominal areas are palpated before proceeding to the pelvic limb.

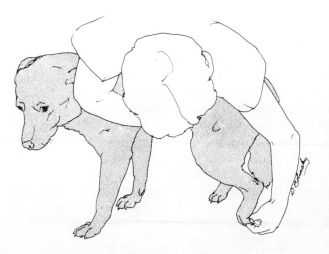

FIGURE 1–2. Conscious proprioceptive response is elicited while the dog is standing with the limbs in a normal position. The dog is supported while the toes are turned over and released. A delay or absence of the dog's quickly returning the toes to a normal position may mean neurological rather than orthopedic problems.

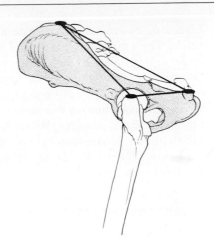

FIGURE 1–3. If imaginary lines are drawn between the wing of the ilium, tuber ischii, and trochanter major, a triangle is formed.

Pelvic Limb

PELVIS ■ Landmarks to note on the pelvic limb are the iliac crests of the ilium, trochanters major, tubers ischii, extensor mechanism (quadriceps, patella, patellar ligament, and tibial tubercle), femoral condyles, distal tibia, fibular tarsal bone, and Achilles tendon.

Asymmetry of the bones of the pelvis could mean pelvic fracture, hip dislocation, femoral head fracture, or chronic coxofemoral arthritis. If imaginary lines are drawn from the wings of the ilium, trochanters major, and tubers ischii, a triangle is formed (Fig. 1–3). With craniodorsal coxofemoral dislocation, the triangle becomes more acute (Fig. 1–4), the trochanter major more prominent, and when the rear quarters are elevated, the toes on the dislocated side appear "shorter." With unilateral ilial fracture and overriding segments, the trochanter major may be closer to the wing of the ilium than the opposite side. In addition, the lateral musculature is swollen. The muscles of the cranial and caudal thigh, and gastrocnemius are palpated.

STIFLE ■ The stifle joint is frequently affected with degenerative, congenital, and traumatic conditions that include cruciate ligament rupture, patellar luxation, OCD, and physeal fracture. Stifle palpation begins with locating the tibial tubercle and following the patellar ligament proximally. Abnormal deviation of the tubercle from the midline plane should be noted and occurs with patellar

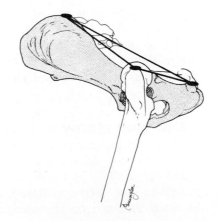

FIGURE 1–4. With hip dislocation, the triangular shape becomes altered when compared with the other normal hip of the dog (compare with Fig. 1–3).

luxation. Normal patellar ligaments should be taut and approximately pencil thick. The cranial two thirds of the pencil-like ligament can be grasped. With stifle injury, swelling from the joint pushes forward around the caudal and lateral aspects of the patellar ligament, making the ligament less distinct and more "band-like" than "pencil-like." The patella is found 1 to 4 cm proximal to the tubercle, but may be better examined in the recumbent animal when joint manipulation is possible. With chronic stifle swelling and osteophyte formation, the diameter of the femoral condylar ridges is enlarged. This is assessed 1 to 2 cm behind the patella. In addition, there may be joint swelling medially between the femur and tibia.

HOCK ■ The tarsocrural joint is affected with traumatic and congenital conditions. Swelling of the hock joint is detected on the standing animal by palpating between the distal tibia and the fibular tarsal bone. Normally, only skin, subcutaneous tissue, and bone are present. Joint swelling from increased fluid accumulation or fibrosis is detected as a firm, soft tissue mass between those two landmarks. Additionally, swelling may be detected cranially or medially. The Achilles tendon is examined above the calcaneus for swelling and continuity.

Recumbent Examination

The animal is placed in lateral recumbency to thoroughly examine previously noted abnormalities. This allows patient restraint and limb manipulations but precludes simultaneous palpation of the opposite side. Most maneuvers discussed do not produce pain in normal animals. Pain production gives the diagnostician clues as to the location of the problem. It may be best to examine the normal side first to relax the animal and to learn individual responses to certain maneuvers. The veterinarian is looking for instability, crepitus, painful regions, and altered ranges of motion. Animals usually do not mind gentle manipulation of abnormal areas. Often, animals do not indicate when a painful area is manipulated, which creates a diagnostic challenge at times. In general, it is well to examine from the toes proximally. Known abnormal areas or maneuvers that may produce pain should be examined last to ensure patient cooperation. Maneuvers producing painful responses should be carefully and gently repeated while immobilizing surrounding tissues to reduce the possibility of misinterpreting the origin of the pain.

Crepitus (a sound or palpable friction sensation) occurs when bone rubs bone, cartilage rubs bone, or subcutaneous tissues move over air pockets or foreign materials such as wires, pins, or suture material. The sensations palpated are characterized as clicks, snaps, clunks, crackling, grinding, or grating. Normal laxity of the carpal, tarsal, or shoulder regions produces innocent clicks that are mistaken as crepitus. In some thin dogs, elbow flexion produces clicks as the ulnar nerve moves over a prominent humeral epicondyle.

Forelimb

PAW AND ELBOW ■ The digits are flexed, extended, and examined for swelling, crepitus, and pain. The interdigital webbing and foot pads are examined for discoloration, abrasions, etc. The proximal sesamoid bones are palpated for swelling on the palmar aspect of the paw at the metacarpophalangeal junction. The carpus is flexed, extended, and a valgus/varus stress applied. Swelling detected on the standing examination is better identified when the exact location of the joint space can be identified. This helps to rule out joint problems from distal radial swelling seen with neoplasia or hypertrophic osteodystrophy. The radiocarpal joint space lies at the same level as the base of the accessory carpal bone.

The elbow is similarly placed through a range of motion. Hyperextension of the elbow may produce pain in dogs with ununited anconeal process, while internal and external rotation with digital pressure applied at the medial joint line may produce pain accompanying conditions such as OCD or fragmented coronoid process.

SHOULDER ■ Swelling of the shoulder joint unfortunately cannot be appreciated because of its depth under musculature. The shoulder is examined for pain by flexing and extending the joint while grasping the forearm with one hand while the other hand stabilizes the front of the shoulder. OCD usually produces pain with this maneuver. Bicipital tendinitis or rupture is painful when the tendon is stretched. To produce diagnostic discomfort, the elbow is extended and the entire limb is pulled caudally along the thoracic wall while digital pressure is applied to the proximal medial humeral region over the tendon (Fig. 1–5).

Fractures of the acromion can cause discomfort and possibly crepitus when the acromion is manipulated. Shoulder instability may be appreciated, usually in the sedated or anesthetized patient, by applying a medial and lateral sliding motion at the joint level.

LONG-BONE PALPATION ■ All areas of the limb are gently squeezed. Long-bone palpation is reserved for the last part of the examination because pain from bone tumor or panosteitis is exquisite at times. To avoid production of pain from pressing normal muscle, it is well to find muscle planes where the fingers can reach bone. These locations include the distal radius, the proximal ulna, and the distal and proximal humerus. Once the fingers touch the bone, a gentle pressure is applied.

Neurofibromas or neurofibrosarcomas must be considered in older dogs with severe progressive foreleg lameness. In these special cases, deep digital pressure in the axilla may detect a mass and produce exquisite pain. In addition, ocular signs of Horner's syndrome (unilateral miosis, ptosis, and enophthalmus) may be present. The "mass" may be compared to the other side in the standing animal.

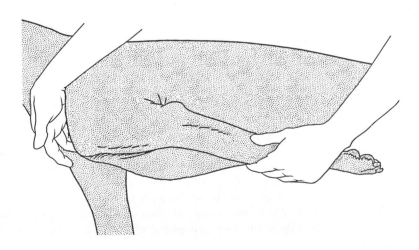

FIGURE 1–5. To detect bicipital tendon pain, the tendon is stretched by extending the elbow and bringing the entire limb parallel to the thorax. Digital pressure is applied to the tendon in the proximal medial humeral region.

Rear Limb

PAW AND HOCK ■ The digits and paw are examined similar to the foreleg. The tarsal region is stressed in extension, flexion, varus, and valgus angles. Instability, pain, and crepitus may be produced with fracture, tendon and ligament breakdown (seen especially in collies and shelties), and OCD of the talus. Achilles tendon continuity is palpated during flexion and extension of the tarsocrural joint.

STIFLE ■ The stifle joint is commonly affected with luxating patellas and cruciate ligament disease, as well as physeal fractures of the distal femur. With fracture, the stifle is quite swollen with a history of young animals sustaining trauma. Swelling also occurs with inflammatory joint conditions, and OCD. Localized swelling occurs with avulsion of the origin of the long digital extensor tendon.

Patellar Luxation ■ With some animals, there is normal mediolateral movement within the trochlea of the femur. Luxation out of the trochlea is abnormal and can cause lameness. Subluxation (patella rides on the trochlear ridge, and "catches" during flexion) occasionally causes lameness. Luxation may be medial or less commonly lateral and occasionally both directions. Luxation of a patella is normally not a painful maneuver. The examiner should stand caudally to the animal. To begin the examination, the tibial tubercle is located and its position noted. Noting the medial location of the tibial tubercle helps avoid misinterpreting a medial luxation (ectopic) that is replaced into the trochlea (i.e., reduced) from a reduced patella that can be luxated laterally. Cat tubercles are not as prominent as dog tubercles. The patella may be found 1 to 4 cm proximally. In small dogs or cats with ectopic patellas, the patella is palpated as a small pea-like bump on the medial (or lateral) femoral condyle. It may or may not move with flexion, extension, and digital pressure. It may or may not be reducible. To luxate a reduced patella medially, the stifle is extended, the toes are internally rotated, and digital pressure is applied to the patella in a medial direction (Fig. 1–6). Conversely, to luxate a patella laterally, the stifle is flexed slightly, toes are externally rotated, and pressure is applied in a lateral direction (Fig. 1–7). Sometimes an unstable patella may be luxated just by internally or externally rotating the paw. A patella that has been luxated upon examination should be reduced. The stifle should *always* be examined for cruciate ligament instability and with the patella reduced.

Cruciate Ligament Instability ■ Palpation for cruciate ligament instability can produce pain and should be performed gently in the relaxed patient. Sedation may be needed if no abnormality can be detected in the tense animal. Drawer movement is the sliding of the bony tibia in relation to the femur. Normally, there is no cranial or caudal drawer movement in the adult animal. Some large puppies have "puppy" drawer, which lasts up to 10 to 12 months of age due to normal joint laxity. Some rotary motion of the tibia is normal and is occasionally mistaken as drawer movement. In a fresh, fully torn cruciate ligament in a relaxed medium-sized animal, the tibia may slide 5 to 10 mm (grade 4). Relatively, larger dogs have less drawer movement than small dogs. Other factors that diminish full drawer movement are chronicity, animal tenseness, partial ligament tear, and the presence of a meniscal injury. Increased drawer movement occurs with multiple ligament tears in the traumatized animal or in Cushingoid dogs. If there is patellar luxation, the patella should be reduced if possible before examining for cruciate instability.

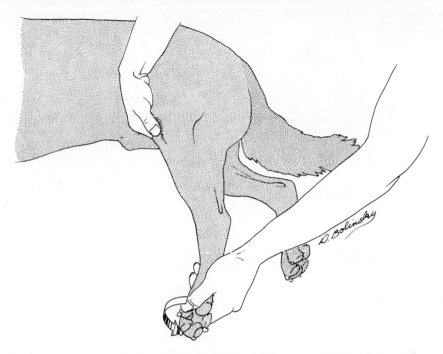

FIGURE 1–6. To luxate the patella medially, the stifle is extended and the toes rotated medially while the patella is pushed medially.

The tibial compression test (indirect drawer movement) compresses the femur and tibia together, and when there is cranial cruciate ligament incompetence, the tibia slides forward in relation to the femur. It can be elicited by holding the stifle in a slightly flexed position while the paw is alternately dorsiflexed as far as possible and then relaxed. The index finger of the opposite hand lies

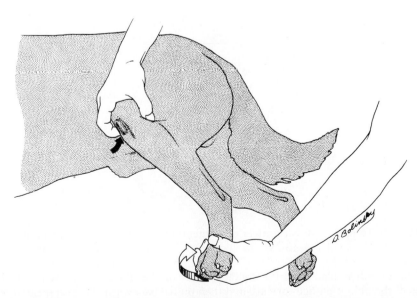

FIGURE 1–7. To luxate the patella laterally, the stifle is partially flexed and the toes are rotated laterally while the patella is pulled laterally.

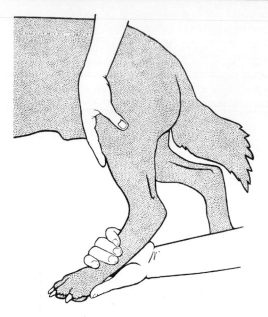

FIGURE 1–8. The tibial compression test produces indirect drawer movement. With the stifle angle held in slight flexion, the metatarsal region is dorsiflexed as far as possible. The index finger of the opposite hand detects the forward movement of the tibial tuberosity if drawer movement is present. It is repeated several times.

cranial to the femur, patellar ligament, and tibial tubercle and detects the tubercle sliding forward (Fig. 1–8). It is repeated several times quickly but gently.[1] Interpretation of this maneuver is more subjective than direct drawer movement, but has the advantage of producing little pain in animals with ruptured cranial cruciate ligaments.

Direct drawer movement (Fig. 1–9) is examined by placing the fingers as close as possible to bone and not soft tissue. The index finger of one hand is

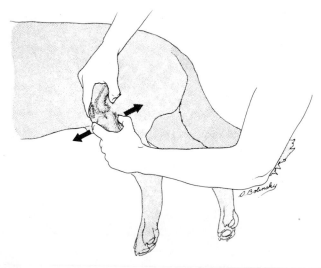

FIGURE 1–9. To palpate direct drawer movement, the index finger of one hand is placed on the proximal patellar region while the thumb is placed caudal to the lateral fabella. The index finger of the opposite hand is placed on the cranial aspect of the tibial crest, while the thumb is placed on the caudal aspect of the fibular head. With the femur stabilized, the tibia is pushed forward and then pulled backward. This is repeated several times and is performed gently but quickly to detect 1 to 10 mm of movement of the tibia in relation to the femur.

placed on the cranial proximal patellar region while the thumb is placed caudally on the lateral fabella. The index finger of the opposite hand is placed on the cranial aspect of the tibial crest while the thumb is positioned caudally on the fibular head. With the wrists held straight and not bent, the femur is held stable while the tibia is pushed forward (and not rotated) and then pulled backward. This is repeated quickly and gently several times. At first the stifle is held firmly in slight extension, and then repeated with the stifle held in extension, and then in flexion.

Interpretation of Instability ■ With cranial cruciate ligament rupture, the cranial end point is "soft" with no sudden stoppage, because the secondary restraints of the stifle become taut. When the tibia is pulled caudally, a sudden "thud" is palpated as the normal caudal cruciate ligament becomes taut. Conversely, with rare caudal cruciate rupture (usually grade 2 or less of motion), when cranial force is applied, there is a sudden "thud" that is not present when caudal force is applied. "Puppy" drawer (grade 2 or less of motion) has a sudden end point cranially and caudally. It usually disappears by 6 to 9 months of age unless chronic painful conditions of the hip, stifle, or hock exist.

Five common mistakes are made by inexperienced palpaters of the stifle. If the wrists are bent or if just the fingertips alone touch bone, proper force cannot be applied. Thirdly, if the fingers are placed laterally/medially instead of cranially/caudally, the skin moves and is misinterpreted as drawer. If drawer movement is performed slowly, detection of 1 to 2 mm of motion is impossible. Lastly, tibial rotary movements, which may be normal or excessive, are misinterpreted as drawer.

Collateral Ligament Instability ■ When the collateral ligaments *and* joint capsule are torn, the stifle will have medial, lateral, or combined instability. Cutting either of these ligaments alone without cutting the joint capsule will not produce much instability in research animals. The cruciate ligament(s) is (are) invariably torn in clinical cases of collateral instability. To detect this instability, the stifle should be held in "neutral" drawer while a valgus (stifle inward) or varus (stifle outward) force is applied. The thumb is placed on the fibular head while the index finger is placed along the medial joint line to perceive the joint opening abnormally with its respective instability.

Meniscal Injury ■ Meniscal injury is suspected when the owner hears a click when the animal walks, or the animal has a severe three-legged lameness several weeks after acute onset of stifle lameness. In addition, a worsening of an improving lameness several weeks to months after cruciate rupture with or without surgical repair sometimes indicates meniscal involvement. Meniscal injury is suspected when flexion, extension (with and without rotation about the stifle), and direct and indirect drawer manipulations produce a click, snap, clunk, or grating. Definitive diagnosis is made upon visualizing the unstable caudal horn or a part of it malpositioned after arthrotomy (see Chapter 17).

HIP JOINT AND PELVIS ■ The hip joint and pelvis are commonly affected with trauma, and congenital conditions such as Legg-Calvé-Perthes, and hip dysplasia. Manipulations may cause pain, crepitus, and instability. The femur is grasped at the stifle and the hip flexed and extended several times. If pain or crepitus is not produced, external hip rotation is added to the flexion and extension maneuvers. This maneuver frequently elicits pain with Legg-Calvé-Perthes. Fine crepitus may be heard when the examiner's ear or stethoscope is placed on the trochanter major during these manipulations. Pressing the femur

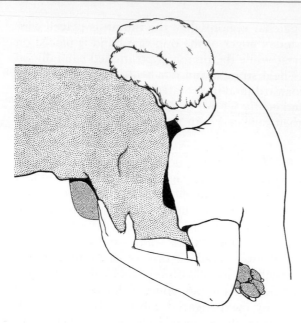

FIGURE 1–10. To hear finer crepitus from coxofemoral arthritis, the examiner's ear is placed on the trochanter major during flexion, extension, abduction, and adduction of the hip joint. Proximal pressure during these movements accentuates the sounds.

into the acetabulum accentuates the crepitus (Fig. 1–10). This crepitus must be distinguished from hair-coat noises. Suspected fracture and dislocation are further evaluated by radiography.

The sacroiliac joint is examined for instability by gentle manipulation of the wing of the ilium. The tuber ischii is pressed to detect instability and crepitus. A rectal examination may detect pubic and ischial fractures.

Hip laxity seen with hip dysplasia may be detected by three methods. The sign of Ortolani is a noise or palpable "thud" produced when an unstable hip is replaced into the acetabulum.[2] To produce this while the dog is in lateral recumbency, the hip is subluxated proximally by grasping the adducted stifle and pushing proximally while the other hand stabilizes the pelvis. When the stifle is abducted, downward pressure is applied across the trochanteric region

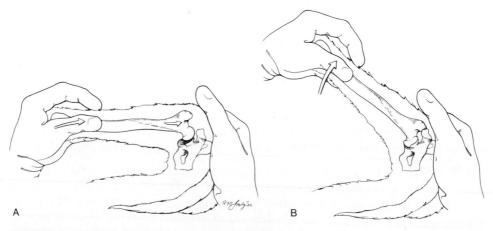

A　　　　　　　　　B

FIGURE 1–11. The Ortolani sign is the sound produced when the subluxated hip is suddenly reduced into the acetabulum. To subluxate the hip joint, the stifle joint is adducted while proximal pressure is applied (*A*). Reduction of the subluxation occurs when the stifle is abducted, which reduces the hip creating a "thud" (*B*).

and a noise is produced as the femoral head glides over the rim into the ace-tabulum (Fig. 1–11). This can also be done bilaterally with the dog in dorsal recumbency. The stifles are adducted, pushed proximally, and then abducted to produce the "thud" (see Fig. 20–8C, D, E). A third way to detect this instability is to place the dog in lateral recumbency. One palm stabilizes the pelvis with two fingers on the trochanteric region while the other hand grasps the distal femur and positions it parallel to the table or floor. The femoral head is alter-nately levered laterally and relaxed while the fingers on the trochanter major are alternately relaxed and then pressed downward. The amount of subluxation in millimeters may be detected. However, this maneuver is often painful even in normal animals due to the force applied on the thigh muscles. Muscle tension often masks the instability.

DIAGNOSTIC TOOLS

Beyond the physical examination, there are several tools available for diag-nosing and evaluating orthopedic diseases and treatments. These include ra-diography, fluoroscopy, arthrography, myelography, diagnostic ultrasonography (DUS), computed tomography (CT), magnetic resonance imaging (MRI), nu-clear imaging, arthroscopy, force plate analysis, kinematic gait analysis, explor-atory surgery, biopsy, clinical pathological tests, arthrocentesis with joint fluid analysis, serology, and hormonal assay. A brief description of each of these modalities follows along with their uses.

RADIOGRAPHY ■ By far, the most common diagnostic tool used to inves-tigate orthopedic disease is radiography. The history and physical examination should suggest the area of the body involved. Radiography is also used to rule out other concurrent common diseases such as a large dog with cruciate liga ment rupture with concurrent hip dysplasia. It is very useful in detecting and evaluating fractures, joint dislocations, osteoarthrosis, neoplasia, joint incon-gruities, and congenital joint conditions (such as OCD and hip dysplasia). It is also useful in evaluating fracture fixation and healing as well as following pro-gress of joint treatments. In general, two orthogonal (90 degrees to each other) views of an area are taken. Special views are discussed elsewhere under each disease. Many times, animals even with fractures may be positioned for radi-ography without sedation if enough personnel are available. If personnel are unavailable or state laws prohibit their exposure to radiation, then sedation or anesthesia may be required using appropriate positioning and restraining devices.

FLUOROSCOPY ■ Another modality using radiation is fluoroscopy with or without image intensification. It is occasionally used to detect instability (e.g., shoulder luxation), retrieve metallic foreign materials (pins, wires, bullets), ob-serve contrast material used in arthrography, confirm needle placement for mye-lography and angiography, and aid placement of surgical implants. Fluoroscopy is a "movie" of radiographic images, and image intensification enhances the signal to reduce the amount of radiation necessary to see the images. Spot hard-copy films can be made from selected images.

ARTHROGRAPHY ■ An arthrogram is a radiograph of a joint after a con-trast substance such as an iodine solution, air, or both have been injected. In-jection techniques are discussed later. The most frequent joint undergoing arthrography is the shoulder joint. Interruption of contrast material flow occurs with bicipital tendonitis or rupture. It is useful in identifying obscure OCD cartilaginous flaps. The contrast solution we prefer is a half-and-half mixture of sterile water and 60 percent Hypaque (diatrizoate meglumine and diatrizoate sodium, used for intravenous pyelograms). The shoulder of a 30-kg dog should have 2 to 3 ml of this mixture injected and radiographs taken within 5 to 10 minutes after which the ionic solution is resorbed or diluted with synovial effusion and loses its contrast quality. In a recent study, nonionic contrast agents were found to have superior radiographic imaging qualities owing to their decreased absorption rate and/or joint fluid influx. However, they are also more costly.[3]

MYELOGRAPHY ■ Myelography is the process of injecting the spinal intrathecal space with a water-soluble nonionic sterile iodine solution to detect abnormal obstruction or deviation of contrast material flow due to spinal neoplasia, degenerative disk disease, or vertebral trauma and instability. Contrast agents, such as iohexol and iopamidol, are used for myelography.

COMPUTER TOMOGRAPHY ■ CT is specialized radiography in which cross-sectional images of a body structure are reconstructed by a computer. A CT unit is an apparatus in which the x-ray source moves in one direction while the x-ray detector moves in synchrony in the opposite direction (Fig. 1–12). This allows detailed vision without obscuration from superimposed structures. With computer configuration, serial "slices" as small as 1.5 mm in width may be made through a body part. These machines cost between $350,000 and $1,100,000, and some veterinary teaching hospitals have these machines or have access to them at human hospitals. Its primary use in small animals is examination of the spine, skull, and brain. It can also be used in conjunction with contrast agents. It is very helpful in diagnosing fragmented coronoid process disease in dogs (see Chapter 11). It is useful in guiding a surgeon trying to locate a radiodense foreign body, or discovering subtle joint fractures. Two

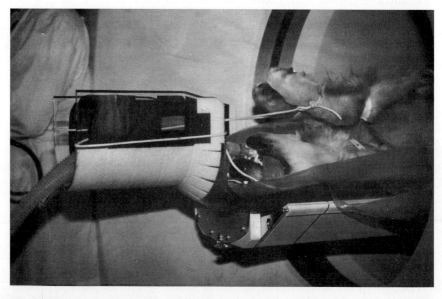

FIGURE 1–12. An anesthetized dog is placed into the gantry of a CT machine. The black circular region contains the ionizing radiation source.

disadvantages of this diagnostic modality is that anesthesia must be used, and it is not particularly useful for soft tissue conditions.

MAGNETIC RESONANCE IMAGING ■   MRI is another newer imaging piece of equipment even more expensive than CT ($750,000 to $2,000,000) which, in addition, needs a special dedicated room for its use. MRI produces computer images of internal body tissues from magnetic resonance of atoms within the body induced by the application of radio waves. Again, animals must be anesthetized and the study usually performed at human hospitals. Its biggest advantage in human orthopedics is that soft tissue and articular cartilage can be studied. It is *the* best noninvasive technique for diagnosing meniscal and cruciate injuries in humans.

NUCLEAR IMAGING ■   Nuclear imaging uses radioactive pharmaceuticals that when given intravenously accumulate in certain organs based upon their chemical structure and the carrier to which they are bound. These radioactive materials accumulate in vascularized tissues, and can be compared with contralateral limbs to detect increased vascularity seen with inflammation, trauma, or neoplasia. Radioactive decay emits gamma radiation that is detected by a scintillation crystal (gamma camera; Fig. 1–13) and transmitted to a dedicated computer for image production. In animals, technetium-99m methylene diphosphonate (^{99m}Tc MDP) is used for bone scans, and is distributed in soft tissues for imaging within 4 to 8 minutes. Bone uptake may be imaged 2 to 8 hours following intravenous injection. Both phases are scanned with the animal under sedation. The animal must be housed in special holding facilities while radiation decay occurs. Gamma cameras cost over $2000, but the computer that creates the image and hard copy can cost over $300,000. In humans, it can be used to detect stress fractures, while in the horse it is helpful in identifying the anatomic origin of occult lameness. In small animals, its use is becoming more popular to detect early neoplastic, inflammatory, and traumatic lesions.

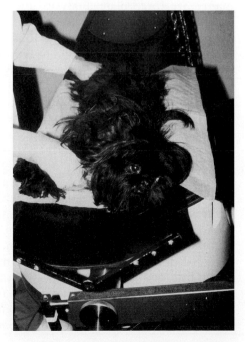

FIGURE 1–13. A sedated dog is positioned over the radiation detector or gamma camera (white object) for nuclear imaging.

DIAGNOSTIC ULTRASONOGRAPHY ■ DUS is infrequently used for musculoskeletal problems in small animal medicine. It has been used somewhat successfully in diagnosing bicipital tendonitis in dogs, although it was less reliable than arthrography.[4] It may be useful for other problems such as the evaluation of soft tissue masses and OCD. The application of DUS in skeletal evaluation is poor due to absorption of sound waves by bone.

ARTHROSCOPY ■ Arthroscopy involves puncturing a joint with a specialized endoscope after distention with a liquid or gas for the purpose of exploration and surgical repair if indicated. This modality is extremely useful in human medicine because there is less surgical trauma resulting in less pain, shorter hospitalization, less time off work or physical activity, quicker healing time, and less adhesion formation. When appropriate arthroscopic equipment became available to perform therapeutic manipulations, it became more than a diagnostic tool. Many surgeons became trained in its use and it is cost effective. Arthroscopy is also extremely useful in horses with loose bone and/or cartilage bodies in joints where open surgery and its long rehabilitation would cause an economic loss in the performance individual. Pet owners frequently ask if small animal veterinarians have the capability to perform arthroscopy, and the answer at this point is that it is impractical, although a few referral centers have used it.[5,6] Other surgical manipulations such as ligament reconstruction, internal fixation of bony fragments, and meniscal repair require more sophisticated equipment and surgical training. Dogs ordinarily do not get the joint stiffness that people get from open surgery, probably due to their high pain tolerance. Dogs that could benefit from the commonly available equipment are those suffering from loose OCD or coronoid fragments. However, these dogs use their legs immediately after conventional open surgery, thereby minimizing the apparent advantages of arthroscopy. Additionally, there are no savings in anesthesia or patient preparation time.

FORCE PLATE ANALYSIS AND KINEMATIC GAIT ANALYSIS ■ Two relatively new research tools used in veterinary medicine to evaluate gait performance are force plate analysis[7] and kinematic or motion analysis.[8] They are included in this chapter because they are a more objective means than clinical impression to evaluate function following certain orthopedic treatments. Some recent reports compare different treatments for specific conditions (e.g., different cruciate ligament repairs, total hip replacement versus excisional arthroplasty) using these modalities. These tools detect altered gait that may not be apparent upon visual observation.

Briefly, *force plate* analysis is a system where the magnitude of weight-bearing (ground-reactive) force can be measured as the animal steps onto a sensor plate during gait (Fig. 1–14). Multiple passes are completed across the force plate to acquire representative data. Assessment of lameness grade may now be quantitated. However, it only measures the force on that single step as the animal strikes the plate. It does not measure problems that owners see such as stiffness upon arising, or lameness after running 3 to 4 miles.

Motion analysis has the advantage of allowing multiple measurements of successive motions during locomotion. Multiple markers are placed on the skin at different joint levels. During locomotion, these markers move and are detected by video cameras whose signals are sent to a computer (Fig. 1–15). Limb movements may be calculated at 60 to 100 measurements per second, which allows precise definition of normal versus lame gait. Different joint angles and the duration of stance and swing phases of the gait cycle vary with the joint

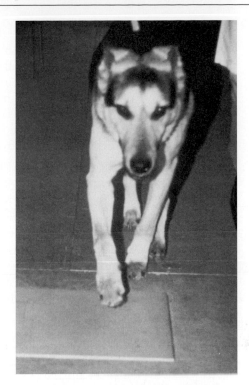

FIGURE 1–14. A dog is stepping one foot on the rectangular force plate.

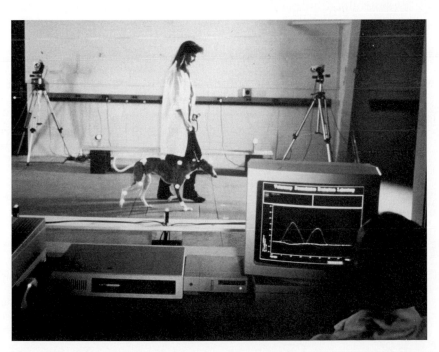

FIGURE 1–15. Kinematic motion analysis. Multiple markers are attached to the animal and then gaited between video cameras that send marker location signals to a computer. As many as 100 measurements per second can be made. Joint angles and duration of gait phase may be analyzed. (Courtesy of Dr. Charles DeCamp.)

affected. Thus, a dog's gait with hip dysplasia may be characterized.[9] During most of the stance phase, hip extension is quicker, but has increased extension compared to normal. Coxofemoral flexion is more rapid in the early swing phase, but slower in the middle of swing phase. There are also distal alterations in the stifle and tarsus. Medical or surgical treatments may then be compared to the individual's baseline data. Perhaps in the future it will be helpful in distinguishing which area is the cause of lameness when multiple abnormalities are found in the same limb (e.g., elbow arthrosis, calcification of the supraspinatus, possible bicipital tendonitis).

EXPLORATORY SURGERY ■   Exploratory surgery is often used to totally assess a condition or to discover the origin of joint, muscle, or bone problems. For example, a mature dog with a swollen stifle without drawer movement or patellar instability may have a partial cruciate tear, an old OCD lesion, inflammatory joint disease, synovial tumor or synovial chondromatosis. It allows gross inspection of the joint as well as the opportunity to obtain biopsy specimens. Tissues removed should be of sufficient volume to be representative and to allow for histopathology, microbiology, or both.

ARTHROCENTESIS ■   Arthrocentesis involves puncture and aspiration of joint fluid. Fluid may be grossly inspected, cultured, or analyzed for cell types and numbers (see Table 6–3), protein, viscosity, and glucose content. In addition it allows instillation of medications, dye, or air for arthrography. With all joint injections, the hair is clipped and surgical scrub applied. Spinal needles (18- to 22-gauge) are used. Care must be taken to avoid scratching the articular surfaces and make a "clean" puncture to avoid blood contamination. The appearance of joint fluid confirms proper needle placement. If no fluid appears, the needle is reintroduced in the same region, moved slightly, or approached from the other side of the joint if possible. Often with swollen inflamed joints (rheumatoid arthritis), there is little extracellular fluid present.

The techniques for various arthrocentesis sites are as follows:

Coxofemoral joint—the needle is introduced just cranioproximal to the trochanter major, aimed slightly ventrally and caudally (Fig. 1–16).

Stifle—with the stifle flexed, the needle is introduced medial or lateral to the patellar ligament midway between the femur and tibia. Lack of fluid could mean the needle is in the fat pad or cruciate ligaments (Fig. 1–17). Alter-

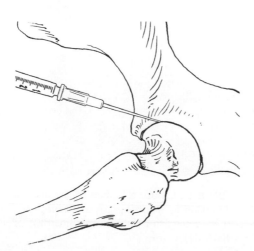

FIGURE 1–16. Arthrocentesis of the coxofemoral joint. The needle is introduced proximal and cranial to the trochanter major, with the needle directed somewhat ventrally.

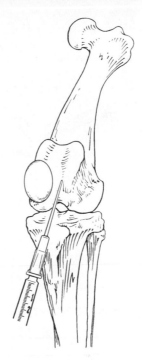

FIGURE 1–17. Arthrocentesis of the stifle joint. With the knee flexed, the needle is introduced just medial or lateral to the midportion of the straight patellar ligament.

natively, the needle may be aimed carefully toward the femoral condyle just below the patella. There is less fat pad interference, but the needle may scratch the femoral surface.

Tarsocrural joint—with the tarsocrural joint hyperextended (that distends the joint caudally), the needle is inserted lateral or medial to the fibular tarsal bone and aimed cranially toward the middle of the joint (Fig. 1–18). If swelling appears to be more cranially, then a cranial approach can be used.

Shoulder joint—the needle is inserted about 1 cm distal to the acromion process and just slightly caudal to it (Fig. 1–19). If fluid is not found, the needle should be "walked" in different directions from the same skin punc-

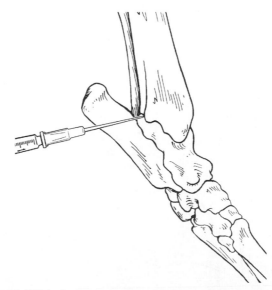

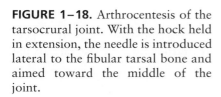

FIGURE 1–18. Arthrocentesis of the tarsocrural joint. With the hock held in extension, the needle is introduced lateral to the fibular tarsal bone and aimed toward the middle of the joint.

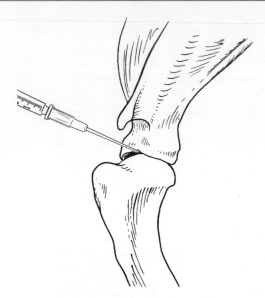

FIGURE 1–19. Arthrocentesis of the scapulohumeral joint. The needle is introduced about 1 cm distal to the acromion process of the scapula. If no fluid is obtained, an assistant may gently pull the forearm distally to "open" the joint space.

ture site. If the forearm is pulled distally (separating the humerus from the scapula), sometimes the needle is introduced in the center of the joint rather than under the capsule lateral to the humeral head.

Elbow joint—the elbow is hyperextended to allow the joint to distend caudally. The needle is introduced lateral to and alongside the olecranon and inserted cranially toward the middle of the joint until contact is made with the humeral condyle (Fig. 1–20).

Carpal joint—the carpal joint is located with thumbnail pressure during joint motion. This joint is located on the same level as the *base* of the accessory carpal bone. The needle is introduced from the dorsal cranial aspect of the joint (Fig. 1–21).

Other tests that may help diagnose systemic musculoskeletal disorders include testing for infections affecting muscle and joints (e.g., toxoplasmosis, Lyme dis-

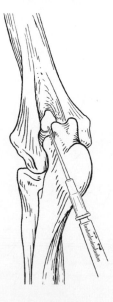

FIGURE 1–20. Arthrocentesis of the elbow joint. With the elbow in extension, the needle is introduced just lateral to the olecranon.

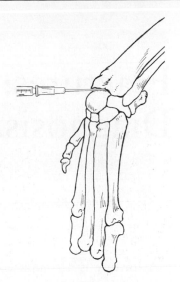

FIGURE 1–21. Arthrocentesis of the carpal joint. The joint lies on the same level as the base of the accessory carpal bone. With the joint flexed, the needle is introduced at the midline of the joint.

ease), endocrine myopathies (hyperadrenocorticism, hypothyroidism), immune-mediated myopathies, and immune-mediated joint disease (rheumatoid arthritis or systemic lupus erythematosis). These tests include hematology, serology, histochemical staining of muscle, serum enzymes, electromyography, and cytology of swollen tissues.

References

1. Henderson RA, Milton JL: The tibial compression mechanism: A diagnostic aid in stifle injuries. J Am Anim Hosp Assoc 14:474–479, 1978.
2. Chalman JA, Butler HC: Coxofemoral joint laxity and the Ortolani sign. J Am Anim Hosp Assoc 21:671–676, 1985.
3. van Bree H, Van Ryssen B: Positive contrast shoulder arthrography with iopromide and diatrizoate in dogs with osteochondrosis. Vet Radiol Ultrasound 14:203–206, 1995.
4. Rivers B, Wallace L, Johnston GR: Biceps tenosynovitis in the dog: Radiographic and sonographic findings. Vet Comp Orthop Trauma 5:51–57, 1992.
5. Lewis DD, Goring RL, Parker RB, et al: A comparison of diagnostic methods used in the evaluation of early degenerative joint disease in the dog. J Am Anim Hosp Assoc 23:305–315, 1987.
6. van Bree H, Van Ryssen B, Desmidt M: Osteochondrosis lesions of the canine shoulder: Correlation of positive contrast arthrography and arthroscopy. Vet Radiol Ultrasound 33:342–347, 1992.
7. Anderson MA, Mann FA: Force plate analysis: A noninvasive tool for gait evaluation. Compend Cont Educ Pract Vet 16:857–867, 1994.
8. Allen K, DeCamp CE, Braden TD, et al: Kinematic gait analysis of the trot in healthy mixed breed dogs. Vet Comp Orthop Trauma 7:148–153, 1994.
9. Bennett RL, DeCamp CE, Flo GL, et al: Kinematic gait analysis of canine hip dysplasia. J Am Vet Res 7:966–971, 1996.

2

Fractures: Classification, Diagnosis, and Treatment

A fracture is a complete or incomplete break in the continuity of bone or cartilage. A fracture is accompanied by various degrees of injury to the surrounding soft tissues, including blood supply, and by a compromise of locomotor system function. The examiner handling the fracture must take into consideration the patient's local and overall conditions.

CLASSIFICATION OF FRACTURES

Fractures may be classified on many bases, and all are useful in describing the fracture.[1-3] These bases include causal factors, presence of a communicating external wound, location, morphology and severity of the fracture, and stability of the fracture following axial reduction of the fragments.

Causal Factors

Direct Violence Applied to the Bone ■ Statistics indicate that at least 75 to 80 percent of all fractures are caused by car accidents or motorized vehicles.

Indirect Violence ■ The force is transmitted through bone or muscle to a distant point where the fracture occurs (e.g., fracture of the femoral neck, avulsion of the tibial tubercle, fracture of the condyles of the humerus or femur).

Diseases of Bone ■ Some bone diseases cause bone destruction or weakening to such a degree that trivial trauma may produce a fracture (e.g., bone neoplasms, or nutritional disturbances affecting the bone).

Repeated Stress ■ Fatigue fractures in small animals are most frequently encountered in bones of the front or rear foot (e.g., metacarpal or metatarsal bones in the racing greyhound).

Presence of a Communicating External Wound

Closed Fracture ■ The fracture does not communicate to the outside.

Open Fracture ■ The fracture site communicates to the outside. These fractures are very apt to be contaminated or infected, and healing at best may be complicated and delayed (see Fig. 2–3A).

TABLE 2–1. THE AO VET ALPHANUMERIC MORPHOLOGICAL FRACTURE CLASSIFICATION SYSTEM*

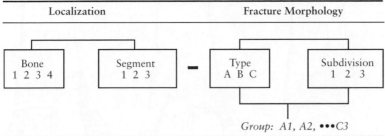

Localization		Fracture Morphology	
Bone 1 2 3 4	Segment 1 2 3	Type A B C	Subdivision 1 2 3

Group: A1, A2, •••C3

*Redrawn from Unger M, Montavon PM, Heim UFA: Classification of fractures of the long bones in the dog and cat: Introduction and clinical application. Vet Comp Orthop Trauma 3:41–50, 1990.

Location, Fracture Morphology, and Severity

The system used here for long-bone fractures is based on the classification system adopted by AO Vet, which was developed to allow fractures to be alphanumerically coded for easy data retrieval via computer.[3] It is based on the system used by the AO/ASIF group for documentation of human fractures.[4] It permits grading of the complexity of fracture configuration and relative stability following reduction, thus providing information regarding appropriate treatment and prognosis (Table 2–1).

Localization of the fracture is provided by numbering each long bone (*1, humerus; 2, radius/ulna; 3, femur; 4 tibia/fibula*) and dividing each bone into *1, proximal; 2, shaft;* and *3, distal zones.* As a measure of severity each fracture is typed as *A, simple; B, wedge;* or *C, complex* (Fig. 2–1). Each grade is further grouped into three degrees of complexity (e.g., *A1, A2, A3*) depending on the type and extent of bone fragmentation. Thus, the simplest shaft fracture of the humerus would be characterized as 1 2 A1. Proximal and distal zones may require individual descriptions to accommodate the specific bone morphology (Fig. 2–2).

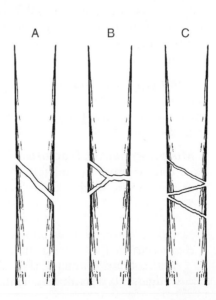

FIGURE 2–1. Diaphyseal fracture types. (*A*) Simple fracture. (*B*) Wedge fracture. (*C*) Complex fracture. (Redrawn from Unger M, Montavon PM, Heim UFA: Classification of fractures of the long bones in the dog and cat: Introduction and clinical application. Vet Comp Orthop Trauma 3:41–50, 1990, with permission.)

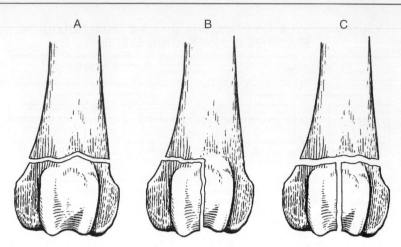

FIGURE 2–2. Proximal and distal long-bone fracture types. (*A*) Extra-articular fracture. (*B*) Partial articular fracture. (*C*) Complete articular fracture. There are some special cases in the proximal humerus, radius/ulna, and femur due to their specific anatomy.

Additional specific *nomenclature* can be applied to each of the above descriptions in order to convey more information. The orientation of the fracture line relative to the bone's long axis allows the following descriptions:

Transverse Fracture ■   The fracture crosses the bone at an angle of not more than 30 degrees to the long axis of the bone (Fig. 2–3*D*).

Oblique Fracture ■   The fracture describes an angle of greater than 30 degrees to the long axis of the bone (Fig. 2–3*E*).

Spiral Fracture ■   This is a special case oblique fracture where the fracture line curves around the diaphysis (Fig. 2–3*F*).

The extent of damage can be described as:

Incomplete Fracture ■   Most commonly used to describe a fracture that only disrupts one cortex, and is called a *greenstick* fracture in young animals because of the bending of the nonfractured cortex (Fig. 2–3*B*). *Fissure* fractures exhibit fine cracks that penetrate the cortex in a linear or spiral direction. In skeletally immature animals the periosteum is usually left intact (Fig. 2–3*C*).

Complete Fracture ■   This fracture describes a single circumferential disruption of the bone. Any fragmentation that results in a defect at the fracture site must be smaller than one third of the bone diameter after fracture reduction (Fig. 2–3*D*).

Multifragmental Fractures ■   Also known as *comminuted* fractures, these have one or more completely separated fragments of intermediate size. These fractures can be further described:

> *Wedge fracture.* A multifragmental fracture with some contact between the main fragments after reduction (Figs. 2–1*B*, 2–3*G*).
> *Reducible wedges.* Fragments with a length and width larger than one third of the bone diameter (Fig. 2–3*G*). After reduction and fixation of the wedge(s) to a main fragment, the result is a simple fracture.

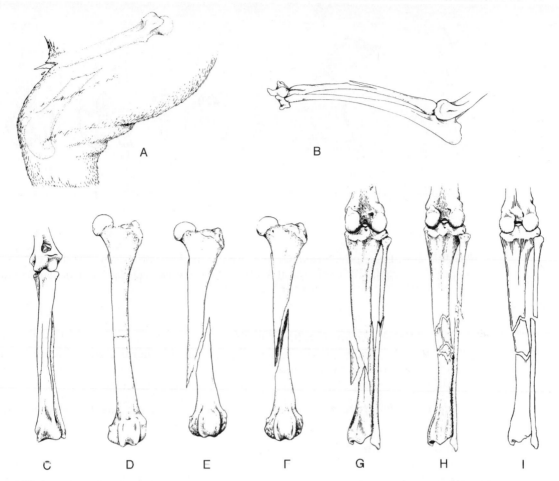

FIGURE 2–3. Descriptive nomenclature of diaphyseal fractures. (A) Open. (B) Greenstick. (C) Fissure. (D) Transverse. (E) Oblique. (F) Spiral. (G) Reducible wedge. (H) Nonreducible wedges. (I) Multiple or segmental.

Nonreducible wedges. Fragments with a length and width less than one third the bone diameter, and that result in a defect between the main fragments after reduction of more than one third the diameter (Fig. 2–3H).

Multiple or segmental fracture. The bone is broken into three or more segments; the fracture lines do not meet at a common point (Fig. 2–3I). This is a special case of a reducible wedge fracture.

Proximal and distal metaphyseal zones require specific nomenclature to describe the wide variety of extra- and intra-articular fractures seen here:

Extra-articular Fractures ■ The articular surface is not fractured, but is separated from the diaphysis (Fig. 2–2A). These are commonly called *metaphyseal* fractures. In a *physeal* fracture the fracture-separation occurs at the physeal line or growth plate. This type occurs only in the young, growing animal (Fig. 2–4C).

Partial Articular Fractures ■ Only part of the joint surface is involved, with the remaining portion still attached to the diaphysis (Fig. 2–2B). *Unicondylar* fractures are the most common example (Fig. 2–4D).

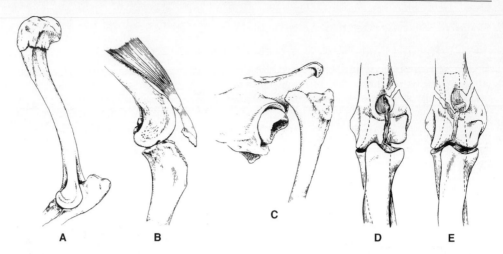

FIGURE 2–4. Descriptive proximal and distal zone fracture nomenclature. (*A*) Metaphyseal, impacted. (*B*) Metaphyseal avulsion. (*C*) Physeal. (*D*) Partial articular or unicondylar. (*E*) Complete articular or bicondylar.

Complete Articular Fractures ■ The joint surface is fractured and completely detached from the diaphysis (Fig. 2–2*C*). Humeral *T* or *Y* fractures are representative of this type (Fig. 2–4*E*).

Additional descriptive terms are applied to certain fractures:

Impacted Fracture ■ The bone fragments are driven firmly together (Fig. 2–4*A*).

Avulsion Fracture ■ A fragment of bone, which is the site of insertion of a muscle, tendon, or ligament, is detached as a result of a forceful pull (Fig. 2–4*B*).

Stability Following Replacement in Normal Anatomical Position

Stable Fracture ■ Fragments interlock and resist shortening forces (e.g., transverse, greenstick, impacted). The primary objective of fixation is to prevent angular and/or rotational deformity.

Unstable Fracture ■ The fragments do not interlock and thus slide by each other and out of position (e.g., oblique, nonreducible wedges). Fixation is indicated to maintain length and alignment and to prevent rotation.

BLOOD SUPPLY AND HEALING OF BONE

Until about 1940, almost all fractures were reduced closed, and stabilized by external means such as coaptation splints, plaster of Paris casts, and Thomas splints. The various methods of internal fixation were introduced and developed in the same time period as were aseptic technique in veterinary surgery, open approaches to the various bones and joints, and open reduction of fractures. In order to properly handle tissues and implement reduction and fixation to best advantage, an understanding of blood supply and bone healing is essential.

Normal Vascularization of Bone

An adequate blood supply is necessary for bone to carry out its normal physiological function. Clinically, most vascular problems arise in the long bones. Blood supply to these bones is derived from three basic sources: the afferent vascular system, the intermediate vascular system of compact bone, and the efferent vascular system.[5,6] The afferent system carries arterial blood and consists of the principal nutrient artery, the metaphyseal arteries, and the periosteal arterioles at muscle attachments (Fig. 2–5). The periosteal arterioles are minor components of the afferent system and supply the outer layers of the cortex in the vicinity of firm fascial or muscle attachments.

The vessels in compact bones are intermediate between the afferent and efferent systems and function as the vascular lattice where critical exchange between the blood and surrounding living tissue occurs. This system consists of the cortical canals of Havers and Volkmann and the minute canaliculi, which convey nutrients to the osteocytes.

Venous drainage (the efferent system) of cortical bone takes place at the periosteal surface. Blood flow through the cortex is essentially centrifugal, from medulla to the periosteum. Other venous drainage from the marrow cavity is present; however, this is connected with the hematopoietic activity of the marrow cavity.

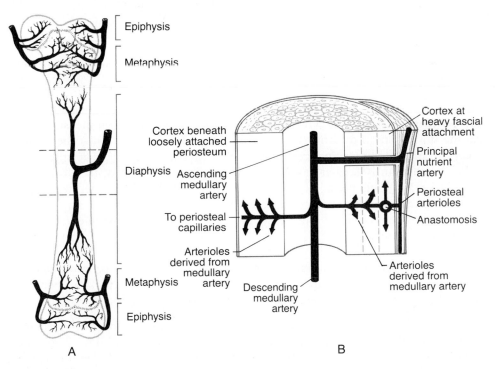

FIGURE 2–5. Normal blood supply to bone. (*A*) Schema of afferent blood supply to immature bone. After the growth plate closes (adult bone), the metaphyseal and epiphyseal vessels anastomose. (*B*) Section of diaphysis showing schema of normal afferent blood supply to compact bone. (From Rhinelander F, Phillips RS, Steel WM, et al: Microangiography in bone healing. J Bone Joint Surg 50-A:643, 1968, with permission.)

Response of Vascularization Following Fracture

Disruption of the normal blood supply to bone varies with the complexity of the fracture. The afferent vascular components are stimulated and respond by hypertrophy, increasing in both diameter and number. In addition, a new blood supply is developed, termed the extraosseous blood supply of healing bone,[5,6] from the immediate surrounding soft tissues. This is separate from the normal periosteal arterioles. It furnishes blood to detached bone fragments, devitalized cortex, and the developing periosteal callus. When stability at the fracture site and continuity of the medullary circulation are established, the extraosseous blood supply regresses. Fortunately, the regenerative powers of the medullary arterial supply are rapid and enormous under favorable circumstances, since this must be re-established for healing of cortical bone.

Some of the factors that may deter vascular response and, thus, bone healing are (1) trauma in connection with the original accident, (2) careless or improper surgical handling of the soft tissues, (3) inadequate reduction, and (4) inadequate stabilization of bone fragments. Intramedullary nails may temporarily damage the medullary afferent system, whereas plates may block the venous outflow. Either blood supply to the bone may be partially compromised, but both must be present to an adequate degree for bone healing.

Bone Healing

The pattern of bone healing varies according to the mechanical conditions present within the fracture line following reduction and stabilization of the fracture. Four basic mechanical situations can be observed, and all may be present in one fracture.[7]

1.   Bone immediately adjacent to a compression plate or lag screw may experience very high static (stabilizing) load, with very little dynamic (destabilizing) component.

2.   A site farther from a compression plate, or a fracture stabilized with a very stiff external fixator, will experience moderately high compressive static loading with a small dynamic component. This situation could also be present in certain intramedullary pin/cerclage wire fixations.

3.   A site slightly farther from a compression plate or screw, fixation with a buttress or bridging plate, or a fracture stabilized with a moderately stable external fixator will experience more even distribution between static and dynamic components. This would also be typical of many intramedullary pin fixations.

4.   At the cortex opposite a plate or a unilateral external fixator, in some buttress or bridging plate situations, and in some intramedullary pin fixations, a gap is continuously present due to varying dynamic loads (tension, bending, shear) that continuously exceed the stabilizing compressive loads.

In areas of intermittent bone contact there will be resorption of the fracture surfaces to enlarge the gap, followed by *indirect bone union* (Fig. 2–6). The sequence of events in this case may be very briefly stated as (1) hemorrhage in the area, (2) clot formation, (3) inflammation and edema followed by (4) proliferation of pluripotential mesenchymal cells, (5) cartilage and bone formation, and (6) remodeling of callus back to normal bone. The sequence of events results in a progressive replacement of the tissue in the fracture gap with stiffer and stronger tissue, going from granulation tissue to connective tissue to fibrous tissue to cartilage to mineralized cartilage to lamellar bone to cortical bone. This entire process is under the direction and control of a host of cellularly produced active mediators such as chemoattractants, and angiogenetic and growth factors.[8]

Callus formation may be subdivided on the basis of location as medullary bridging callus, periosteal bridging callus, or intercortical bridging callus (Fig. 2–6). The pattern of callus formation will vary markedly in response to circumstances and stimuli present. In general, stabilization of fractures by external splintage, the external fixator, buttress (bridging) plates, and intramedullary pins is characterized by the formation of callus in all three areas. Stability of the fracture fragments is not absolute and micromotion is present. The developing callus is responsible for early stabilization of the fracture and results in relatively early clinical union; that is, the point at which the bone is able to assume normal weight-bearing forces without dependence on the fixation device. Contrarily, excessive dynamic loading is responsible for *delayed union*, where the transformation of callus from cartilage to bone is delayed due to the poor blood supply within the areas of excessive motion. Other than in the young growing animal, the amount of callus is in inverse relation to the degree of stability at the fracture site.

Healing in areas of contact and high compression forces, and in very small stable gaps (<0.1 mm), is described as *direct bone union* (Fig. 2–7). This type of union bypasses most of the steps described above and goes directly to cortical remodeling. Union of the cortices is achieved by internal remodeling of the Haversian systems without resorption of the fracture surfaces. This intense remodeling at the fracture surface may be radiographically confused with resorption, as it results in slight loss of density in the fracture zone. Thus, stabilization of fractures by use of compression plates and screws is characterized by no visible intercortical callus and small amounts of medullary bridging callus. Healing in areas of mixed compressive and dynamic loads can exhibit all three types of healing patterns.

Successful healing in areas of direct contact of the bone fragments or in areas of very small fracture gaps depends on absolute stability because *strain* on individual cells filling the fracture gap is magnified by any motion at the site, and can easily cause rupture of these cells. As can be seen from Table 2–2, there is a dramatic difference in the tolerance to strain by the three major cell types found in the healing fracture gap. Figure 2–8 illustrates the effect of micromotion in a small fracture gap.[10] Thus it becomes obvious that if close reduction and interfragmentary compression is chosen, it becomes imperative to provide absolutely stable fixation. If this cannot be guaranteed, then it is better to not reduce the fragments too closely in order to ensure survival of the tissues in the fracture gap in the presence of the micromotion inevitable in such a mechanical situation. This is the basis of the concept of bridging osteosynthesis discussed below.

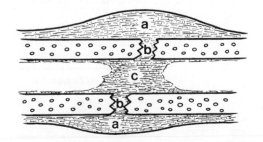

FIGURE 2–6. Callus formation in bone healing. (*A*) Periosteal bridging callus. (*B*) Intercortical bridging callus. (*C*) Medullary bridging callus.

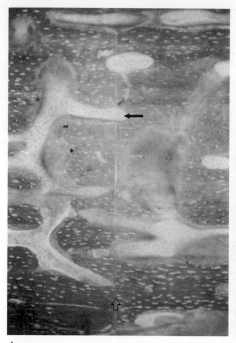
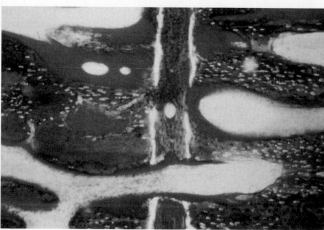

A   B

FIGURE 2–7. Direct (primary) bone union. (*A*) Contact healing at 4 weeks of an osteotomy stabilized by a compression plate. A thin zone of necrotic bone can be seen in the center of the section. There is extensive Haversian remodeling of the bone ends with osteons growing across both living and dead cortex and bridging the osteotomy. (*B*) On the side opposite the plate there is a small fracture gap. This space is invaded by capillaries and accompanied by osteoblasts that deposit osteoid. Bone lamellae form initially parallel to the fracture line and then are replaced by axially oriented osteons to complete the remodeling. This type of direct bone healing without the intermediate steps of fibrous tissue and cartilage formation is possible under conditions of good stability and a gap up to 0.3 mm wide. (Courtesy of Dr. Robert Schenk.)

In summary, bone healing depends on and is influenced by blood supply at the fracture line, reduction of the fracture fragments, and the degree of stabilization of the fracture fragments.

DIAGNOSIS OF FRACTURES AND PRINCIPLES OF TREATMENT

The history and clinical signs usually indicate the presence of a fracture; however, radiographs are essential for precise determination of its nature.

The first consideration is preserving the patient's life; repair of tissues and restoration of function are secondary. Treatment for shock, hemorrhage, and

TABLE 2–2.   TOLERANCE TO INTERFRAGMENTARY STRAIN[9]

Tolerance to Elongation		Tolerance to Bending
Granulation tissue	100%	40 degrees
Cartilage	15%	5 degrees
Bone	2%	0.5 degree

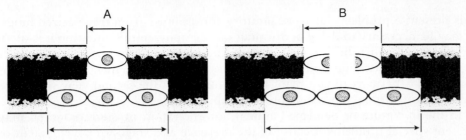

FIGURE 2–8. The concept of interfragmentary strain in a small fracture gap. (*A*) One granulation tissue cell is seen within the 10-μm fracture gap and three cells within the 30-μm gap. (*B*) Increasing the gap 10-μm (not perceptible to the eye) causes a 100 percent strain and rupture of the cell in the small gap, while only a 33 percent strain on the cells in the larger gap. Thus the resorption of fragment ends seen in areas less than totally stable is an attempt to protect the soft tissues by widening the gap. (Redrawn from Rahn BA: Bone healing: Histologic and physiologic concepts. In Sumner-Smith G (ed): Bone in Clinical Orthopaedics. Philadelphia, WB Saunders Co, 1982, pp 335–386.)

wounds of the soft tissues, if present, should be instituted immediately, and the patient should be made as comfortable as possible.

Examination of an animal with a fracture or suspected fracture should include:

1. Assessment of the animal's general health.
2. Determination of whether tissues or organs adjacent to the fracture or other parts of the body have been damaged and to what extent.
3. Examination to ascertain whether fractures, ligamentous instability, or dislocations are present in other parts of the body.
4. Precise evaluation of the fracture or fractures. (See Chapter 1 for a more complete discussion on physical examination of the locomotor system.)

Clinical Signs

Even though they are not always readily detectable, visible signs at the fracture area include one or more of the following:

1. Pain or localized tenderness.
2. Deformity or change in angulation.
3. Abnormal mobility.
4. Local swelling. This may appear almost immediately or not until several hours after or a day following the accident. It usually persists for 7 to 10 days owing to disturbed flow of blood and lymph.
5. Loss of function.
6. Crepitus.

Radiographic Examination

Radiographs of at least two views at right angles to each other are essential for accurate diagnosis and selection of the best procedures for reduction and immobilization.

Reduction and Immobilization

Because movement of fracture fragments results in pain to the animal, these radiographs usually require sedation or short-acting general anesthesia. Should this present a problem due to respiratory compromise from traumatized lungs, it may be necessary to delay performing radiography. In this situation it is often helpful to take just the one view that can be taken without anesthesia in order to confirm the location and severity of the fracture. This then allows the formation of a basic treatment plan. Bear in mind that the second view should be taken before attempting reduction and stabilization.

In the immature or deformed animal, interpretation of the radiograph may present special problems because of the presence and stages of development of various osseous growth centers. Radiographs of the opposite limb are usually helpful.

Treatment

The goal of fracture treatment is early ambulation and complete return of function.

Return to Function

The principles of fracture treatment have been best articulated by the AO/ASIF group.[11-13] They are:

1. *Anatomical reduction* of fracture fragments, especially in articular fractures.
2. *Stable fixation*, suitable to the biomechanical and clinical situation.
3. *Preservation of the blood supply* to the bone fragments and surrounding soft tissues through atraumatic reduction and surgical technique.
4. *Early active pain-free mobilization* of muscles and joints adjacent to the fracture in order to prevent development of fracture disease.

The interpretation and emphasis of these principles has undergone a gradual change in recent years as the concept of *biological fixation* has been championed by AO/ASIF. Primary in this concept is the protection of the soft tissues and the blood supply of the fracture fragments. This means that anatomical reduction in the sense of total reconstruction of all fracture lines is only insisted upon for articular fractures or shaft fractures treated by interfragmentary compression by means of lag screws or cerclage wires, which are then protected by a neutralization plate. Direct bone union without callus is to be expected under this protocol. Other shaft fractures are treated by leaving the fragments undisturbed to protect their blood supply. The fracture zone is either spanned by a bridging plate that is attached to each end of the bone, or stabilized by an external skeletal fixator or interlocking medullary nail. Healing in this case is by the indirect route, with early callus formation being responsible for much of the stabilization. Hulse and Aron have proposed the term "bridging osteosynthesis," which seems very descriptive, and will be used throughout this text.[14] Anatomic reduction in this circumstance means restoring axial alignment in both the frontal and sagittal planes, eliminating torsional deformity, and maintaining bone length to the extent possible, although the latter is not of so much consequence in quadripeds as in bipeds.

The concept of stable internal fixation has also to be re-evaluated in consideration of the aims of bridging osteosynthesis. All fixation must maintain axial alignment and length, and provide rotational stability. Stabilization by interfragmentary compression demands absolute stability of the small remaining fracture gap in order for direct Haversian bridging to occur (see section Bone Healing, above). When the objective is bridging osteosynthesis the fixation only need be as strong as needed to allow callus formation. *Small* amounts of inter-fragmentary motion are not only probable but even desirable for callus formation, which actively enters into the role of stabilizer of the fracture, thus protecting the internal fixation from mechanical overload and failure. How much fixation is needed in a given situation is difficult to define succinctly, but will be addressed in depth in coming sections of this chapter as well as when dealing with specific fractures in later chapters.

The concept of atraumatic technique can be seen to have received increased emphasis in the employment of bridging osteosynthesis strategies, especially as applies to preservation of blood supply to bone fragments. Providing sufficiently strong internal fixation to allow early pain-free mobilization of the limb has always been of primary importance to the veterinary orthopedic surgeon, and continues to be sought after. Not only is bone healing aided, but the soft tissue integrity of the limb is better maintained, and nursing care of the animal is greatly simplified.

Reduction and Fixation

Reduction and fixation of the fracture should be undertaken as soon as the patient's condition permits.[15,16] Delay makes reduction more difficult because of spastic contraction of the muscles and inflammatory thickening of the soft tissue. In some cases, fixation can be accomplished when the patient is presented; in others, it may be advisable to delay for a day or longer until the patient becomes an acceptable anesthetic risk. It is inadvisable to wait until the swelling has subsided before going ahead with reduction and fixation. By this time, organization of the hematoma and callus formation are well under way. The latter also obscures fracture lines, nerves, and blood vessels. Surgical hemorrhage is also markedly increased as a result of increased circulatory response in the area. This circulatory response is usually evident around the fourth day after trauma. Surgery prior to this time is accompanied by less hemorrhage.

RATE OF BONE UNION AND CLINICAL UNION

The moment a fracture occurs, changes in the tissue in the immediate area set the stage for its repair, and the rapidity of the process of repair may be influenced by many factors. The surgeon can do little to alter such factors as age, character of the fracture, state of the soft tissues in the surrounding area, and certain systemic or local bone diseases. Unfavorable factors such as poor reduction, inadequate immobilization, excessive operative trauma, or lack of aseptic procedures in surgery, however, are within the control of the surgeon. These factors may slow or even interrupt the healing process. When all other factors are equal and the fracture is optimally treated, age of the patient is the most influential single factor affecting the rate of healing.

Clinical union refers to that period of time in the recovery process of a fracture when healing has progressed to the point in strength so that the fixation can be removed. Average periods of anticipated healing time for the typical uncomplicated fracture treated in optimal fashion are listed in Table 2–3. These healing times vary somewhat, depending on the type of fixation used. Fractures immobilized with external fixation, skeletal fixation, and intramedullary pins heal with the development of an external and internal bridging callus. The bridging callus does give added early strength to the fracture site. Fractures immobilized with rigid fixation (bone plate) heal primarily by direct union and

TABLE 2–3.   RATE OF UNION IN TERMS OF CLINICAL UNION

Age of Animal	External Skeletal, and Intramedullary Pin Fixations	Fixation with Bone Plates
Under 3 months	2–3 weeks	4 weeks
3–6 months	4–6 weeks	2–3 months
6–12 months	5–8 weeks	3–5 months
Over 1 year	7–12 weeks	5 months–1 year

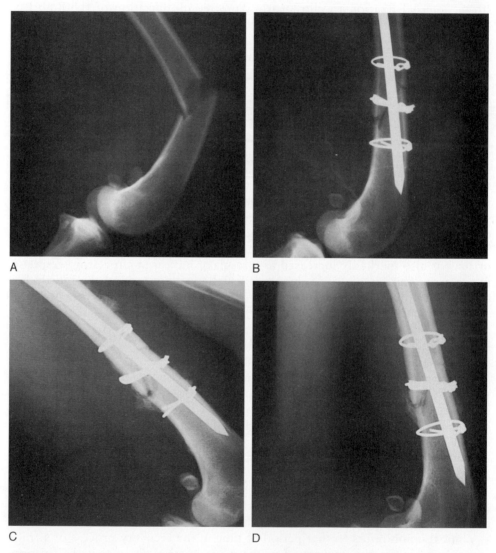

A   B

C   D

FIGURE 2–9. Fracture healing in various forms. Table 2–4 summarizes this process. *Indirect healing* is illustrated in parts *A–J*. (*A, B*) Type A2 simple diaphyseal fracture of the femur stabilized with a Steinmann pin, two cerclage wires to prevent propagation of fissure fractures, and an interfragmentary skewer-pin and wire. The fracture lines are clearly visible postoperatively. (*C*) At 4 weeks the fracture line is less visible and there is patchy mineralization of unstructured bridging callus. (*D*) The fracture line is faintly visible at 7 weeks, and callus is smoothing and becoming uniform in density. The Steinmann pin was removed. *Figure continued on opposite page*

some internal callus, and fractures treated by this method should have the fixation in place for a longer period of time.

Table 2–3 is not to be interpreted as an indication that one method of fixation is superior to another. Each method has its place, indications, and contraindications as will be described below.

Radiographic evaluation of fracture healing (Fig. 2–9) should be routinely

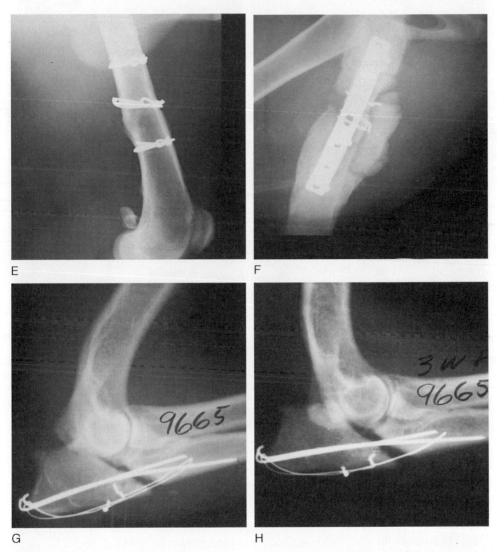

FIGURE 2–9. *Continued*   (*E*) By 14 weeks only a faint hint of the fracture line remains, and the dense callus is being remodeled on the periosteal and endosteal surfaces. (*F*) Florid periosteal callus in a skeletally immature dog 4 weeks postoperatively. This extreme callus is not due to instability, but rather to intraoperative trauma to the active periosteum. Note the absence of callus cranially at the fracture site, which was the area most devitalized by intraoperative handling. This area later bridged with callus. (*G, H*) To illustrate the widening of the fracture gap seen due to vascularization of the fracture edges, compare the postoperative gap seen in (*G*) with the situation 3 weeks later in (*H*). This is a more dramatic than normal response due to the fact that the fracture was 3 weeks old at the time of surgery and the fracture fragment edges were more devascularized than in a fresh fracture. *Figure continued on following page*

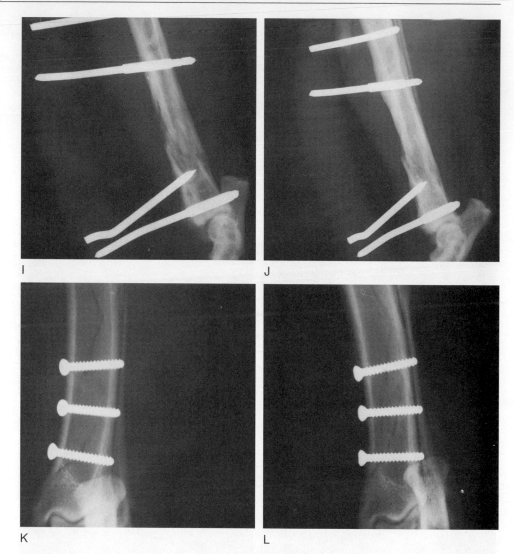

FIGURE 2–9. *Continued* (*I*) This type A3 complex distal tibial extra-articular tibial fracture was stabilized by external fixator and closed reduction (biological osteosynthesis) 20 weeks previously. Fracture lines are faintly visible, with remodeling of callus and cortical bone evident. The fixator was destabilized at this time by removing some of the proximal fixation pins. (*J*) At 32 weeks cortical remodeling is almost complete and the fixator was removed. *Direct healing* is illustrated in parts *K–M*, a type A1 simple extra-articular tibial fracture stabilized with lag screws and external coaptation. (*K*) Postoperatively the double-spiral fracture line is obvious despite the perfect reduction. (*L*) Fracture lines are becoming hazy and fading proximally at 6.5 weeks. No callus is present except at the fibular fracture. *Figure continued on opposite page*

performed at the time of expected union as indicated in Table 2–3. The mnemonic AAAA has proven useful for evaluation of such radiographs (E. Egger, P. Schwarz, personal communication, 1994).

1. *Alignment.* This is basically an assessment of the restoration of the bone as a whole, and is evaluated relative to angular and torsional displacement relative to normal. Return to normal alignment is necessary for normal long-term function.

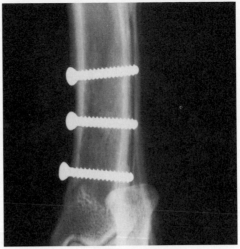

FIGURE 2–9. *Continued* (M) At 10 weeks, the fracture lines have disappeared in most areas and are obviously well bridged in those areas where they can be identified. (Radiographs courtesy of Dr. Richard Park.)

M

2. Apposition. Looking more directly at the fracture site, we are here evaluating the degree of realignment of the fracture fragments. A certain degree of apposition is required for routine bone healing, but this degree is highly dependent on the type of fixation employed; thus no single definition can be used in all situations.

3. Apparatus. Is the fixation device functioning as intended to maintain stability of the fracture until healed? Were applicable protocols for the device followed? Is there evidence of loosening of implants? Is there evidence of impending failure of the implant such as bending or screw loosening?

4. Activity. This is the biological activity of the bone in response to the fixation used. In order to evaluate this it is necessary to know the age of the animal, the length of time since the fracture was stabilized, and the degree of functional use of the limb. It is also useful to consider such things as pre-existing infection, and open wounds or other devascularizing injuries. This is the area where the type and amount of callus formation is evaluated. Signs of infection such as bone lysis or periosteal new-bone formation must be searched for. Bone resorption is evaluated to decide if this represents normal revascularization of bone fragment edges or whether it indicates infection or loosening of an implant. Typically observed radiographic signs of healing are detailed in Table 2–4.

REDUCTION OF FRACTURES

Reduction of a fracture refers to the process of replacing the fractured segments in their original anatomical position. Fractures can be reduced by either closed reduction with traction and manipulation of the fragments, or by open reduction and direct visual reconstruction of the bone. Bones with their muscles attached may be likened to a system of levers with springs attached. Muscles are constantly contracting (normal tonus). Flexors oppose extensors, counterbalancing the part at the joint. When a bone is fractured, all opposing muscles contract maximally, and overriding and shortening of the bone occur. Spastic contraction of the muscle is intensified by injury to soft tissues of the region.

TABLE 2–4. RADIOGRAPHIC SIGNS OF FRACTURE HEALING ASSUMING NORMAL ADULT FRACTURE SITUATION WITH STABLE FIXATION AND GOOD VASCULARITY TO THE FRACTURE FRAGMENTS

Radiographic Sign	Postoperative Time
Sharp fracture margins (Fig. 2–9A, B)	1 week
Indistinct fracture margins and widening of fracture gap (Fig. 2–9G, H)	2 weeks
Unstructured and patchy mineralization of bridging callus; fracture line still visible (Fig. 2–9C, F)	4–6 weeks
Bridging callus of even density and smooth borders; fracture line faintly visible (can remove some of fixation; e.g., pins from external fixators) (Fig. 2–9D)	6–9 weeks
Dense callus of reduced size; fracture line barely visible, early corticomedullary remodeling (stage of early clinical union) (Fig. 2–9E)	8–12 weeks
Further condensation of callus; distinct corticomedullary separation due to remodeling; fracture line not visible (Fig. 2–9I, J)	10 weeks>>>

The pull caused by the muscle spasm is constant and continuous, even under general anesthesia. Initially, the contraction and overriding are primarily muscular and are responsive to general anesthesia, countertraction, and some of the muscle-relaxing drugs. After several days, inflammatory reaction in the area with its accompanying proliferating changes brings about contraction of a more permanent nature; thus, more difficulty is encountered when attempting reduction.[2]

Gas anesthesia (halothane, methoxyflurane, or isoflurane) is superior to the barbiturates in bringing about relaxation of muscle spasm. The addition of muscle relaxants is helpful in overcoming spastic contraction when used in addition to general anesthesia and within the first 3 days after a fracture occurs. Succinylcholine (0.44 mg/kg) or pancuronium (0.05 to 0.1 mg/kg) has been used in small animals. The former drug is preferred. At these doses, they also produce respiratory paralysis, and assisted respiration is a necessity. The duration of action is about 20 to 30 minutes.

To a large extent, healing is influenced by the handling of the soft tissues, blood supply to the fracture segments, accuracy of reduction, and efficiency of immobilization. All may be influenced or altered by the surgeon.

The ideal is anatomical replacement of the fracture segments, because this gives the possibility of maximum stability when fixation is applied. Anatomical apposition is always preferred but not always necessary, particularly in fractures of the diaphysis. Rotational alignment must be restored between the joints proximal and distal to the fracture to ensure good function. Axial bending in the cranial-caudal direction (sagittal plane) is well tolerated unless the limb becomes excessively shortened. Moderate medial angulation in the frontal plane (varus) of the distal segment is quite well tolerated, but lateral angulation (valgus) usually produces significant functional problems.

When a joint surface is involved in a fracture, the articular fragments must always be reduced anatomically to restore joint congruency and thus to eliminate or at least minimize abnormal wear and secondary osteoarthrosis. The secret of reduction is the application of continual steady pressure over a period of time. This fatigues the muscles, bringing about relaxation and lengthening.

Closed Reduction

Closed reduction is usually accomplished by manipulation along with the application of traction and countertraction. This is ideal, provided that it can be accomplished and maintained with minimal tissue trauma, and many fractures are so treated in man. This should not influence the veterinary surgeon unduly, as the problems we face in matters of patient cooperation and aftercare cannot be compared to those in man. Closed reduction is the norm when external fixation devices such as casts and splints are employed. This method is most useful below the elbow and stifle, where soft tissues are not a hindrance in palpating the bone to aid in determining reduction. This is also the region where casts and splints are most applicable in animals.

Success of the method is greater in small and relatively long-legged breeds than in large, chondrodystrophied, or heavily muscled breeds. Closed reduction should be attempted as soon as the patient's condition will permit general anesthesia, as delay increases muscle spasm and contracture and increases the difficulty of obtaining reduction. Do not wait for the swelling to go down, as it will not regress until reduction restores normal circulation. Initially the contracture and overriding is primarily muscular in nature and responds to traction, general anesthesia, and muscle-relaxant drugs. After 2 to 3 days, inflammatory reaction and its proliferative changes cause a much more permanent and difficult-to-overcome contracture.

Methods of Closed Reduction

The guiding principle in any method of closed reduction is to apply slow, continuous traction to the fragment that can be controlled, aligning it with the less manageable fragment. It is important to perform all manipulations with a mind to the possibility of laceration, perforation, or compression of a major vessel or nerves. Apply traction *slowly* to relax muscles and not cause irritation.

Traction can be obtained by manual force (Figs. 2–10, and 2–11) or by gravity (Fig 2–12). Manual traction is facilitated if a gauze or soft rope loop is placed around the axillary or groin region and anchored to the edge of the table near the animal's back. Another gauze or rope is placed around the carpal or tarsal area and traction is applied against the first rope. The Gordon extender is a mechanical device that allows similar traction to be exerted without as much force being exerted by the surgeon (Fig. 2–13). Relaxation of muscle is best accomplished by slow progressive increase of traction tension over 10 to 30 minutes.

To use gravity to obtain traction, place the animal on its back, and place gauze, tape, or soft rope around the paw of the affected limb, then attach this to an infusion stand or to a ceiling-mounted eyebolt (Fig. 2–12). The length of the attaching material is adjusted to raise the animal slightly off the table, so that a portion of the body weight is being supported and thus producing trac-

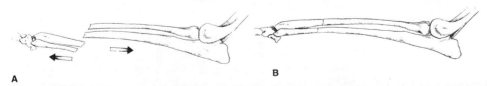

A   B

FIGURE 2–10. (*A, B*) Application of traction, countertraction, and manipulation.

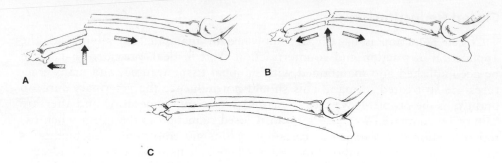

FIGURE 2–11. (A–C) Application of traction, countertraction, and toggeling or bending.

tion on the limb. Ten to 30 minutes will adequately fatigue the muscles and aid in reduction.

Skeletal traction, where sterile pins or ice tong–like devices are attached to the distal fragment and traction is exerted on the device, is a method not widely used in veterinary surgery but has merit, as it allows for a straight pull on the bone fragments, whereas the other methods all cause some distraction of bone ends due to muscle pull. The Gordon extender is useful as the method of producing traction.

Following adequate traction it may be possible to directly reduce the fragments by direct manipulation of the more movable fragment (Fig. 2–10). More likely is the necessity of resorting to toggeling, or angulation of the bone ends (Fig. 2–11). Here the bone fragments are angulated to form a V so the ends

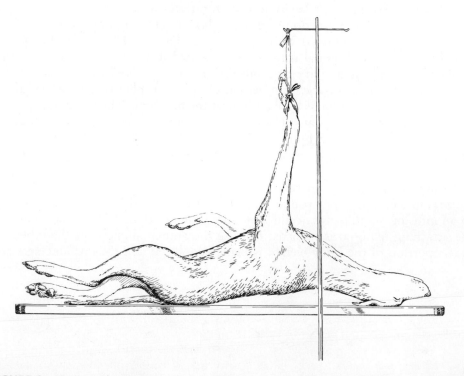

FIGURE 2–12. Use of animal's weight to apply traction and countertraction in fatiguing spastically contracted muscles.

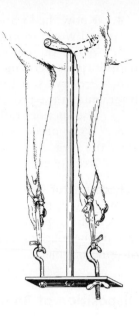

FIGURE 2–13. Use of the Gordon extender. Gradual turning down of the wing nut increases traction on the affected limb. The wing nut is tightened at about 5-minute intervals to increase traction.

can be brought into contact, then the ends are maintained in reduction while the angle formed by the bones is forcefully reduced by pressure at each end of the bone. Maintenance of this pressure fatigues the muscle to allow restoration of length.

Open Reduction

Open reduction is the method of choice in many cases. The fragments are reduced under direct vision, and usually some type of internal fixation is applied to ensure that the position is maintained. (Internal fixation is discussed under the section Immobilization and in the chapters covering treatment of specific fractures.)

Open reduction technique is usually used in a high percentage of fracture cases, particularly in those that are unstable and more complicated, those of more than several days' duration, those involving an articular surface, and those for which internal fixation is indicated. Many of the more common open approaches are described in connection with the treatment of fractures involving the various bones. The book *An Atlas of Surgical Approaches to the Bones and Joints in the Dog and Cat* is the standard reference for these approaches.[17] The surgeon should strive continually to improve soft tissue handling techniques. The following are some of the principal points to follow:

1. Attain strict hemostasis. Active bleeding must be controlled if the operative field is to be clearly visualized. Control of hemorrhage may also be critical in preserving the life of the animal, and it reduces some of the possible complications in postoperative healing. Electrocoagulation is invaluable, as it is efficient in sealing small bleeding points and shortens operating time.

2. Follow normal separations between muscles and fascial planes.

3. If a muscle needs to be severed for exposure, do this near its origin or insertion to minimize trauma and hemorrhage, facilitate closure, and minimize loss of muscular function.

4. Know the location of major blood vessels and nerves. Locate these structures and work around them.

5. Avoid putting excess traction on nerves because this may bring about temporary or permanent injury.

6. Preserve soft tissue attachments (and, therefore, blood supply) to bone fragments in the process of exposure, reduction, and application of fixation.

7. Use suction, rather than blotting, to minimize soft tissue trauma.

8. When necessary, blot with moist gauze sponges (Ringer's solution) to help clear the area. Avoid wiping.

9. Irrigate copiously to remove blood clots and debris.

Each fracture is unique and may require a different maneuver or combination of maneuvers to bring about reduction. Again, the preferred technique in most cases is the application of gradual progressive pressure over a period of time to fatigue the muscles and bring about sufficient relaxation to allow the reduction of bone fragments.

Disposition of Bone Fragments at the Fracture Site

The presence of various bone fragments in the fracture area is frequently encountered. As a general rule, all fragments are kept whether or not they have soft tissue attachment. The exact disposition of these fragments depends on what scheme of internal fixation will be employed. As will be discussed below in the section Immobilization, there are the possibilities of either trying to achieve anatomical reconstruction of the fragments, or of leaving the fragments untouched in order to preserve their blood supply. If anatomic reconstruction is chosen, all fragments with soft tissue attachments are carefully handled to maintain this attachment. The pieces that are too small for internal fixation with bone screws, wires, or Kirschner wires are maneuvered back into position as best as possible with minimal disruption of soft tissue attachments. In most cases, the surrounding soft tissue maintains or even improves the position of these pieces as the process of healing begins. Large fragments, with or without soft tissue attachment, are usually fixed in place with lag screws, wires, or Kirschner wires.

As a general rule, these fragments aid in restoring the original bone substance and function as an autogenous bone graft. They only form sequestra when contamination or infection is present, and even under these circumstances, they may enter into callus formation.

Removal of fragments in many cases results in delayed union, nonunion, or a decrease in diameter of the bone in that area. Generally, if removed, they should be replaced by a bone graft. That is particularly true if rigid fixation (plate) is applied, or if any conditions are present (aged animal, devitalized surrounding tissue, architecture deficits after reduction, and so forth) that result in slow healing. See Chapter 3 for further discussion of bone grafting.

Methods of Open Reduction

The following are presented as suggestions:

1. Application of levering by use of some instrument such as an osteotome, bone skid, periosteal elevator, or scalpel handle (Fig. 2–14).

2. Application of direct force (using bone-holding forceps) on one or more of the bone fragments (Fig. 2–15).

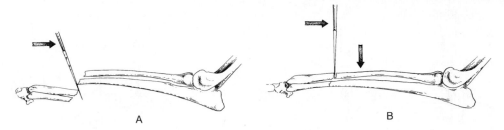

FIGURE 2–14. (*A*, *B*) Application of levering by use of an osteotome.

3. Direct application of force on both of the bone fragments (Fig. 2–16*A*, *B*). After they are reduced by the application of traction, countertraction, and corrective rotation, self-holding bone forceps may be used to temporarily maintain reduction while fixation is applied (Fig. 2–16*E*).

4. Application of distraction force through the bone-holding forceps (Fig. 2–16*C*, *D*). If the overriding muscle forces are strong enough, it may be difficult to get the last small amount of distraction to allow complete reduction by simple traction as illustrated in Figure 2–16*A*, *B*. If the bone-holding forceps is applied with finger pressure across the bone at an angle, it can then be rotated to force each bone fragment into the reduced position. This maneuver depends on the friction between the bone and forceps being greater than that between the bone fragments. Apply this method cautiously in young animals, as the bone may be crushed before adequate friction is created between the bone and forceps.

5. Direct application of force on both of the bone fragments combined with the use of levering (Fig. 2–17).

6. Use of the fracture distractor (Synthes Ltd. [USA], Paoli, PA; Jorgensen Laboratories, Loveland, CO) (Fig. 2–18). In multifragmentary fractures it is often difficult to restore length through direct distraction forces, and the distractor is invaluable here. Fixation pins are applied through both cortices, then attached to the distractor with finger nuts. Wing nuts on a threaded rod allow the fracture to be slowly distracted until the fragments can be secured with bone-holding forceps, Kirschner wires, or cerclage wires. Definitive fixation, usually a bone plate or external fixator, can be applied at this time. Some angular deformity develops as distraction progresses, and this will have to be reduced during application of the definitive fixation.

7. Use of the Steinmann pin as a fracture distractor (Fig. 2–19). This is a simple alternative to the fracture distractor applicable to fractures of the hu-

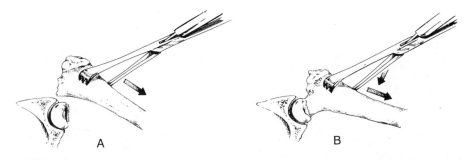

FIGURE 2–15. (*A*, *B*) Application of direct force (using bone-holding forceps) on one or more bone fragments.

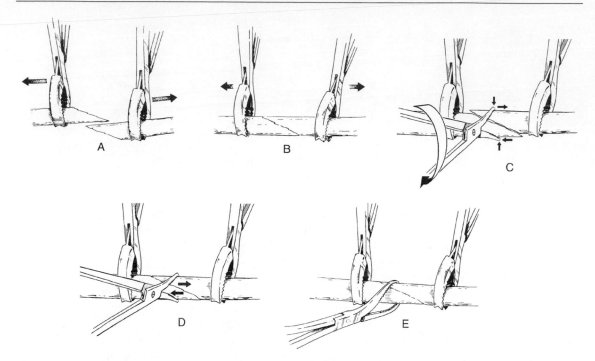

FIGURE 2–16. Open reduction of fractures. (*A, B*) Direct application of force to the bone fragments. (*C*) Oblique fracture overriding can be reduced by grasping the fragments with a bone-holding forceps that is angulated so that each jaw is towards the end of the bone fragment. The forceps is not locked, but held by finger pressure only. (*D*) By rotating the forceps in the direction shown in *C* while applying enough pressure to cause the forceps to grasp the cortex, the fragments will slide into reduction. (*E*) After reduction, a locking bone-holding forceps is used to maintain temporary reduction of the fragments while fixation is applied.

merus and femur. A Steinmann pin with a diameter of 50 percent of the medullary canal is introduced into the bone in either a normograde or retrograde manner. It is then driven across the fracture line(s) into the distal fragment. This is facilitated if the distal fragment is angulated to restore axial alignment by means of a bone-holding forceps. While the proximal fragment is secured with a bone-holding forceps to allow force to be applied in a proximal direction, the pin is driven against the distal metaphyseal area without any rotational drilling action, thus producing distraction. Once adequate length is attained, the frag-

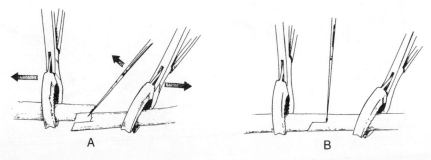

FIGURE 2–17. (*A, B*) Direct application of force on both bone fragments combined with the use of levering.

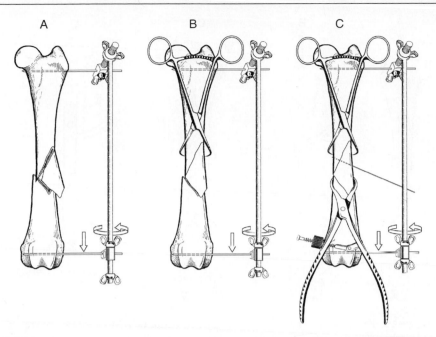

FIGURE 2–18. Use of the fracture distractor to aid in reduction is particularly helpful in femoral fractures in large-breed dogs. (*A*) Fixation pins are placed through both cortices of the proximal and distal fragment in locations that will cause minimal interference when fixation is applied. In most cases these pins are placed through the skin outside the open approach. Clockwise rotation of the wing nut will cause distraction of the fracture. (*B*) As length is regained, individual fragments can be reduced and held with bone-holding forceps. (*C*) When length is totally restored it is possible to completely reduce the fracture and stabilize it with a bone-holding forceps. Kirschner wires are also useful for temporary fixation. If bone plate fixation is used, the plate can be molded and clamped to the bone before the distractor is removed.

ments are secured with bone-holding forceps, Kirschner wires, cerclage wires, or a bone plate, and the pin is withdrawn.

Note: Bone fragments must be handled with care because too much force may result in additional fragmentation. In skeletally immature animals, the bone is easily crushed by bone-holding forceps.

IMMOBILIZATION (FIXATION)

Immobilization involves fixing the bone fragments so that they are motionless with respect to each other during the healing process. The objectives are to stabilize the fragments and to prevent displacement, angulation, and rotation. Ideally, the method used should (1) accomplish uninterrupted stabilization at the time of the original surgery, (2) permit early ambulation, and (3) permit the use of as many joints as possible during the healing period.

The peculiarities of each fracture will dictate or suggest the method of immobilization to be employed. Some fractures lend themselves to a variety of methods, whereas in others, the methods may be very limited for a successful outcome.

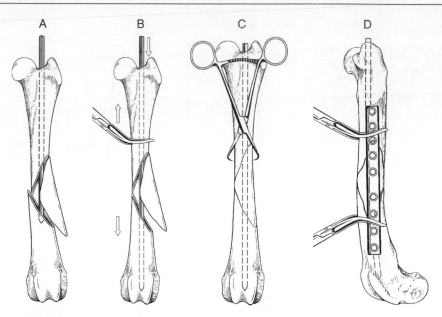

FIGURE 2–19. Fracture distraction with an intramedullary (IM) pin. (*A*) A Steinmann pin is placed in the normograde manner and driven distally across the fracture site, and the pin is maneuvered into the medullary canal of the distal fragment. If the IM pin will not be used for final fixation, the pin diameter can be smaller than usual. (*B*) The distal fragment is brought into axial alignment by bone-holding forceps and traction through the proximal tibia while the stifle is flexed 90 degrees. The pin is driven distally by pressure without rotation until it seats in the distal metaphysis. As pressure is applied to the pin with counterpressure on the proximal fragment via a bone-holding forceps, the distal fragment is gradually reduced. (*C*) Bone-holding forceps are used to hold reduced fragments. (*D*) If bone plate fixation is used, the plate is molded and clamped to the bone before the IM pin is removed.

Methods of Fixation

The methods of fixation may be classified as follows:

1.   Limb splintage (coaptation splints, casts, modified Thomas splint).
2.   Bone splintage (intramedullary pin, external skeletal fixator, bone plate).
3.   Compression (lag screw, cerclage/interfragmentary wire, tension band wire, tension band/compression plate).

Fixation by *splinting* stabilizes the bone either indirectly as with casts and splints, or directly as with pins, fixators, or bone plates that are attached to the bone. There is a certain amount of motion at the fracture site due to the inherent flexibility of these types of devices. The surgeon must ensure that the amount of motion at the fracture site is still within the limits consistent with callus formation. Fixation by *compression* utilizes interfragmentary friction produced by relatively small implants to produce stability of the bone surfaces. The compression may be static in nature, as with a lag screw or cerclage wire, in which case the compression is not expected to change with time. Dynamic compression, on the other hand, does change cyclically with loading of the limb as limb function periodically loads and unloads the bone surfaces. Functionally induced tension of the bone fragments is transformed into compression forces by the tension band wire or plate.

Temporary Splintage

If for some reason there is a delay in reduction and fixation, temporary splintage (e.g., Robert-Jones dressing, coaptation splint, Thomas splint) of the limb may be indicated to reduce additional trauma. This is true particularly for fractures distal to the elbow and stifle. In most other fractures, the animal is more comfortable simply with cage rest and mild sedation/analgesia. The objective in most fracture cases is early reduction and fixation.

Coaptation Splints and Casts

External casts, splints, and bandages are often called coaptation fixation devices, the word "coapt" meaning to approximate. This is accomplished by simply immobilizing muscles, as with a bandage, or by transmitting compression forces to the bony structures by means of the interposed soft tissues as with casts and splints. Such pressure must be uniformly distributed throughout the cast or splint to avoid circulatory stasis and swelling.

Casts are generally considered to be molded tubular structures that, if removed, would form a mold from which a casting of the limb could be made. A splint is something less than a full cast and typically is molded only to one aspect of the limb. A wire frame structure such as the Schroeder-Thomas splint is a special case, using soft bandage materials to suspend the limb within the wire frame.

As a general rule, molded casts and splints are more efficient stabilizers of the bones and joints than premade ones or the Schroeder-Thomas splint, although good use can be made of both of the latter methods. The advantage of molded devices is that they custom-fit the animal perfectly and therefore cause fewer soft tissue problems and are better tolerated by the patient. For many years, plaster of Paris was the only moldable material available, but many such materials have become available. Of these, two types have proved especially useful, the thermomoldable and the fiberglass/resin materials. X-Lite (AOA Kirschner Medical Corporation, Marlow, OK) is a thermomoldable plastic material, impregnated onto an open-mesh fabric. When heated to 160° to 170°F, it becomes very soft and self-adherent and then hardens within a few minutes as it cools to room temperature. It is available as precut splints or rolls in 3-, 4-, and 6-inch widths. X-Lite is most useful in small animal patients for making splints. Veterinary Thermoplastic (VTP) (Imex Veterinary Inc., Longview, TX) is similar in application, but is a solid homogenous material rather than an open mesh, and is available in rolls of varying widths. Because these materials are self-adherent they can be made as stiff as necessary by adding layers to effect.

Fiberglass materials have a resin/binding material impregnated into the roll of knitted fiberglass tape. They are popular because of ease of application and relatively few complications. The resin is activated by a 10- to 15-second immersion in water of room temperature, following which the material cures and hardens within a few minutes at room temperature. Fiberglass has proved very useful for full-cylinder casts, although it can also be used for splints. Cast-cutting saws are essential for removing cylinder casts. All of these products are lightweight, strong, and waterproof. Since wider width material generally makes stronger casts, use the widest roll consistent with the animal's size.[18] To obtain maximal usefulness, use them with polypropylene or other synthetic stockinet and cast padding, both of which shed water. Because these materials all "breathe" and do not retain water, there are few soft tissue problems such as maceration of skin. Pressure sores are still possible when casts are incorrectly applied, but even this problem occurs less frequently than when cotton padding materials are used. Synthetic orthopedic felt used over bony prominences will do much to reduce pressure sores. In general, the middle and distal phalanges of the middle toes should be left exposed to monitor swelling.

Owners should be instructed to observe the protruding toes twice daily, looking for signs that the toenails are spreading apart. Such a sign indicates swelling and requires that the cast be removed immediately to prevent pressure necrosis. Reapplication of the cast with less pressure can follow immediately, or the limb can be placed in a Robert-Jones bandage for a few days to allow swelling to be resorbed. The animal should be kept indoors to minimize damage to the external fixation device. If taken outside for eliminations in wet or damp conditions, a plastic bag or similar impervious material should be temporarily placed over the foot to keep the cast/splint or bandage material clean and dry. An electric hair dryer can be applied to hasten drying in case the limb becomes wetted. The owner should be instructed to have the device checked regularly at 7- to 10-day intervals or at any sign of foul odor, drainage, loosening, chafing, instability, or obsessive licking or chewing on the appliance. Such signs are indications for removal of the device and evaluation of the soft tissues, with appropriate treatment. Reapplication of the cast/splint may require some revision to prevent recurrence of the problem. The thermomoldable materials are reheated and reapplied as originally. Do not remove a cast or splint simply because a certain amount of time has gone by and you are curious to see the soft tissues; if the animal is tolerating the device well and it is still functional it should be left undisturbed until the appropriate time for removal.

Because of the pain created by manipulating broken bones, and the muscular relaxation needed for most reductions, general anesthesia is almost always indicated when applying these devices.

INDICATIONS FOR COAPTATION ■ Consider the forces acting on the bone and how well the proposed immobilization will neutralize them: angulation or bending, rotation (shear), shortening or overriding (shear), and distraction. The following generally fall within the range of casts and splints:

1.   Closed fracture below elbow or stifle. In Figure 2–20, a', b', c', and d' indicate the length of cast/splint needed for fractures in zones a, b, c, and d.
2.   Fractures amenable to closed reduction as discussed above.
3.   Fractures in which the bone will be stable after reduction relative to shortening or distraction; classified above as type A or B fractures (see Table 2–1].
4.   Fractures in which the bone can be expected to heal quickly enough that cast/splint will not cause severe joint stiffness/muscle atrophy (fracture disease).
5.   Specific indications:

Greenstick fractures.
Long-bone fractures in young animals where periosteal sleeve is mostly intact.
Impaction fractures.

LONG-LEG CYLINDER CAST ■ A long-leg cast is one that extends from the toes to the axilla or groin (Fig. 2–21). Plaster of Paris or fiberglass/resin tape are the most commonly employed materials. A variety of casting tapes made of knitted fiberglass substrate and impregnated with various resins are now available, and are utilized much in the same manner as plaster of Paris. These products are strong, lightweight, waterproof, and porous, but cannot be molded as

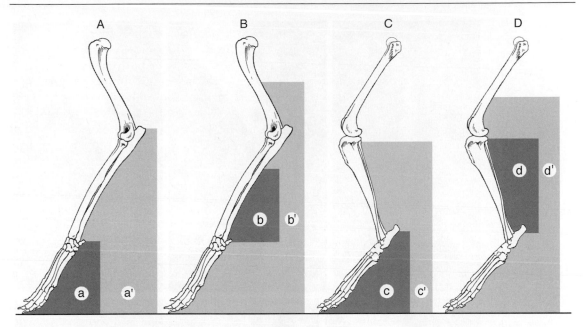

FIGURE 2–20. (A–D) Optimal splint or cast length for fractures in the dark shaded areas are shown by the length of the light shaded areas.

perfectly as plaster. These casts have to be removed with a cast-cutting oscillating saw whether they are made of plaster of Paris or fiberglass.

The cast can be bivalved after it has hardened for ease of inspection and redressing. To prevent the padding from sticking to the resin it is covered with a sheet of thin polyethylene film (as used for food storage) while the cast material is applied. After hardening of the resin, the cast-cutter saw is used to split the cast into halves along either the saggital or frontal planes. The plastic film is removed after separating the two halves, which are then reapplied and held together with nonelastic white tape. Future cast changes are accomplished by cutting the tape, removing the half shells, repadding the limb, and reapplying the half shells. Care must be taken to apply the same amount and type of padding as was used originally in order to prevent either undue pressure or looseness when the cast is reapplied.

Indications ■ Immobilization of the elbow and stifle, the radius and ulna, and the tibia and fibula.

SHORT-LEG CYLINDER CAST ■ A short-leg cast extends only to the proximal tibia or radius (Fig. 2–22). The elbow and stifle joints are free to move normally.

Indications ■ Immobilization of the carpus and metacarpus and the tarsus and metatarsus. As a general rule, short-leg casts are used primarily in large, active animals to provide more stabilization than short-leg splints.

SPICA SPLINT—FORELEG ■ Although this splint can be constructed with wood, rigid plastics, or aluminum, the molded splint is better tolerated and gives better immobilization (Fig. 2–23). This splint is named for the method of attaching it to the body by a spica (figure-of-8) bandage. In the dog the bandage

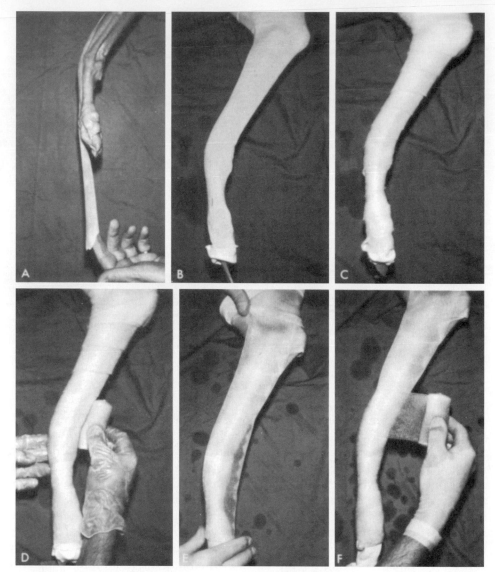

FIGURE 2–21. A long-leg cylinder cast extends from the toes to the axilla or groin. Application here is to the forelimb with fiberglass material. (*A*) Adhesive tape stirrups are applied to the lower limb and extend several inches beyond the toes. (*B*) Polypropylene stockinet is applied to the limb. The material should be long enough to extend distally beyond the toes and well into the axilla proximally. (*C*) Two to three layers of polypropylene cast padding are applied to the limb starting at the toes and proceeding proximally. (*D*) After the fiberglass tape is immersed in water at room temperature for 12 to 15 seconds and gently squeezed of excess water, the roll of fiberglass is spiraled onto the limb; rubber or vinyl (as recommended by the manufacturer) gloves are used to protect the hands. This material should be rolled on smoothly using even pressure, which is facilitated by rolling continuously around the limb in a spiral fashion and not raising the roll away from the skin. Two layers of cast material are produced by overlapping the spirals by half the width of the roll. The distal end of the cast should be at the level of the base of the distal phalanx of the middle toes. (*E*) A longitudinal splint is applied to both the medial and lateral sides. This material is cut from the roll and applied over the spiraled material. Mechanical testing has revealed that these splints add more strength to fiberglass casts when applied cranially and caudally.[18] (*F*) A second spiral layer is applied over the splints, resulting in four spiraled layers plus the medial and lateral splints. Very large breeds may require six layers. *Figure continued on opposite page*

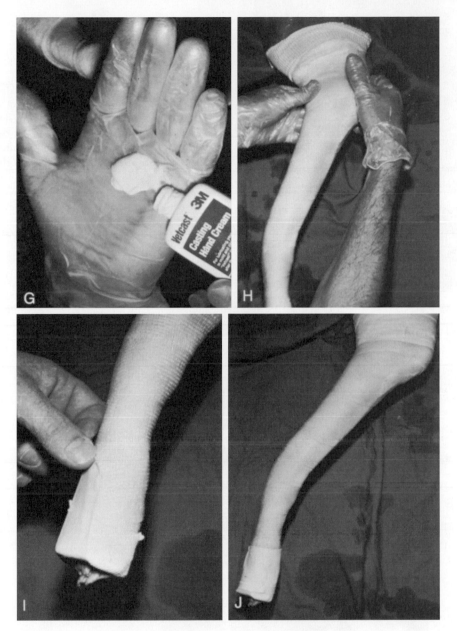

FIGURE 2–21. *Continued* (*G*) Hand lotion or lubricating jelly is used to treat the gloves to prevent them from sticking to the fiberglass resin. Some products do not require the use of lotion. (*H*) After use of the lotion or jelly on the gloves, it is possible to smooth the fiberglass and conform it to the limb. The material begins to harden in 4 to 5 minutes under average temperature conditions. (*I*) After hardening of the fiberglass, the ends of the cast are dressed by folding the stockinet over the end of the fiberglass. At the distal end, the tape initially applied to the skin is folded over the end of the cast. This tape and the stockinet are secured with circular wraps of tape. The proximal end of the cast is similarly taped. (*J*) The completed cast. Note that both the elbow and the carpus have been maintained in moderate flexion.

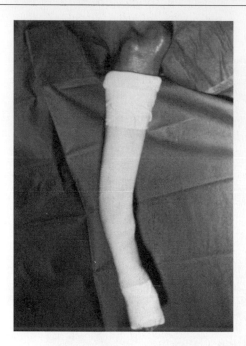

FIGURE 2–22. A short-leg cylinder cast is made in the same manner as the long-leg cast but does not cover the elbow or the stifle. In this case, the cast has been applied to the forelimb and ends just distal to the elbow joint.

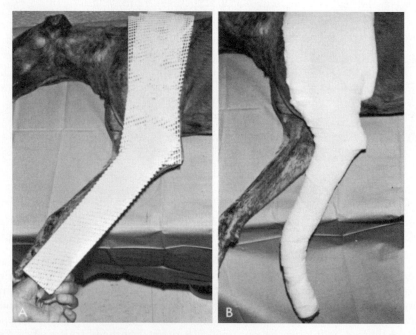

FIGURE 2–23. Spica splint for the foreleg. (A) Precut X-Lite splints are laid over the limb, and the area of overlap is noted. Veterinary Thermoplastic can be applied in one piece, since it comes in long rolls. Three to six thicknesses are used, depending on the size of the animal and the degree of rigidity required. (B) The limb has been padded with two or three layers of polypropylene cast padding to the axilla, and sheet cotton is placed over the proximal humerus, shoulder joint, and scapula. This padding should extend dorsally to the midline. *Figure continued on opposite page*

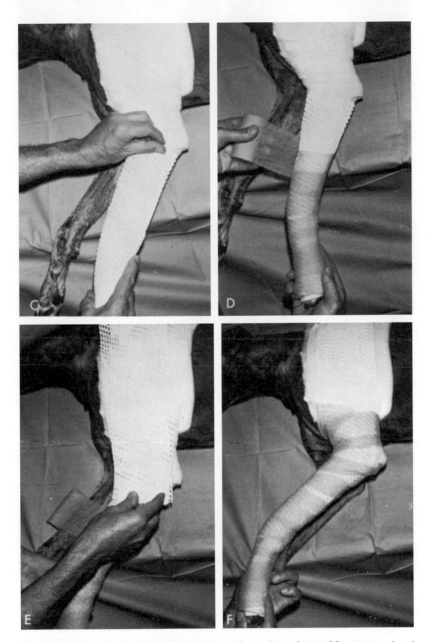

FIGURE 2–23. *Continued* (*C*) The distal splints have been heated by immersion in water at 170°F and are being placed over the lower limb, then molded by hand. (*D*) Conforming gauze is used to hold the softened splint material against the limb while it hardens. The proximal end of the splint is left exposed for attachment to the upper splints. (*E*) The upper splints have been heated and are placed over the shoulder and onto the more distal splints. The material will adhere to itself and form a continuous splint. These splints are then molded by hand to conform to the limb. (*F*) Conforming gauze has been rolled proximally to the axilla to complete molding of the proximal splints. The upper end of these proximal splints can be molded over the shoulder by hand pressure until sufficiently cooled to harden. *Figure continued on following page*

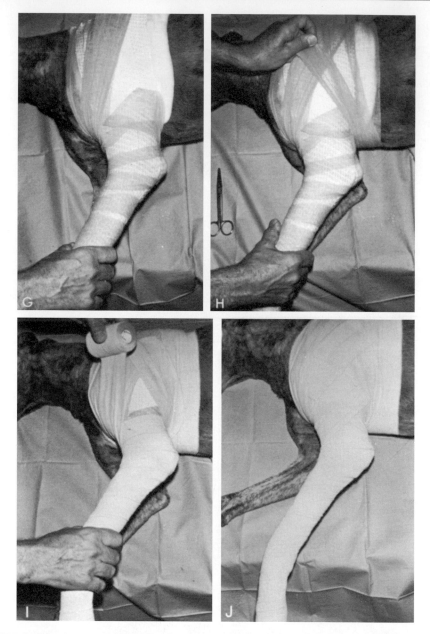

FIGURE 2–23. *Continued* (G) Conforming gauze is used to attach the splint to the chest wall. This gauze creates a half figure-of-8 around the splinted limb but is carried behind the opposite axilla. (H) Bandaging has been completed. (I) The bandage is covered with wide elastic tape, applied in a pattern similar to that of the gauze. If short-term immobilization is contemplated, white tape can be substituted. (J) Bandaging has been completed.

is modified to be only half of a figure-of-8. It can be applied to the hip, but bandaging in this region is very difficult, especially in the male dog, and ambulation is awkward.

Indications ■ Immobilization of the shoulder, humerus, and elbow.

LONG LATERAL SPLINT ■   This splint is shorter than a spica, but otherwise it is constructed and attached similarly from the axilla or groin distally (Fig. 2–24).

Indications ■   Immobilization of the elbow and stifle joints.

SCHROEDER-THOMAS SPLINT ■   This versatile splint has been widely used for immobilization of fractures (Fig. 2–25). Considerable artistry is required to construct a functional, well-tolerated, and effective splint. Widely used in the past,[19] it has been largely superseded by molded splints and casts. Nevertheless it remains useful for those versed in its application.

Indications ■   Immobilization of the elbow, stifle, carpus, and tarsus; the radius and ulna, and the tibia and fibula. It is perhaps the most effective device for immobilization of the stifle joint at a functional angle. Care must be taken to keep the splint as short as possible, in order to allow active weight bearing; this is accomplished by placing all joints at functional (standing) angles.

SHORT LATERAL SPLINT—HIND LEG ■   Although this type of molded splint (Fig. 2–26) can be applied to any surface of the lower hindlimb, the lateral surface has resulted in fewer soft tissue injuries.

Indications ■   Immobilization of the tarsus and metatarsus.

SHORT CAUDAL SPLINT—FORELEG ■   This splint (Fig. 2–27) replaces the preformed rigid plastic and metal "spoon" splints in wide use. Such splints are not suitable for long-term use because of the incidence of soft tissue problems and poor immobilization. The only way a curved limb can be put in a straight premolded splint is with copious padding, and this destroys rigid immobilization. A properly made molded splint can often be left on for 6 weeks with no soft tissue problems.

Indications ■   Immobilization of the carpus and metacarpus.

PHALANGEAL SPLINT ■   This bivalved splint (Fig. 2–28) is designed to protect the toes while leaving the antebrachiocarpal or tarsocrural joints free to move normally.

VELPEAU SLING ■   This bandage is generally well tolerated by most animals (Fig. 2–29). In addition to its main use for shoulder and scapular injuries, it can serve as a substitute for hard casts or splints when the objective is simply to prevent weight bearing of the foreleg, although the carpal flexion bandage is much easier to apply (see below).

CARPAL FLEXION BANDAGE ■   The flexion bandage is intended purely to discourage weight bearing while maintaining passive motion of the shoulder and elbow joints. It is useful following lateral shoulder luxation, supraspinatus, and biceps brachii surgery. The carpus is less than fully flexed while two or three layers of wide white tape are applied from the distal third of the radius/ulna to the metacarpal region. Narrower tape is used in the middle to keep the bandage from slipping off the leg. Although usually well tolerated when applied as illustrated (Fig. 2–30), some animals will develop skin irritation on the cranial surface of the antebrachium, and will need to have cast padding applied between the skin and tape.

EHMER SLING ■   Primarily used to partially immobilize and stabilize the hip joint (Fig. 2–31), this bandage can also be used to prevent weight bearing of

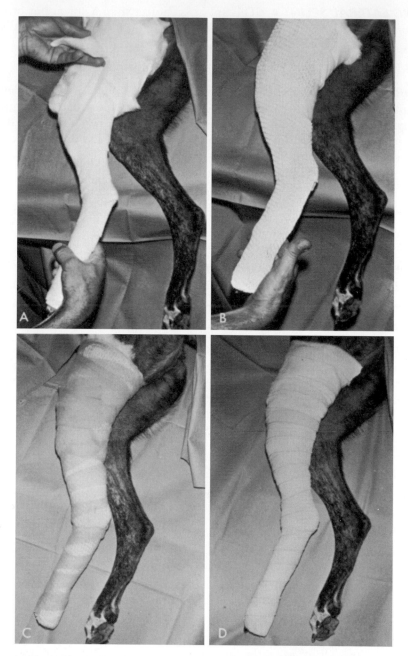

FIGURE 2–24. A long lateral splint applied to the hindlimb. (*A*) The lower limb is padded with two to three layers of polypropylene cast padding to the level of the stifle, and sheet cotton is applied from the stifle to the level of the hip joint. The cast padding overlaps the lower end of the sheet cotton to help fix it in place. (*B*) Overlapping precut X-Lite splints, or full-length Veterinary Thermoplastic splints are applied proximally and distally, with three to six thicknesses, depending on the size of the animal and rigidity required. The splints will stick together where they overlap, and the splints are initially molded by hand to conform to the limb. (*C*) The softened splints are covered with conforming gauze bandage to hold the splints conformed to the limb while they harden. (*D*) Following hardening, the splint material is covered with wide elastic tape to complete the splint.

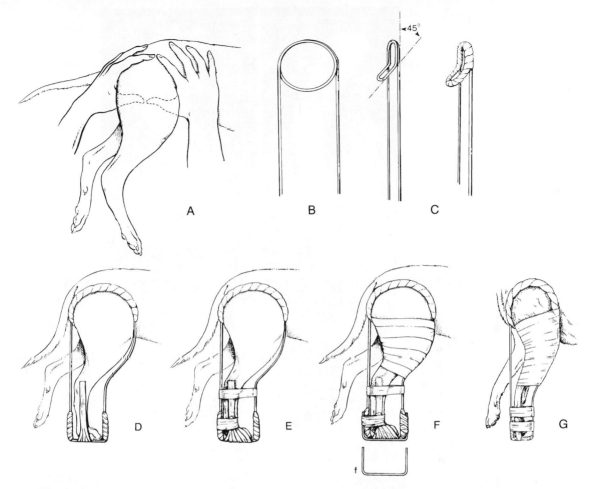

FIGURE 2–25. Fabrication of the modified Thomas splint. After the diameter of the thigh is approximated (*A*), the aluminum alloy rod is bent, forming 1½ circles (*B*). (*C*) The lower half of the ring is bent at a 45-degree angle to accommodate the thickness of the thigh and to avoid femoral vessel pressure; foam, cotton, or cast padding is added, followed by gauze and tape. (*D*) With the splint pushed firmly up in the inguinal region, the caudal bar is first bent to approximate the length of the leg with the limb in normal standing angulation and the toes flexed to simulate standing. Next the cranial rod is bent to approximate normal angulation of the limb with the toes flexed to simulate standing. The distal ends of the bars are then taped securely together. (*E*) Splint is again pushed firmly up in the inguinal region; foot is anchored with adhesive tape. (*F*) If a dog weighs more than 25 pounds, a walking bar (*f*) is applied. A layer of cotton is placed around the upper leg, then both are anchored as one to the cranial bar with a layer of gauze and tape. Anchoring the tape to the bar in the inguinal area holds the padding for the thigh in place; otherwise it slips distally and serves no useful purpose. (*G*) The forelimb splint is reversed from the hindlimb to accommodate the normal joint angles.

any joint of the hindlimb. The ASPCA sling (see below) is probably better tolerated when prevention of weight bearing is the primary objective.

ASPCA SLING[20] ■ This sling (Fig. 2–32) is very effective in preventing weight bearing on the hindlimb, yet allows passive motion of the hip and stifle joints. It is better tolerated and has fewer complications than the Ehmer sling.

ROBERT-JONES BANDAGE ■ This highly padded bandage (Fig. 2–33) is very versatile, being useful not only in immobilization distal to the elbow or

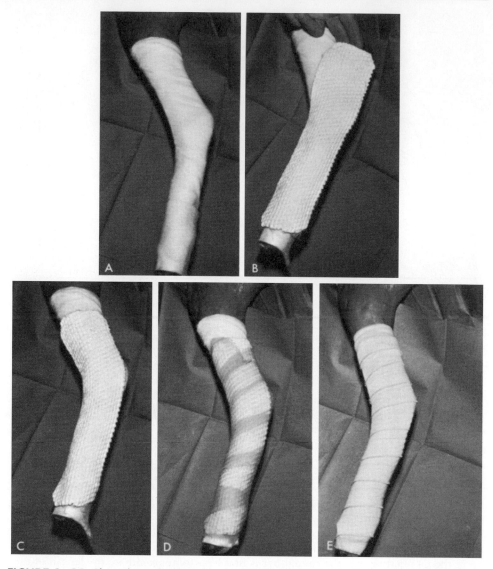

FIGURE 2–26. Short lateral splint for the hindleg. (*A*) The limb is padded with two to three layers of polypropylene cast padding to the level of the tibial tubercle. A small piece of orthopedic felt is placed on the tuber calcis and is secured by the cast padding. Additional thicknesses of cast padding can be substituted. (*B*) Four to six thicknesses of precut X-Lite splints or full-length Veterinary Thermoplastic splints are placed on the lateral side of the limb. The distal end of the splint extends to the level of the base of the distal phalanx of the middle toes. (*C*) The splint is molded to the standing angle of the hock while the material is placed laterally to slightly dorsolaterally on the hock region. If the splint material extends more than 180 degrees around the limb, it should be trimmed. (*D*) The splint is held in position by a conforming gauze bandage while the material hardens. (*E*) The splint is completed by covering with elastic tape.

stifle but also in decreasing or preventing edema. It is well tolerated, but because of the large volume of cotton, it can absorb considerable quantities of water and cause maceration of skin or contamination of surgical incisions. It is generally used only for short-term immobilization. Additional rigidity can be obtained by adding a wire frame or molded splints to the bandage.

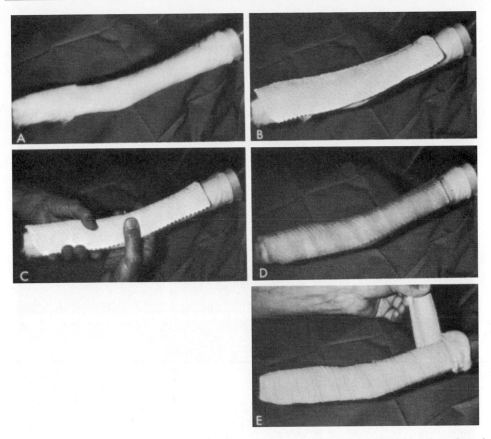

FIGURE 2–27. Short caudal splint for the foreleg. (A) The dog is positioned in dorsal recumbency to expose the caudal surface of the lower limb, which is padded with two to three layers of polypropylene cast padding. (B) Three to six precut X-Lite splints or full-length Veterinary Thermoplastic splints are heated and applied to the caudal surface of the limb. If the splint material extends more than 180 degrees around the limb, it should be trimmed. (C) The splints are conformed to the limb with the desired degree of carpal flexion. The distal end of the splint should extend to the level of the base of the distal phalanx of the middle toes. (D) The softened splints are held in position by a conforming gauze bandage. This bandage material must not be rolled too tightly, for it will create soft-tissue pressure sores along the edge of the splint. (E) After the splint hardens, it is completed by covering with conforming tape.

General Considerations

When a coaptation splint or cast is used, the following points should be considered:

Padding ■ If closed reduction is used, the hair is usually not clipped. A light padding (cast padding, stockinet, cotton, sheet wadding, felt) should be applied to protect the soft tissues, with particular emphasis given to bony prominence (e.g., accessory carpal pad, tuber calcis, olecranon process, dewclaw). This is best accomplished by increased padding in the depressed areas over and less over the prominences. Avoid overpadding because it may allow movement of bone fragments inside the coaptation splint or cast.

Fixation ■ Anchor in place to avoid shifting on the limb. This is particularly applicable if the leg is swollen when the cast is applied. This may be accom-

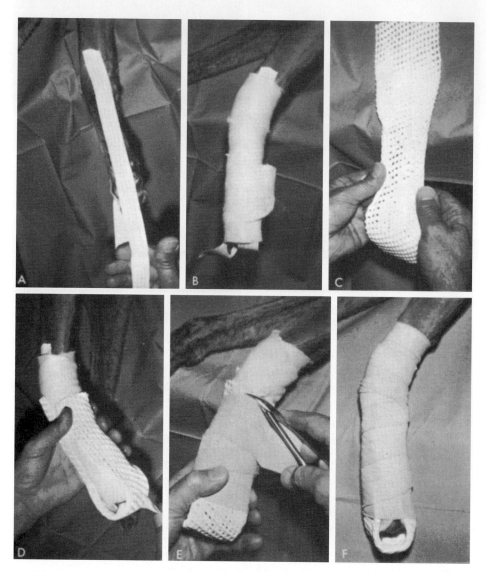

FIGURE 2–28. A phalangeal splint applied to the front foot. On the hindfoot, the splint extends proximally to the level of the distal tarsal bones. (A) Adhesive tape is attached to the medial and lateral surfaces of the paw. (B) The paw and lower limb are covered with three to four layers of polypropylene cast padding to a point just proximal to the carpus. (C) Two to three thicknesses of precut X-Lite splints or full-length Veterinary Thermoplastic splints are heated to soften. The middle portion is then crimped on each edge to make the splints slightly narrower at this point and to create extra thickness at the end of the splint. (D) The soft splint material is applied on the dorsal and palmar sides of the foot with the splint material folded over the toes. There should be room to insert a finger between the toes and the end of the splint. The splint is conformed by hand pressure while the material cools and hardens. (E) The splint is covered with elastic tape. A portion of the proximal end of the palmar portion of the splint is trimmed when necessary to avoid pressure caused by flexion of the carpus. Wire-cutting scissors can be used for this trimming. (F) Elastic tape is applied over the splint and proximally to the end of the padding.

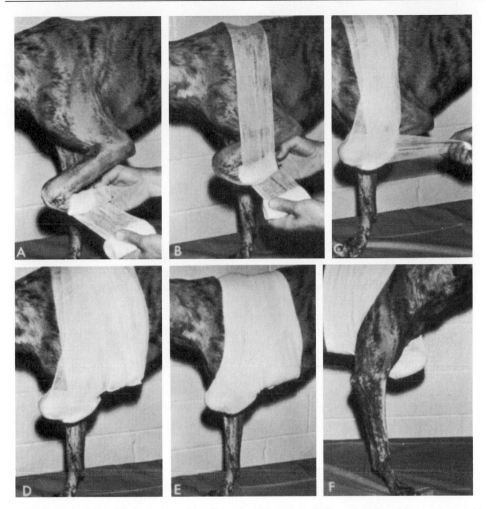

FIGURE 2–29. A Velpeau sling bandage used to immobilize the shoulder region. (*A*) Conforming gauze bandage material is wrapped loosely around the paw in a lateral to medial direction. (*B*) With the carpus, elbow, and shoulder all flexed, the gauze is brought from the paw over the lateral aspect of the limb and shoulder, over the chest, and behind the opposite axilla. It then continues under the chest, back to the starting point. (*C*) Several more layers of gauze are applied in a similar manner, and a few layers are brought around the flexed carpus to prevent extension of the elbow. Such extension could force the lower limb out of the bandage. (*D*) Gauze bandaging is completed. (*E*) Wide elastic tape is used to cover the gauze in a pattern similar to the gauze application. (*F*) On the opposite side of the animal, both gauze and adhesive tape are brought behind the opposite axilla.

plished with use of adhesive tape and by molding the cast to the contour of the limb.

Radiographs ■ Check reduction radiographically before and after application and again in several days.

Extent ■ Distally, the toes may be covered or preferably the center two digital pads exposed.

Patient's Tolerance ■ Usually, coaptation splints are reasonably well tolerated by the animal, if they are accomplishing their mission, the cast is kept

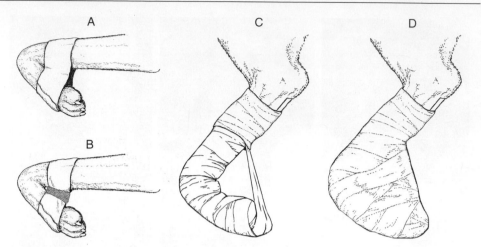

FIGURE 2–30. Carpal flexion bandage. (A) The carpus is flexed while 2-inch white tape encircles the distal radius and ulna and the metacarpal region. (B) Narrow tape is applied to the middle area of both sides of the encircling tape to prevent the tape from slipping over the carpus. (C) Another method involves covering the lower limb with padding and tape, then flexing the carpus with several thicknesses of tape from the dorsal surface of the toes to the proximal antebrachium. (D) The entire bandage is covered with tape.

dry, and activity is limited. Indications of complication include pain, elevation of temperature, swelling, edema, numbness, foul odor, cyanosis of digits, loss of appetite, systemic depression, irritated areas, and chewing on the cast.

EXTERNAL SKELETAL FIXATION*

Use of the external fixator for immobilization of long-bone fractures requires transcutaneous insertion of two to four pins in each of the proximal and distal bone fragments, which are then connected by one or more external bars or rods (see Figs. 2–36, and 2–42 through 2–44).[2,21–24] The entire apparatus is referred to as a splint or a frame, while the bone and attached frame are called a construct or montage. Fixators can be used on all of the long bones, the mandible, and for bridging joints, but are not adaptable to most intra-articular fractures.

Indications or Uses[2,21–36]

The external fixator is adaptable to:

1. Stable and unstable fractures.
2. Open fractures.
3. Gunshot fractures.
4. Osteotomies.
5. Delayed unions and nonunions.
6. Arthrodesis of certain joints.

---

*The author (DLP) would like to gratefully acknowledge the contributions of a colleague, Dr. Erick Egger, to this section.

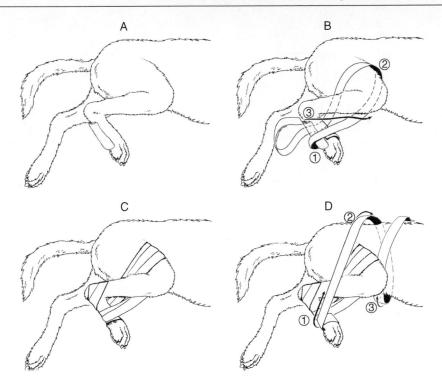

FIGURE 2–31. Ehmer (figure-of-8) sling. (*A*) Application of the sling begins with placing some padding on the plantar surface of the metatarsus. (*B*) Conforming roller gauze bandage is wrapped around the metatarsus (*B1*) from lateral to medial, being sure to include most of the metatarsal pad. After several wraps to secure it, the gauze is carried medial to the flexed stifle (*B2*) and over the cranial surface of the thigh. This internally rotates the limb at the hip joint. Finally (*B3*) the gauze is brought medial to the tibia and tarsus and over the plantar surface of the tarsus. Several more circuits are made in the same manner. (*C*) The gauze is continued in a figure-of-8 fashion around the flexed hock and paw to secure it. The entire bandage is then covered with elastic adhesive tape that overhangs the gauze to anchor the sling to the hair. Although some construct the bandage without any gauze by starting with adhesive tape applied to the skin, this invariably leads to considerable skin irritation on the cranial thigh region as well as the difficulty of removing the large amount of tape. (*D*) It is difficult to keep the sling from slipping down over the stifle on short-legged breeds. One solution is to attach wide adhesive tape to the paw area of the completed sling (*D1*), then carry the tape upwards over the back (*D2*) and then around the belly (*D3*). This is simple in the bitch or cat, but care must be taken to avoid the sheath in the male dog.

    7. Stabilization of certain joints following ligament or tendon reconstruction.

The advantages of the external fixator include (1) ease of application; (2) its usefulness in treating fractures reduced by either open or closed methods; (3) if applied in connection with an open approach, minimization of the approach; (4) fixation pins that can usually be inserted some distance from an open wound; (5) an open wound is readily accessible for dressing; (6) its compatibility for use in conjunction with other internal fixation devices; (7) toleration by both dogs and cats; (8) in most cases, removal without placing the animal under general anesthesia; and (9) reasonable cost.

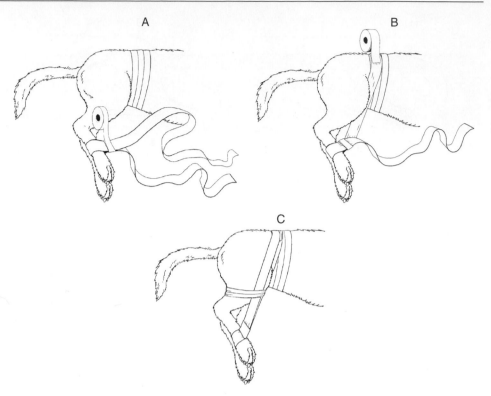

FIGURE 2–32. ASPCA (Robinson) off-weight-bearing sling.[20] (*A*) Six to 8 feet of 2-inch white tape is folded at the center and the adhesive sides pressed together. This double-thickness tape is secured to the tarsus by wrapping with 1-inch tape. A belly wrap of adhesive tape is applied. (*B*) The inner section of double-thickness tape is passed medial to the stifle and is secured to the belly wrap with additional adhesive tape. The length of this section is adjusted to shorten the limb just enough to prevent weight bearing. (*C*) The outer section of double-thickness tape is passed lateral to the stifle and secured to the belly band. The double-thickness tape is stabilized by a wrap of tape approximately halfway between the hock and stifle joints.

Components of the External Fixator

There are an amazing variety of fixators available throughout the world, most of them having been developed for human use. Because of their size and cost, most are not practical for veterinary use, although some are adaptable, especially those designed for hand or forearm use in man. In North America the traditional devices commercially available (Imex Veterinary, Longview, TX; Osteo-Technology International Inc., Hunt Valley, MD; Gauthier Medical, Rochester, MN) are based on the Kirschner-Ehmer adaption of the Roger Anderson splint.[22] The earlier Stader apparatus did not achieve lasting popularity.[21] Similar devices are available from various manufacturers in Europe. The clamps used in these fixators are rather simple in design, and although they have some inherent deficiencies relative to stability, nevertheless they function adequately if properly applied, and provide a relatively economical method of stabilizing a wide variety of fractures. Unless otherwise noted, all frames depicted in this text are of the Kirschner-Ehmer variety.

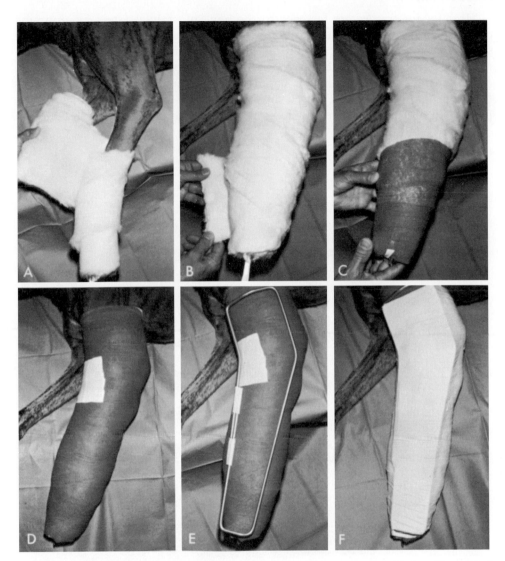

FIGURE 2–33. Robert-Jones bandage. Application of the cotton for this heavily padded bandage is simplified by splitting a 1-pound roll of cotton into two narrower ½-pound rolls. (A) Adhesive tape stirrups have been applied to the lower limb and are used for traction while cotton is spiraled proximally. The tape is carried as high as possible into the axilla or groin. (B) One-half to 2 pounds of cotton are necessary to complete the padding, depending on the size of the animal. (C) Vetrap (3M Animal Care Products, St. Paul, MN) is used to compress the cotton. The tape applied to the limb is folded back and incorporated into the 4-inch-wide Vetrap. The first layer of Vetrap is used to conform and compress the cotton, and the second layer is used to further compress and firm the cotton padding. (D) Adhesive tape is used to secure the end of the Vetrap. (E) Additional stability can be obtained by bending an aluminum splint rod to conform to the Robert-Jones bandage. (F) The splint rod is attached to the Robert-Jones bandage with nonelastic tape. X-Lite or Veterinary Thermoplastic splints can also be used to stiffen the bandage by molding one or more layers over the lateral side in place of the aluminum rod.

Fixation Pins

Most fixator frames are fastened to the bone by stainless steel fixation pins that must penetrate both the first and second cortices. These pins may be either smooth, partially threaded, or fully threaded in design. The latter are not widely used due to their lack of stiffness. Partially threaded pins are either end-threaded or center-threaded. Threads can be cut from the stock of the pin (negative-thread-profile), or built up (raised-thread, enhanced-thread, or positive-thread-profile) to a larger diameter than the pin shaft (Fig. 2–34). Negative-thread-

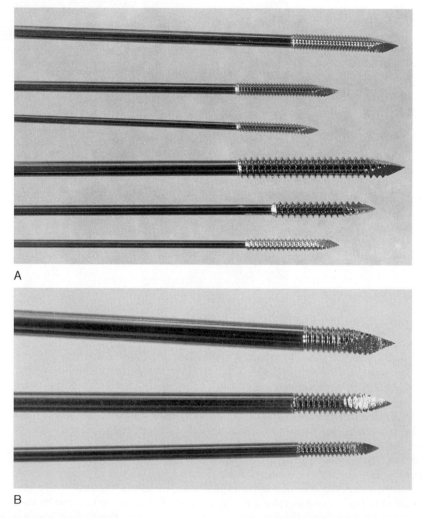

A

B

FIGURE 2–34. External fixator components. (*A*) Fixation half pins with positive thread profile in large (³⁄₁₆-inch; 4.8-mm), medium (⅛-inch; 3.2-mm), and small (⁵⁄₆₄-inch; 2.0-mm) diameters. The upper three pins have cortical threads and the lower three pins have cancellous threads. (*B*) Partially threaded pins with negative cortical thread profile. The threads penetrate the second cortex and the smooth part of the pin rests in the first cortex. *Figure continued on opposite page*

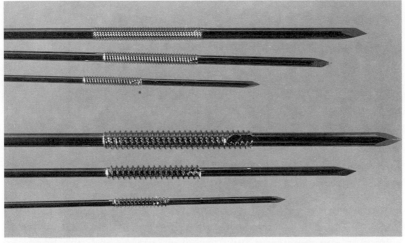

C

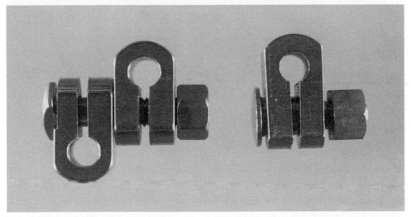

D

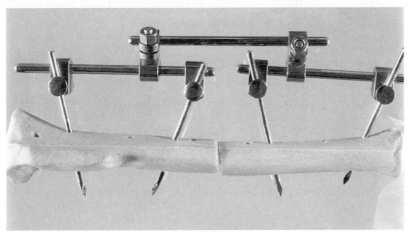

E

FIGURE 2–34. *Continued.* (C) Fixation full pins with positive thread profile in large (3/16-inch; 4.8-mm), medium (1/8-inch; 3.2-mm), and small (5/64-inch; 2.0-mm) diameters. The upper three pins have cortical threads and the lower three pins have cancellous threads. (D) Kirschner-Ehmer double and single clamps. (E) The original Kirschner-Ehmer splint utilizing both double and single clamps.

profile pins usually have a fine thread; that is, a relatively high number of threads per unit of length and are designed for cortical bone insertion. Positive-thread-profile pins are available in both the cortical thread and in a coarser, flatter pitch thread intended for insertion into cancellous bone such as found in the metaphyses of long bones. Typically, a mixture of threaded and smooth pins are used in most frames. Kirschner-Ehmer clamps allow the use of pin diameters up to $\frac{5}{64}$ inch (2.0 mm) in small clamps, to $\frac{1}{8}$ inch (3.2 mm) in medium clamps, and to $\frac{3}{16}$ inch (4.8 mm) in large clamps. An important consideration in the fabrication of frames using positive-profile-threaded pins is that the threads of these pins will not slide through Kirschner-Ehmer clamps, so they must always be inserted into the clamps from the unthreaded end unless oversized clamps are used. Some other available systems utilize clamps that allow them to be attached after the fixation pin is placed. Smooth pins are typically Steinmann pins of the appropriate diameter cut to length after insertion into the bone. Ring fixators use Kirschner wires placed under tension as fixation pins.

If the fixation pin penetrates only one skin surface and two bone cortices it is called a *half pin*, and is the only pin used in type I frames. Those pins that penetrate two skin surfaces and two bone cortices are called *full pins* and are the basis of type II frames. A minimum of two pins is required in each major bone fragment to ensure stability, but more often three or more pins are indicated, as will be discussed in the section Biomechanical Considerations.

Connecting Bars

The connecting bar, or rod, functions to connect the fixation pin clusters attached to the bone fragments, the resulting bone-frame construct providing enough stability to allow the bone to heal while maintaining functional use of the limb. These bars are typically solid stainless steel circular rods with a diameter between $\frac{1}{8}$ and $\frac{1}{4}$ inch (3.2 and 6.5 mm) (Fig. 2–34). Traditionally, the connecting rod has been used only as a straight rod, but as will be illustrated below, there are many instances when it is useful to contour the rod. Although hollow rods are more rigid, they cannot be contoured and their cost has not made them feasible for veterinary use.

Acrylic materials can often be used to mold a connecting bar between the fixation pin clusters. This method is particularly applicable to bones such as the mandible and maxilla, and in transarticular applications, where it can be difficult to drive all the fixation pins in the same plane.[24]

Clamps

Single clamps grip the fixation pin and connecting bar and are rotatable in two axes: that of the fixation pin and that of the bolt (Fig. 2–34). They are the only clamps required for one-plane frames (see below). Where two connecting bars need to be connected to each other, *double clamps* are used, in which two clamps rotate around the bolt axis (Fig. 2–34). The design of this clamp allows construction of multiplane frames, and these clamps are integral to the type IA double-clamp frame that was the basic design used by Ehmer.[22] Because double-clamps are not inherently as stiff (resistant to deformation when subjected to loading) as single clamps, they have been relegated to an ancillary role in fracture fixation but are still useful in fixation of corrective osteotomies in young dogs, where bone healing is vigorous and the need for long-lasting stability is only moderate. The use of two connecting bars between the pin clusters significantly stiffens type IA double-clamp frames.

Classification of Frame Configurations

For many years the various types of frames were described and named in a variety of ways, but gradually some uniformity of nomenclature is emerging, and this is necessary for easy communication. It is probably naive to believe that everyone will ever agree on a single system, so here we will utilize the two most commonly used nomenclatures, as described by Roe.[37] As used here the terms "unilateral" and "bilateral" refer to the insertion of fixation pins through either one or two skin surfaces, while the term "plane" references the projected plane formed by the fixation pin clusters.

Type I/Unilateral (Fig. 2–35A, B)

Although type I splints can be used in either one or two planes, perhaps the most widely used frame is the type I/unilateral half-pin splint, which is applicable to all long bones. Such a splint can be further described using either the alphanumeric descriptor "IA," or the adjectival form "one plane." Further de-

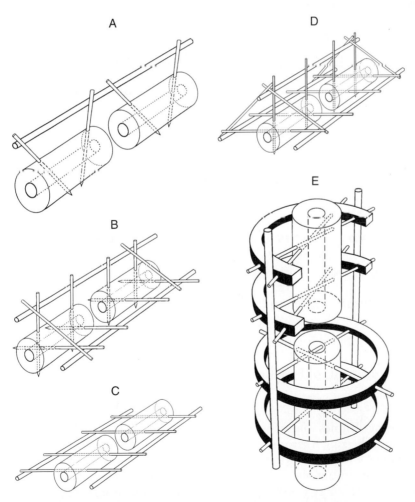

FIGURE 2–35. Classification of external fixator frame configurations. (*A*) Type IA/one plane unilateral. (*B*) Type IB/two plane unilateral. (*C*) Type II/bilateral one plane. (*D*) Type III bilateral two planes. (*E*) Ring fixator, showing complete and partial rings.

scription requires the use of the adjectives double or single to specify the type of clamps or number of connecting bars.

IA/ONE PLANE ■   Three subtypes of frames are included within this group.

Double Clamp (see Fig. 2–47) ■   This was the original veterinary device, commonly referred to simply as the Kirschner-Ehmer pin splint.

Single Bar (see Fig. 2–42*A*) ■   It is assumed that only single clamps are used for attaching the fixation pins to the connecting bar in this frame. This form is widely applicable, and is responsible for the renewed interest in the external fixator stimulated by Brinker and others in the 1970s.[23]

Double Bar (see Fig. 2–43*E*) ■   As with the single-bar frame, the use of only single clamps is assumed in this frame design.

IB/TWO PLANE (see Figs. 2–35*B* and 2–45*B*) ■   This frame is simply two type IA single-clamp frames applied at an angle of 60 to 90 degrees to each other. Interconnecting the connecting bars increases torsional rigidity and decreases pin loosening.

Type II/Bilateral One Plane (Fig. 2–35*C*)

Because they utilize full pins, these frames are applicable only to the lower limbs, distal to the elbow or stifle. They are particularly suitable for closed reduction and stabilization of radial and tibial fractures. Various combinations of full and half pins are used in these frames.

IIA/FULL PINS (see Fig. 2–44*F*) ■   Widely applied to tibial fractures in man, there are some technical problems in driving all the pins in the same plane to allow attachment to the connecting rods which will be described in the section on fundamentals of application, below. These frames are very versatile and useful not only in fractures of the lower limbs but also in transarticular fixation of lower limb joints.

IIB/FULL AND HALF PINS (see Fig. 2–44*D*) ■   The problem of getting more than two full pins driven in the same plane is eliminated in this design, at the price of a slight loss in stiffness compared to the full pin frame.

Type III/Bilateral Two Plane (see Figs. 2–35*D* and 2–46)

The strongest frame design, as well as the most complicated and costly, this frame is used only in situations of extreme instability of the fracture and where slow healing is anticipated. Tibial fractures are the primary application, but it can also be adapted to the radius.

Ring (Fig 2–35*E*)

Unlike other frames that depend on stiff fixation pins for stability at the bone-pin interface, the ring fixator pioneered by Ilizarov[38] utilizes small-diameter flexible Kirschner wires as fixation pins. Stiffness of these pins is created by placing them under tension as they are attached to the rings. By use of threaded connecting rods the rings can be adjusted to align the bone fragments, and to provide either compression or tension on the fragments. Its primary veterinary application is in corrective osteotomy for angular deformity or limb lengthening (see Chapter 22).

Biomechanical Considerations (see Figs. 2–42 through 2–44)

An approximation of the strength, or stiffness, of fixator frames is suggested by the numbers of the classification system, with I being the weakest and III being the strongest. Matching the required fixator strength to the clinical situation is partly art and partly science. The art portion is only acquired by experience, but the science can be explained and studied. In general, fractures that are expected to heal readily, with abundant callus formation, will heal consistently with type I frames. Contrarily, those fractures in which delayed union is the norm are best fixed with type II or III frames. A specific plan for choosing the appropriate form of fracture fixation for a given situation will be discussed later in this chapter in the section Selection of Fixation Method.

Mechanical studies have elucidated a great deal of knowledge regarding the mechanical characteristics of external fixators and the fixator-bone construct, from which we can gain insight to the clinical situation.[30–35,39] Based on these studies, the following generalizations can be made:

OVERALL FRAME STIFFNESS ■ As stated above, stiffness in compression and torsion increases from type IA to IB to type II to type III. Bilateral splints are two or more times as stiff as unilateral splints. All frames are stiffest in the plane of their application; therefore, bilateral type II frames are stiff in medial-lateral bending, while unilateral type IA splints lose stiffness when the bending is toward the side of the splint. However, type IB splints are stiffer in bending than type II splints. Medium Kirschner-Ehmer frames are a mean 85 percent stiffer than small frames.[40]

FIXATION PIN NUMBER, SPACING, ANGLE OF INSERTION ■ The pin-bone interface is subjected to very high stress loads that can lead to bone resorption around the pins and subsequent pin loosening. *Increasing the number of fixation pins from the minimum of two pins per major fragment increases the area of the pin-bone interface, consequently decreasing the incidence of bone resorption and subsequent pin loosening, which is the major postoperative complication seen.* This is the most important factor to understand in clinical application of external fixators. Increasing the number of fixation pins also stiffens the frame, which further decreases the incidence of pin loosening, but the effect is probably not important once four pins per major fragment is reached.

Widening the spacing between pins to place them as close as practical (one half the bone diameter) to the ends of the bone and to the fracture line (see Fig. 2–42C, F) stiffens the construct in the bending plane perpendicular to the pins. Angling smooth pins 20 degrees relative to the long axis of the bone stiffens the frame and helps prevent accidental dislodgement of the pins by the patient. Angling of fixation pins is not important when positive-profile-threaded pins are used and simplifies application.

FIXATION PIN DESIGN, SIZE, TYPE ■ Threaded pins have better holding power than smooth pins (roughly tenfold acutely and even more chronically), and most frames should be constructed with either all fixation pins threaded or with a combination of smooth and threaded pins. Negative-thread-profile pins are weakest at the junction of the threaded and unthreaded portions, this area acting as a stress concentrator and being susceptible to fatigue failure due to repetitive bending. The Ellis pin depicted in Figure 2–34 has a short negative-profile-threaded tip to allow the threaded end to penetrate the second cortex while the junction of threaded and unthreaded portion is protected within the medullary cavity. Positive-thread-profile pins offer the most holding power, and end-threaded half pins do not suffer from loss of stiffness at the junction of threaded and unthreaded areas. In type I unilateral frames it is optimal to place these pins at each end of a pin cluster. Centrally threaded positive-thread-profile pins are advisable for at least the most proximal and most distal full pins in type II and III frames.

Larger pins are stiffer than smaller pins by a direct relationship to the fourth power of the radius, thus a small increase in diameter produces a large increase in stiffness. However, pin diameters larger than 20 to 25 percent of the bone diameter weaken the bone and should be avoided.

Type II bilateral frames offer some technical difficulties in full pin placement. Insertion of the most proximal and distal pins and attaching them to the connecting bars is not difficult, but placing additional full pins is hindered by the need to place these pins in the same plane as the first pins. Half pins can be substituted for full pins in this situation (see Fig 2–44A, B, D), but at a cost of some loss of stiffness. One method for placing the intermediate pins is as follows:

1.   With the end pins placed, the medial and lateral connecting bars, with the appropriate number of empty clamps placed on each, are positioned in the end clamps.

2.   The fracture is reduced and held by any means in the reduced position while the four end clamps are tightened.

3.   A third connecting bar with the same number of empty clamps is attached to the end pins on the most convenient side.

4.   The intermediate fixation pins are placed through the clamps attached to the double connecting bars and drilled through the bone to emerge on the opposite side. The fracture must be reduced satisfactorily before these pins are drilled.

5.   Because all three connecting bars are in the same plane, the fixation pins will line up with the clamps on the opposite side, where the pins are secured by tightening the clamps.

6.   When all the fixation pins are placed and secured in their clamps, the temporary connecting bar and clamps are removed.

CONNECTING BARS, CLAMP CONFIGURATION ■   Stiffness of the connecting bar is of greatest concern in type I unilateral splints, where it is the limiting factor in frame stiffness. Adding a second bar to unilateral splints (see Fig. 2–43D, E, F) nearly doubles frame stiffness. Conforming the connecting bar to keep it as close to the bone as possible (see Fig. 2–48C) is helpful in increasing frame stiffness because it decreases the working length of the fixation pin. Stiffness of the pin is inversely proportional to the third power of the length, so keeping the length as short as possible is desirable. For similar reasons clamps should be positioned on the connecting bar with the bolt inside the connecting bar (see Fig. 2–41B), as this also shortens the working distance of the fixation pin.

Acrylic connecting bars offer good mechanical characteristics, such as easy conformation of the bar to the skin surface, thereby maximizing fixation pin stiffness. In mechanical testing a ¾-inch (19-mm) column of molded methyl methacrylate displayed more strength and stiffness than the ³⁄₁₆-inch (4.6-mm) stainless steel rod typically used in the medium Kirschner-Ehmer frame.[41] Additionally, acrylic connecting bars offer more freedom of fixation pin placement to accommodate the fracture and the anatomy, and allow the use of positive-thread-profile fixation pins anywhere in the frame.

Fundamentals of Application

The first consideration in applying an external fixator is the decision about which basic approach will be taken toward reduction of the fracture. Because of its versatility, the external fixator lends itself to either (1) open approach, anatomic bone reconstruction and rigid fixation, or (2) closed or minimal open approach with reduction aimed at aligning the diaphysis relative to angular and rotational deformity, and little or no reduction of bone fragments by direct manipulation. The first method represents the traditional rigid fixation approach to internal fixation, while the latter represents the *biological fixation* or *bridging osteosynthesis* approach discussed earlier. Consideration should always be given to finding a way to reduce the major fragments sufficiently to allow load sharing between the bone and fixator, even if it requires some shortening of the bone. This will allow the use of a simpler frame and will reduce the possibility of premature pin loosening and loss of fixation due to high stress loads at the pin-bone interface.

The following guidelines are suggested[2,3,23,24,42–44]:

1. *Use aseptic technique.* This includes preparation of the patient, the operating room, the equipment, the surgeon, and postoperative care.

2. *Use proper bone surface location for insertion of pins.* Complications can be minimized if the splint is located on the bone surface that allows insertion of the fixation pins through the skin and directly into the bone. This minimizes the length of pin between the fixation clamp and bone, thus maintaining maximum pin stiffness. It also minimizes soft tissue irritation; pins penetrating through muscle and skin are more irritating than those penetrating skin alone. The proper surface for the unilateral splint on the tibia is medial; for the radius, craniomedial or medial; for the humerus, craniolateral, and for the femur, lateral (Fig. 2–36). In order to insert the pins in the humerus and femur, it is necessary to penetrate both skin and underlying muscle; however, the aforementioned surfaces keep muscle thickness to a minimum.

3. *Use the most suitable configuration of the splint.*[22,23,28–30,34,35] Guidelines relative to this decision in specific clinical situations will be discussed later in this chapter in the section Selection of Fixation Method. General guidelines are that type I unilateral configurations can be used on all of the long bones and the mandible, while biplanar and bilateral configurations are limited in use to fractures of the tibia, radius and ulna, and mandible to avoid interfering with the body wall. Although static strength and stiffness evaluations of the various frame configurations (starting from the lowest) places them approximately in the order of (1) type IA unilateral one plane, (2) type IB unilateral two plane, (3) type II bilateral one plane, and (4) type III bilateral two plane, it must be remembered that clinical performance is dependent on many variables mentioned above such as the diameter and contouring of the connecting bars, diameter and number of fixation pins, angle and location of pins in the cortical bone, length of the pins from the fixation clamps to the bone, and the inherent stability at the fracture site. The importance of the latter is difficult to overemphasize; if *load sharing* can be achieved between the bone and frame, as in type A simple or type B wedge fractures, then the frame can be less stiff as compared to the situation where there is no load sharing, as in type C complex

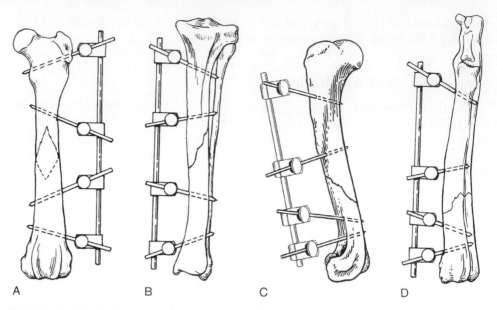

FIGURE 2–36. Preferred location of the unilateral external fixator in relation to the bone surface and associated soft tissue. (*A*) Lateral surface of femur. (*B*) Medial surface of tibia. (*C*) Craniolateral surface of humerus. (*D*) Craniomedial or medial surface of radius.

fractures, and the fixator must function as a *buttress*. Clinical experience supports the statement that the stiffness produced by the type IA unilateral configuration—one connecting bar with two to four pins per bone fragment—is adequate in type A simple and most type B wedge fractures where load sharing can be achieved and when supplemented with appropriate auxiliary fixation as indicated. Because fractures vary widely in type, stability, condition of soft tissue, animal activity, and size of the patient, no single configuration is best suited for all fractures; however, the simple configurations serve very well on most fractures.

4.   *Auxiliary fixation should be used when indicated.* If the goal of fracture treatment is rigid uninterrupted stabilization of the main fracture fragments, then auxiliary fixation (which may include use of lag screws, intramedullary pins, Kirschner wires, and cerclage or interfragmentary wire configurations) may be helpful in maintaining reduction during insertion of the fixation pins and in aiding rigid stabilization (Fig. 2–37). However, rigid devices such as lag screws and cerclage wire should be used cautiously in combination with the less stiff type IA unilateral frames, since they can act as stress concentrators and cause secondary fractures or loosening of the implant due to bone resorption. An additional consideration is the disruption of fracture biology caused by their placement. They are safest in situations where good stability can be achieved and rapid bone healing is anticipated.

5.   *The fracture should be reduced and maintained in reduction during application of the splint.* With the fracture reduced, the soft tissues are restored to their normal anatomical position, and the pins can be inserted without distorting the soft tissues. This helps to minimize tissue irritation and discomfort to the animal. If at any time reduction is lost during pin insertion, it should be regained before proceeding. Fractures of the radius/ulna and the tibia can often be reduced closed by applying the splint while the limb is suspended overhead

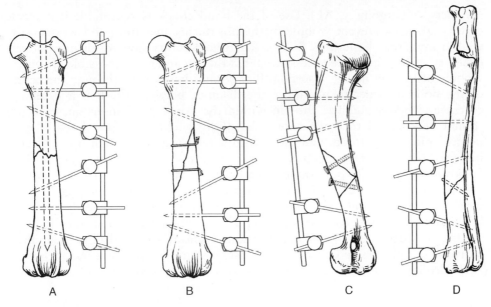

A   B   C   D

FIGURE 2–37. Auxiliary fixation commonly used with the external fixator. (*A*) Intramedullary pin. (*B*) Cerclage wire. (*C*) Lag screws. (*D*) Diagonally inserted Kirschner wire.

as illustrated in Figure 2–12. Suitable draping technique includes a sterile cover for the suspending tape or rope that extends far enough upwards to preclude accidental contamination of the surgeons.

6. *Insert pins through soft tissue in a manner that does not distort the tissue.* A short (¼-inch; 2- to 3-mm) stab incision is made in the skin. If the pin is inserted through muscle, tunnel bluntly through the muscle with a hemostat and then spread the hemostat jaws to allow the pin to be placed through the tunnel into contact with the bone. Placing the pins between muscle bellies and tendons to the extent possible will do much to reduce postoperative problems (see below). If an open reduction is being done the pins should not be placed through the incision and it is important to remove all retractors from the incision before pins are placed in order to prevent soft tissue distortion. At the conclusion of the procedure, extend the original pin incisions as necessary to relieve any skin wrinkling. If there is no alternative to inserting pins through the incision, it must be done in a manner that allows penetration of the muscles without distortion of the muscle, and relief incisions must be made in the skin to allow it to return to its normal position.

7. *Pin drilling technique is critical.*[2,3,30,31,42] Use a slow-speed power drill (150 rpm or less) for pin insertion, as a higher speed power drill creates an undue amount of heat, which can cause bone necrosis and pin loosening. Rechargeable battery-powered drills operate at these low speeds and have sufficient torque to make them an economical substitute for true surgical drills. The technical problem in the use of these drills is the issue of sterilizing them, as they cannot be steam sterilized. Ethylene oxide sterilization is a simple and satisfactory solution, if available, and the drill can be handled as any other sterile instrument during surgery. If ethylene oxide sterilization is not an option, sterile fabric shrouds to cover the drill and an extended shaft and detachable and sterilizable chuck are needed (Extend-a-Chuck drill extension and shroud, Animal Clinic

Products, Montgomery, AL). Use of the hand chuck is acceptable if extreme care is taken to prevent wobble of the pin during insertion, and works quite well in immature bone (Fig. 2–38). Hand-held rotary bone drills are not satisfactory, as they generate excessive heat at the pin and it is impossible to control wobble of the pin during insertion. Pins should be inserted through the center of the bone in order to maximize the distance between the first and second cortex and better stabilize the pin within the bone. After insertion, each pin should be checked to make sure it is solidly anchored in the bone. Trocar pointed pins are favored, and those with a relatively long point are preferred because they penetrate the bone faster and are easier to insert (Fig. 2–39). Positive-thread-profile pins should not be inserted directly into bone, as they produce microfractures of the cortex at the entry and exit points, particularly with cancellous thread pins. This damage can be reduced by predrilling a pilot hole in the bone 10 percent smaller than the pin diameter. Such drilling requires the use of a drill sleeve to protect the soft tissues if a twist drill is used; alternatively, the pilot hole can be drilled using a smooth pin or Kirschner wire. After drilling pilot holes it is safest to then insert positive-thread-profile pins

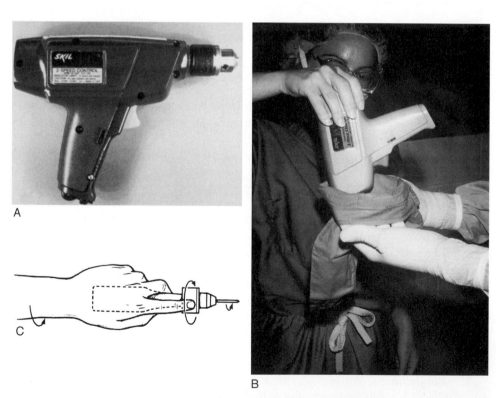

FIGURE 2–38. (*A*) Fixation pins are inserted with a standard low-speed (150 rpm) orthopedic or battery-powered drill. (*B*) Nonsterile battery-powered electric drill being dropped into a sterile shroud being held open by the surgeon. The shroud is secured by hook and eyelet material to keep it closed over the drill. A sterile Jacob's chuck and extension tube is then screwed into the drill through a small opening in the shroud. Care must be taken to prevent the shroud from becoming wetted and allowing bacterial strike through. Alternatively, the drill can be sterilized in ethylene oxide gas. (*C*) The correct method of holding the pin chuck to minimize wobbling is with the wrist straight and the elbow flexed so that the forearm, pin chuck, and pin are rotated as a unit around a constant axis.

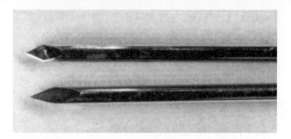

FIGURE 2–39. Trocar-pointed Steinmann pins. The relatively long point is preferred over the short point; it penetrates faster and easier.

using a hand chuck, as this will minimize bone damage such as accidental stripping of the threads.

8. *Insert pins through both cortices of the bone.* Invariably, any pin that is not fully inserted through both cortices loosens and thus does not accomplish its mission. With few exceptions, the pin point can be palpated on penetration of the far cortex. When using a power drill, a definite change in the pitch of the drill motor sound will be detected as the pin penetrates through the second cortex. When inserting pins by hand, there will be an increased amount of torque needed as the point of the pin penetrates the second cortex, followed by a sudden decrease in resistance as the tip of the pin clears the cortex. The pin should penetrate about the length of the trocar point. If pins should penetrate too far on insertion, they should be left in position if possible, as withdrawing the pin causes the pin-bone interface to be weakened and pull-out strength diminished.[42] Even overly long protruding pins rarely cause any clinical problem.

9. *Insert smooth and negative-thread-profile pins at an angle of 70 degrees to the long axis of the bone*[23,24,40] (Fig. 2–40). Pins inserted at this angle give maximum stiffness to the fixator along with maximum pull-out resistance from the bone. This angularity is not important with positive-thread-profile pins, thereby simplifying insertion of an adequate number of pins per fragment.

10. *Insert all related fixation pin clusters in the same plane.* This has two advantages: (1) all pins can be attached to a common connecting bar, thus

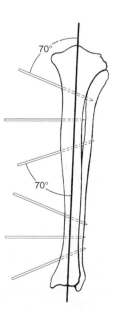

FIGURE 2–40. For maximum stiffness, the end fixation pins in each group should be inserted at a 70-degree angle to the long axis of the bone.

eliminating the need for the less stiff double clamps; and (2) if postoperative swelling occurs, the fixation clamps can be loosened and readily adjusted without affecting reduction at the fracture site. The procedure for application using one connecting bar is shown in Figure 2–41.

11. *Insert pins in the proper location of the bone fragment.* Experimental[34,39] and clinical studies indicate that maximum stability is accomplished by inserting the pins near the proximal and distal ends of the bone fragment rather than by inserting both pins near the ends or near the fracture site (Fig. 2–42). The pins should be kept one half the bone diameter distant from the fracture line, and fissures in the cortex must be avoided. Because the cortex is normally quite thin in the proximal metaphyseal region of the humerus and tibia and the distal metaphysis of the femur, it is advantageous to avoid placing smooth or negative-thread-profile pins in these areas, as cancellous bone has very little holding power on the pins. Cancellous positive-thread-profile pins should be used in these areas, after drilling a pilot hole.[44]

12. *Insert two to four pins in each major bone fragment.* Until the early 1970s, two pins per bone fragment were used in most cases. Studies since that time definitely indicate that three or four pins per fragment increase the stiffness of the construct[24,30,34,35,39,40] (Figs. 2–43 and 2–44). How much stiffness is needed to heal a specific fracture is unknown, but general guidelines are presented below in the section Selection of Fixation Method. Biomechanically, it appears that one of the major advantages of using more than two pins per fragment is a decrease in pin-bone stress forces to which the pins are subjected during healing. This appears to hold true in clinical use because bent pins and loosening are much less frequently encountered when three to four pins per fragment are used. All fractures require a minimum of two pins on each major

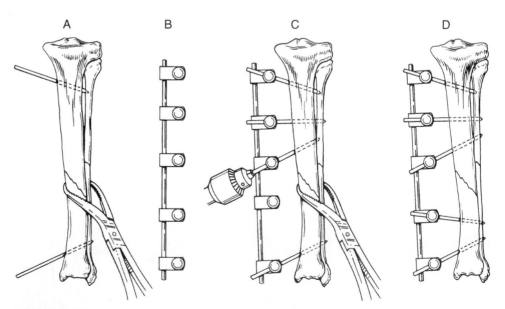

FIGURE 2–41. Unilateral (type IA) external fixator, one connecting bar, 3/2 pins. (*A*) The fracture is first reduced, and reduction is maintained during the application procedure. The proximal and distal pins are inserted. (*B*) The fixation clamps are assembled on the connecting bar. (*C*) The fixation clamps are attached to the proximal and distal pins. The remaining three pins are inserted through the clamps and bone. (*D*) All clamps are tightened, and the incision is closed.

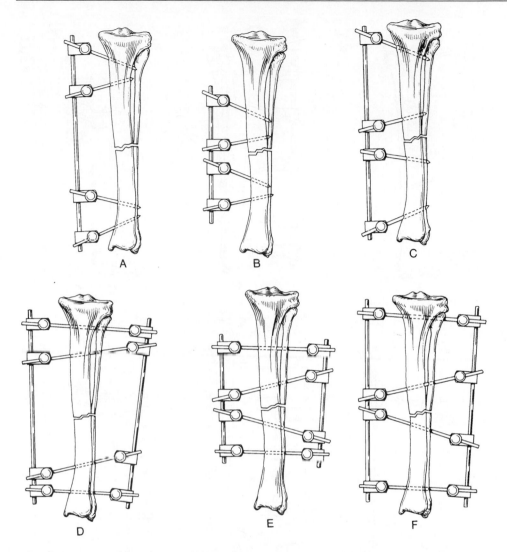

FIGURE 2–42. Unilateral (type IA) configuration (*A–C*) and bilateral (type IIA) configurations (*D–F*). Maximum stability is accomplished by inserting the pins near the proximal and distal ends of the bone fragment (*C, F*) in preference to both pins near the proximal end (*A, D*) or the fracture site (*B, E*).

bone segment. If healing is anticipated to be slow as a result of fragmentation, contamination, old age, and so forth, more pins per segment are useful.

13.   *Choose optimal size fixation pins and connecting bars.* The appropriate size of both varies with the size of the bone involved. In the United States, the Kirschner-Ehmer splint is the apparatus used almost exclusively in small animals (Figs. 2–45 through 2–47). The medium-size fixation clamps accommodate a ³/₁₆-inch (4.6-mm) connecting bar. The use of two connecting bars (Fig. 2–43) approximately doubles the stiffness of the splint and may be indicated for use in some large- or giant-breed dogs. The medium-size fixation clamps accommodate ³/₃₂- and ¹/₈-inch (2.4 to 3.2-mm) fixation pins. The ¹/₈-inch pins are used most frequently; however, the ³/₃₂-inch pins may be used on animals in the 18- to 25-pound (8- to 11-kg) range. The small Kirschner-Ehmer clamps accommodate a ¹/₈-inch connecting bar, and fixation pins can range up to ⁵/₆₄ inch

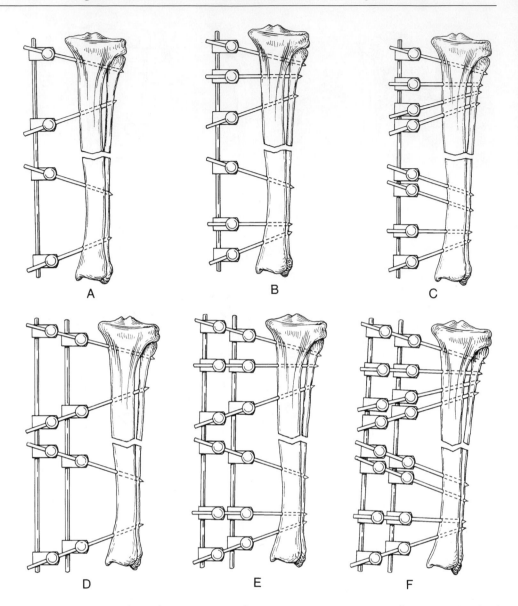

FIGURE 2–43. Unilateral (type IA) configurations. One connecting bar: (*A*) 2/2 pins/ fragment, (*B*) 3/3 pins/fragment, (*C*) 4/4 pins/fragment. Two connecting bars: (*D*) 2/2 pins/fragment, (*E*) 3/3 pins/fragment, (*F*) 4/4 pins/fragment. Using two connecting bars approximately doubles the stiffness of the splint; however, this is usually only indicated in the very large dog. *Note*: The "fracture gap" is for artistic clarity.

(2.0 mm) diameter. In clinical settings, the largest practical pin size is used because this gives stiffness to the apparatus, bends less at the pin-bone interface on cyclic loading, and is less apt to loosen during the healing period. However, in general, the fixation pin should not exceed one fourth of the diameter of the bone because weakening and fracture can occur. Pins should be cut as close to the clamp as possible, with a pin (bolt) cutter or saw, in order to minimize the overall dimensions of the splint.

14. *Place the connecting rods an optimal distance between the fixation clamps and the skin.* This distance at the time of application varies with both

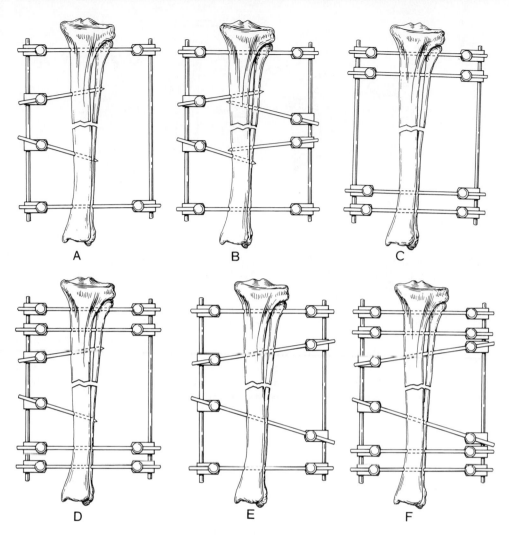

FIGURE 2–44. Various bilateral (type II) configurations. On the basis of stiffness response, starting from the least and progressing upward, the ranking is A through F. Stiffness is improved by through-and-through pins instead of half pins, using angled pins, or increasing the number of pins. *Note*: The "fracture gap" is for artistic clarity.

the size of the animal and the anticipated postsurgical swelling. The distance is usually ³⁄₈ to ½ inch (10 to 13 mm) (Fig. 2–48). The thickness of the small finger is a good approximation in most people. Contour the rod to fit the skin/ muscle surface where necessary to minimize the clamp-bone distance (Fig. 2–48C). Postsurgical swelling, which usually occurs within the first 10 days, may necessitate readjustment and moving the fixation clamps outward on the pins because contact pressure will result in necrosis of the soft tissue. Regions of tissue movement (e.g., near joints) swell more than do regions of little motion.

15. *Bone graft significant cortical deficits.* Because rigidity of fixation using the external fixator is usually less than that when using plates, the body is stimulated to produce more bridging callus. If there are definite architectural deficits present, however, they should be filled with a bone graft. This is partic-

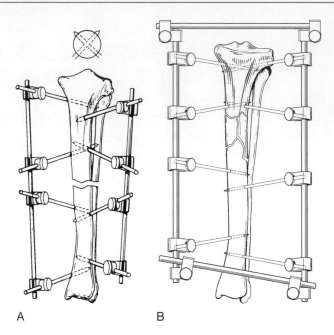

A   B

FIGURE 2–45. (*A*) Biplanar type I configuration. One unilateral external fixator is placed on the medial surface of the tibia or radius, and another is placed on the cranial surface. Their connecting bars or the end pins (see *B*) may be bridged by two or more connecting bars. (*B*) Modifications of this configuration work well on very proximal or distal fractures. *Note*: The "fracture gap" is for artistic clarity.

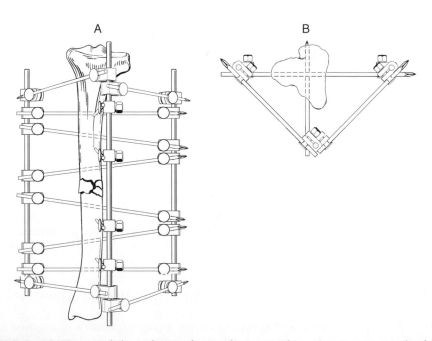

FIGURE 2–46. Type III bilateral two-plane splint. (*A*) This splint is most applicable to the tibia, although it can also be adapted to the radius. (*B*) The tent-like configuration can be seen in this proximodistal view.

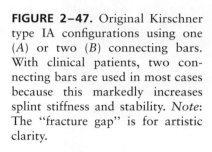
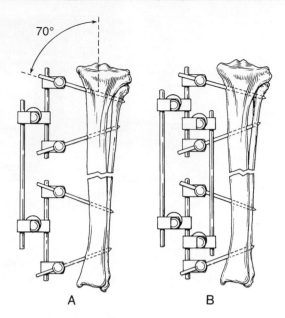

FIGURE 2–47. Original Kirschner type IA configurations using one (*A*) or two (*B*) connecting bars. With clinical patients, two connecting bars are used in most cases because this markedly increases splint stiffness and stability. *Note*: The "fracture gap" is for artistic clarity.

ularly true in mature and older animals, osteotomies of diaphyseal bone, and nonunions.

Aftercare

Following surgery, a compressive (Robert-Jones) bandage is applied to protect the incision and minimize swelling in fractures of the radius/ulna and tibia (Fig. 2–49). Any open wounds and all incisions are covered with a sterile nonad-

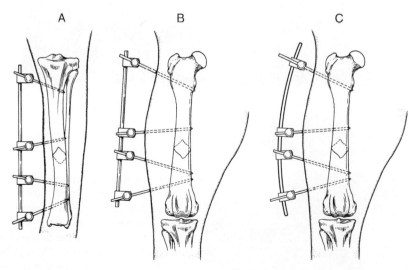

FIGURE 2–48. The distance between the fixation clamps and the skin is usually ⅜ to ½ inch. (*A*, *B*) This distance varies with the size of the animal and anticipated postsurgical swelling. If swelling causes the skin to press against the fixation clamps, readjustment and movement of the clamps outward on the pins are indicated because contact pressure will result in necrosis of the soft tissue. (*C*) In some situations it is useful to gently contour the connecting rod to follow the skin/muscle surface.

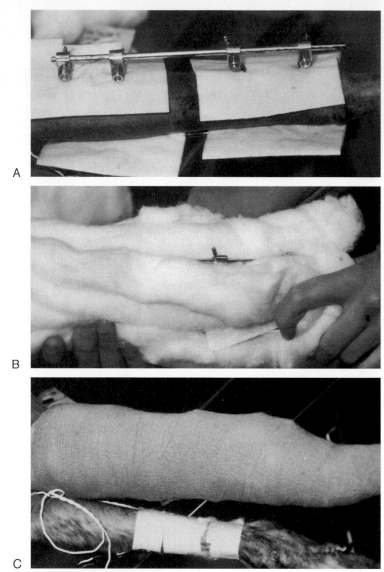

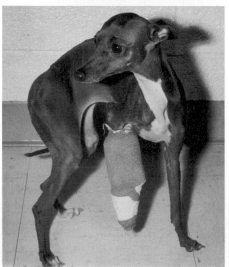

FIGURE 2–49. Postoperative dressing of an external fixator. (*A*) Nonadherent dressings are partially cut to allow them to be positioned over the pin-skin sites. (*B*) Roll cotton, cotton fluffs, or other bulky dressing material is positioned on the skin along the fixator and distally to the toes. (*C*) Starting at the toes, elastic bandage material (Vetrap here) is applied with moderate compression to cover all the cotton padding. (*D*) The dressing and the patient 24 hours postoperatively. This dressing is usually left in place 3 to 4 days.

herent dressing, and roll cotton or cast padding is packed around the pins and under the connecting bars. Additional cotton or padding is rolled on the leg from the toes to the frame. The padding is then compressed with an elastic conforming bandage (Vetrap, 3M Animal Care Products, St. Paul, MN; Flexus, Kimberly-Clark Corporation). It is important that the padding and wrapping start at the toes and then proximally to cover the frame. Covering only the frame with this type dressing will cause severe swelling of the limb distal to the frame. In most cases this bandage is removed after 2 to 5 days. This step is not possible with humeral and femoral fractures. With open fractures or with severe soft tissue injury, the wound is often debrided, lavaged, and rebandaged every 2 to 3 days until it is covered with granulation tissue. Because of the stability the fixator provides, such frequent bandage changes can be performed without traumatizing early vascular granulation tissue and callus formation.

The compressive bandage is replaced with a gauze and Vetrap cover, which encloses only the connecting clamps and bars, and protruding ends of the fixation pins of the fixator (Fig. 2–50). This cover protects the animal and the owner from the sharp ends of the fixation pins and decreases the chance of catching the apparatus on fixed objects. Flexible plastic caps can also be fitted on the ends of the fixation pins, which are usually quite sharp as a result of being cut with a pin (bolt) cutter. The cover should be applied so it does not contact the skin, but allows air circulation around the skin-pin interface. Do not use adhesive tape for this cover, as it is very difficult to remove from the metal frame components. Gauze can be used as a first layer, which is then covered by adhesive tape, but the tape is not brought into contact with the frame components. This type cover for the frame is done immediately postoperatively in the case of humeral and femoral fractures.

The use of a broad-spectrum antibiotic is indicated for contaminated open or infected fractures until a culture and sensitivity can direct more specific therapy. Because of the soft tissue trauma attending even most closed fractures, we tend to use a broad-spectrum antibiotic such as cephalexin for 4 to 7 days following surgery, until the body defenses are mobilized.

The animal is released with instructions to limit exercise to leash walking for elimination only and to take particular care to avoid fencing or other similar structures that might catch the apparatus. Protection of the apparatus with a cover should be maintained until the device is removed. The owners are in-

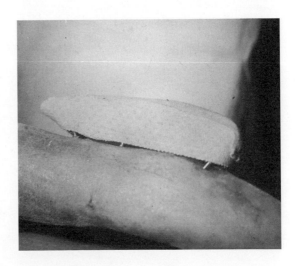

FIGURE 2–50. Protective cover for the fixator is applied after the postoperative dressing is removed. The objective of the cover is to help prevent the fixator from becoming "snagged" on fences, bushes, etc. The cover shown here is fashioned from gauze and elastic tape, but can also be covered with Vetrap. Do not allow the gauze padding to contact the skin at the pin sites, and do not adhere adhesive tape directly to the splint.

structed to inspect the apparatus daily and advised to expect a small amount of dry crust to develop at the skin-pin interface. In the absence of complications (see below) we advise no or minimal cleaning or treatment of the pin sites. Others advise a rigorous regimen of postoperative care that includes daily cleaning of crusts and exudate around the pins, treatment of the pin sites with a topical antibacterial medicine, and a dressing to both cover the splint as well as to compress and immobilize soft tissues under the splint with gauze padding placed between the skin and splint. This dressing is changed every few days, depending on the amount of exudate present around the pin tracks (see below).[43,44]

Complications

The most common cause of morbidity following external skeletal fixation is drainage from the fixation pin tracks (Fig. 2–51). This problem is associated with excessive skin and deeper soft tissue movement causing pressure against the pins, or with loose pins. This tends to be a somewhat closed-loop series of events, since one of the causes of loosening of fixation is muscle motion against the pin. Constant motion of soft tissues around the pin, or motion of the pin relative to soft tissues, prolongs the debridement phase of wound healing and results in continual exudation of the pin track.[43] There is inevitably a degree of bacterial contamination from the skin and environment, and these bacteria propagate within the pin track and add further to the exudation. Careful placement of the pins through nondisplaced soft tissue and avoiding large muscle masses will minimize this problem in most cases. The use of the bulky splint dressing with pressure on the soft tissues advocated by Aron and Dewey is aimed at both immobilizing soft tissue and minimizing bacterial contamination.[43] In some locations, such as the distal femur, soft tissue movement against the pins is unavoidable and some drainage is to be expected. In this situation activity restriction and periodically cleansing the pin site with 2 percent hydrogen peroxide or organic iodine solution is recommended first. If this is not effective in controlling drainage, then the padded bandage of Aron and Dewey is used.

Moderate drainage from pin sites is not associated with significant loss of function as long as the skin around the track is healthy and the pin remains

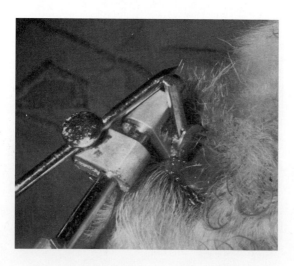

FIGURE 2–51. Drainage from pin track caused by motion of the soft tissues relative to the fixation pin. Swelling of soft tissue has caused the clamp to become very close to the skin, adding further to the skin exudation.

stable. If function of the limb is impaired in the absence of a loose pin and the drainage does not respond to the simple measures outlined above, then true infection of the pin track, although rare, should be suspected. The surrounding skin will appear tense and erythematous, and may be tender to touch. Steps should be taken to ensure drainage around the pin by incising skin for 1 cm on each side of the pin. Topical antibacterials and mechanical cleansing by lavage should be done at least daily. Systemic antibiotics given for several days are useful in controlling the infection. Bacterial culture and antibiotic sensitivity testing are not usually helpful due to many skin organisms being present in the sample. It is safe to assume *Staphylococcus* spp. as the cause of the drainage and to choose the antibiotic on this basis. Only rarely does such infection affect the bone, although radiograpic signs of bone reaction are often seen.[45]

Loosening of fixation pins is most often caused by soft tissue interference as detailed above, or with instability of the fracture and resultant motion due to an overly flexible fixator frame and/or too few fixation pins. Such motion of the bone results in high stress loads at the pin-bone interface, leading to bone resorption and pin loosening. Correct choice of frame type and number of fixation pins for the clinical situation is the only help for preventing this problem. Loosening of the fixation pin at the pin-bone interface will commonly result in drainage and potentially infection of the pin tract. Once a pin becomes loose, the only effective treatment is removal. The drainage will usually resolve rapidly. Aside from the nuisance of drainage, loosening of pins may cause a decrease in limb function. If too many pins loosen too quickly, stability may be lost and delayed or nonunion can follow, although this is a rare problem.[45] If the fracture is not yet healed and the loss of a loose pin appears to significantly weaken the fixator, additional fixation pins must be inserted to maintain adequate stability. While this requires general anesthesia and aseptic technique, it can be done by closed insertion of a new pin at a new site. Selection of an appropriate frame type, use of three or four pins per fragment, and use of positive-thread-profile pins will prevent most pin loosening and subsequent drainage or infection.

Another uncommon source of drainage and loosening of pins is the ring sequestrum that forms around a pin after insertion with a high-speed drill or with undue pressure that caused excessive heat generation (Fig. 2–52). Bone death occurs in a circular pattern around the pin, with secondary infection, drainage, and pin loosening. The radius is the most common site of this problem, as placing pins in the frontal plane of the bone requires drilling through primarily cortical bone due to the elliptical cross section and small medullary cavity of this bone. Treatment is removal of the pin and sequestrum, curettage of the tract, and replacement of the pin, if needed for continuing stability.

A relatively rarely encountered problem is iatrogenic fracture of the bone through the fixation pin holes. This usually occurs when oversized fixation pins (>33 percent of bone diameter) are used, when fixation pins are placed too close together, or when fixation pins are placed in fissure fractures. The latter problem is usually avoided if pins are not placed closer than one half the bone diameter from the fracture line. Unrestricted postoperative activity can also result in fractures through pin holes, particularly if the holes are enlarged by loose pins. Such problems are managed by replacement of pins in intact bone.

Removal of Frames

When radiographic and clinical signs of bone union are confirmed, the fixator can be removed. In many cases this can be done with little or no sedation; if

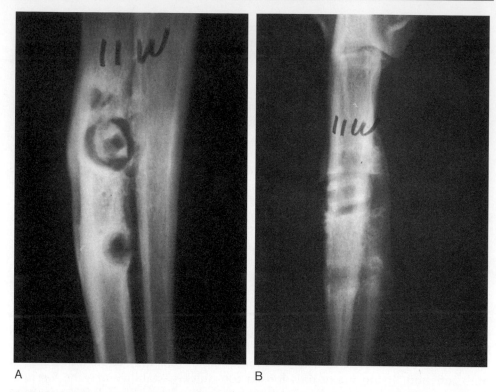

A   B

FIGURE 2–52. Ring sequestrum caused by thermal necrosis during insertion of the fixation pin. (A) In this mediolateral view of the proximal radius, the sequestrum appears doughnut shaped due to the lucency of the pin hole and the area of detachment from surrounding bone. (B) Three lucent zones are seen in the craniocaudal view.

the animal is apprehensive or excitable, a narcotic-tranquilizer combination by injection is usually adequate. Very often the pins are somewhat loose by the time of clinical union due to the increasing activity of the animal; this is especially true with smooth fixation pins.

Clamps are loosened and connecting bars are removed. Loose half pins often can be removed with the fingers without any signs of pain. If resistance is encountered, or if threaded pins are present, a Jacobs chuck with handle is attached to the pin and it is unscrewed from the bone. This may cause slight pain, as periosteum can be stimulated. Full pins are cut close to the bone on one side and the short protruding end is disinfected, after which the pin is removed by pulling the short end through the bone.

Some bleeding accompanies pin removal, and this is cleaned and the pin sites are covered with sterile gauze dressings and a light bandage, which is maintained for 48 to 72 hours. Even pin sites that have enlarged to 2 cm diameter due to skin motion heal very quickly without visible scarring. Do not suture pin holes, as this can result in entrapment of exudate and lead to abscessation.

Acrylic Frames[24,36,41,46,47]

Replacement of the conventional clamp and connecting bar system with a plastic material potentially offers some significant advantages in the clinical application of external skeletal fixation. The ability to conform the connecting bar to any shape allows placement of pins in multiple planes in order to make best use of whatever bone is available for their placement and to allow orientation of the pins to avoid soft tissue entrapment. Although applicable to any external skeletal fixation application, this method is especially advantageous in the areas of the mandible, in the long bones of toy and miniature breeds, and in transarticular applications in the carpus and tarsus. Eliminating the need for fixation clamps also reduces the cost of the apparatus, always a consideration in veterinary applications.

The material most commonly used for the plastic connecting rod is methyl methacrylate, an acrylic resin that has been used for many years in the production of tray molds for the fabrication of dental prostheses, and in veterinary applications for hoof wall repair (Orthodontic resin, L.B. Caulk Co., Division of Dentsply International Inc., Milford, DE; Technovit hoof acrylic, Jorgensen Laboratories, Loveland, CO). In a sterile and much more costly form it is also used for anchoring varying types of metal and plastic prostheses to bone in both man and animals. There is no difference in strength between the sterile and nonsterile forms and therefore for economic reasons the nonsterile form is most commonly used, although careful planning is needed to allow most fixator applications to be performed without the need for sterile cement.

Solid methyl methacrylate is created by mixing a volatile liquid monomer solvent with methyl methacrylate powder, which initially creates a liquid stage not unlike a flour/water batter. This liquid stage lasts 2 to 3 minutes and is followed by a doughy, moldable phase (4 to 5 minutes) that hardens into a very strong mass 7 to 10 minutes after initial mixing. There are slight variations in these times due to ambient temperatures, higher temperatures lowering and cool temperatures lengthening the cure time. There is considerable exothermic heat liberated by the polymerization reaction of the last 2 to 3 minutes of the cure cycle, but this does not seem to present a real danger. A $\frac{3}{4}$-inch (19-mm) column of solid methyl methacrylate has been shown to have superior mechanical characteristics to the $\frac{3}{16}$-inch (4.6-mm) rod commonly used with the medium Kirschner-Ehmer splint.[41]

Fundamentals of Application

The exact sequence followed depends upon the choice of using the liquid or the moldable stage methyl methacrylate. Liquid methyl methacrylate can be injected with a catheter-tip 60-ml-dose syringe into flexible plastic tubing that has been impaled over the fixation pins, while the doughy stage requires hand molding of a column that is pressed onto the pin clusters. A useful method applicable to nonsterile acrylic fixator frames is the *biphase technique*. If nonsterile acrylic is to be used during an open reduction, the fracture must be reduced and the soft tissues closed before the connecting acrylic column can be attached to the fixation pins. This may make it difficult to maintain fracture reduction during attachment of the connecting columns. Even during a closed reduction it can be difficult to maintain reduction during attachment of the columns. The biphase technique utilizes a temporary frame using normal clamps and connecting bars to maintain reduction while the acrylic column is attached.

Phase 1 involves reduction of the fracture by either open or closed methods and insertion of fixation pins as previously described. The fixation pins are not cut short, but are left long enough to attach clamps and a connecting bar 1.5 to 2-inches (3.8 to 5 cm) from the skin surface. It is seldom necessary to attach all fixation pins to this temporary connecting bar. This phase can be done aseptically, thus the bone can be reduced and stabilized under open reduction. Following closure of the open reduction radiographic confirmation of the reduction can be obtained if desired.

Phase 2 is the joining of all pin clusters by an acrylic column, as will be further described below. If nonsterile methyl methacrylate is used, the incision must be closed at this point. After the acrylic is hardened the fixation pins are cut close to the column and the temporary clamps and bar are discarded. It may be useful to dress the protruding cut pins with a file or rotary burr in order to reduce the sharpness of the end produced by the pin cutter and to reduce the chances of the protruding pin hanging up on clothing and so forth.

LIQUID STAGE APPLICATION ■

Methyl methacrylate powder and liquid monomer are mixed with a tongue depressor in a disposable paper (*not* polystyrene) cup in the approximate ratio of three parts powder for dental acrylic, or two parts powder for hoof acrylic, to one part liquid. Mix smoothly, without "whipping," to avoid trapping air bubbles in the mixture, and as soon as the powder is well mixed with the liquid, pour the mixture into the barrel of a catheter-tip dose syringe, and then replace the plunger.

Thin-wall flexible tubing of appropriate inner diameter (3/4 inch for medium fixation pins, 1/2 inch for small fixation pins) is used as a mold for the liquid. Disposable plastic adult anesthesia breathing circuit tubing works well for the larger size column, and polyvinyl or rubber medical tubing or pediatric breathing circuit tubing is useful for the smaller sizes. The tubing is impaled over the fixation pins, taking care to avoid tearing large holes in the tubing. Short incisions are necessary in polyvinyl and some rubber tubing. If the biphase technique is to be used, the clamps and connecting bar are now attached to the fixation pins outboard of the tubing. Note that the tubing would need to be sterilized if this part of the procedure were being done in conjunction with an open approach. An open procedure could continue nonaseptically from this point once the incision was closed. The lower end of the tube is plugged with cotton wadding or a sponge to prevent leaking and the liquid acrylic is injected in the opposite end to fill the tubing. Following hardening of the acrylic the pins are cut close to the column and dressed as described above.

A commercially available kit contains all the components needed to apply type II biphase fixators of either the small or medium size (APEF System, Innovative Animal Products, Rochester, MN) (Fig. 2–53). An advantage of this kit is that the materials are all sterile, thus allowing the entire fixation under direct vision during an open approach.

MOLDABLE STAGE APPLICATION ■

This method eliminates the need for tubing molds and simplifies the use of the biphase technique with nonsterile methyl methacrylate powder. Mixing of the liquid and powder proceeds as described above, but mixing is continued until the mixture becomes doughy and no longer sticks to the surgical glove. The dough is removed from the cup to a flat surface, where it can be rolled to a rod of appropriate diameter with the palm of the hand. This soft rod is then impaled on the fixation pins and molded firmly around the pins by digital pressure. Following hardening of the acrylic the pins are cut and dressed as discussed above. It is also possible to inject liquid-stage acrylic into soft tubing such as a Penrose drain, allow it to reach the doughy stage, and then impale it on the pins.

Further refinements of either method are useful in order to allow a more firm adhesion of the acrylic to the fixation pins. Notches can be produced in the ends of the pins with a pin cutter to provide a roughened surface. Stainless steel wire can be attached between fixation pins to provide a foundation for the

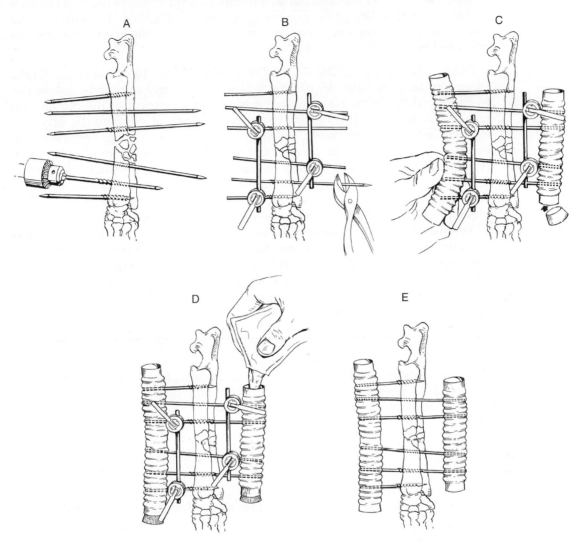

FIGURE 2–53. APEF biphase method. (*A*) Pin placement and size can be optimized for fracture stability and minimal soft tissue interference. Any combination of positive-thread-profile or smooth pins can be used. Predrilling pin holes for threaded pins is simplified because no drilling or pin placement is done through fixation clamps. (*B*) The fracture is reduced and temporary stabilization is achieved by use of two connecting bars and APEF alignment frame clamps, which are placed at skin level. If an open reduction was done, the soft tissues are closed, or a closed reduction can be radiographically verified. Fixation pins are cut 1.5 to 2 inches (4–5 cm) from the skin. (*C*) The corrugated plastic tubing that will mold the connecting bars is pushed over the fixation pins and pushed toward the clamps. Fixation pins too long to allow the tubing to rest against the clamps without penetrating the outer wall of the tubing must be recut to shorten them. The dependent ends of the tubing are plugged. (*D*) Prepackaged acrylic is mixed within its plastic bag, the corner of the bag cut, and the liquid phase acrylic poured into the open ends of the tubes. Leakage of acrylic at pin sites is controlled with cotton balls or sponges. Biplanar configurations are interconnected by pins placed through the connecting bar tubing while the acrylic is still in liquid phase. (*E*) After hardening of the acrylic, 10 to 12 minutes from the start of mixing, the frame alignment clamps are loosened and removed with the temporary connecting bars. Excess length of the connecting bars can be removed by saw. (From Innovative Animal Products, Rochester, MN, with permission.)

bridging acrylic column. An extension of this concept involves bending the ends of fixation pins to bridge the gap between pins (see Fig. 20–10). Both of these latter two techniques can complicate removal or adjustment of the frame, as discussed next.

REMOVAL OR REVISION OF ACRYLIC FRAMES ■ Removal of an acrylic frame can be done either by cutting fixation pins to free the acrylic column or by cutting the column between each pin to allow removal of the pin and attached column as a unit. Cutting the pins between the skin and the acrylic is the simplest method in theory, but may be difficult to execute because of insufficient clearance between the skin and the column to allow use of a pin cutter. A hand-held hacksaw can be used for cutting the pins in this situation. Cutting of the acrylic column is most easily done with an oscillating cast saw if there is no wire or fixation pin to be cut. In the latter case, or in the absence of an oscillating saw, the hacksaw works well to cut the acrylic.

At times it may be necessary to alter the reduction after the column has hardened, or to replace a loose pin. Revision of the frame begins by removing a segment of the acrylic column bridging the area to be realigned, or by cutting on each side of the pin to be removed. After cutting away several centimeters of the column, several small holes approximately 1 cm deep are drilled into the opposing cut ends and around the circumference of the end of the column. The purpose of these holes is to key the patch to the existing column to increase the adhesion of the patch. Methyl methacrylate is mixed to the doughy stage and handpacked and molded into the existing gap in the column while the desired reduction is maintained, or after the pin has been replaced. Using similar methods, acrylic frames can be revised to different type frames, adding or removing portions of the frame as circumstances dictate.

Ring Fixators

Although ring fixators were originally employed for fracture fixation, they are more costly and complex than conventional fixators and seem to have very little application in fracture repair. The technique for their use will be discussed in Chapter 22.

Bone Healing with External Skeletal Fixation

The concept of *biological fracture fixation* or *bridging osteosynthesis* has been mentioned earlier in this chapter, wherein some degree of interfragmentary motion or loading is accepted if the fracture can be stabilized in a manner that minimally disrupts soft tissues and bone vascular supply. Reliance is placed on early bridging callus to stabilize the fracture and allow continued healing. Placement of external skeletal fixation with closed reduction or with minimal open exposure is ideally suited to such a strategy.

Fracture healing can be manipulated in the presence of an external skeletal fixator in a unique strategy called "dynamization."[48] This concept involves modification of an initially rigid frame to allow axial compressive loading of the fracture with physiological weight bearing once early healing has occurred. This should enhance callus hypertrophy and remodeling of the fracture while providing protection from excessive stress, which might cause refracture. This concept would be most useful in those unstable fractures that initially require a relatively rigid frame to maintain reduction. An undesirable situation can arise when very stiff fixators are left in place too long, in which bone healing proceeds by direct Haversian remodeling, as is commonly seen with bone plate fixation. Although there is no question that the bone will heal, clinical union is much slower than when healing is by the indirect route and external callus is present. This means that the fixator must be maintained for a longer period, with its attendant cost and morbidity; thus it is optimal to have callus form when using external skeletal fixation. Experimental studies have indicated that around 6 weeks after surgery is the optimal time for dynamization of fractures in dogs. This can be achieved by removing the connecting bars and pins from one side of a type II or two sides of a type III splint to create a type I splint, which allows increased compressive loading while still protecting from bending loads. Removing alternate fixation pins of a type I splint accomplishes the same effect, although these splints are rarely stiff enough to require such manipulation.

INTRAMEDULLARY PINS*

Intramedullary (IM) pin (or nail) fixation for fracture treatment in small animals started in the 1940s.[2,49–52] It slowly gained popularity largely through the advent of safe general anesthesia, aseptic technique, antibiotics, and awareness by veterinarians and clients alike that successful repair could be accomplished in the majority of cases. Despite its limitations, it remains worldwide as the most common form of internal fixation in veterinary orthopedic surgery. In recent years, largely due to a better understanding of the biomechanical considerations necessary for successful bone healing, and in combination with cerclage and tension band wire techniques and with external fixators, intramedullary pinning has entered a new phase.

The key element for successful application of both pinning and wiring techniques is an *acute awareness of their shortcomings* in stabilizing fractures. Once these deficiencies are recognized and counteracted, pins and wires can be successfully used in a high percentage of routine fractures, with a minimum of complications.

General Considerations[52]

Advantages of Intramedullary Fixation

There are many potential advantages of pin and wire fixation over bone plates for the veterinary surgeon. Pin and wire fixation is much less expensive than bone plate fixation when the cost of implants, the large inventory of equipment needed, maintenance, and repair costs for bone plating equipment are compared to pinning costs. The issue of cost is less important when comparing intramedullary fixation to external skeletal fixation, but it is true that less inventory is needed for pin fixation. However, as will be developed below, pin fixation cannot be applied to its maximum advantage without the availability of external skeletal fixation. Most equipment needed for pins and wires is readily available from many manufacturers and is basically the same as that used for external skeletal fixators. For a small investment, newer wire tighteners and pin cutters will update existing equipment. Most pin and wire equipment will last a lifetime

*The author (DLP) gratefully acknowledges the contributions of a colleague, Dr. SJ Withrow, to this section.

of heavy usage, whereas plating requires periodic replacement of taps and drill bits. Most pin and wire fixations require less surgical exposure than for bone plates, resulting in less tissue trauma and vascular damage and resultant enhancement of healing. In general, pins and wires can be applied in less time than is needed for plates. This time factor saves money and decreases anesthesia time.

Pins are usually much easier to remove than plates, often being done under simple sedation and local analgesia. Plate removal, on the other hand, necessitates a second major invasive procedure with its attendant costs. Pins and wires have minimal effect on medullary blood supply and therefor on bone healing. Except in cases where active reaming for seating of large intramedullary nails (not widely practiced in animals) has taken place, total destruction of the medullary supply does not occur. The use of a Steinmann pin will decrease this medullary blood supply initially, but will by no means destroy it. Hypertrophy of medullary vessels will take place around the pin unless the pin completely fills the cavity or when the inner cortex has been reamed (as with Küntscher-type nails in man). Serious interference with medullary blood supply is most likely when a large pin fills the medullary cavity of a straight femur, as found in toy/miniature breeds and cats. When plates (or any implant) are applied there is some interference with cortical blood supply under the plate, which can lead to weakening of the bone. The problems created are postplate removal fracture or, eventual cycling, fatigue and fracture of the plate if the fracture is delayed in healing. Pins and wires only rarely result in this vascular interference.

Disadvantages of Intramedullary Fixation

Pins and wires definitely have some disadvantages compared to plates. Most of them relate to the biomechanical factors discussed below. If bone fragments are too small to be reduced and stabilized, then pin and wire fixation may not be as stable as a plate. Pin and wire fixation is not designed to maintain bone length (act as a buttress), since there is no load sharing between the round pin and the bone. Plates, on the other hand, can and do have the capability to prevent compressive forces from causing collapse (shortening) of a multifragment fracture that cannot be anatomically reconstructed. This is referred to as the *buttress effect*. Without plates, the best method of achieving a buttress effect is with external skeletal fixators.

It has been stated that IM pinning of open fractures may disseminate infection up or down the medullary cavity. This is surely theoretically possible, but is a rare occurrence. If any internal fixation is used in treatment of open fractures, it must produce very stable fixation, as bone will heal in the face of infection if it is stablized.

Biomechanical Factors

An understanding of how pins resist the various stresses or forces of bending, compression, and rotation acting on a long-bone fracture is necessary. Bending stress from any direction is well counteracted when a round pin of adequate diameter is well anchored both proximally and distally in the bone. Bone can still bend around an undersized pin, however, and the diameter of the medullary canal may be too small (e.g., the radius) to allow a suitable pin to be introduced. Rotational and compressive forces are counteracted only by frictional force between the bone and the pin, which is too small to be effective in the clinical situation. Although transverse fractures have minimal tendency to override or shorten, spiral and multifragment fractures need ancillary support as listed below to stop axial collapse. Likewise, a pin has virtually no ability to resist rotational forces. On occasion, if the fracture interdigitates, and the muscles pull the bone ends together, rotation may be stopped. In general, however, some means of antirotation must be utilized with the pin. The interlocking nail, widely used in human orthopedics,[53] is capable of resisting both compression and rotational forces, and is being introduced to veterinary orthopedics.[54] Distraction forces are not present in shaft fractures, but are present in areas of musculotendinous attachment such as the tuber olecranon and calcaneus. In such bones a pin alone will rarely adequately stop distraction. These fractures typically require the use of a pin and a tension band wire, or a lag screw.

The most common forms of *ancillary fixation* employed with intramedullary pins to counteract rotational and compressive forces are:

- Cerclage or interfragmentary wire (see Fig. 2–56A, B, G, H).
- External skeletal fixation (see Fig. 2–56C, D).
- Stack pins (see Fig. 2–56F). Multiple Steinmann pins are not very effective, as will be discussed below.
- Lag screw fixation (see Fig. 2–56E). Although lag screw fixation is very effective and will be discussed below, the limitation of bone size required to place both a screw and pin within the medullary canal limits the application of this technique.

These fixation methods will be discussed in detail below. Proximal pin migration postoperatively is a definite indication of motion due to insufficient stability at the fracture site, as motion of the pin relative to the bone causes bone resorption and subsequent loosening of the pin. Distal pin migration into the joint means, with very few exceptions, that the pin penetrated distal articular cartilage at the time of insertion. This can usually be corrected at surgery by retracting the point of the pin back into the medullary cavity, then angling the distal fragment in a slightly different direction before advancing the pin. Do not simply retract the pin and leave it in its original pin track.

External coaptation is sometimes combined with intramedullary fixation, but should only be necessary in intramedullary fixation of metacarpal and metatarsal bones, and never in long-bone fractures, since it defeats the main goal of internal fixation (i.e., early return to functional limb usage). Immobilizing the elbow or stifle joint in the presence of a long-bone fracture has an unacceptably high risk of loss of joint motion due to periarticular and intra-articular fibrosis. Fixation of the joints distal to the fracture has the effect of increasing the disruptive lever arm forces acting at the fracture site.

In discussing the pros and cons of pinning it is assumed that one adheres to the fundamental principles of the technique. Any technique will fail if not properly performed. In retrospect, very few nonunions or delayed unions are free of error at the surgery table.

Pin Types

STEINMANN PINS, KIRSCHNER WIRES ■ Both Steinmann pins and Kirschner wires (K-wires; pins that look like Steinmann pins but are smaller in diameter: 0.035, 0.045, and 0.062 inch, or 0.9 to 1.5 mm) are circular in cross section and either smooth or with partial or fully negative-thread-profile shanks (Fig. 2–54A). Steinmann pin diameters vary from $\frac{1}{16}$ inch (1.5 mm) to $\frac{1}{4}$ inch (6.5 mm). The threads probably offer little stability and are actually weaker than the standard smooth pins. This weakness is especially pronounced in the partially threaded pin where the thread meets the shank. This is an area

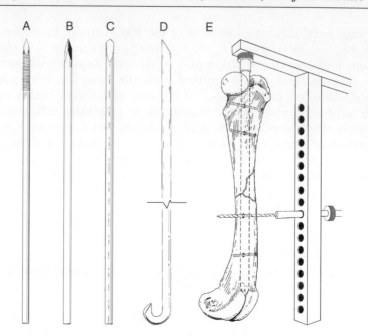

FIGURE 2–54. Intramedullary pin types. (*A*) Steinmann pin, partial negative-profile-thread, trochar point. (*B*) Steinmann pin, trochar point. (*C*) Steinmann pin, chisel point. (*D*) Rush pin. (*E*) Interlocking nail and drill jig for placing bone screws through the pin.

of stress concentration, and if this junction falls at or near the fracture site and is subjected to repetitive bending forces, these pins will often break. If a partially threaded pin binds against the bone during placement, the threads may cause the shank to be twisted completely off, just as a screw that is overtorqued will shear off at a thread.

The major reason that the threads do not achieve any extra stability initially is that the point of the pin is as wide as the outside thread diameter, and in placing the pin no threads are cut in bone. That is to say, the point produces a glide hole rather than a tap or thread hole. The threaded or partially threaded pin can in no way be equated to a bone screw (see the section Bone Screw Fixation for more information). Mechanical testing of the force required to pull out smooth and partially threaded pins from bone showed insignificant differences.[55] Upon removing a threaded pin after fracture healing it is sometimes necessary to "unscrew" them, but this is because bone has grown into the threads rather than the pin being threaded into the bone.

The tip of a Steinmann pin is designed to cut bone as it is inserted with a drilling motion. The most common tip is the three-sided *trochar* point, with a very sharp end that allows the pin to be started into bone at some angle to the bone (Fig 2–54B). The four-sided *diamond* or *chisel* point is more effective in cutting through very dense bone but not as easy to start without slipping on the bone surface (Fig. 2–54C). In the smaller sizes of K-wires the chisel point tends to bind and twist on itself in areas of dense cortical bone, so the trochar point is to be preferred in these pins. The most desirable type Steinmann pin is smooth shanked and furnished with a trochar point on one end and chisel point on the other end. This allows the choice of the most efficient point for drilling: it makes no difference which point is used once the pin is seated in the bone.

RUSH PINS ■ Whereas Steinmann pins are passive intramedullary splints, exerting no mechanical force on the bone, Rush pins (Fig 2–54D) are dynamic intramedullary splints, since they exert continuous compression forces at two or three points on the bone due to their becoming flexed during introduction. This flexion is induced by introducing the pin at an angle of about 20 degrees to the axial axis of the bone, rather than on the axial axis as with the Steinmann pin (Fig. 2–55A). As long as this flexion does not exceed the elastic limits of the metal, the pin will react to the bending by trying to return to its original shape. In this manner it locks itself to the bone at the point of entry, where it deflects off the opposite cortex, and in some cases, where the tip comes to rest on the original cortex.

To enable the Rush pin to be used in the manner described it has a noncutting beveled point that glides rather than cutting when it encounters bone. The opposite end is hook shaped to allow close approximation of this end with the bone, and to allow positive control of the direction of the flexion during introduction.

KÜNTSCHER NAIL ■ Although it was one of the early forms of intramedullary fixation[50] in the dog due to its wide use in man at the time, this pin has never achieved wide application in small animals. The **V** cross-section shape requires close contact of the pin through a considerable length of the bone to ensure stability. Because dog bones rarely are true cylinders, and because the cortex is too thin for reaming to a uniform diameter as is done in man, this device is not very useful in dogs or cats.

INTERLOCKING NAIL ■ The intramedullary reaming required to insert Küntscher nails in human patients was recognized as extremely nonphysiologic because of the damage done to the medullary blood supply, and the unreamed interlocking nail was developed to replace the Küntscher nail.[53] An interlocking nail is basically an intramedullary pin secured in position by proximal and distal transfixing screws that secure the bone to the nail to provide torsional and axial stability. Because this technique in man generally involves insertion by closed technique on a distraction table under fluoroscopic control, it seemed to be beyond any practical application in veterinary orthopedics. The recent introduction of the IN System (Innovative Animal Products, Rochester, MN) has provided a method for insertion of the interlocking nail without the need for specialized equipment (Fig. 2–54D).[54] With a minimal medullary canal diameter of 6 mm required its application is limited to femoral, tibial, and humeral fractures in large breeds.

Indications for Intramedullary Fixation

Because of the variety of intramedullary devices, it is not possible to list indications without qualifying the fixation device to be used. Fracture types are listed in Table 2–1, and for discussion of the fracture patient score mentioned below see the section Selection of Fixation Method later in this chapter

STEINMANN PIN ■ When used *without any ancillary fixation*, the list is quite short:

1. Stable fractures that do not have a tendency for axial shortening or rotation. These will primarily be type A fractures with a high fracture patient score.

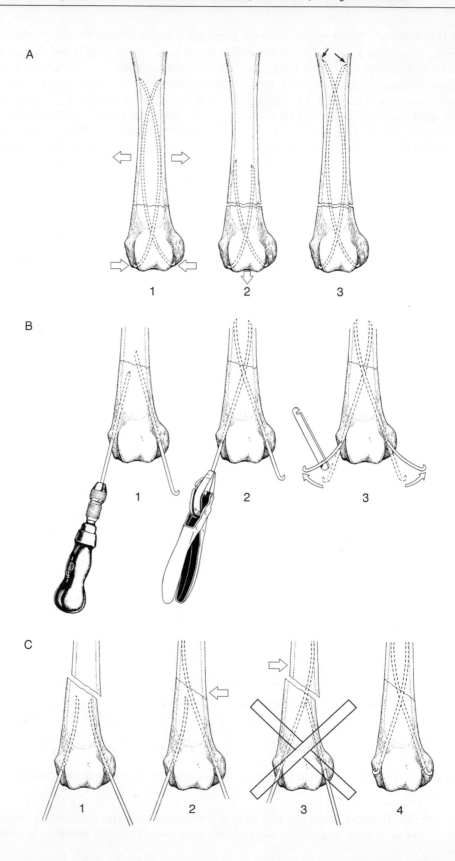

2.   In skeletally immature animals, especially puppies and kittens less than 4 months of age, type B and some type C fractures can be successfully treated due to the rapid callus formation seen in these animals.

When used in combination *with ancillary fixation*, virtually all fracture types can be handled, although perhaps not as efficiently as other fixation methods in type C fractures with a low fracture patient score.

Steinmann pin fixation can be accomplished by either an open or closed method. The closed technique is restricted to simple fractures, those of recent origin, and those that can be easily and accurately reduced. The latter is influenced by the size of the animal, time since injury, and the experience of the operator.

RUSH PIN ▪ The use of Rush pins for diaphyseal fractures in dogs and cats has not been well evaluated, although one of us (DLP) has long used them in place of Steinmann pins with good results in tibial fractures. The primary application for these pins is in proximal or distal fractures, where the double pin configuration provides good stability. When there is an intra-articular component, the Rush pin is easily combined with lag screw fixation.

INTERLOCKING NAIL ▪ All diaphyseal fracture types in the humerus, femur, and tibia are amenable to this fixation as long as the medullary canal diameter is at least 6 mm.

Methods of Application

Steinmann Pins

Specific landmarks for pin insertion in the various bones will be given in later chapters covering fractures in individual bones. The following remarks are general in nature and apply to all bones.

PIN CHUCKS AND POWER DRILLS ▪ Steinmann pins are most commonly inserted with a hand chuck; that is, a Jacobs keyed chuck to grip the pin, which

---

FIGURE 2–55. Rush pin principles. (A) Proper length of pins, usually two thirds to three fourths the length of the bone, allow the pins to glide off the opposite cortex and bend back toward the cortex of insertion, as in A^1. The elasticity of the pins causes them to exert dynamic forces on the bone as indicated by the arrows. If the pins are too short (A^2) their elasticity will cause distraction of the fracture. If the pins are too long (A^3) the tips of the pins may impinge the cortex sufficiently (*arrows*) to prevent complete reduction of the fracture. (B) The pilot hole is drilled with a Steinmann pin or bone awl at an angle of approximately 20 degrees to the long axis of the bone (B^1), and both pins are seated before being alternately driven across the fracture line (B^2). If inserted at the correct angle the pins will deform and glide on the opposite cortex with moderate force. If the condyle is too wide to allow insertion at the proper angle the pins are stress relieved by gentle bending (B^3), to allow easier bending at the opposite cortex. If bent too far, the pin will lose its dynamic force on the bone. (C) When double pinning an oblique fracture (C^1) it is important to drive and partially seat first the pin that forms a V angle with the fracture line (C^2), as this pin will create some compression force at the second cortex and will cause minimal displacement of the short distal fragment. If the pin that forms an X angle with the fracture line is seated first (C^3), it will cause marked angular displacement of the short fragment. Alternating the advancement of the pins until they are seated close against the bone (C^4) maintains good reduction.

is attached to a handle. The pin is inserted into the bone with a back-and-forth rotational motion while exerting force on the chuck. Care should be taken to avoid describing an arc with the handle, as this will cause the bone hole to be enlarged (see Fig. 2–38B). Power drills allow easy pin insertion but do have significant drawbacks. With too much speed and forceful insertion, thermal necrosis of surrounding bone can easily occur, resulting in loosening of the implant with time. These drills can be safely used if low-speed drilling (150 rpm) is performed. When properly used, power drills offer the advantage of less wobble during pin insertion, thus preventing enlargement of the entrance hole through cortical bone. They also significantly increase the ease of insertion of Kirschner wires, which tend to bend easily when inserted with a hand chuck. See the section above on pin insertion methods for external fixators for further discussion of power drills.

PIN DIAMETER ■ It has been said in the past that a goal of pinning is to fill the fracture site with pin or pins, as this gives the most stiffness to the pin-bone construct. One must, however, weigh this goal against its possible drawbacks. If you are dealing with a straight bone (cat), then filling the cavity will still allow anatomic reduction, although an overly large pin in a straight bone does increase the risk of significant interference with re-establishment of the medullary blood supply, with resultant delayed union. In curved bones, however (most dogs), to fill the fracture site with the pin will often mean inability to achieve anatomic reduction. For midshaft fractures try to fill about 60 to 75 percent of the medullary cavity at its narrowest point. If in doubt, use a smaller pin, since you can always replace it with a bigger one. If you go from a big pin to a smaller one, you will have a big hole at the entry site that does not "bind" the smaller pin. If the fracture is in the location of the narrowest diameter you can estimate pin size directly, but if the fracture is proximal or distal to the narrowest diameter, it must be estimated from the radiograph.

STACK PINNING ■ This method of pinning involves the use of several pins rather than one pin to fill the cavity. It is rarely needed, except in the very big dog where the biggest pin (¼ inch) is not large enough. It will only be necessary for the humerus or femur as a general rule. The theoretical advantages include better rotational stability, and more points of bone contact; however clinical results do not bear this out, with a 50 percent complication rate and generally unsatisfactory results reported in one study.[56] Another study did not find statistically significant differences in mechanical torsional strength studies comparing single, double, and multiple pin fixation of femoral fractures.[57] Disadvantages include: (1) greater tendency for pins to migrate due to the difficulty of firmly seating all pins distally; (2) potential problems with many pins exiting in one place (e.g., greater chance of hitting sciatic nerve in femur fractures); and (3) difficulty of cutting multiple pins at the entrance site short enough to prevent soft tissue irritation.

SEATING OF PIN ■ Landmarks are given later for each bone on how far to seat a pin, but they are only "rough estimates" and variance from this is common. Always watch the fracture as the pin is driven; if distraction of the fracture is seen, the pin is probably engaging the distal cortex and pushing the bones apart. The pin should then be retracted, the fracture reduced again, and additional counterforce applied to resist the tendency to distract. This can be either in the form of manual pressure from some point distal to the fracture, or with bone clamps if the fracture allows. In this situation the pin should be rotated without too much pressure, to allow it to cut into the bone without distracting the fracture. Driving the pin too far results in penetration of the distal cortex, often with resulting intra-articular pin placement. When this happens the pin must be redirected from the fracture site into the distal fragment, as simply retracting the pin often results in late migration of the pin back into the joint. As one approaches final pin placement, be sure that no crepitus (pin on bone) is present in the joint (elbow, stifle, hock). Use another pin of similar length, matched to the protruding end of the working pin, to confirm the position of the point of the pin within the bone.

CUTTING OF PIN ■ The most practical method of cutting is usually a bolt cutter or specialized pin cutter. Metal saws can be used but are awkward and deposit considerable amounts of metallic particles into the skin wound. Watch the fracture during and after the pin is cut with bolt cutters. With large pins, considerable movement of the pin occurs with resultant movement at the fracture. Except for small size pins it is often difficult to cut the pins short enough with bolt cutters. The usual goal is to cut the pin as short as possible (~5 mm) above the bone. This prevents large seromas and impingement on nearby structures (sciatic nerve, femoral condyles), lessens postoperative pain, and keeps the pins more stable by avoiding muscle and tissue action on the exposed pin end. One method of keeping pin ends short when they cannot be easily cut is depicted in Figure 18–1: (1) seat the pin the proper depth; (2) withdraw it about 2 cm; (3) cut off as close as possible (usually about 2 to 3 cm from bone); and (4) impact the pin with a punch and mallet, being careful to stabilize the fracture carefully before impacting.

PIN PLACEMENT IN LONG BONES ■ Pins are placed in long bones by either retrograding (i.e., driving pins from fracture site, out one end of the bone and then back into opposite fragment) or normograding, where the pin is placed from one end of the bone, into and through the medullary canal, and into the other fragment (Figs. 16–1 and 16–2). Depending on the bone, one or both methods may be acceptable, and these will be discussed in the appropriate chapters.

Rush Pin

INSTRUMENTATION ■ These pins are generally available in diameters from $\frac{1}{16}$ inch (1.5 mm) to $\frac{1}{4}$ inch (6.6 mm). The latter is too large for any small animal application; $\frac{3}{32}$ inch (2.4 mm) and $\frac{1}{8}$ inch (3.2 mm) are the most useful sizes in dogs. Pins are available in a variety of lengths proportional to their diameter (Osteo-Technology International Inc., Hunt Valley, MD), as they cannot be cut to length at the surgery table. Because these pins are often used in pairs and because they are precut in length, it is probably worthwhile, although not absolutely necessary, to have a double set of pins. The only other special equipment necessary for use of Rush pins is an impactor, which is used to seat the pin. Passably useful substitutes for Rush pins can be fabricated from Steinmann pins with a metal saw and file, but obviously this has to be done preoperatively.

TECHNIQUE ■ Unlike the Steinmann pin, which is static in the medullary canal, the Rush pin is put into the bone so that the pin is forced to bend as it is inserted (see Fig. 2–55A). The pin is inserted at an angle of approximately 20 degrees to the long axis of the bone. If the forces produced on the bone are properly manipulated they can be used to increase the stability of the fixation.

The technique is somewhat more demanding than Steinmann pinning and will require some practice to perfect, but it is well worth doing so.

1.   Since Rush pins do not have cutting points, a pilot hole must be drilled with a twist drill or Steinmann pin of the same size as the Rush pin (Fig. 2–55B1). With the fracture reduced, the pin is started into the bone while held at the hooked end in a pair of pliers. The hook provides a means of keeping the gliding point properly oriented to strike the second cortex. When double pins are used for proximal or distal fractures the pin length is chosen to approximate two thirds to three fourths of the bone length (Fig. 2–55A). Pin diameter is based on bone size and the age of the patient. In skeletally immature animals a pin that is too stiff (because of its diameter) will tend to break through the second cortex rather than bend and glide. For cats and small breed dogs $\frac{1}{16}$ inch (1.5 mm) is appropriate; $\frac{3}{32}$ inch (2.4 mm) for animals to 30 pounds (15 kg); and $\frac{1}{8}$ inch (3.2 mm) for larger animals.

2.   When resistance is felt as the pin contacts the opposite cortex, the pin is driven with a mallet and a special Rush pin driver or impactor which is very much like a nail-set, although the pliers will provide sufficient force to insert the smaller pins (Fig. 2–55B2). The double pins are alternately driven a short distance, until both are fully seated. The impactor or pliers are used to seat the hook end of the pin tightly against the entry cortex, where it provides some compression and stability against rotation of the pin. If the pin resists moderate driving force, it can be prebent slightly to relieve some bending strain and allow easier insertion without the chance of damaging the bone (Fig. 2–55B3). This bend must not be so severe as to preclude the pin being further bent as it is inserted: to do so would make the pin behave in a passive rather than a dynamic mode, and stability would be compromised.

3.   When a Rush pin crosses an oblique fracture, its dynamic characteristics will cause either distraction or compression of the fracture line, depending on the orientation of the pin relative to the obliquity of the fracture (Fig. 2–55C). When driving double pins it is important to lead with the pin that will tend to reduce the fracture, and follow with the pin that displaces the fracture.

4.   Because of the hook end lying close to the bone, Rush pins are usually not removed following bone union, as they create very little soft tissue irritation. When used across physeal lines they may cause growth arrest in animals under 5 months of age. This can be prevented by removing the pins 3 to 4 weeks postoperatively, or by cutting the hook off after the pin is seated.

CERCLAGE WIRE

The term cerclage means to encircle or wrap into a bundle. This procedure refers to a flexible wire that completely (see Fig. 2–59H) or partially (see Fig. 2–59I) passes around the circumference of a bone and is then tightened to provide *static interfragmentary compression* of bone fragments. The latter method is also known as hemicerclage. Cerclage or hemicerclage wire is *never used* as the sole method of fixation on any type of diaphyseal fracture. To do so routinely causes a pathological fracture at the most distal wire, which acts as a stress concentrator for bending forces. Current clinical use of cerclage wiring is based on the work of Rhinelander,[58] who showed that the small diameter of the tightly placed wire did nothing to disturb the centripetal flow of blood from medullary canal to periosteum. The key in preserving cortical blood supply is that the wires be tight, as a moving wire will disrupt the periosteal capillary network, devascularizing the underlying bone and disrupting periosteal callus formation.

Indications

These wires are used primarily on long oblique, spiral, and certain comminuted or multiple fractures. They are used as ancillary fixation with intramedullary pins (Fig. 2–56A, B), external skeletal fixators (Fig. 2–56C, D), and bone plates (Fig. 2–57). Additionally, they are used intraoperatively to aid in holding fracture segments in the reduced position while primary fixation is applied (Fig. 2–57).

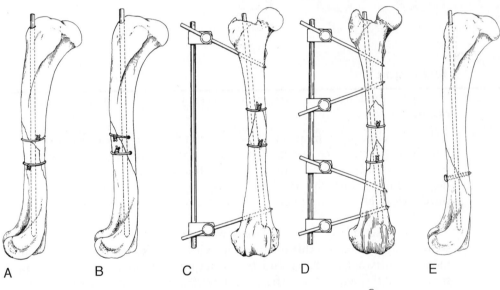

A   B   C   D   E

FIGURE 2–56. Auxiliary fixation used with an intramedullary pin. (A) Two cerclage wires. (B) Two hemicerclage wires. (C) External fixator 1/1 pin (half-Kirschner splint) and cerclage wires. (D) External fixator, 2/2 pins, and cerclage wires used in a multiple fracture. (E) Lag screws. Their use is usually limited to larger dogs. (F) Two intramedullary pins used in a serrated short oblique fracture. (G, H) Interfragmentary wire crossed around intramedullary pin as auxiliary fixation in a serrated transverse fracture.

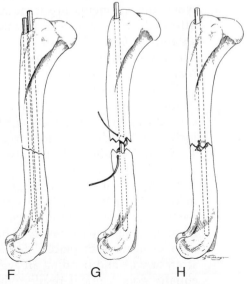

F   G   H

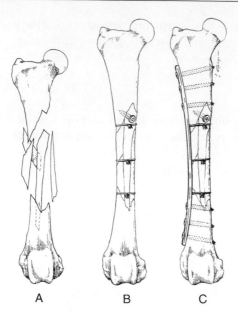

FIGURE 2–57. Cerclage wire and bone plate. (*A*) Comminuted fracture of the femur. (*B*) Comminuted area reconstructed and compressed using cerclage wires and a lag screw. (*C*) Neutralization plate applied.

A   B   C

Technique

Several fundamentals must be observed if these wires are to be used with optimal success.

1. Cerclage wire fixation should be restricted to those fractures where the length of the fracture line is at least twice the diameter of the bone or longer (see Fig 2–59D). This ensures that the fracture line describes an angle of 45 degrees or less with the axial axis of the bone and thus tensioning of the wire produces stable interfragmentary compression rather than shear forces (see Fig. 2–59E).

2. Restrict use of wires to areas where the cylinder of bone can be reconstructed anatomically; this means that, with rare exceptions, there should be no more than two fragments and two fracture lines in the transverse plane described by the wire. Three fracture lines/fragments should only be attempted when the fragments are large and interdigitate well, so that the compression afforded by the wire will maintain reduction (see Fig. 2–59F). Cerclage wires *should not be used to surround multiple unreduced fragments* (see Fig. 2–59G). These wires will become loose and disrupt vascular supply, and are one of the main causes of nonunion.

3. Use monofilament stainless steel wire of sufficient strength for immobilization. Wire of 22 gauge (0.025 inch, 0.64 mm) is suitable for toy breeds and cats, 20 gauge (0.032 inch, 0.81 mm) for average dogs, and 18 gauge (0.040 inch, 1.0 mm) diameter for large breeds. For giant breeds 16 gauge (0.049 inch, 1.25 mm) is indicated. It is always safest to err on the side of too large wires, rather than too small.

4. Apply all wires tightly to bring about rigid fixation of the fracture segments. Anything short of this allows movement of the implant and bone fragment, with subsequent devascularization, and demineralization of bone. Placement of a tight wire involves both tensioning the wire around the bone and then securing it in place. There are two methods in common use, twisting a straight wire and bending an eyelet wire (see Fig. 2–59A, B), and both produce equally good clinical results when properly performed. The eyelet wire tech-

nique results in less soft tissue irritation from the bent end, is less technically demanding than the twist method, but is slightly more expensive. Although more tension is produced in the wire by the eyelet method, the yield point, where the wire begins to deform due to tension forces, is lower for the eyelet than the twisted wire.[59,60] This difference can be negated by using the next size larger wire when using the eyelet method. With either method it is important to try moving each wire on the bone after placement. There should be no movement with the application of any reasonable force. Twisted wires can be given additional twists to further tighten them, but this is not possible with bent eyelet wire; they must be replaced if not tight enough on the first try.

TWIST METHOD ■ Instruments required for placing twist wires are quite simple (Fig. 2–58A, B, C). Almost any type of pliers will suffice, but needle holders are only useful with the smallest wire. The threaded collar device in Figure 2–58 is the most consistent and easiest to use. Wires should be twisted under tension preload so as to produce a uniform twist of both wires (Fig. 2–59B); this requires that the position of the twisting device be continuously adjusted to produce the correct twist. Excessive movement of the twisting instrument, or twisting one wire only (Fig. 2–59C) results in fracture of the wire before it is tight. The twisted end can either be cut seven or eight twists from the bone and bent flat while continuing to twist slightly, or left upright and cut three or four twists from the bone. The latter results in the least loss of tension,[59] but can only be done where the wire is covered by an adequate thickness of soft tissue.

BENT EYELET WIRE METHOD ■ Although there are several types of tighteners available for eyelet wire, including those with built-in tension gauges, the simple type illustrated here (Fig. 2–58C) produces equally good results clinically and experimentally.[60] The tensioning and bending method is illustrated in Figure 2–60.

5. In applying the wire, avoid destruction of periosteal blood supply resulting from detachment of soft tissue in areas where muscle or ligaments attach

A   B   C

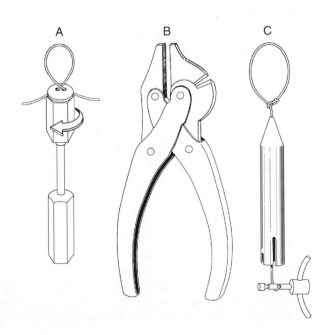

FIGURE 2–58. Wire-tightening instruments. (*A*) This twisting instrument secures the wire between a fixed double-perforated tip and a large nut that is tightened (arrow) on a threaded shaft. (*B*) Parallel jaw pliers work well for twisting and are available at hardware stores. (*C*) Eyelet wires are tightened by wrapping the long end of the wire around a rotating key inserted into a hollow bullet-nosed tube.

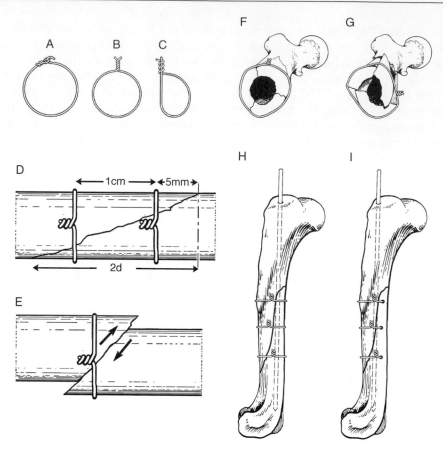

FIGURE 2–59. Cerclage wire principles. (*A*) Tightening and securing an eyelet wire. See also Figure 2–60. (*B*) Tightening and securing a twisted wire. Note that each wire is equally twisted at a uniform angle and that there are at least three twists below the cut ends. (*C*) An improperly tightened twisted wire. This wire will loosen when loaded, and will quickly fatigue and break with continued attempts to tighten it. (*D*) For compression to be produced by a cerclage wire, the length of the oblique fracture line must equal at least twice the bone diameter. Wires are placed approximately 5 mm from the end of the fracture, and spaced about 1 cm apart. There is no mechanical advantage to closer spacing (d = diameter). (*E*) If the length of the fracture line is less than twice the bone diameter, tightening the wire produces shearing rather than compression forces. (*F, G*) Stability of cerclage fixation requires that the tubular shape of the diaphysis be reconstructable, and that there are a maximum of three fragments included. If the fragments are not completely reduced, or do not interlock when compressed, the wire will become loose as the fragments move. (*H*) An ideal cerclage wire fixation: a long oblique two-piece fracture, used in support of a Steinmann pin. (*I*) Placing part of the wire through a bone tunnel does not change the mechanical function of the wires, and is a good method of preventing displacement of wires in a tapering bone.

to periosteum. Avoid entrapping muscle or nerves by passing the wire very close to the bone. The wire passer (Fig. 2–61) serves very well for placing the wire around the bone with a minimum of trauma. The end of the wire can also be bent into a half circle of appropriate size and passed directly around the bone with a needle holder. This method works best with the larger wire sizes. The wire must be placed so that it will be perpendicular to the axial axis of the bone when tightened; an angled wire will loosen just as a too large ring on the

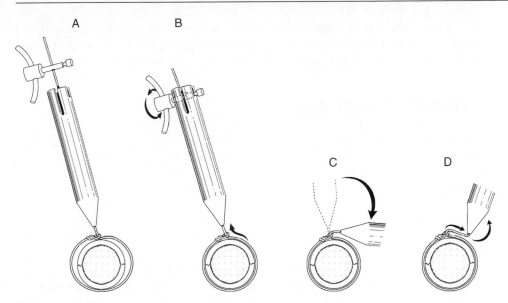

FIGURE 2–60. Tightening and securing eyelet cerclage wire. (*A*) The free end of the wire is secured in the rotating key of the tightener. (*B*) Tension is produced in the wire as the key is turned. The angular bend of the wire, indicated by the arrow, must not be too acute or the wire will fatigue and easily break. (*C*) After attaining sufficient tension, the tightener is rotated 90 degrees to secure the wire. (*D*) Loosening the tightener and rotating it back to the upright position allows the bent wire to be pressed closely to the bone and then cut.

finger will be loose. Avoid placing wire in an area where it will increase the fracture gap when tightened.

6.   If a relatively long fracture area is to be covered, the cerclage wires should be placed approximately ¼ inch (5 mm) from the ends of the fragments, then spaced approximately 1 to 1.5 cm apart. Placement closer than this may result in unnecessary devitalization of the bone (caused by detachment of soft tissue in placing the wires) and delay of union, and does not increase the fixation stability. The number of cerclage wires used is in direct relation to the length of the fracture, but is never less than two. A single wire acts as a fulcrum to concentrate all bending loads but cannot supply enough interfragmentary compression to prevent bending. Single wires are used only for fissure fractures.

7.   When placing a full cerclage on a bone that is conical, or tapering, in shape (e.g., proximal femur), precautions need to be taken to prevent the wire from slipping towards the smaller diameter and so becoming loose. Often the natural surface irregularities of the bone accomplish this, but it may be necessary to notch the bone or drive a small Kirschner wire perpendicular to the bone to trap the wire. One end of the Kirschner wire is bent 90 degrees to discourage late migration of the implant.

FIGURE 2–61. AO/ASIF wire passer (Synthes Ltd. [USA], Paoli, PA). This instrument makes it possible to insert the cerclage wire around the bone with a very minimum of soft tissue detachment.

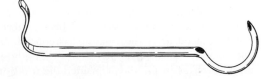

8.   Above all, stabilize the main bone fragments with stable, uninterrupted primary fixation. Depending on the type of fracture, this may be accomplished with an intramedullary pin, an external fixator, or a bone plate.

INTERFRAGMENTARY WIRE

These techniques are typically utilized to prevent rotation of short oblique or transverse fractures, to secure bone fragments, and to stabilize fissure fractures. As the name implies, the wire does not encircle the bone, but rather passes through and partially around the bone. This is the *least secure and consistent* form of internal fixation, and should not be depended upon for long-lasting stability when subjected to high dynamic loading forces. It should be reserved for smaller dogs and cats, or for immature animals who can be expected to form callus early and abundantly. If the fracture line is suitable for cerclage wiring, this is always a better choice relative to stability produced.

The most commonly used patterns are shown in Figure 2–62. The holes in the bone are made with K-wires or twist drills and the wire passed through. If the wire enters the medullary canal, it is best to first drill the bone, place the wire into both bone segments, reduce the fracture, then seat the pin and tighten the wire. It makes little difference if the pin is encircled, as in Figure

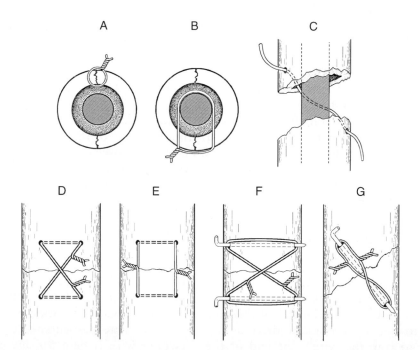

FIGURE 2–62. Various interfragmentary wire patterns. (*A*) Simple interfragmentary "suture" placed through holes drilled from the cortex to the medullary cavity. The wire must be positioned before the fracture is reduced. (*B, C*) Wire placed around the pin. In some situations this may pull the pin tightly against the cortex, which increases stability of the fixation. (*D, E*) Interfragmentary wires place through bone tunnels tangential to the medullary cortex. These patterns offer increased rotational stability and can be placed after the fracture is reduced. (*F, G*) Combining interfragmentary wires with K-wires may be simpler than drilling bone tunnels. Crossing the fracture line with the K-wire, as in *G*, adds considerable rotational stability.

2–62B, C, unless the pin is small enough to deform and be brought into contact with the cortex. The cruciate and horizontal mattress patterns shown in Figure 2–62D, E, and F are more effective in preventing rotation than are simple patterns (Fig. 2–62A).[61] Even so, they are not very efficient, merely changing the rotational point from the central axis of the bone to the cortex secured by the wire. The opposite side of the bone remains unstable unless the fracture lines interdigitate sufficiently. Maximum rotational stability is provided by the transfixation pin and wire technique shown in Figure 2–62G.

TENSION BAND WIRE

According to the tension band principle, active distracting forces are counteracted and converted into compressive forces.[62] The tensile forces exerted by contraction of muscles on fractures such as those involving the olecranon process, trochanter major, tuber calcis, or detached tibial tuberosity can be overcome and converted to compressive forces by inserting two K-wires and a tension band wire (Fig. 2–63). The K-wires are needed to neutralize shear forces at the fracture line, while the tension band wire not only neutralizes bending loads, but actually converts them to compressive forces. The cortex that forms the bending point must be intact for this method to work. The wire is usually placed in a figure-of-8 fashion to ensure that the longest possible lever arm, between the bending point and the wire, is maintained. This fixation device is more stable when the animal is weight bearing than when at rest, surely a useful thing for the veterinary surgeon.

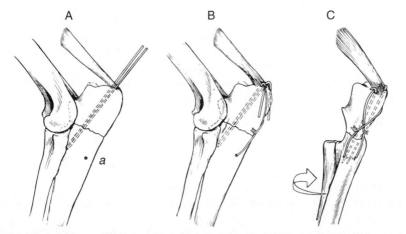

FIGURE 2–63. Tension band wire and Kirschner wire fixation. (A) Olecranon fracture. Kirschner wires placed at caudomedial and lateral corners of triceps tendon insertion. Ideally, the pins contact the cranial ulnar cortex distal to the coronoid process. A transverse hole (a) is drilled through the caudal cortex. (B) The tension band wire is positioned and twisted tight on both sides of the figure-of-8. The wire should pass through the triceps tendon close to the olecranon proximally. The Kirschner wires are bent caudally, cut, and (C) rotated 180 degrees so that the ends are buried in soft tissue. If the fragments of the above fracture do not interlock or if comminution is present, plate fixation is indicated.

Technique

The technique is illustrated here on the olecranon, one of the most common applications. The usual procedure in repairing a fracture or osteotomy of the olecranon process requires first reducing the fracture, then inserting two pins that are started on the caudomedial and caudolateral areas of the tuber. Such placement interferes less with the triceps tendon, and bending of the pins can be accomplished more effectively. If the pins can be inserted diagonally to engage the cranial cortex distally, they do a better job of securing the fragments and countering rotational and shearing forces than if they just go down the medullary canal. The pins should be as parallel to each other as possible to allow for compression of the fracture line as the wires are tightened.

A transverse hole is then drilled through the diaphysis distal to the fracture site (Fig. 2–63A). This hole is positioned to place the crossing point to the figure-of-8 wire near the fracture line, and so maintain the lever arm. The wire is inserted in a figure-of-8 fashion and tightened by twisting each side of the figure-of-8. Avoid overtightening, because this will create a gap at the articular notch if the fracture is in this area (Fig. 2–63B). Note that the wire is passed through the triceps tendon close to the bone to avoid cutting the tendon when tightening the wire. Alternatively, the wire can be placed through a second hole in the bone to prevent interference with soft tissues, as is done in the tuber calcis (Fig. 2–64D). Use monofilament stainless steel wire of sufficient strength for immobilization. Wire of 22 gauge (0.025 inch, 0.64 mm) is suitable for toy breeds and cats, 20 gauge (0.032 inch, 0.81 mm) for average dogs, and 18 gauge (0.040 inch, 1.0 mm) diameter for large breeds. For giant breeds, 16 gauge (0.049 inch, 1.25 mm) is indicated. It is always safest to err on the side of too large wires, rather than too small. Eyelet wires can be used in place of twisted wire, but due to the stiffness of the wire some difficulty will be noted in the 1.0- and 1.25-mm sizes in getting both halves of the figure-of-8 equally tight.

The K-wires are then bent down the caudal surface of the ulna, cut, and rotated so that the ends are buried in soft tissue (Fig. 2–63C). If properly inserted, these implants do not interfere with movement of soft tissue and usually do not need to be removed after healing.

Other situations in which the tension band wire principle can be used to advantage include the following:

1.   Avulsion fracture or osteotomy of the trochanter major of the femur (Fig. 2–64A).
2.   Avulsion fracture of the tibial tubercle (Fig. 2–64B).
3.   Fracture or osteotomy of the medial malleolus of the tibia (Fig. 2–64C).
4.   Fracture of the tuber calcanei (Fig. 2–64D).
5.   Fracture or osteotomy of the acromial process of the scapula, usually in large dogs (Fig. 2–64E).
6.   Fracture or osteotomy of the greater tuberosity of the humerus (Fig. 2–64F).
7.   Arthrodesis of the proximal intertarsal joint (Fig. 2–64G).

BONE SCREWS

There are two basic types of bone screws: cancellous (Fig. 2–65) and cortical (Fig. 2–66).[62,63] Figure 2–67 details the typical assortment of bone screws avail-

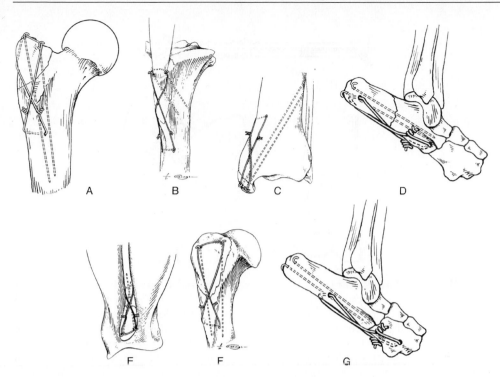

FIGURE 2–64. Conditions in which the tension band wire principle can be used to advantage. (*A*) Avulsion fracture or osteotomy of the trochanter major of the femur. (*B*) Avulsion fracture of the tibial tubercle. (*C*) Fracture or osteotomy of the medial malleolus of the tibia. (*D*) Fracture of the tuber calcanei. (*E*) Fracture or osteotomy of the acromion process of the scapula. (*F*) Fracture or osteotomy of the greater tuberosity of the humerus. (*G*) Arthrodesis of the intertarsal joint.

able to the veterinary surgeon. Bone screws are usually employed to provide static interfragmentary or plate/bone compression by means of the *lag screw* principle. Interfragmentary compression is produced when the head of the screw bears on the first cortex and the threads of the screw are engaged only in the second cortex. Tightening of the screw converts that torque force to interfragmentary compression. Partially threaded screws automatically function as lag screws if their threads do not cross the fracture line (Fig. 2–65*B*, *C*). Fully threaded screws require special insertion technique in order to function as interfragmentary lag screws (Fig. 2–66*B*, *C*). Fully threaded screws provide plate/bone compression because the screw threads do not engage the plate and are anchored in the bone only, usually in two cortices. A secondary function of bone screws is to hold fragments in a fixed position without interfragmentary compression, where it is called a *position screw*. Such use is rare, usually being applied to prevent a small bone fragment or graft from displacing into the medullary canal.

Cancellous screws are used to compress fragments of epiphyseal and metaphyseal bone. The screw may be partially or completely threaded with relatively few threads per unit length; threads are quite deep, and the pitch of the threads is relatively high. Although very useful in human osteoporotic bone, there is much less need for this type thread in canine and feline bone, since even the metaphyseal zones are covered in dense cortical bone, where cortically threaded screws hold well. Partially threaded screws suffer from an inherent weakness at

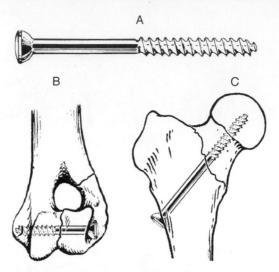

FIGURE 2–65. Partially threaded lag screws. (*A*) Partially threaded screws most commonly have a thread designed for cancellous bone. The junction of the smooth shank and the threads is a potential stress raiser, where bending loads concentrate. Both fragments are drilled the diameter of the screw shank. This will allow tapping of the screw threads in the second fragment. (*B*) Lateral part of the humeral condyle stabilized by lag screw fixation. In order for compression to be produced, it is critical that all the threads be across the fracture line from the screw head. This may position the shank/thread junction close to the fracture line and predispose to breakage of the screw. (*C*) In this femoral neck fracture it can be seen that the shank/thread junction is some distance from the fracture, with little chance of screw breakage.

the junction of the threaded and unthreaded zones, where there is a dramatic change in stiffness of the screw shaft. This produces a stress-concentrating effect and makes this area subject to stress fracture when subjected to repetitive bending loads. Because of this it is well to try to ensure that this junction is as far from the fracture line as possible.

Cortical screws were designed to be used primarily in the dense diaphyseal bone (Fig. 2–66). The screw is fully threaded with more threads per unit length than cancellous screws; threads are shallower and more flatly pitched than cancellous screws. By proper application these screws can be made to function as lag screws (Fig. 2–66*B–I*). Because fully threaded screws are of uniform diameter throughout their length, they do not suffer from the stress-accumulating effect described above for partially threaded screws, and are less prone to breakage when used in heavily stressed fractures such as the lateral aspect of the humeral condyle.

Indications and Principles of Insertion

Primary Fixation in Certain Fractures

These fractures are usually in the metaphyseal or articular areas of the bone rather than in the diaphysis. Either partially threaded cancellous screws or fully threaded cortical screws can be used. To accomplish interfragmental compression, cancellous screws are inserted so that the thread of the screw does not cross the fracture line (Fig. 2–65*B, C*). The fracture segments are first reduced; after the appropriate diameter *tap hole* (equivalent to the screw core diameter

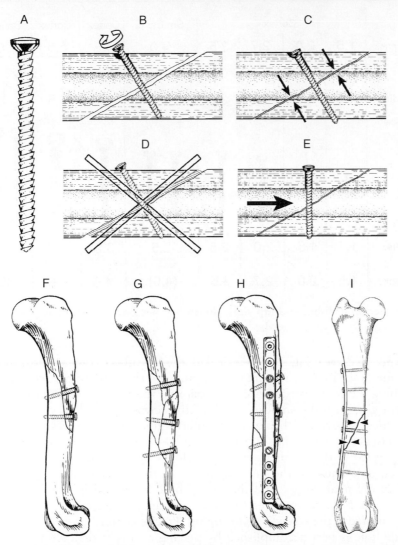

FIGURE 2–66. Fully threaded lag screws. Although these illustrations show diaphyseal bone, the same principles apply in metaphyseal fractures as shown in Figure 2–65. (*A*) Fully threaded screws typically are designed for use in cortical bone, although this does not diminish their usefulness in canine and feline metaphyseal regions. (*B*) In order for fully threaded screws to function as lag screws and produce interfragmentary compression, the hole in the first cortex (fragment) must be equal to the diameter of the screw threads, allowing the screw to glide within the hole. The hole in the second cortex is the diameter of the core of the threads, allowing the threads to engage or tap into the bone. (*C*) Because of the glide hole in the first cortex the bone is pulled into compression between the screw head in the first cortex and the distal threads engaged in the second cortex. (*D*) If both cortices are threaded (or tapped), the bone cannot glide on the screw and no compression is generated. Continued tightening of the screw will strip the threads in the bone. (*E, F*) Although a lag screw perpendicular to the fracture line, as in *C*, produces maximal interfragmentary compression, a screw perpendicular to the cortex is better able to resist axial loading. In shaft fractures it is ideal to combine both positions if the fracture line is long enough to accommodate two screws. (*G, H*) This complex fracture was completely stabilized by interfragmentary lag screw compression, then a neutralization plate was applied to protect the screw fixation from bending, rotational, and axial forces. (*I*) When the plane of the fracture line allows, interfragmentary compression can be applied by a lag screw placed through a plate hole. As in *G* and *H*, the plate functions as a neutralization plate.

Screw: —Type	Cortex				Sm.Canc.	Cortex	Cortex	Cancellous
—Diameter (mm)	1.5	2.0	2.7	3.5	4.0	4.5	5.5	6.5
Drill Bit dia. for Gliding Hole	1.5	2.0	2.7	3.5	none	4.5	5.5	in hard bone 4.5
Drill Bit dia.	1.1	1.5	2.0	2.5	2.5	3.2	4.0	3.2
Tap for	1.5	2.0	2.7	3.5	(4.0)	4.5	5.5	(6.5)

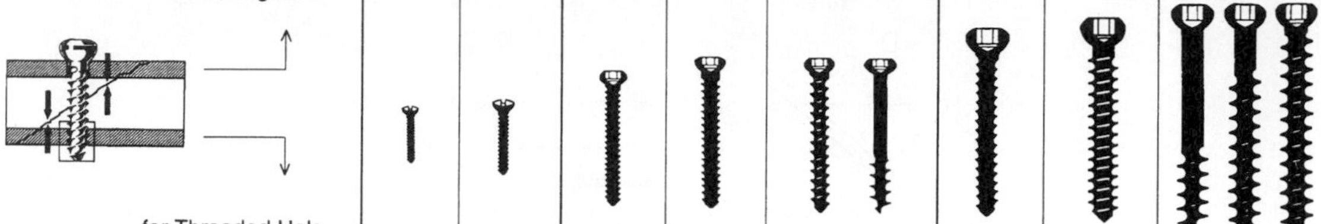

FIGURE 2–67. Screw, drill bit, and tap sizes. (From Synthes Ltd. [USA], Paoli, PA.)

in the threaded area; Fig. 2–67) is drilled, the thread is cut using the appropriate tap. Some cancellous screws are self-tapping and thus do not require pretapping. Tightening the screw produces compression of the fracture segments as the near fragment glides on the smooth shank of the screw.

A cortical screw will bring about interfragmentary compression when it is inserted to accomplish a lag effect, and can also be used to repair these fractures when inserted in the manner described below (Fig. 2–66). This requires that an oversized hole equal to the outer diameter of the screw threads (*glide hole*) be drilled in the near cortex and that a tap hole be drilled in the far cortex and tapped so that the screw thread becomes engaged on insertion. The latter step can be omitted if the screw is self-tapping. Precise centering of the tap hole with the glide hole is best accomplished by placing an insert drill sleeve in the glide hole. Alternatively, the tap hole is first drilled through both cortices and then the first cortex hole is enlarged to glide hole diameter. Tightening the screw allows compression to be exerted between the two cortices, as the first cortex can move on the screw due to the glide hole not engaging screw threads (Fig. 2–66C). When threads are engaged in both cortices no gliding can occur, hence no compression is produced (Fig. 2–66D). Maximum interfragmentary compression is secured when the axis of the screw is perpendicular to the fracture line, hence an attempt is always made to orient the screw as close to this axis as bone contour and exposure will allow.

Screws are *never* used as the primary fixation in shaft fractures. They are always supplemented with a plate, pin, or external skeletal fixator. Primary fixation of shaft fractures with screws always results in fracture at a screw hole or failure of the screw unless the limb is immobilized in an external splint/cast, thus negating the advantages of internal fixation.

Aid in Reduction and Auxiliary Fixation

With long oblique, spiral, or multiple fractures of the diaphysis, cortical bone screws inserted with a lag effect to accomplish interfragmentary compression may be used as an aid in accomplishing reduction and serve as auxiliary fixation

(Fig. 2–66F). Two adjoining fragments are reduced and usually held in the reduced-compressed position during drilling, tapping, and insertion of the bone screw. The bone screw should be inserted at a distance from the fracture line at least equal to the screw diameter, so the center of the hole must be 1.5 diameters from the fracture line. When the fracture is multiple in nature and the bone segments are of sufficient size, the entire bone or portions of it may be reconstructed anatomically by reducing and fixing two fragments at a time until reconstruction is complete (Fig. 2–66G). A neutralization plate (see below) is one choice for final fixation (Fig. 2–66H). Plate screws can also be inserted for lag effect when the fracture line is properly oriented to the plate (Fig. 2–66I). Whenever possible, lag screws should be used in preference to cerclage wire to accomplish interfragmental compression and to aid in reduction and auxiliary fixation. Lag screws are more reliable than cerclage wires in producing interfragmentary compression because there are fewer potential technique errors possible during insertion. Additionally, insertion of a lag screw causes less disruption of soft tissue and periosteal blood supply than does placement of a cerclage wire, and if a screw should loosen, it does not cause the vascular disruption of the cerclage wire.

BONE PLATES

One of the primary objectives in the treatment of fractures is early return to full function of the injured limb. Bone plates are ideal for accomplishing this goal because they have the potential to restore rigid stability to the reconstructed fractured bone when properly applied.[62–64] Bone plates are adaptable to many situations:

1. Most long-bone fractures.
2. Multiple and complex fractures.
3. Fractures in the larger dogs and semidomesticated animals (especially the femur) because postoperative complications are less frequent and postoperative care is reduced when the fixation apparatus is covered with soft tissue.

Although many designs and sizes of plates are available, the ASIF (Association for the Study of Internal Fixation, Synthes Ltd., [USA], Paoli, PA) system (see Fig. 2–68) will be used to illustrate the principles because it is the system with which the authors are most familiar. Several manufacturers now produce plates and screws very similar in design and function to the ASIF implants. For optimum results in the use of bone plates, a scientific understanding of the following areas is a prerequisite:

1. Anatomy (e.g., structure of bone; location of blood and nerve supply; muscle separations; and attachments of muscles, tendons, and ligaments).
2. Principles of active forces (knowledge of compression, tension, and torsional and bending forces as they affect the bone).
3. Understanding of the mechanics of fixation in detail and viewing and planning its application in three dimensions.
4. Proper selection of a surgical approach and method of internal fixation best suited for the individual fracture.
5. Bone healing patterns (see also previous discussion in this chapter). It is important to be able to interpret the biological response with *rigid fixation*, where primary or direct bone union is anticipated. Development of a cloudy

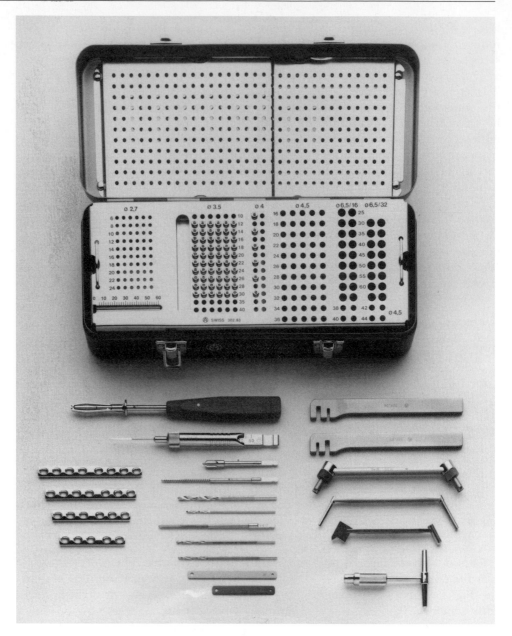

FIGURE 2–68. Basic bone-plating equipment and plates. (From Synthes Ltd. [USA], Paoli, PA.)

irritation callus is a warning sign and indicates some movement occurring at the fracture site and the potential for delayed or nonunion. When two vascular, anatomically reduced bone fragments are rigidly fixed under compression so that no shearing or torsional forces can act on them, no resorption of bone at the fracture line takes place, and a direct bony union occurs without any radiologically visible periosteal callus.[65,66] On the other hand, if a *bridging osteosynthesis* approach was adopted to stabilize the fracture, considerable periosteal and endosteal bridging callus is anticipated, and its absence would be cause for concern.

Terminology

Plates may be inserted to function as a compression plate, a neutralization plate, bridging plate, or a buttress plate. Such names do not imply anything about the physical characteristics of the plate, but only its function.

Compression (Tension Band) Plate

When the plate is applied so that it is under tension and the fracture fragments are under compression, it is referred to as a compression plate, or alternatively a tension band plate. Long bones (e.g., the femur) are subject to eccentric loading and may be compared to a bent column. The lateral side is subject to distracting or tension forces; the medial side, to impacting or compressive forces (Fig. 2–69A, B). It is vital that the plate be applied on the side of the bone that is most frequently under a distracting or tension force (Fig. 2–69C). Clinically these surfaces are the lateral surface of the femur, medial or cranial surface of the tibia, cranial or lateral surface of the humerus, and the craniomedial or cranial surface of the radius.

When a plate is applied to the lateral surface of the femur, it counteracts all tension forces and creates compressive forces along the fracture line, thus providing rigid internal fixation (Fig. 2–69C). If it were applied on the medial surface, it would not give long-lasting fixation because the plate would be under excessive bending stress and subject to fatigue fracture (Fig. 2–69D). It is also

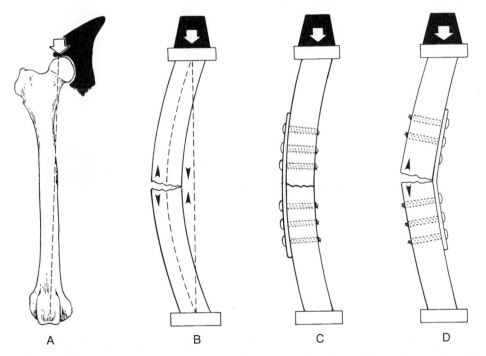

A	B	C	D

FIGURE 2–69. Principle of a compression plate. Insert the plate only on the tension side of the bone so that the bone will receive compressive forces. Because long bones are subject to eccentric loading, the side of the bone to be under tension must be known to determine where to apply the plate. The femur (A), for example, can be compared to a bent column (B). The plate that is applied to the outer or convex side can then counteract all tension forces (C) and provide rigid internal fixation. If it were applied on the inner or concave surface, it would not provide fixation (D); such a plate would come under excessive bending stresses and would soon show a fatigue fracture.

critical to long-term stability and prevention of plate failure that the cortex opposite the plate be intact in order to prevent compression forces on that cortex from becoming bending forces being applied to the plate (Fig. 2–69B). The cortex opposite the plate in this situation acts as a buttress against the compression forces.

Production of tension in the plate was originally accomplished by use of a tensioning device (Fig. 2–70D) that was temporarily applied to the plate and attached to the bone, but the self-compressing plate has totally replaced the tension device in practice. Axial compression is accomplished at the fracture site with these plates, and the dynamic compression plate (DCP) introduced by Synthes, and discussed further below, has been the pattern for these plates (Figs. 2–70 and 2–71).[67] Compression plates are used on type A stable fractures, osteotomies, and arthrodeses.

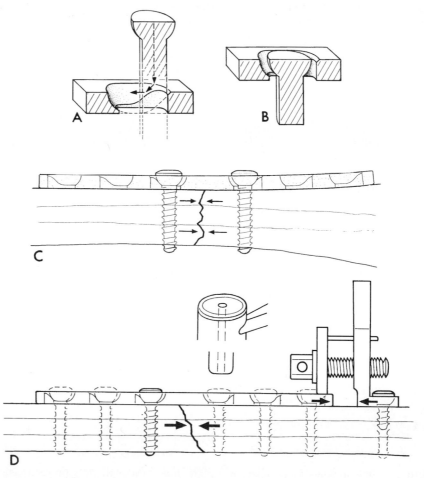

FIGURE 2–70. Self-compressing plate (DCP). (*A*, *B*) Sagittal sections of a screw and screw hole in a DCP show the mechanical principle. (*C*) The first screws on either side of the fracture line are inserted eccentrically (load position) and alternately tightened to produce compression. (*D*) If there is a wide fracture gap, additional compression can be accomplished by the use of a tension device. (From Müller M, et al: Manual of Internal Fixation, 2nd ed. Translated by J Schatzker. New York, Springer-Verlag, 1979, with permission.)

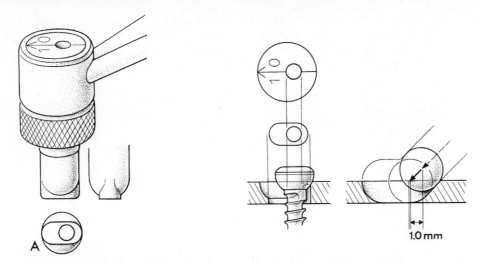

FIGURE 2–71. Drill guides for insertion of the self-compressing plate (DCP). (*A*) Load guide. The guide is inserted in the screw hole of the plate with the arrow pointing to the fracture line. The screw is located eccentrically so that in tightening, it moves 1 mm (it also moves the bone fragment 1 mm). (*B*) Neutral guide. The screw is located slightly eccentrically so that in tightening it moves 0.1 mm. (*C*) For oblique fractures, a lag screw may be inserted at an angle through the plate. (*D–F*) When multiple fracture lines are present, the first fracture line is compressed as the second screw in the load position is tightened. The second fracture line is compressed as the third screw in the load position is tightened. (From Allgöwer M, et al: The Dynamic Compression Plate. New York, Springer-Verlag, 1973, pp 15, 24, 34, with permission.) *Figure continued on following page*

Neutralization Plate

This plate is applied on the tension side of the bone to neutralize or overcome torsional, bending, compressive, and distraction forces on fracture lines that have been stabilized by interfragmentary compression supplied by lag screws and cerclage, hemicerclage, or interfragmentary wire (Fig. 2–66C). If possible, the plate is applied to exert some axial compression. Neutralization plates are used on osteotomies or type B and some type C unstable fractures that can be anatomically reconstructed using lag screws or cerclage wire.

Buttress or Bridging Plate

This nomenclature can be somewhat confusing, as the term "bridging plate" is a latecomer that was developed to signify a buttress plate used for bridging osteosynthesis of diaphyseal fractures. The buttress plate functions to shore up a fragment of bone, thereby maintaining length and the proper functional angle in fractures such as those involving the proximal tibial plateau (Fig. 2–72A, B). The bridging plate may be considered to splint or bridge the fracture area to maintain length of the bone when the fragments are left unreduced or are missing and replaced with cancellous bone graft (Fig. 2–72C).

Application of Bone Plates

Number of Screws

Clinical data indicate that an absolute minimum of two screws (four cortices) should be used in the bone segments on each side of the fracture in small

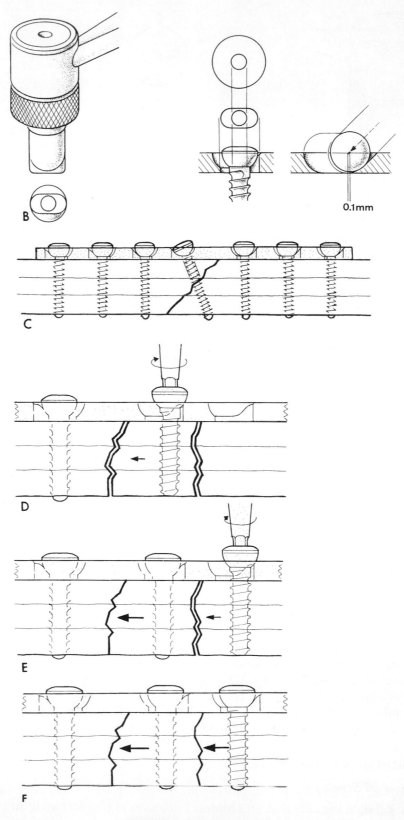

FIGURE 2-71. *Continued*

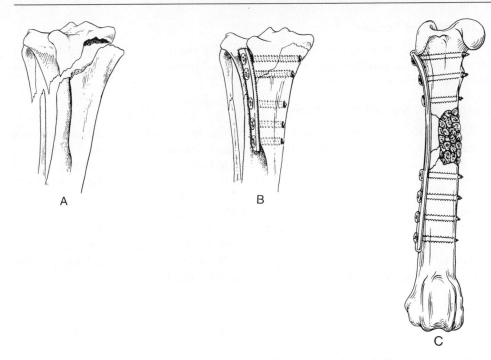

FIGURE 2–72. Buttress plate. (*A*) Fracture of the proximal tibial plateau. (*B*) Buttress plate fixation shores up the fragment, maintaining length and proper functional angle. (*C*) Bridging plate bridges a defect, filled with bone graft in this case.

animals. However, a minimum of three to four screws (six to eight cortices) is ideal for compression and neutralization plates and is mandatory for bridging plates in small animals (Fig. 2–73). These numbers do not vary much with the size of the animal, as the plate sizes vary to allow approximately the same number of screws per unit of bone length. The number of screws is a function of plate length, which is discussed below.

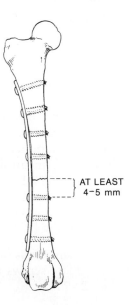

FIGURE 2–73. Plate fixation: number of screws and screw placement. Although two screws (four cortices) are an absolute minimum on each side of the fracture line, three to four screws (six to eight cortices) are more ideal and are mandatory for larger breeds. Minimal distance between fracture lines and screws is 4 to 5 mm.

AT LEAST
4–5 mm

Placement of Screws

Clinical and experimental data indicate that the minimal distance between screw hole and fracture line should be 4 to 5 mm, or at least equal to the diameter of the screw used (Fig. 2–73).[62,63]

Length and Size of Bone Plate

Bone plates are made in a variety of sizes to mate with the various diameter bone screws (Fig. 2–68). Both length and thickness are proportional to the size screw intended for use with the plate. A long plate is much more effective than a short plate in neutralizing forces to which the fractured bone may be subjected because it increases the working length of the implant and distributes destabilizing forces over a larger surface. The ideal in most cases is to use a plate that is just short of the entire length of the bone (Fig. 2–73). See Figure 2–74 for plate size guidelines relative to the bone involved and the size of the animal. Because the number of screw holes is directly proportional to the length of the plate, with the longer plate, more screws can be used.

Contouring the Plate

If anatomical reduction of the bone fragments is to be maintained during application of the bone plate, it is mandatory that the plate be contoured to closely fit the bone surface to which it is to be applied. In some cases, this is accomplished by bending; in others, by a combination of bending and twisting. The plate should be bent between the screw holes (Fig. 2–75). Prestressing (underbending) the plate is advisable in most cases because it aids in minimizing the gap on the far cortex and aids in compression when the screws are finally tightened. This usually amounts to a 1-mm gap between the bone and plate at the fracture site (Fig. 2–75B, C).

Insertion of a Lag Screw Through the Plate

In some cases, the fracture line lends itself to interfragmentary compression by inserting the lag screw through the bone plate (Fig. 2–66A).

Dynamic Compression Plate

The design of the screw holes in this plate is based on the spherical gliding principle developed by the ASIF and patented by Synthes. As the screw is tightened, the spherical screw head glides toward the center of the plate until the deepest portion of the hole is reached (Fig. 2–70A, B). The result is that the bone fragment into which the screw is being driven is displaced at the same time and in the same direction; that is, toward the center of the plate and the fracture line. By alternate tightening of the screws on each side of the fracture line, the fragments are compressed (Fig. 2–70C). The tension device may be used for additional compression, although it is rarely needed (Fig. 2–70D). Two drill guides (neutral and load) are used in drilling the holes in the proper position. The load guide has the potential of moving the fragment 1.0 mm and the neutral guide 0.1 mm in the 4.5-mm plate (Fig. 2–71A, B). In general, all of the principles that apply to the insertion of regular plates apply to the DCP; however, the DCP has these additional advantages[62,63]:

1. Cancellous bone screws may be inserted in any plate hole.
2. Plate screws may be applied at varying angles when used as lag screws (Fig. 2–71C).

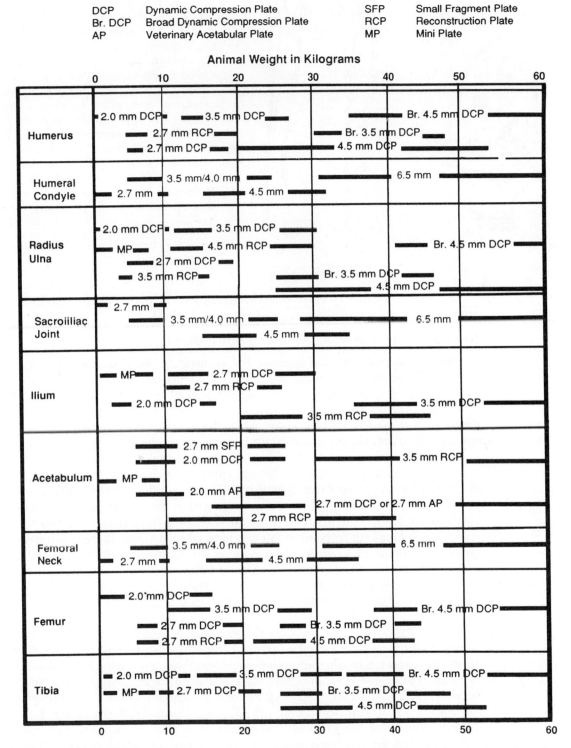

FIGURE 2–74. A guide for selection of plates with respect to animal weight and fracture location. (From Synthes Ltd. [USA], Paoli, PA.)

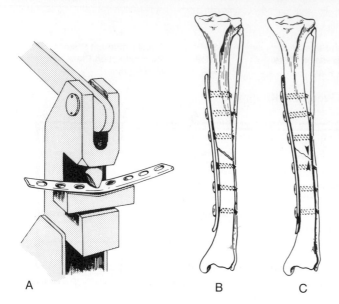

FIGURE 2–75. Plate fixation: contouring the plate. (*A*) The plate must be contoured so that it approximately fits the bone surface to which it is applied. Using the bone plate bending press, gently bend the plate between the screw holes. (*B*) Prestressing (underbending) the plate supplies added compression to the far cortex. In a curved bone, the plate is contoured to leave a 1-mm gap between plate and bone at the fracture site. In a straight bone, the plate is bowed slightly to produce the 1-mm gap. (*C*) Tightening the prestressed plate causes added compression on the cortex opposite the plate.

A   B   C

3. With a fracture of three or more segments, the plate has the potential of compression at each of the fracture lines (Fig. 2–71D–F).

Selection of Proper Bone Plate and Screw Sizes

One of the problems confronting the surgeon is the choice of the size of implant to use on the various fractures in patients of different sizes. Various factors may be considered in choosing the size of implant, such as type and location of the fracture, age, activity, size of bone, weight of animal, and condition of soft tissue.[63,68,69] However, when the basic fundamentals of implantation are observed, the most consistent factor in choosing the size of the implant is the weight of the patient. To provide guidelines in selecting proper bone plate and screw size, data were compiled on approximately 1000 bone plate cases and 300 screw fixation cases in which they were used as the primary method of fixation.[68] The summation of data collected is presented in Figure 2–74. Corrections have been made and included for implants that were too weak (resulting in breaking or bending) or too large. As expected, there is some overlapping of appliance sizes for given weights. In addition to the size of the implant, some of the more common causes of failure include bone plates that are too short in length, an insufficient number of bone screws, vascular impairment, infection, and failure to bone graft.

Special Plates

Since most plates are manufactured for use in human beings, there are many anatomical areas in small animals where no suitable plate exists, hence a variety of bone plates have been designed for application in small animals in special circumstances (Synthes Ltd. [USA], Paoli, PA). These include C-shaped plates for use on the dorsal acetabular rim; T-shaped mini-DCP plates for 1.5- to 2.0-mm screws for use on distal radial fractures; straight mini-DCP plates for 1.5- to 2.0-mm screws; hook plates for intertrochanteric osteotomy (see Chapter 15), and cuttable plates. Other manufacturers have similar devices available.

VETERINARY CUTTABLE PLATE ■ Although a fairly recent development, variable cuttable plates (VCPs) have rapidly become popular in small animal use because they fill a very real gap in previously available implants for long-bone fractures in small breeds, and in small-bone fractures in larger breeds. The previously available miniplates for 1.5- to 2.0-mm screws are often too weak or too short, while the 2.7-mm plate is either too thick or does not have enough screw holes per unit of length. Additionally, the 2.7-mm diameter screw may exceed 25 percent of the bone diameter and so weaken the bone. The VCP (Fig. 2–76) is 300 mm in length, 7 mm wide, and either 1.0 mm thick (1.5- or 2.0-mm screws), or 1.5 mm thick (2.0- or 2.7-mm screws). The screw holes are all round and the spacing of the holes is identical in both size plates, allowing the stacking or sandwiching of two plates to increase stiffness as required for the situation. The plates are easily cut at a screw hole with a small pin or wire cutter, allowing one plate to be used for several cases, and are very economical compared to other plates. A small amount of bone compression can be obtained by drilling the screw holes slightly eccentric (away from the fracture line) to the plate hole.

Stacking of plates allows for a total of five thicknesses: 1.0, 1.5, 2.0, 2.5, and 3.0 mm. Two identical length plates are stacked if the increased stiffness is desirable over the full length of the plate. In some cases it may be desirable to allow slightly more flexibility at each end of the bone, and the top plate can be shortened to between one half and three fourths the length of the base plate.[70] Stacked plates should be contoured simultaneously by placing a screw through both plates at each end of the plates to prevent sliding of the plates relative to each other during contouring. Mechanical studies have demonstrated that the VCP is more resistant to bending force than 1.5- to 2.0-mm miniplates, and less resistant than 2.7-mm plates.[71] Stacking plates yielded a stiffness slightly less than the sum of stiffness for each plate, and two thick plates had a stiffness of approximately two thirds that of the 2.7-mm plate. Screw size did not have a pronounced effect on stiffness.

Reports of clinical application of the VCP have been uniformly encouraging.[70,72,73] Primary use has been in multifragmental type C long-bone fractures in small breeds, pelvic fractures, and metacarpal-metatarsal fractures in large breeds. The ability to place many screws within a short distance is very useful in multifragmental fractures, and often makes the bone-plate construct stronger than a larger plate with fewer screws.

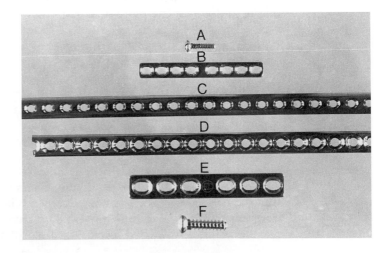

FIGURE 2–76. Mini-plates and screws (Synthes Ltd. [USA], Paoli, PA). (*A*) 2.0-mm screw. (*B*) 2.0-mm DCP. (*C*) 1.5-mm/2.0-mm cut-to-length plate, 1.0-mm thick. (*D*) 2.0-mm/2.7-mm cut-to-length plate, 1.5 mm thick. Note the increased number of screw holes available compared to the standard 2.7-mm DCP shown in *E*. (*F*) 2.7-mm screw.

Removal of Bone Plates in Small Animals

Indications for Removal

Bone plates should be removed under certain conditions[63,74]:

1.   When the plates become nonfunctional (e.g., loose, broken, or bent), they are no longer serving a useful purpose and some cause discomfort.

2.   The plate may be acting as a thermal conductor. A small number of owners have observed that their animals show some favoring of the leg after being out in the cold for a period of time. However, normal function returns after the animal comes back into the house. Lameness has been most frequently noted with plate fixation of the radius and tibia. This is thought to be caused by a difference in expansion and contraction of the plate and bone when subjected to change in temperature, and by the thermal mass of the plate chilling adjacent periosteum. Removal of the bone plate, after clinical union, has corrected this temporary lameness.

3.   The bone plate may cause bone beneath the plate to become osteoporotic due to remodeling associated with vascular interference by the plate on the bone surface. These changes are the result of a local periosteal circulatory disturbance brought about by plate-bone contact.[75] We have not seen these changes to be as severe as are seen in man, probably because the surface of the dog bone is quite irregular and there is not close plate-bone contact over large areas of the bone. One situation in which serious problems can arise as a result of remodeling osteoporosis is where a rather stiff plate ends in the middiaphyseal region. Plating of a proximal femoral fracture is an illustration, as is plate fixation of a stifle joint arthrodesis. Under these circumstances the end of the plate acts as a stress concentrator, focusing all bending loads that the bone normally distributes over a much larger area. Concentrating these loads where there is a dramatic transition from normal bone to osteoporotic bone can be a cause of pathological fracture.

4.   Interference with bone growth may occur in the young animal. Many shaft fractures in the young can be treated by closed reduction and fixation or simple intramedullary pinning, since they heal rapidly and because most axial deformities correct themselves by the active remodeling present during bone growth. Nevertheless, open reduction and internal fixation are indicated when congruent articular surfaces or leg length cannot be obtained and maintained by these means. In our experience, altered bone growth in the young has not been a problem when bone plates have been removed at the time of clinical union, and where the plate does not cross a growth plate.

5.   The plate may cause irritation. Occasionally, an implant just beneath the skin gives rise to a lesion characteristic of a lick granuloma. Plate removal after clinical union has occurred has cleared up the condition. Late lameness is occasionally seen 1 or more years after plate fixation. Radiographic signs of implant loosening (bone resorption around screws, evidenced by a black halo) or infection are absent. Plate removal causes the lameness to disappear, but the reason is unclear.

6.   Infection may occur. If infection is present, it is difficult to clear it up totally until the plate is removed. As a rule, if the plate is not loose, it is left in place as long as immobilization is indicated. When clinical union is achieved, it is removed and the infection usually clears up with appropriate treatment (see Chapter 5). Plate removal in these circumstances is also indicated because most fracture-associated sarcomas in animals have a history of a metallic implant, infection, and a disturbed fracture healing pattern.[76]

7. The plate may also impede full functional performance in field and racing animals, for reasons that are not entirely clear. This situation may be similar to the late lameness described in item 5 above.

Suggested Policy in Regard to Plate Removal

1. Leave all pelvic plates in place unless specific complications indicate removal. Relatively small plates are used, and to date no evidence of stress protection has been noted.

2. Leave plates in place in skeletally mature animals that have undergone uncomplicated healing. Those cases that have experienced complications such as infection, delayed union, or nonunion probably should have plates removed.

3. In skeletally immature animals, remove all plates on the long bones at the time of clinical union.

4. Ideally, it is best to remove all plates on long bones, although the economic realities of veterinary practice make this difficult to accomplish. Call the owner's attention to the potential reasons for removal at the time of discharge and give an approximate time for recheck and plate removal. Needless to say, it is difficult to get an animal back for plate removal when all appears to be going well. If complications occur after clinical union, it is best to have talked to the owner about recheck and plate removal.

Suggested Timing of Plate Removal

Data were collected covering patient age and plate removal time in more than 300 cases[74] and is collated in Table 2–5, which suggests timing of bone plate removal. The time until removal may need to be increased in more complex cases or problem cases.

Surgical Removal of Implant

Radiographs should be taken prior to and after plate removal. This will add to one's knowledge of bone healing and radiographic interpretation, and it will help to avoid repeating surgical errors. The procedure is performed as follows:

1. A standard approach is made to the bone involved.
2. The cicatrix encasing the plate is opened over its entire length.
3. In some animals, a portion of the plate will be covered with a layer of bone. An osteotome is usually required for its removal over the surface of the plate. Bone filling empty screw holes will usually fracture if the plate can be levered away from the bone.
4. Following bone plate removal, active hemorrhage (which is usually minimal) is controlled, the wound is closed in layers, and a pressure dressing is applied. Associated cerclage wires and lag screws are routinely left in place.

TABLE 2–5. REMOVAL
OF BONE PLATES

Age	Postoperative Time for Plate Removal
Under 3 months	4 weeks
3–6 months	2–3 months
6–12 months	3–5 months
Over 1 year	5–14 months

Refracture

Refracture is a fracture of normal bone occurring in the region of a previous fracture that appears to have undergone sound union both clinically and radiographically.[63,69,74,76,77] An incidence of less than 1 percent has been encountered in our fracture cases. Most refractures result from premature implant removal, poor anatomical reduction, or osteoporotic bone. They can be kept very minimal if the basic fundamentals of applying and removing implants are followed, with particular emphasis on anatomical reduction, proper implant size, and bone grafting of architectural defects.

Plate removal from the radius of toy and miniature dogs is somewhat worrisome due to the delicate nature of this bone and the tendency for these breeds to jump off of furniture. The holes left after screw removal may be large enough relative to the bone to weaken it. Autogenous cancellous bone grafting of the screw holes is one way to hasten return of normal bone strength. The limb can also be lightly splinted for 3 weeks, with provisions to leave the foot exposed to allow active weight bearing while protecting the bone from excessive bending loads.

Postoperative Care Following Plate Removal

The appearance of the radiographs and the activity of the patient are usually the determining factors in postoperative care. Treatment usually involves the following:

1. Application of a compression bandage over the operative area for 2 to 3 days to help prevent possible hematoma or seroma formation.

2. Supportive measures (such as a coaptation splint, external fixator, or intramedullary pin) if bone healing on the radiograph following plate removal appears to be less than adequate, or if the bone appears to be markedly osteoporotic under the plate. If the thickness or density of the bone in the fracture area is markedly altered, bone grafting may be indicated.

3. Restriction of activity for 1 to 4 weeks. This may range from confinement to the kennel or house, walking on a leash, or restricting play.

SELECTION OF FIXATION METHOD

Fracture Treatment Planning

Decision making regarding an appropriate method of treatment for a specific fracture in a specific patient can be either straightforward or very difficult, depending on many factors. As in many other areas of veterinary practice, it is partly science and partly art. One cannot simply look through the following chapters to find a fracture that looks like the one under consideration and then blindly copy the method of fixation depicted. To do so ignores the fact that the fracture is attached to an animal that is part of a milieu composed not only of its fracture but also other injuries, body weight, general health, physical environment, owner's care, and the owner's expectations for the long-term function of the animal.

Most commonly it is with diaphyseal/metaphyseal fractures that we must make choices between several possible methods of fracture fixation. As has been seen in a previous section, there is very little choice of fixation methods for treating intra-articular fractures, while a seeming myriad of possibilities exists for treatment of shaft fractures. Furthermore, the basic indications for many of these methods overlap considerably, leading to varying degrees of uncertainty about the best choice. Regarding the overlap of indications, we must remember that many roads may lead to the same point and that there probably is not any single way to treat a given shaft fracture. There is nothing wrong with choosing a particular approach to a specific situation as long as the decision is rationally based and good results are obtained.

Factors considered in choosing a fixation method cover a wide gamut. The answers to many of these questions are self-evident, but some will require considerable probing before the repair is attempted. The *type of bone* involved determines the healing pattern and relative stability needed for healing. Cortical bone is the most demanding of stability and is represented by fractures of the shaft of long bones, the mandible, the tuber calcis, and the olecranon. In corticocancellous bone, as in flat bones and metaphyseal bone, stability is less critical.

Location of fracture in the bone determines the forces acting on the fracture and fixation device. In the shaft the primary forces are bending and shear (rotation and shortening). The femur is the most highly loaded bone during weight bearing. In the metaphysis the primary loads are bending and shear. This is also the area of insertions of ligaments/tendons and these create their own shear and tension forces. Articular fractures are usually subjected primarily to shear and tension. Location of the fractures also determines the potential suitability of various classes of fixation. Coaptation is only suitable for long-bone fractures distal to the elbow/stifle, the scapular body, and some fractures of the metacarpal/metatarsal bones. Internal fixation is the best choice for everything else.

The *type of fracture* is critical in determining fixation methods, as many methods are very limited in their ability to neutralize forces acting on the fracture fragments. See below in this section for further discussion of this aspect.

Concurrent injuries of either the musculoskeletal system or soft tissues may dictate more rigid forms of internal fixation in order to achieve early ambulation of the patient and thereby ease the problem of postoperative care for the animal. Open and infected fractures need early stabilization with rigid internal fixation.

Age of the patient determines stability and length of time fixation may be needed to achieve healing. Skeletally immature animals produce abundant and early periosteal/endosteal callus, which equals early stability. Aged animals typically produce minimal periosteal/endosteal callus, and clinical union is slower. Therefore, types of fixation that do not achieve long-lasting stability (IM pins, casts) may become unstable before clinical union is achieved.

Size, breed, and temperament are secondary factors in fixation choice, in the sense that exactly the same basic principles will govern the choice, but we will always favor the most stable of the range of choices when dealing with a large, active, or excitable animal. Likewise, when considering the fracture type it is well to score it very conservatively in these animals.

The *degree of function* needed is also important in choosing a fixation method. The activity levels of our patients vary considerably. Consider the functional demands on the bone in the large working/sporting breed versus the small sedentary pet. Likewise, the owner's expectations of function are critical. We would be more likely to use a very stable form of fixation when a high level of function is mandatory.

The *environment* of the animal and expected *control of animal* by the owner may well influence the choice of fixation. An external fixator may not be the best choice for an animal kept on a chain in the yard, nor would it be a good choice for an owner that will not follow instructions for care and rechecks faithfully. Inquire very carefully into the housing conditions of the animal and the owner's attitudes before the repair, not after.

Equipment available and experience level of the surgeon must be considered and we must be scrupulous in our self-evaluation. When possible, a timely referral may be in order to ensure the best outcome for the patient and owner.

Economic constraints are a fact of life that must be faced in veterinary medicine and may tend to override other concerns. This must be handled on a case-by-case basis, but we must not be forced into doing a procedure that we know will fail simply because it is what the client can afford. It is a commonly held opinion that external casts and splints are less expensive to apply than is internal fixation. While this may be true in some cases, it is not uniformly so. If we rigorously evaluate costs of coaptation in terms of cost of materials, time involved in not only application but also rechecks and replacement, and most importantly in results achieved, we will often see that simple forms of internal fixation are very competitive with coaptation.

Choice of Fixation

An elegant method of compiling many of the considerations discussed above has been devised by Palmer et al.[78,79] (Table 2–6). The routine use of this or a similar method of evaluation will force the surgeon to consider the "mechanical, biological, and clinical variables affecting fracture healing and return to function in a given patient."[78] Each line should be scored if applicable and the results totaled and divided by the number of scorable factors to obtain an average. With practice one will be able to mentally assess the score without the arithmetic, but the exercise will force consideration of all the factors listed. This type of evaluation is of value primarily in diaphyseal fractures, where many fixation methods might be considered. It is of less use in most other fractures, where the choices of fixation are much more pragmatic due to anatomical and mechanical considerations. The best examples of this are the articular fractures, where the fixation method for a specific fracture will not vary much from patient to patient.

Scores from Table 2–6 can be correlated with fixation methods as follows.

TABLE 2–6. FRACTURE PATIENT SCORING SYSTEM*

Score	1	2	3	4	5	6	7	8	9	10
Mechanical Factors										
Non–load-sharing			Neutralization possible					Good load sharing		
Large, obese patient			Medium patient					Small patient		
Multiple limb injury/disease								Single-limb injury		
Biological Factors										
Local Factors										
High energy fx-wedges			Two-piece fracture					Low-energy–greenstick		
Long open reduction								Short open reduction; closed reduction		
Open fx—degree 3				2					1	
Gunshot fx—grade 3				2					1	
Systemic Factors										
Geriatric			Mature					Immature		
Debilitated/ill								Healthy		

*Data from Palmer et al. (1993) and Palmer (1994).

- Score 9–10
  Fracture—transverse or short oblique; type A:
  1. Cast/splint
  2. IM pins in many, but not all cases; may be combined with interfragmentary wires.
  3. Compression plate.
  4. External fixator, type IA.

- Score 8(7)–9
  Fracture—long oblique or spiral; type A and B1 one reducible wedge:
  1. IM pins/cerclage-hemicerclage wires.
  2. Neutralization plate.
  3. External fixator, type I, II (may be combined with cerclage wires/lag screws).

- Score 4(3)–7
  Fracture—wedge; type B:
  1. Neutralization plate.
  2. External fixator, type IA double bar or IB, II (may be combined with cerclage wires/lag screws).

- Score 1–3
  Fracture—complex; type C:
  1. Buttress/bridging plate.
  2. External fixator, type II or III.

OPEN FRACTURES

Open fractures usually occur in about 5 to 10 percent of the total fracture cases seen. The term "compound fracture" is obsolete in North America but is still widespread in other areas. An open wound overlying a fracture practically always means contamination, reduction in local host defense mechanism by the presence of foreign material and debris, devitalized necrotic tissue, and dead space. All these factors increase the potential for infection in the open wound and prevention of such infection is the most overriding concern with these injuries. Aggressive *early internal fixation* of the fracture is key to controlling infection.

Classification

Degree I.   The skin is penetrated from the inside by a sharp bone fragment, which then usually retracts under the skin and is no longer visible. The wound typically is less than 1 cm in diameter and surrounding tissues are only mildly contused.

Degree II.   Wounding of the skin occurs from the outside, leaving a variably sized soft tissue deficit and more severe contusion of surrounding tissues (Fig. 2–77A). Foreign material may be carried into the wound at the time of injury or later.

Degree III.   Extensive skin, subcutaneous tissue, and muscle injury from the outside is present and the bone is usually fragmented due to high-energy injury (Fig. 2–77B, C). There is often soft tissue avulsion, degloving, and neurovascular injury. High-velocity bullet wounds and traumatic partial amputations are common examples.

Prognosis for first- and second-degree injuries is little different from similar closed fractures, but third degree injuries carry a less favorable outlook. Treatment of these injuries is both extensive and expensive, but if aggressively man-

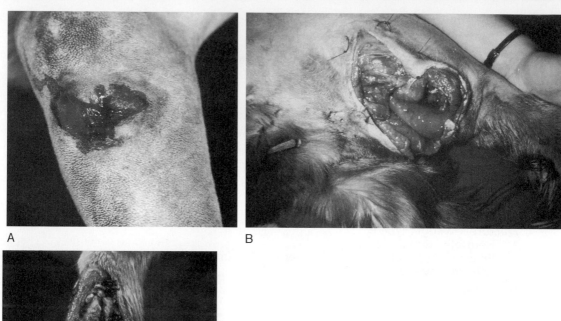

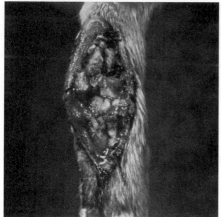

FIGURE 2–77. Open fracture classification. (*A*) Degree II, wounding from outside with moderate soft tissue injury. (*B*) Degree III, extensive skin and muscular injury in the brachial region. (*C*) Degree III, degloving abrasion injury of paw.

aged they represent an acceptable risk for most owners, since amputation is often the only alternative.

Treatment

Principles

The following principles apply to the treatment of open fractures.[63,80,81]

1. Prevention or minimization of contamination from time of occurrence of injury until initiation of surgical treatment.
2. Thorough cleansing and aseptic surgical debridement to remove nonviable and devitalized tissue.
3. Preservation of vascularity to both soft tissue and bone.
4. Stable fixation.
5. Early active mobilization of the limb.

Emergency Treatment

First aid by the owner should be directed toward stopping hemorrhage and preventing contamination. Covering the area with a clean bandage applied with minimal pressure usually accomplishes this objective. An open fracture is always considered an emergency and is treated as such. At the hospital it should immediately be covered by a large sterile dressing, which should remain until debridement is possible. A soft splint is useful in the distal limbs.

After and/or during thorough physical and orthopedic exam to expose and evaluate concurrent injuries particular attention is given to the cardiovascular system regarding perfusion and circulating red blood cell volume. The animal is stabilized as necessary with fluids and other supportive therapy. It is a good rule to take chest radiographs of all fracture patients as soon as their general condition permits. A thorough physical and radiographic orthopedic examination is essential for diagnosis, prognosis, and determination of the type of fracture treatment.

It may be necessary to clip hair in order to appreciate the presence of a first-degree injury. Cultures should be taken from the wound at this time for sensitivity testing. Systemic antibiotics (usually a cephalosporin) should be started immediately. Staphylococci account for 60 percent of the infection at our hospitals, with most of the rest equally divided between *Streptococcus* and *Escherichia coli*. *Pseudomonas*, *Proteus*, and *Klebsiella* are found rarely. For many first-degree injuries, clipping of hair, cleansing the wound, and bandaging are all that is necessary prior to fracture stabilization. For second- and third-degree injuries, adequate surgical debridement and primary fracture fixation are urgent and are done as soon as the animal will tolerate general or regional anesthesia.

Definitive Surgical Treatment

CLEANSING AND DEBRIDEMENT ■ Utmost care in aseptic technique is indicated because most strains of bacteria found in wounds are indigenous to the hospital in which treatment was performed rather than to the scene of the accident. Cleansing and debridement are carried out under general anesthesia. Caps, masks, and gloves should be worn to clip and wash the area. The open area is covered with sterile lubricating jelly, and the surrounding surgical area is clipped and surgically scrubbed. Loose hair from the clippers will be trapped in the jelly and rinsed away. Debridement should be done in the operating room or a clean area using aseptic technique. Careful removal of obviously dead tissue and foreign material is aided by copious lavage with saline or Ringer's solution. Addition of chlorhexidine to make a 0.5 percent solution, or 100 ml of 10 percent povidone-iodine solution (or whirlpool concentrate) per liter of irrigating fluid is advocated by some for added disinfection. If the wound must be enlarged to allow for adequate debridement, some thought must be given to blood supply, as additional compromise could predispose to infection.

Debridement must be meticulous to remove all devitalized tissue and not damage vessels and nerves. Very large wounds present difficulties in this regard and need to be left open to allow progressive debridement over several days. It is best to initially be conservative in evaluating skin viability as it is easily removed in later sessions if it does not survive. Nonviable muscle is a good culture medium and recognition is difficult: loss of contractility, lack of bleeding when cut, and pale color are the most useful criteria. Cortical bone fragments stripped of their soft tissue attachments are removed unless they are part of a joint surface or essential for stabilization of the fracture. Resulting bony defects are filled with autogenous cancellous bone graft. Large devascularized cortical fragments left in situ may become sequestra and require removal if the wound becomes infected.

The importance of removal of all dead or devitalized material in the prevention of deep-seated wound infection cannot be overemphasized.

FRACTURE FIXATION ■   Stabilization of the fracture must be addressed following debridement. It is critical to success to do the fracture fixation at this point because stabilizing the fracture also stabilizes soft tissues, preserving existing blood supply and allowing capillary invasion to establish new blood supply. Thus, stabilizing the fracture is the best defense against infection of both the bone and the soft tissues. Open reduction can be performed through the wound if it is correctly placed, or through a separate incision. Consideration must be given to a second incision's effect on skin blood supply.

First-degree injuries are treated as closed fractures. Second-degree injuries require different initial care, but stabilization and poststabilization care is similar to closed fracture treatment. Stabilization of third-degree injuries is primarily done with external skeletal fixation, although the interlocking nail may prove to be an important method. The following types of fixation may be used; each has its indications and limitations.

1.   Splints and casts are usually reserved for those cases with minor puncture wounds; those treated within the first 6 to 8 hours; and stable fractures of the distal half of the radius and ulna, carpus, tarsus, and foot.

2.   Internal fixation involves these methods:

    a.   Intramedullary pins are usually restricted to stable, first degree fractures treated within 6 to 8 hours. Secondary fixation (such as an external fixator) may be added for more stability.

    b.   Bone screws and/or plates have the advantage of stable uninterrupted fixation; however, an extensive open approach is required for application. They are particularly applicable when the fracture involves an articular surface, and on the femur of dogs, where postoperative limb function is not optimal with the external fixator.

    c.   External skeletal fixation has the advantage of minimal application time, and the fixation pins can usually be applied proximal and distal to the fracture and skin wound area, leaving the traumatized area freely accessible for treatment as an open wound. This type of fixation is particularly adaptable to infected fractures, gunshot fractures, and the more severely traumatized cases. Because of its ease of application on the tibia and radius/ulna, it is the first choice for open fractures of these bones.

Whatever type of fixation is used should remain in place until clinical union is achieved, as long as it is secure and accomplishing stabilization of the fracture segments. Healing is routinely delayed in third-degree fractures and fixation should be chosen with this in mind. Loose implants should be replaced if clinical union has not been achieved.

BONE GRAFTING ■   Bone grafting is usually indicated in open fracture cases in which bone is missing and in some of the more severely fragmented fractures. For more complete details, refer to Chapter 3. Autogenous cancellous grafts can be used at the time of surgery, after debridement, reduction, and fixation. If the graft cannot be covered with soft tissue, it is usually covered with petrolatum-impregnated gauze. If infection, suppuration, and questionable vascularity are present, however, it is usually advisable to delay grafting until suppuration has ceased and healthy granulation tissue is present. The granulation tissue is elevated and the graft packed into the bony deficit.

Cortical grafts should not be used in an infected area because they are slow to become vascularized and usually become sequestered. If a cortical graft is indicated, the procedure should be delayed until the infection has cleared.

WOUND CLOSURE ■ Closure of the wound should only be considered in first- and second-degree injuries where the minimal soft tissue injury can be adequately debrided and the skin closed without tension. It is important to cover vessels, nerves, and tendons, but bone can be left exposed if necessary as can bone plates. Transposition of muscle bellies often allows soft tissue coverage of vital structures when skin is not available. Theoretically, contaminated wounds do not become infected for 6 to 8 hours—the "golden period"—and can be successfully closed after debridement without the need for drainage. However, some wounds are so heavily contaminated or devitalized that the golden period is considerably shortened. *When in doubt, leave the wound open*, which is more successful than surgical drainage in our hands. If no suppuration develops, delayed primary closure can be done in 4 to 5 days. If there is suppuration, secondary closure can be done after healthy granulation is established, or the wound can be left to heal by second intention.

AFTERCARE ■ Systemic antibiotics are continued several days postoperatively, or as long as there is suppuration, and may be changed to suit the sensitivity report. Open wounds are kept under sterile dressings, with saline-soaked sterile natural gauze sponges packed into the wound. Dressings are changed daily until secretion and suppuration slows, then as needed. Once granulation has become well established, the frequency of bandage changes can be reduced. Keeping the wound covered during the epithelialization period will keep the tissue moist and prevent overgrowth of granulation tissue. See Chapter 5 for further details regarding infected fractures.

Early active, but limited, use of the limb stimulates both soft tissue and bony repair. Radiographic evaluation of bone healing is done at monthly intervals until healing is obvious. External fixator removal can often be staged to allow a more gradual return to normal stress patterns in the bone.

Case Studies

CASE 1 ■ Figure 2–78A shows a grade 2 open type B wedge fracture in a 1-year-old, 55-pound dog that was struck by a car bumper. The open area was covered with a clean bandage immediately and presented for treatment within 8 hours. Fixation was performed using an intramedullary pin and a two pin type I external fixator (Fig. 2–78B). The wound was treated as an open lesion with nitrofurazone dressings. The skin lesion closed within 2 weeks (Fig. 2–78C). The external fixator was removed in 1 month, and the intramedullary pin was removed at the time of clinical union (2 months).

CASE 2 ■ Figure 2–79A shows a grade 2 open type C, complex gunshot fracture, in a 2-year-old, 60-pound dog. Fixation was done using a bone plate (Fig. 2–79B). The fracture healed; however, minor fistulous tracts opened up intermittently during the healing period (Fig. 2–79C). These cleared up promptly after removal of the bone plate and a sequestrum 11 months after injury. The defect in the shaft was the sequestrum site (Fig. 2–77D).

CASE 3 ■ Figure 2–80A depicts a grade 3 open infected type B wedge fracture in an 8-month-old, 15-pound dog 6 days after trauma. The end of the distal segment was still protruding from the skin; the dog's temperature was 105°F. A type I external fixator was applied (Fig. 2–80B), and the local area was treated with numerous nitrofurazone dressings. The animal was placed on a systemic antibiotic. The local and systemic infection cleared, and healing was

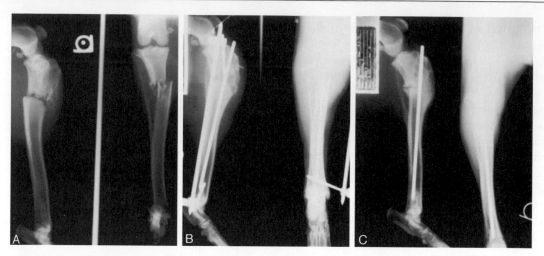

FIGURE 2–78. (*A*) Grade 2 open comminuted fracture that resulted when a 55-pound, 1-year-old dog was struck by a car bumper. Open area was covered with a clean bandage immediately and presented for treatment within 8 hours. (*B*) Fixation using an intramedullary pin and unilateral external fixator, 1/1 pin. (*C*) Intramedullary pin shown at time of clinical union (7 weeks). The external fixator was removed at 4 weeks and the intramedullary pin at 7 weeks.

delayed, although without sequestra formation (Fig. 2–80C, D). The fixator was removed at 4 months.

GUNSHOT FRACTURES

Gunshot fractures of the limbs cause multisystem wounding that can be the cause of massive destruction of soft and hard tissues and result in complicated and delayed healing of both. With judicious treatment the rates of success and complications are very acceptable for the less complicated fractures, while more guarded prognoses are indicated for the most difficult fractures.[82] Although the treatment of gunshot fractures shares much with that of open fractures, it is important to know something of the type of wounding missile, specifically, the ballistics of the bullet/pellet. No knowledge of firearms is necessary, and the information needed is gained from physical examination of the wound and examination of the radiographs.

Pathophysiology

When tissues are struck by a missile, whether it be a bullet or an automobile bumper, the kinetic energy of the wounding object is converted into work on the tissues and results in plastic and elastic strain (deformation) and dissipative energy in the form of heat. This kinetic energy is described by the formula: $KE = MV^2/2$. Because the energy developed is greatly influenced by the velocity raised to the second power, most attention has been devoted to the muzzle velocity of the bullet. While it is true that when the bullet weight is constant, raising the velocity is a good way to increase the wounding energy available, it is also true that sheer mass can have a significant effect.[83] Table 2–7 illustrates that the kinetic energy of the 30-06 Springfield bullet (a common hunting rifle) is almost double that of the M16 (current military weapon), although the square

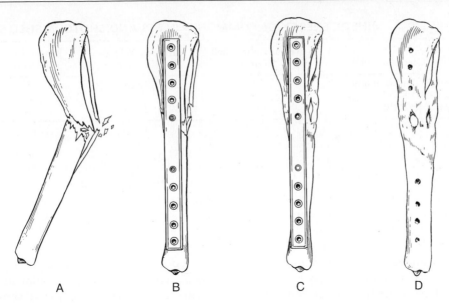

FIGURE 2–79. (A) Grade 2 open gunshot fracture in a 60-pound dog. (B) Fixation using a bone plate. (C) Fracture had healed (11 months after injury); however, intermittent minor draining tracts were still present. (D) After removal of the plate and sequestra, the draining tracts disappeared. The defect in the diaphysis was the site of sequestra. In retrospect, a better choice of stabilization would have been a unilateral external fixator.

of its muzzle velocity is only 72 percent of the M16. The kinetic energy of the small bullet of the M16 is highly dependent on its high muzzle velocity, while the bullet of the 30-06 has sufficient mass to be a significant contributor to the wounding energy. The effect of mass is most dramatically illustrated by the shotgun: as seen in Table 2–7 the 12-gauge shotgun has a muzzle velocity of only 1300 ft/sec, but because of the tremendous mass of the pellets (700 grains) the kinetic energy available is 2700 foot-pounds. Although this amount of

FIGURE 2–80. (A) Grade 3 open infected fracture, 6 days after trauma, in a 15-pound dog 8 months of age. End of distal segment still protruding from skin, temperature 105°F. (B) Unilateral external fixator was applied. (C, D) Local and systemic infection cleared; healing was delayed, although without sequestra formation. Splint removed at 4 months.

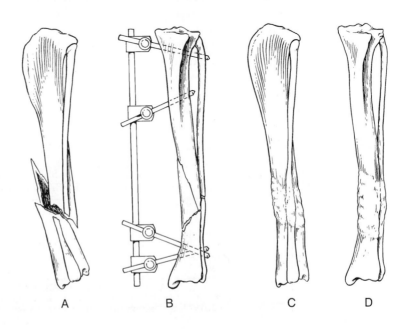

TABLE 2–7. KINETIC ENERGY OF COMMON BULLETS AND SHOTGUN SHELLS

Type Cartridge/Shell	Weight Bullet/Shell (grains)	Muzzle Velocity (feet/sec)	Kinetic Energy (foot-pounds)
12-gauge, 3-inch magnum	701	1315	2726
M16 (AR-15)	55	3250	1290
30-06 Springfield	150	2750	2519

energy is only available in short-range situations, where the pellets are still tightly enough grouped to act as a single missile, the shotgun does have a tremendous wounding potential. In the following text the terms "high energy" and "low energy" will be used in place of the commonly used "high velocity" and "low velocity" descriptors.

The location of gunshot injuries of the dog varies with the environment in which the pet lives. In metropolitan settings the dog is commonly an apartment dweller who confronts an intruder. Here, head wounds with mandibular and maxillary fractures are common, almost always caused by handguns at short range. In suburban and rural settings wounds are more commonly inflicted by hunting rifles at longer range, and the location of fractures is much more random. It is interesting to note the relatively high incidence of humeral fractures, probably due to the heart/chest being a common aiming point. Fortunately the incidence of short-range shotgun injuries is low. Long-range shotgun injuries are usually confined to shallow wounding by a few pellets.

A classification system to characterize the various types of gunshot fractures is helpful in developing a treatment protocol. Such a scheme is described in Table 2–8. *Low-energy type 1 fractures* (Fig. 2–81A) produce predictable penetrating wounds of the soft tissues, and there is often no exit wound. Soft tissues are disrupted along the path of the missile, and fracture patterns are simple. The severity of bone damage varies with the location of the bone; obviously much more of the initial energy of the bullet is already expended by the time the bullet strikes the midshaft of the femur as compared to the tibia, hence tibial fractures are routinely more complicated. Most of the bullet fragments remain in situ and are usually quite large, although some smaller dust-like fragments are present.

High-energy type 3 fractures (Fig. 2–81C) are much more complicated, with both an entry and an exit wound present. The exit wound is often not on line with the entry wound if the bullet ricochets off a bone. As the bullet's energy is transferred to the soft tissues they expand around the missile, creating a temporary cavity which then immediately collapses. Hydrostatic shock waves are created that injure tissues within a radius as much as 30 times the diameter

TABLE 2–8. CLASSIFICATION OF GUNSHOT FRACTURES*

	Kinetic Energy	Fracture Type	Soft Tissue Injury
Type 1	Low	A, few B	Minimal
Type 2	Medium	A, B, few C	Moderate
Type 3	High	C	Extensive

*Adapted from Schwach RP, Park RD, et al: Gunshot fractures of extremities: Classification, management, and complications. Vet Surg 8:57–62, 1979, with permission.

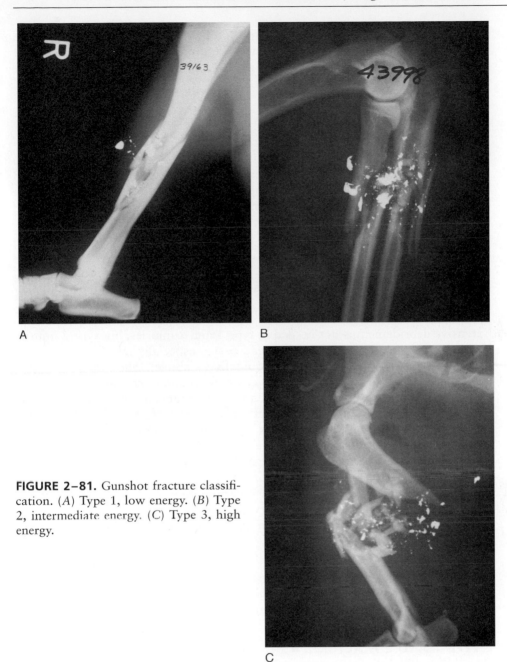

FIGURE 2–81. Gunshot fracture classification. (A) Type 1, low energy. (B) Type 2, intermediate energy. (C) Type 3, high energy.

of the bullet.[82] Bone is shattered into small pieces and the bullet is reduced to myriad dust-like fragments; probably most of the bullet continues through the exit wound, where it can produce a secondary injury in adjacent tissues. Extensive devascularization of bone is produced not only by fragmentation but also by soft tissue detachment and thrombosis of canaliculi in cortical bone. The exact type of bone injury varies with the location of the impact and the type of bone (cortical versus metaphyseal) involved. *Type 2 fractures* (Fig. 2–81B) exhibit characteristics of both types 1 and 3, depending on the specific wounding missile. These wounds are generally produced by low- to medium-velocity bullets that are relatively heavy; the lead fragments seen radiographically are a combination of the large type 1 fragments and the dust-like type 3 fragments. Similarly, the fracture patterns are more fragmented than in type 1 fractures, but the fragmentation is neither as severe nor as extensive as with the type 3 injuries.

Surgical Protocol[82]

Initial Evaluation and Wound Treatment

Treatment of gunshot fractures is basically the treatment of type 2 and 3 open fractures. All are considered contaminated and type 3 injuries have the greatest potential for infection to become established. Antibiotic therapy should be started immediately after culturing the wound for antibiotic sensitivity testing. After stabilization of the patient as indicated by clinical signs, and performing a complete physical and neurological examination, definitive fracture treatment can be considered. Radiographic examination, preferably under general anesthesia, is necessary to establish the exact fracture type and plan further treatment.

Wounds are cleansed and debrided as described above for open fractures. Extensive debridement is not needed in type 1 and 2 injuries, but type 3 injuries require more attention to removing dead tissue, especially muscle that is completely devitalized (see debridement guidelines, above). Short-range shotgun wounds result in massive soft tissue injuries and require extensive debridement. Hair, small detached bone fragments, and lead fragments that are readily accessible are all removed. It is not strictly necessary to remove lead fragments, so extensive probing and dissection is to be avoided; however, intra-articular lead should always be removed. Leave all bone fragments with soft tissue attachments, and all large fragments regardless of soft tissue integrity. As with open fractures, be cautious about primary closure of the wounds; it is much safer to allow open drainage until a determination can be made about the presence of infection. Delayed primary closure or healing by granulation are always preferable to wound disruption due to exudation.

Fracture Fixation

As with open fractures, immediate stabilization of the fracture is helpful in treating the soft tissues. With the exception of a few type 1 fractures of the radius/ulna and the tibia, the remaining gunshot fractures require internal fixation.

TYPE 1 AND 2 FRACTURES ▪ Treatment is similar to closed fractures of type A, B, or C. Either an anatomical reconstruction with stable internal fixation or a biological osteosynthesis approach may be taken with these fractures.

TYPE 3 FRACTURES ▪ Because of the extensive bone devascularization involved in these complex type C fractures, very delayed healing is to be expected. The fixation must therefore be capable of long-lasting stability, and because of the fragmentation the fixation must be capable of acting as a bridging or buttress device. The choices are thus limited to bone plates, interlocking IM nails, or external fixators. Experience has shown that the bridging osteosynthesis approach is preferable in these fractures. They are reduced either closed or with a minimal open approach. No attempt is made to reduce fragments, rather, the emphasis is on restoring axial and rotational alignment and maintaining as much length as possible. To attempt extensive manipulation and stabilization of small fragments not only further devascularizes them but also rarely results in adequate stabilization. The severe nature of the wounding process is actually helpful in establishing the cascade of humoral and local factors needed for early callus formation, and to the extent that the area is invaded and further disturbed we can slow this healing reaction.

These criteria for reduction and fixation are most ideally met *in the dog* by the external fixator for fractures of the humerus, radius/ulna, and tibia. Consult the External Skeletal Fixation section for the splint types appropriate to these bones. Because dogs often do not function well with external fixators on the femur, the interlocking IM nail or bone plate may be a better choice for this bone. As above, the goal is restoration of axial and rotational alignment and maintaining length to the extent possible. In placing the bridging plate the emphasis is on simply attaching it proximally and distally, with minimal disturbance of the fracture site and fragments. This is facilitated by contouring the plate from a radiograph of the contralateral bone. Likewise, with placement of the interlocking nail, the open approach is only sufficient to allow guiding the nail across the fracture area into the distal fragment. The availability of cinefluoroscopy would eliminate the need for any open approach, as is common in human applications.

If bone plates or interlocking nails are not available, there should be no hesitation to use the external fixator on canine femoral fractures, but there is a tendency to delayed bone healing and soft tissue tiedown problems in the stifle joint. Aggressive physiotherapy during the healing period may minimize these problems. *Cats* do not exhibit the tendency toward poor limb function with the external fixator applied to the femur, hence it can be readily used on all bones in this species.

Healing Time, Prognosis

Type 1 and 2 fractures generally heal as would closed fractures of the same type; that is, between 6 and 10 weeks. Type 3 fractures routinely exhibit delayed healing times of 12 to 20 weeks. Progressive destabilization of external fixators commencing at 8 weeks is helpful in producing more vigorous callus formation. Overall prognosis was reported as good to excellent for type 1 fractures, fair to good for type 2 fractures, and fair to poor for type 3 fractures by Schwach et al.[82] The prognosis for type 2 and 3 fractures has certainly improved since that report because of the increased sophistication of external fixator applications, but we have no firm figures available.

References

1. Adams JC: Outline of Fractures, 7th ed. Edinburgh, F&S Livingstone Ltd, 1978, pp 4–8.
2. Brinker WO: Fractures. In Canine Surgery. Santa Barbara, American Veterinary Publications Inc, 2nd ed, 1952, pp 548–643; 3rd ed, 1957, pp 548–640; 1st Archibald ed, 1965, pp 777–849; 2nd Archibald ed, 1975, pp 957–1048.
3. Unger M, Montavon PM, Heim UFA: Classification of fractures of the long bones in the dog and cat: Introduction and clinical application. Vet Comp Orthop Trauma 3:41–50, 1990.
4. Müller M: The comprehensive classification of fractures of the long bones. In Allgöwer M (ed): Manual of Internal Fixation; Techniques Recommended by the AO–ASIF Group, 3rd ed. Berlin, Springer–Verlag, 1991, pp 118–150.
5. Rhinelander F: The normal microcirculation of diaphyseal cortex and its response to fracture. J Bone Joint Surg 50-A:784, 1968.
6. Rhinelander F, Phillips RS, Steel WM, et al: Microangiography in bone healing. J Bone Joint Surg 50-A:643, 1968.
7. Perren SM: Basic aspects of internal fixation. In Allgöwer M (ed): Manual of Internal Fixation; Techniques Recommended by the AO–ASIF Group, 3rd ed. Berlin, Springer-Verlag, 1991, pp 18–19.

8. Hulth A: Current concepts of fracture healing. Clin Orthop Rel Res 249:265–84, 1989.
9. Perren SM, Cordey J: The concept of interfragmentary strain. In Uthoff HK (ed): Current Concepts of Internal Fixation. Berlin, Springer-Verlag, 1980, p 63.
10. Rahn BA: Bone healing: Histologic and physiologic concepts. In Sumner-Smith G (ed): Bone in Clinical Orthopaedics. Philadelphia, WB Saunders Co, 1982, pp 335–386.
11. Perren SM : Basic aspects of internal fixation. In Allgöwer M (ed): Manual of Internal Fixation; Techniques Recommended by the AO-ASIF Group, 3rd ed. Berlin, Springer-Verlag, 1991, p 2.
12. Mast J, Jakob R, Ganz R: Planning and Reduction Techniques in Fracture Surgery. Berlin, Springer-Verlag, 1989.
13. Gautier E, Perren SM, Ganz R: Principles of internal fixation. Curr Orthop 6:220–232, 1992.
14. Hulse DA, Aron DN: Advances in small animal orthopedics. Compendium 16:831–832, 1994.
15. Seibel R, LaDuca J, Border JR, et al: Blunt multiple trauma, femur traction, and the pulmonary state. Ann Surg 202:283–395, 1985.
16. Allgöwer M: The scientific basis of aggressive traumatology in lesions of the locomotor system. Dialogue 1:2–3, 1985.
17. Piermattei DL: An Atlas of Surgical Approaches to the Bones and Joints of the Dog and Cat, 3rd ed. Philadelphia, WB Saunders Co, 1993.
18. Wilson DG, Vanderby R Jr: An evaluation of fiberglass cast application techniques. Vet Surg 24:118–121, 1995.
19. Schroeder EF: The traction principle in treating fractures and dislocations in the dog and cat. North Am Vet 14:32–36, 1933.
20. Robinson GW, McCoy L: A pelvic limb sling for dogs. In Bojrab MJ (ed): Current Techniques in Small Animal Surgery. Philadelphia, Lea & Febiger, 1975, pp 567–569.
21. Stader O: A preliminary announcement of a new method of treating fractures. North Am Vet 18:37–38, 1937.
22. Ehmer FA: Bone pinning in fractures of small animals. J Am Vet Med Assoc 110:14–19, 1947.
23. Brinker WO, Flo GL: Principles and application of external skeletal fixation. Vet Clin North Am Small Anim Pract 5:197–208, 1975.
24. Egger EL: External skeletal fixation; general principles. In Slatter D (ed): Textbook of Small Animal Surgery, 2nd ed. Philadelphia, WB Saunders Co, 1993, pp 1641–1656.
25. Wa JJ, Shyr HS, et al: Comparison of osteotomy healing with different stiffness characteristics. J Bone Joint Surg 66-A:1258–1264, 1984.
26. Lewallen DG, Chao EY, et al: Comparison of the effects of compression plates and external fixators on early bone healing. J Bone Joint Surg 66-A:1084–1091, 1984.
27. Rittman WW, Schibli M, et al: Open fractures: Long-term results in 200 consecutive cases. Clin Orthop 138:132–140, 1979.
28. Etter C, Burri C, et al: Treatment by external fixation of open fractures associated with severe soft tissue damage of leg. Clin Orthop 178:81–88, 1983.
29. Behrens F, Searls K: External fixation of tibia: Basic concepts and prospective evaluation. J Bone Joint Surg 68-B:246–254, 1986.
30. Egger EL, Histand MB, et al: Effect of pin insertion on bone pin interface. Vet Surg 15:246–252, 1986.
31. Gumbs JM, Brinker WO, DeCamp CE, et al: Comparison of acute and chronic pull out resistance of pins used with the external fixator (Kirschner splint). J Am Anim Hosp Assoc 24:231–234, 1988.
32. DeCamp CE, Brinker WO, Sautas-Little RW: Porous titanium-surfaced pins for external skeletal fixation. J Am Anim Hosp Assoc 24:295–300, 1988.
33. Matthews LS, Green CA, Goldstein SA: The thermal effect of skeletal fixation-pin insertion in bone. J Bone Joint Surg 66-A:1077–1083, 1984.
34. Brinker WO, Verstraete ME, Soutas-Little RW: Stiffness studies on various configurations and types of external fixators. J Am Anim Hosp Assoc 21:280–288, 1985.
35. Egger EL: Static strength evaluation of six external skeletal fixation configurations. Vet Surg 12:130–136, 1983.
36. Stambaugh JE, Nunamaker DM: External skeletal fixation of comminuted maxillary fractures in dogs. Vet Surg 2:72, 1982.
37. Roe SC: Classification and nomenclature of external fixators. Vet Clin North Am Small Anim Pract 22:11–18, 1992.
38. Cech O, Trc T: Prof. Ilizarov and his contribution to the challenge of limb lengthening. Injury 24(Suppl 2):2–8, 1993.
39. Bouvy BM, Markel MD, et al: Ex vivo biomechanics of Kirschner-Ehmer external skeletal fixation applied to canine tibiae. Vet Surg 22:194–207, 1993.
40. Palmer RH, Hulse DA, et al: Principles of bone healing and biomechanics of external skeletal fixation. Vet Clin North Am Small Anim Pract 22:45–68, 1992.
41. Willer RL, Egger EL, Histand MB: A comparison of stainless steel versus acrylic for the connecting bar of external skeletal fixators. J Am Anim Hosp Assoc 27:541, 1991.

42. Dernell WS, Harari J, Blacketter DM: A comparison of acute pull-out strength between two-way and one-way transfixation pin insertion for external skeletal fixation in canine bone. Vet Surg 22:110–114, 1993.

43. Aron DN, Dewey CW: Application and postoperative management of external skeletal fixators. Vet Clin North Am Small Anim Pract 22:69–98, 1992.

44. Toombs JP: A review of the key principles of external skeletal fixation. Proc (Sm Anim) ACVS Vet Symposium, Washington, DC, 1994, pp 405–406.

45. Johnson AL, Kneller SK, Weigal RM: Radial and tibial fracture repair with external skeletal fixation: Effects of fracture type, reduction, and complications of healing. Vet Surg 18:367–372, 1989.

46. Toombs JP: Transarticular application of external skeletal fixation. Vet Clin North Am Small Anim Pract 22:181–194, 1992.

47. Ross JT, Matthiesen DT: The use of multiple pin and methylmethacrylate external skeletal fixation of the treatment of orthopaedic injuries in the dog and cat. Vet Comp Orthop Trauma 6:115–121, 1993

48. Egger EL, Histand MB, et al: Canine osteotomy healing when stabilized with decreasingly rigid fixation compared to constantly rigid fixation. Vet Comp Orthop Trauma 6:182–187, 1993.

49. Brinker WO: The use of intramedullary pins in small animal fractures: A preliminary report. North Am Vet 29:292–297, 1948.

50. Jenny J: Kuentscher's medullary nailing in femur fractures of the dog. J Am Vet Med Assoc 17:381–387, 1950.

51. Carney JP: Rush intramedullary fixation of long bones as applied to veterinary surgery. Vet Med 47:43, 1952.

52. Rudy RL: Principles of intramedullary pinning. Vet Clin North Am 5:209–228, 1975.

53. Weller S, Höntsch D: Medullary nailing of the femur and tibia. In Allgöwer M (ed): Manual of Internal Fixation; Techniques Recommended by the AO-ASIF Group, 3rd ed. Berlin, Springer-Verlag, 1991, pp 291–366.

54. Dueland RT, Johnson KA, et al: Forty two interlocking nail fracture cases in the dog. Proc Vet Orthop Soc 21:51–52, 1994.

55. Howard PE, Brusewitz GH: An in vitro comparison of the holding strength of partially threaded vs nonthreaded intramedullary pins. Vet Surg 12:119–122, 1983.

56. Gibson KL, vanEe RT: Stack pinning of long bone fractures: A retrospective study. Vet Clin Orthop Trauma 4:48–53, 1991.

57. Dallman MJ, Martin RA, et al: Rotational strength of double pinning techniques in repair of transverse fractures of femurs in dogs. Am J Vet Res 51:123–127, 1990.

58. Rhinelander FW: The normal microcirculation of diaphyseal cortex and its response to fracture. J Bone Joint Surg 50A:784, 1968.

59. Rooks RL, Tarvin GB, et al: In vitro cerclage wiring analysis. Vet Surg 11:39–43, 1982.

60. Blass CE, Piermattei DL, et al: Static and dynamic cerclage wire analysis. Vet Surg 15:181, 1986.

61. Blass CE, Arnoczky SB, et al: Mechanical properties of three wire configurations. Am J Vet Res 46:1725, 1985.

62. Schatzker J: Screws and plates and their application. In Allgöwer M (ed): Manual of Internal Fixation; Techniques Recommended by the AO-ASIF Group, 3rd ed. Berlin, Springer-Verlag, 1991, pp 179–199.

63. Brinker WO, Hohn RB, Prieur WD: Manual of Internal Fixation in Small Animals. Heidelberg, Springer-Verlag, 1984, pp 29–79, 104–107.

64. Perren SM, Russenberger M, et al: A dynamic compression plate. Acta Orthop Scand Suppl 125:31, 1969.

65. Perren SM, Hutzschenreuter P, Steinemann S: Some effects of rigidity of internal fixation on the healing pattern of osteotomies. Z Surg 1:77, 1969.

66. Matter P, Brennwald J, et al: The effect of static compression and tension on internal remodeling of cortical bone. Helv Chir Acta 12(Suppl):5–43, 1975.

67. Perren SM, Allgower M, et al: Clinical experience with a new compression plate DCP. Acta Orthop Scand Suppl 125:45, 1969.

68. Brinker WO, Flo GL, et al: Guidelines for selecting proper implant size for treatment of fractures in dog and cat. J Am Anim Hosp Assoc 13:476–477, 1977.

69. Jiunn–Jerr W, Shyr HS, et al: Comparison of osteotomy healing under external fixation devices with different stiffness characteristics. J Bone Joint Surg 66-A:1258–1264, 1984.

70. Brüse S, Dee J, Prieur D: Internal fixation with a veterinary cuttable plate in small animals. Vet Comp Orthop Trauma 1:40–46, 1989.

71. Fruchter AM, Holmberg DL: Mechanical analysis of the veterinary cuttable plate. Vet Comp Orthop Trauma 4:116–119, 1991.

72. McLaughlin RM, Cockshutt JR, Kuzma AB: Stacked veterinary cuttable plates for treatment of comminuted diaphyseal fractures in cats. Vet Comp Orthop Trauma 5:22–25, 1992.

73. Gentry SJ, Taylor RA, Dee JF: The use of veterinary cuttable plates: 21 cases. J Am Anim Hosp Assoc 29:455–458, 1993.

74. Brinker WO, Flo GL, et al: Removal of bone plates in small animals. J Am Anim Hosp Assoc 11:577–586, 1975.
75. Perren SM : Basic aspects of internal fixation. In Allgöwer M (ed): Manual of Internal Fixation; Techniques Recommended by the AO-ASIF Group, 3rd ed. Berlin, Springer-Verlag, 1991, pp 18–19.
76. Stephenson S, Hohn RB, et al: Fracture-associated sarcomas in the dog. J Am Vet Med Assoc 180:1189–1196, 1982.
77. Noser GA, Brinker WO, et al: Effect of time on strength of healing bone with bone plate fixation. J Am Anim Hosp Assoc 13:559–561, 1977.
78. Palmer RH, Hulse DA, Aron DN: A proposed fracture patient score system used to develop fracture treatment plans (abstr). Proc 20th Ann Conf Vet Orthop Soc, 1993.
79. Palmer RH: Decision making in fracture treatment: The Fracture Patient Scoring System. Proc (Sm Anim) ACVS Vet Symp, 1994, pp 388–390.
80. Bardet JF, Hohn RB, Basinger R: Open drainage and delayed autogenous bone grafting for treatment of chronic osteomyelitis in dogs and cats. J Am Vet Med Assoc 183:312, 1983.
81. Rittmann WW, Webb JK: Compound Fractures. In Allgöwer M (ed): Manual of Internal Fixation; Techniques Recommended by the AO-ASIF Group, 3rd ed. Berlin, Springer-Verlag, 1991, pp 683–688.
82. Schwach RP, Parks RD, et al: Gunshot fractures of extremities: Classification, management, and complications. Vet Surg 8:57–62, 1979.
83. Lindsey D: The idolatry of velocities, or lies, damn lies, and ballistics (editorial). J Trauma 20:1068–1069, 1980.

3

Bone Grafting

Bone grafting was introduced into general surgical practice early in the twentieth century, and the principles of grafting have been well established for over 75 years.[1] Use of banked bone (frozen, freeze-dried, and irradiated) came into general usage in the late 1940s.[2] Infection associated with bone grafting in animals has been minimal when aseptic procedures have been used and the bone has not been introduced into a contaminated, infected, or unstable area. We have not encountered outright rejection by the body or bone sequestrum formation when autogenous or frozen allografts are used, although bone does have an antigenic potential.[3] Freezing decreases the antigenic stimulation of the graft. Introduced bone undergoes varying degrees of osteoconduction (creeping substitution) and is completely or partially replaced by host bone.

INDICATIONS FOR GRAFTING

Bone grafting is recommended in several circumstances:

1. To enhance healing in delayed unions, nonunions, osteotomies, and arthrodeses of joints by stimulating early formation of bridging callus.

2. To bridge major defects in multifragmentary fractures by establishing continuity of bone segments and filling cortical defects, thereby stimulating and enhancing early formation of bridging callus.

3. To replace entire cortical segments lost due to fracture fragmentation or excision due to neoplasia.

4. To fill cavities or partial thickness defects resulting from excision of cysts or neoplasms.

CHARACTERISTICS OF BONE GRAFTS

Sources/Terminology

Grafts originate from three sources:

1. *Autograft or autogenous graft*—from the same animal. Autografts have maximal osteogenetic potential and earliest response, but their collection increases operative time and risk, and the bone available may be insufficient in quantity, shape, and size, or mechanically unsuitable.

2. *Allograft*—from the same species. Formerly known as homografts, these grafts are collected from donor animal and either used fresh, or held in a bone bank (freezer) for future use. Experimentally and clinically, an allograft has

about the same enhancing effect as autogenous bone; however, there is no direct osteogenesis and there is an initial delay in response of about 2 weeks in comparison with the response of an autograft. Availability in sufficient quantity, shape, and size is the main advantage. Additionally, allografts are the only feasible source for large cortical grafts.

3. *Xenograft*—from a different species. This graft has the least osteogenetic potential and is most likely to cause a foreign body reaction. There is little clinical application for this type of graft. The term heterograft is obsolete.

Structure

Grafts may be either *cancellous*, *cortical*, or a combination of both—*corticocancellous*. Cancellous grafts are usually collected from the host's metaphyseal bone and used as fresh autografts. Cortical grafts are most often used as frozen allografts, while corticocancellous grafts can be either fresh autografts or fresh or frozen allografts and are usually collected from the ribs or dorsal iliac crests.

FUNCTIONS OF BONE GRAFTS

Bone grafts serve as a source of osteogenesis and may also serve as a mechanical support.[2,3] Rapid formation of bridging callus is important when fracture fragmentation creates a situation where the bone cannot assume any weight sharing with the implant. Under these circumstances, callus can stabilize the fracture sufficiently to relieve the implant of some of these forces and so minimize chances of premature failure or loosening of the implant. When placed in large deficits resulting from trauma or resection of neoplastic bone, cortical bone grafts can serve as a weight-bearing strut or buttress that resists weight-bearing forces, again sparing the implant of some of these loads.

New bone that is formed on or about a graft can be of graft origin (i.e., *directly from osteoblasts or osteoprogenitor cells* that survive the transfer). At best, survival of cells from the graft is estimated at 10 percent when a fresh autogenous cancellous graft is used and handled under optimum conditions. The second way in which the bone graft may function as a source of osteogenesis is by recruitment of mesenchymal or pleuropotential osteoprogenitor cells in the area, which then differentiate into cartilage- and bone-forming cells, a process called *osteoinduction*. A third osteogenic function of grafts is *osteoconduction*, the three-dimensional process of ingrowth of sprouting capillaries, perivascular tissue, and osteoprogenitor cells from the recipient bed into the structure of a graft. The graft acts as a scaffold or template for new-bone formation, and then undergoes varying degrees of osteoclastic resorption and replacement (*creeping substitution*) by host bone.

Cancellous grafts have many advantages such as rapid stimulation of direct bone formation, early osteoinduction, and early vascularization. Autogenous cancellous bone is the only bone graft that can be safely applied in contaminated areas. Vascular invasion and osteoconduction occur much more slowly in cortical grafts, but these grafts have the advantage of affording some immediate stability to the area. They are prone to sequestration in infected areas.

CLINICAL APPLICATION OF BONE GRAFTS

Collection of Bone for Grafting

Strict aseptic technique is mandatory in grafting procedures that do not involve ethylene oxide (ETO) sterilization.

Autogenous Cancellous Bone

Figure 3–1A–D shows the most common areas for collection in small animals, namely the lateral tubercle of the humerus, the subtrochanteric region or medial condyle of the femur, the proximomedial tibia, and the craniodorsal iliac spine. The selected area is approached through a 2- to 3-cm skin incision. The cortical bone is opened with a trephine or a trocar-pointed Steinmann pin (3/16 to 1/4 inch; 4.8 to 6.5 mm), and cancellous bone is scooped out with an oval curette (Fig. 3–1E). The graft is usually held in a small container (covered with a gauze sponge moistened with Ringer's or saline solution) until time for transfer to the new area (Fig. 3–1F). Do not immerse the graft in the fluid and do not apply antibiotics. A blood-soaked surgical sponge can be substituted for the container. The graft should be implanted immediately after it is collected.

Because of their accessibility, the proximal humerus and tibia are the most commonly used collection sites. One or more of these areas is prepared preoperatively and draping should allow access to them if needed during fracture repair. The proximal humerus yields more bone than the tibia, and cancellous bone is restored more completely than in the tibia, where fibrous tissue fills the graft site.[4] Postoperative hematoma is not uncommon at the donor site, but can be minimized by careful layered closure of the site.

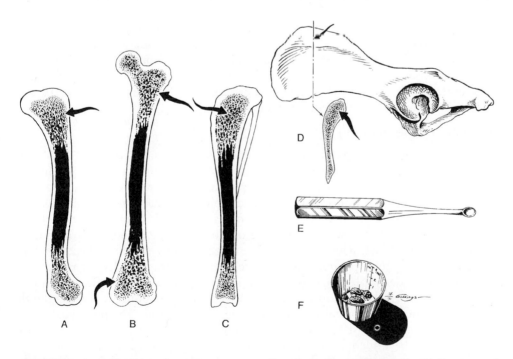

FIGURE 3–1. Collection of autogenous cancellous bone for grafting. (A–D) Sections of a humerus, femur, tibia, and ilium indicating location for collection of bone graft. (E) Curette used to scoop out cancellous bone. (F) Receptacle used for temporarily holding collected graft.

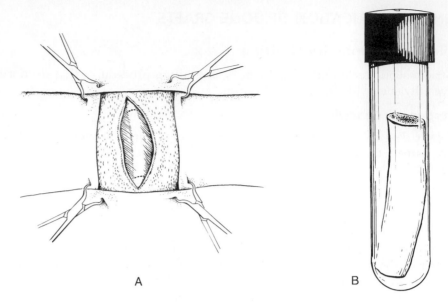

A

B

FIGURE 3–2. Collection of rib grafts for bone bank. (*A*) Ribs are aseptically collected from a donor animal and cleaned of all soft tissue. (*B*) Each rib is placed in a sterile test tube or similar container.

Autogenous Corticocancellous Bone

The ribs and craniodorsal iliac spine are the usual donor sites. The rib collection technique is similar to that illustrated in Figure 3–2 for allografts. An incision through skin and muscle is made directly over the chosen rib. The periosteum is incised and carefully elevated to avoid opening the pleural cavity, and the rib is freed by cutting at both ends. The iliac spine is also approached directly by a dorsal incision of skin and muscle. It is not necessary to elevate periosteum, and a suitable block of bone is freed by osteotome or bone saw. The graft can be either just the lateral cortex or a full-thickness piece of the iliac spine/crest containing both cortices.

Allograft/Bone Banking

Collection technique varies with the method chosen for preservation. The graft can be collected aseptically and preserved by freezing, or collected under clean conditions, sterilized by ETO, and preserved by freezing.[2,3,5]

Bone is collected from a healthy donor animal of the same species, under strict aseptic procedure if ETO sterilization is not used. For corticocancellous bone it is preferable to use a donor from one of the large breeds approximately 4 to 6 months of age. Ribs are the most common source of bone because they have a relatively high proportion of cancellous bone (Fig. 3–2*A*). If more cortical content is desirable, the craniodorsal iliac spine is used as explained above. All periosteum and other soft tissue is removed from the bone by scraping with a scalpel blade or periosteal elevator at time of collection. The harvested bone is placed in a sterile test tube or similar container. A small amount of Ringer's solution may be added to keep the bones moist and to prevent freezer burn (dehydration) in storage. Each bone is usually placed in an individual sterile container or wrap for convenient usage (Fig. 3–2*B*). The sealed and labeled containers are placed in a home-type deep freezer and held at 0°F (−18°C) or lower. Bone preserved in this fashion may be held for approximately 1 year.

Cortical diaphyseal grafts are collected from all the long bones, cutting the diaphyseal portion free at each end with a bone saw. The medullary canal is curetted and flushed to remove soft tissue elements. Packaging and freezing is as described above. Because these grafts will have to match the recipient site quite closely in size, it is well to label them as to size of donor, and also helpful to radiograph the specimen to allow easier matching to the recipient.

ETO sterilization simplifies the collection process in that aseptic technique does not have to be used, although the conditions should be made as clean as possible. After the bones have been cleaned of soft tissue as above, they are double-wrapped in polyethylene instrument sterilization pouches or tubing. Sterilization is by 84 percent ETO (Anprolene, H.W. Anderson Products), for 12 hours, followed by 72 hours aeration, all at room temperature. Following this sterilization the bones are deep frozen as described above.[5] Such sterilization and storage up to 1 year appears to have no effects on cortical bone resistance to compressive, bending, and torsional loads when compared to fresh bone.[6]

Types of Grafts and Placement

The types most commonly used are pure cancellous fragments, corticocancellous bone chips, cortical or corticocancellous onlay or inlay, and cortical tubular intercalary grafts (Fig. 3–3)

Pure Cancellous Fragments

This graft is used immediately after collection by packing the fragments into the desired area and then gently compressing the material. Any graft left after packing into the defect can be spread around the surface of the defect and adjacent bone (Fig. 3–3A). The graft site should be cleaned of tissue fragments

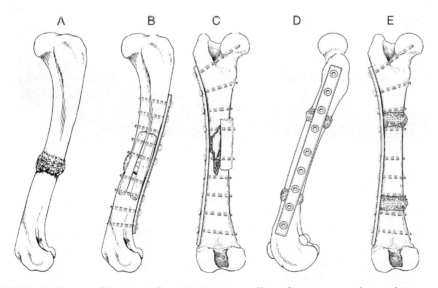

FIGURE 3–3. Types of bone grafts. (A) Pure cancellous fragments or bone chips created by use of a rongeur are packed around the fracture site. (B) Onlay graft (usually a split rib) spans the fracture, and cancellous fragments or chips are packed around the fracture site. (C) Onlay cortical graft acts as a buttress to replace missing cortical bone in the compression cortex opposite the plate. The fragmented area under the plate is grafted with cancellous bone. (D, E) Tubular intercalary allograft used to replace a section of the diaphysis. Autogenous cancellous bone is used at the graft-host junctions.

and blood clots before insertion of the graft. Avoid irrigation of the graft before closing the soft tissues, which should be done immediately. In delayed unions or nonunions, the sclerotic tissue and periosteum are peeled off the host bone segments at the fracture site. This is usually accomplished by using a periosteal elevator or osteotome and mallet (see Fig. 4–3). The bone segments are stabilized by a compression plate, and the graft is placed around the fracture site between the elevated periosteum and cortex.

Corticocancellous Bone Chips[2]

This type graft is usually prepared from banked allograft rib bone. Bone chips of 2 to 5 mm in diameter (Fig. 3–3A) are used in a manner identical to pure cancellous bone, and are useful to increase the volume of graft over that available from pure autogenous cancellous bone, or when an autogenous donor site has not been prepared. The chips are created by using a rongeur to nibble off small bone pieces.

Onlay Bone Graft[2]

Figure 3–3B shows an onlay graft used in treatment of a nonunion fracture. The sclerotic tissue and periosteum are elevated and reflected off the host area. The bone segments are stabilized by a compression plate. The graft is created by splitting a rib bone to expose the cancellous interior, and this side is placed against the recipient bone. One or more onlay grafts are placed on the bone, spanning the fracture site. The graft may be secured in place by bone screws, by cerclage wires, or by suturing the patient's tissue over the area. Rigid fixation of bone segments in the host is much more important than fixation of the transplant. It is usually a good procedure to place autogenous cancellous bone or bone chips around the remaining uncovered portion of the fracture site. Onlay grafts can be used in a similar manner in fresh fractures.

Inlay Graft

This graft is most often cortical bone used as a buttress to replace a portion of missing cortex on the compression side opposite the bone plate (Fig. 3–3C). Its use has declined with the advent of the concept of bridging osteosynthesis (see Chapter 2). In many cases its use is interchangeable with the tubular graft explained below. The graft must be securely stabilized, preferably by bone screws placed through the plate.

Tubular Intercalary Diaphyseal Graft[5,7–9]

Tubular grafts (Fig. 3–3D, E) are indicated chiefly for:

1. Severe multiple or comminuted shaft fractures that do not lend themselves to anatomical reconstruction.
2. Fractures with missing bone segments; bone length can be restored.
3. Replacement of surgically removed segments of neoplastic bone.
4. Reconstruction of certain atrophic nonunion fractures.
5. Correction of malunion.

Good clinical results have been reported for this method. Twenty-five cases followed a mean of 2.1 years yielded normal function in 96 percent of the dogs.[9] Despite these results, the use of this type bone graft in fracture repair has declined with the advent of the concept of bridging osteosynthesis (see Chapter 2), and intercalary grafts are presently used primarily in limb-sparing surgery for bony neoplasia.

The procedure usually consists of squaring off the ends of the viable bone segments, attaching the proper size and length of cylindrical diaphyseal allograft to the center section of the plate, and immobilizing it under compression at both ends by using a dynamic compression plate. Autogenous cancellous graft is used at each end of the graft. There may be an advantage to perforating the graft with small drill holes to encourage vascularization of the medullary canal. Screws should secure a minimum of four cortices in the graft, and six cortices in each end of recipient bone in order to secure adequate stability. Functionally, most animals respond in the same fashion as the patient with an average multiple or segmental fracture stabilized with a bone plate. Replacement of the allograft by host bone is slow and incomplete, with areas of dead graft still present at 8 years in one patient.[10] New bone deposited on the surface of the graft creates clinical union and plates can be removed in 18 to 25 months if indicated.

References

1. Albee FH: Fundamentals in bone transplantation. Experiences in three thousand bone graft operations. JAMA 81:1429–1432, 1923.
2. Brinker WO: Fractures. In Canine Surgery, 2nd ed. Santa Barbara, American Veterinary Publications, 1952, pp 548–643; 3rd ed, 1957, pp 546–640; 1st Archibald ed, 1965, pp 777–849; 2nd Archibald ed, 1975, pp 957–1048.
3. Stevenson S: Bone grafting. In Slatter DH (ed): Textbook of Small Animal Surgery, Vol II, 2nd ed. Philadelphia, WB Saunders Co, 1993, pp 1694–1703.
4. Penwick RC, Mosier DK, Clark DM: Healing of autogenous cancellous bone graft donor sites. Vet Surg 20:229–234, 1991.
5. Johnson AL: Principles and practical application of cortical-bone grafting techniques. Compend Cont Educ Small Anim Pract 10:906–913, 1988.
6. Tshamala M, vanBree H, Mattheeuws D: Biomechanical properties of ethylene oxide sterilized and cryopreserved cortical bone allografts. Vet Comp Orthop Trauma 7:25–30, 1994.
7. Wadsworth PL, Henry WB: Entire segmental cortical bone transplant. J Am Anim Hosp Assoc 12:741–745, 1976.
8. Henry WB, Wadsworth PL: Retrospective analysis of failures in the repair of severely comminuted long bone fractures using large diaphyseal allografts. J Am Anim Hosp Assoc 17:535–546, 1981.
9. Sinibaldi KR: Evaluation of full cortical allografts in 25 dogs. J Am Vet Med Assoc 194:1570–1577, 1989.
10. Wilson JW, Hoefle WD: Diaphyseal allograft: Eight year evaluation in a dog. Vet Comp Orthop Trauma 3:78–81, 1990.

4

Delayed Union and Nonunion

The speed of reunion of bone is in direct ratio to the rigidity with which the two pieces are placed together.

—Richard VonVolkmann (1830–1889)

Delayed union refers to a fracture that has not healed in the usual time for that particular fracture. Table 4–1 details average healing times anticipated for small animals.[1] *Nonunion* refers to a fracture in which all evidence of osteogenic activity at the fracture site has ceased, movement is present at the fracture site, and union is no longer possible without surgical intervention. The term *pseudoarthrosis* is sometimes applied indiscriminately to all nonunions, but should be reserved for those nonunions where sclerotic bone ends are united by a fibrous "joint capsule" filled with serum (Fig. 4–1A). The most common causes of these conditions are local factors:

1. Inadequate immobilization, or failure to maintain immobilization for a sufficient length of time.
2. Inadequate reduction with a large fracture gap and/or interposition of soft tissue.
3. Impairment of the blood supply resulting from the original trauma or surgical trauma.
4. Infection: A fracture may heal in the presence of infection; however, at best, healing is delayed. Implant loosening is common in infected bone.
5. Loss of bone or bone fragments from open trauma or surgery.

General factors such as age, high-dose corticosteroid therapy, or metabolic alteration of osteoblastic activity, such as rickets, are uncommon.

DELAYED UNION FRACTURES

The most common cause of delayed union is inadequate or interrupted fixation of the fracture segments. On radiographic examination (Fig. 4–1B), the fracture line remains evident, has a feathery or woolly appearance, and there is no sclerosis of the bone ends. Evidence of osteogenic activity (callus) is visible, but is minimal and may not bridge the fracture line.

Treatment of delayed union fractures may be approached by various means[2]:

TABLE 4–1.   AVERAGE TIMES TO CLINICAL UNION*

Age of Animal	ESF (type I, some II) IM Pin	Plate Fixation ESF (type III, some II)
<3 mo	2–3 wk	4 wk
3–6 mo	4–6 wk	6–12 wk
6–12 mo	5–8 wk	12–16 wk
>1 yr	7–12 wk	16–30 wk

*Adapted from Hohn RB, Rosen H: Delayed union. In Brinker WO, Hohn RB, Prieur WD (eds): Manual of Internal Fixation in Small Animals. Berlin, Springer-Verlag, 1984, pp 241–254, with permission.

1. If reduction is satisfactory, rigid uninterrupted fixation should be ensured and maintained for an extended period of time. If the original fixation is still deemed adequate, this may involve simply reducing the animal's activity through better owner cooperation, or by use of non–weight-bearing slings (see Chapter 2). The use of external coaptation splints or casts should be avoided in the case of long-bone fractures, as is discussed in Chapter 2.

   If the original fixation is suspect, it should be augmented or replaced. A common scenario is a long-bone fracture (often the femur) treated by intramedullary fixation, with or without cerclage or interfragmentary wire, that is not totally stable in rotation, or perhaps in shear due to collapse with weight bearing. Under these circumstances, closed application of an external fixator is very useful and will usually provide suf-

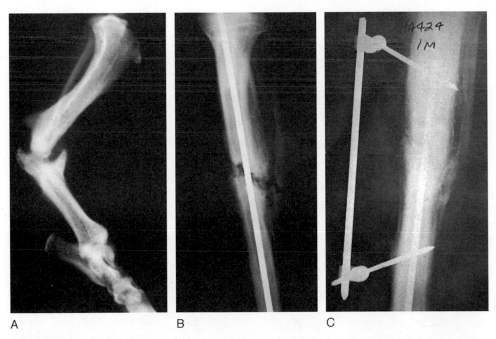

A   B   C

FIGURE 4–1. Delayed and nonunion fractures. (A) Chronic nonunion of the pseudoarthrosis type. The sclerotic bone ends are united by a fibrous "joint capsule" containing serum. (B) Delayed union tibial fracture caused by rotational instability. The fracture line is prominent, with a feathery or woolly appearance. Some nonbridging callus is evident laterally. (C) Four weeks after closed application of an external fixator the fracture has reached clinical union.

ficient stability to allow healing to proceed (Fig. 4–1C). Type I fixators are most commonly used in this situation. Delayed union femoral fractures in large-breed dogs are probably better treated by application of a bone plate (Fig. 4–2A, B), as better limb function can be anticipated than with external fixators.

Bone plate fixation is not immune to problems with delayed union, usually due to instability at the fracture site. Loose screws in bone plates can be salvaged by a variety of means:

a. Replace with larger screws if the plate holes will accept them, or replace cortical threads with cancellous threads.

b. Add a nut to the protruding end of the screw.

c. Fill screw holes with methyl methacrylate. Use liquid cement in a syringe, fill the holes, and insert the screws. After the cement hardens tighten the screws to normal tightness. Do not allow any cement into the fracture area.

d. Substitute cerclage wires for screws. This is the least desirable method, and is used only as a last resort.

2. If there is good end-to-end bone contact, but with malalignment or bending at the fracture site, the bone should be straightened and rigid uninterrupted fixation should be applied. This situation is most commonly a sequel to closed reduction and coaptation fixation. Usually, straightening can be accomplished by careful but forceful pressure with the hands or by applying pressure over a fulcrum point. This is preferable to doing an open surgical correction, as it saves many weeks of healing time (Fig. 4–2C, D). Again, external fixators are often the technique of choice.

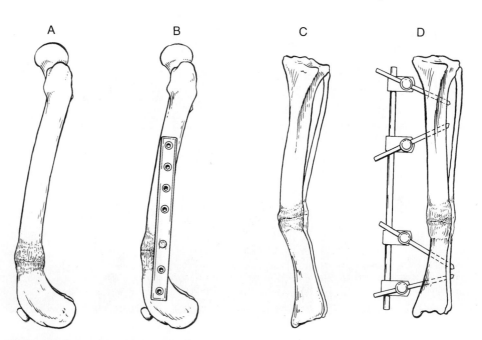

FIGURE 4–2. Delayed union fractures. (A) Satisfactory reduction of delayed union femoral fracture previously treated with an intramedullary pin. (B) Rigid internal fixation provided by a compression plate. (C) Delayed union fracture of a tibia with good contact of bone fragments but with valgus deformity. (D) Bone straightened manually, without surgical exposure. A unilateral external fixator consisting of 2/2 pins was applied for fixation.

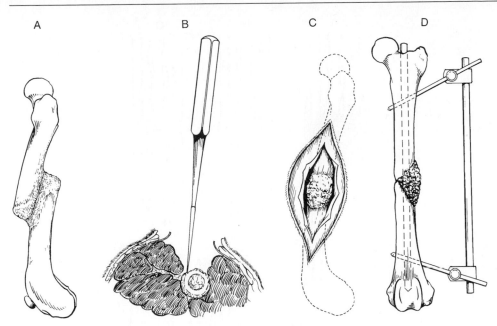

FIGURE 4–3. (*A*) Delayed union fracture with evidence of osteogenic activity, movement at fracture site, overriding of fracture segments, shortening, and favoring the leg. (*B–D*) Open approach, modified periosteal callus layers were reflected away from the cortex as one layer. Reduction and stabilization were achieved by inserting an intramedullary pin and unilateral external fixator (1/1 pins). A cancellous bone graft was added around the fracture site. In cases like this, the medullary space is filled with internal callus; thus, the intramedullary pin fits very snugly and affords excellent stability. The external fixator was added to stabilize against rotation. The other alternative is to use a plate for fixation.

3. If reduction is unsatisfactory, surgical intervention is indicated to correct the deficiencies of reduction and fixation. In the absence of vigorous callus formation autogenous cancellous bone grafting of the fracture site is always indicated (Fig. 4–3).

NONUNION FRACTURES

Two basic types of nonunion fractures, classified by their biological characteristics, were proposed by Weber and Cech, and remain the most useful system for the clinician.[3] All these types may be complicated by the presence of infection.

1. *Viable* (reactive, vascular): This is a biologically active fracture, characterized by a variable degree of proliferative bone reaction with interposed cartilage and fibrous tissue, which is evidenced radiographically and histologically (Fig. 4–4). There are three subtypes within this category, and they represent the types most commonly seen in small animals:
    a. Hypertrophic or elephant foot (Figs. 4–4*A* and 4–5*A*). There is an abundant bridging callus that has not ossified due to motion at the fracture site. What looks like sclerosis of the bone ends is actually abundant appositional bone being deposited and which is unable to bridge the fracture gap due to motion.

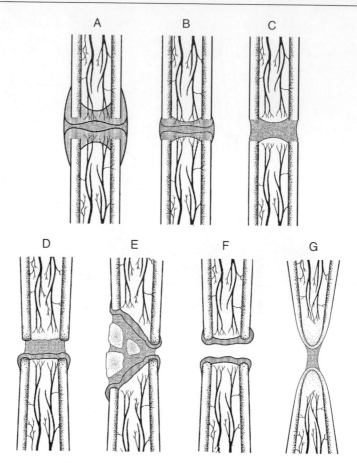

FIGURE 4–4. Classification of nonunion fractures, according to Weber and Cech.[3] *Viable*, or biologically active, nonunions. (*A*) Hypertrophic; elephant foot callus. (*B*) Moderately hypertrophic; horse hoof callus. (*C*) Oligotrophic; callus minimal or absent. *Nonviable*, or biologically inactive nonunions. (*D*) Dystrophic; one or both sides of the fracture line are pooly vascularized. (*E*) Necrotic; devascularized bone fragments (sequestra) remain in the fracture gap. (*F*) Defect; bone fragments missing from the fracture gap. (*G*) Atrophic; resorption and rounding of bone ends and complete cessation of osteogenic activity.

    b.   Moderately hypertrophic or horse hoof (Figs. 4–4*B* and 4–5*B*). Callus is present, but it is not as florid as above.

    c.   Oligotrophic (Fig. 4–4*C*). This type is sometimes difficult to distinguish from the nonviable types described below. Callus is absent or minimal and the fracture gap may simply be bridged by fibrous tissue. The radiographic key is the continued fuzzy or hazy appearance to the bone ends, even if they have become smooth or rounded in outline. This haziness is due to vascularity of the area, as opposed to the sclerotic appearance of devascularized bone.

2. *Nonviable* (nonreactive, avascular). These types of nonunion fortunately are not common, as they represent a much more difficult situation to achieve clinical union.

    a.   Dystrophic (Fig. 4–4*D*). One or both sides of the fracture line are poorly vascularized, sometimes due to a fragment that has healed to one end but has too little blood supply to unite to the other end.

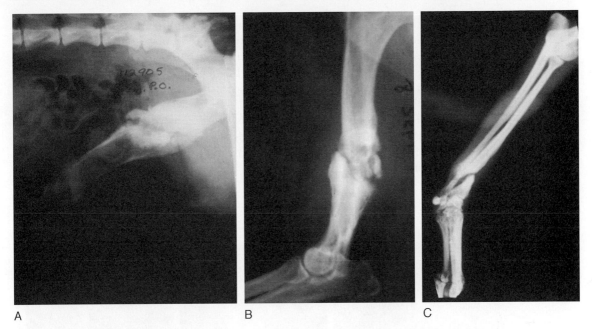

A   B   C

FIGURE 4–5. Radiographic appearance of nonunions. (A) Hypertrophic. (B) Moderately hypertrophic. (C) Atrophic.

Radiographic characteristics include a visible fracture gap, rounded and distinct edges to the bone, and sclerosis extending several millimeters from the bone edges. This type is seen most commonly in distal radius/ulna fractures in toy and miniature dogs.

b. Necrotic (Fig. 4–4F). If bone fragments are not "captured" by invading callus, due to motion or more often infection, they may never become vascularized, and they remain in the fracture gap as sequestra. These fragments will have the same sharp jagged edges as they had in the immediate postfracture radiographs, and will appear more sclerotic with time. The main fragment edges will smooth off as a result of remodeling, and exhibit variable degrees of sclerosis.

c. Defect (Fig. 4–4F). Large fragments may be missing from open fractures, especially high-energy gunshot fractures. If this gap is more than 1.5 times the bone diameter, there may not be enough osteogenetic potential in the local area to bridge the gap with callus, no matter how good the stabilization. This is most common in areas where vascular recruitment is limited due to inadequate soft tissue, such as the distal tibia or radius ulna, or due to local soft tissue and vascular damage.

d. Atrophic (Figs. 4–4G and 4–5C). This is the end point of most nonviable nonunions, with resorption and rounding of the bone ends, with or without disuse osteoporosis, and complete cessation of osteogenic activity.

Treatment

Viable Nonunion

If *reduction is satisfactory*, most patients will respond to stable fixation of any type. Compression at the fracture site (e.g., with a compression plate) is

especially efficacious. Callus should be disturbed as little as possible when applying fixation, even to the point of contouring the plate to accommodate the
callus. Type II and III external fixators can also be employed, especially in the
radius/ulna, and in the tibia. They are the best choice if the nonunion is infected.
Type I external fixators combined with intramedullary pins can be applied in
some situations (Fig. 4–6).

If *reduction is unsatisfactory*, the callus must be divided at the fracture site.
Some callus may need to be resected in order to achieve bone-to-bone contact
and to open the medullary canal with an intramedullary pin, allowing speedy
re-establishment of the medullary blood supply. Appropriate fixation is then

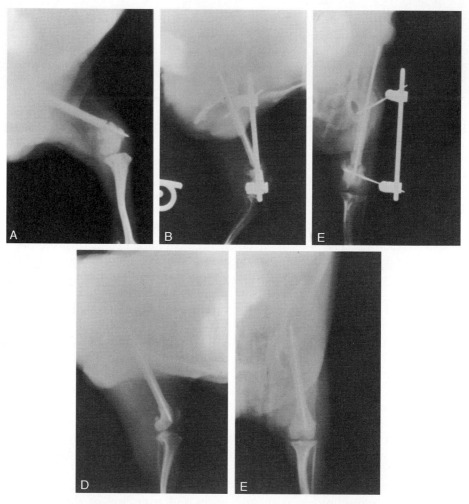

FIGURE 4–6. Moderately hypertrophic nonunion of a supracondylar fracture in a small
Yorkshire terrier immobilized by use of an improperly placed intramedullary pin. There
was rotation at the fracture site. (*A*) Radiographic appearance at 3 months. Clinically,
the area was very painful, and the animal totally refused to use the leg. (*B, C*) A lateral
open approach was used, and an intramedullary pin and unilateral external fixator (1/
1 pin) were applied for stabilization. The external fixator was removed in 6 weeks
because there was sufficient callus to stabilize against rotation. (*D, E*) Clinical union
was present at 3 months, and the intramedullary pin was removed. The animal regained
a full range of movement and function.

applied. Bone grafting is not needed, although pieces of resected callus can be packed around the fracture site.

Nonviable Nonunion

An open approach is made to allow reflection of the covering thickened periosteum with a periosteal elevator or osteotome, and removing the fibrous soft tissue between the bone ends. Sclerosed bone is removed from the bone ends with rongeurs until bleeding is observed from the periosteum and endosteum. Excessive bone length should not be sacrificed to achieve this, however. Additionally, a suitable diameter Steinmann pin or twist drill is used to open the medullary canal. The space between the reflected periosteum and bone is packed with cancellous bone chips, and stable fixation is applied (e.g., a bone plate, external fixator, or an intramedullary pin and external fixator) (Figs. 4–3*B*, *C*, *D* and 4–7). Healing is slow and the fixation will need to remain in place for a prolonged period of time (4 to 6 months). Some of the more indolent conditions may necessitate grafting procedures a second or third time.

Future Treatment Possibilities[4]

Bone morphogenetic proteins (BMPs) function to induce transformation of undifferentiated mesenchymal cells into chondroblasts and osteoblasts and have been shown to induce new-bone formation in vivo and in vitro. BMPs have been isolated from a variety of mammalian tissues and are on the verge of becoming commercially available through recombinant DNA technology in quantities sufficient for clinical application. Potential applications include use as alternatives to bone grafts, promoters of osteointegration of implants, and treatment of nonadaptive bone disease such as stress fractures. Thus BMPs

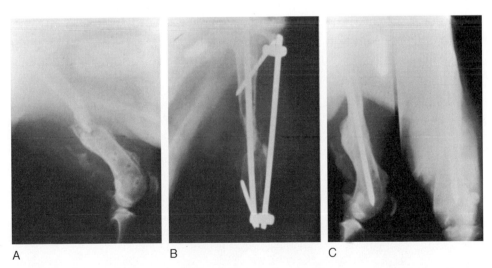

A   B   C

FIGURE 4–7. Nonunion of a fracture of the femur. The markedly comminuted fracture was originally fixed by use of a plate; however, the fracture site deficits were not filled with bone graft. At 15 months, when the animal returned for plate removal, he was favoring the leg. (*A*) Radiograph of femur following plate removal, lateral view. (*B*) Following reflection of the modified periosteum in the fracture site area, an intramedullary pin and a unilateral external fixator (1/1 pin) were applied for fixation, lateral view. A bone graft was applied in the fracture area. (*C*) Clinical union at 4½ months, lateral view. Demineralized bone such as this one responds faster if subjected to stresses; therefore, the intramedullary pin and external fixator were chosen for stabilization.

would appear to have value in the treatment of delayed and nonunion fractures, but their role in this area remains to be defined through clinical trials.

References

1. Hohn RB, Rosen H: Delayed union. In Brinker WO, Hohn RB, Prieur WD (eds): Manual of Internal Fixation in Small Animals, Berlin, Springer-Verlag, 1984, pp 241–254.
2. Brinker WO: Fractures. In Canine Surgery, 2nd Archibald ed. Santa Barbara, American Veterinary Publications, Inc, 1974, pp 949–1048.
3. Weber BG, Cech D: Pseudoarthrosis, Pathology, Biomechanics, Therapy, Results. Bern, Hans Huber Medical Publisher, 1976.
4. Kirker-Head CA: Recombinant bone morphogenetic proteins: Novel substances for enhancing bone healing. Vet Surg 24:408–419, 1995.

5

Treatment of Acute and Chronic Bone Infections

Osteitis or osteomyelitis is defined as a bone inflammation involving the haversian spaces, Volkmann canals, and generally, the medullary cavity and periosteum. Bone infection is usually associated with open fractures, bone surgery (especially those involving metallic implants), or systemic illness. Bite wounds are common causes of osteomyelitis in the lower limbs, mandible, and maxilla in dogs, and of the coccygeal vertebrae in cats.

Acute infection is characterized by a supportive history, localized pain, swelling, erythema, and elevation of body temperature ($\geq$103°F; 39.5°C). In most early cases, radiological signs are not evident. Persistent fever is the most reliable early sign of infection. Postsurgical osteomyelitis signs are usually evident 48 to 72 hours after surgery, but during this period it is difficult to distinguish between incipient osteomyelitis and deep wound infection. Wound disruption and drainage takes several days to develop.

Chronic infection is characterized by a supportive history; draining sinus tracts ($\pm$); muscle atrophy, fibrosis, and contracture; variable lameness; and positive radiographic changes. These changes may include cortical resorption and thinning; osteoporosis; periosteal new-bone formation that may be smooth, expansile, or spiculated[1]; formation of sequestra and involucra; sclerosis; and soft tissue swelling (Fig. 5–1). A *sequestrum* is a piece of dead bone that has become separated from normal bone during the process of necrosis and is surrounded by a pool of infected exudate. Since it has not undergone any resorptive process and is not vascularized, its radiographic density is high, giving the appearance of a very white piece of bone that has very sharp and ragged edges. Most sequestra are found within the medullary cavity or beneath a bone plate. An *involucrum* is a covering or sheath of new-bone formation and fibrous tissue covering a sequestrum.

Most commonly, osteomyelitis implies bacterial infection; however, fungi or viruses can also infect bone and marrow. Staphylococci cause 50 to 60 percent of bone infections in dogs,[1] and historically the organism most commonly reported has been *Staphylococcus aureus*; however, a recent report indicates *Staphylococcus intermedius* to be more common.[2] The significance of this is that most of these were resistant to penicillin because of β-lactamase production. Other common organisms include *Streptococcus*, *Escherichia coli*, *Proteus*, *Klebsiella*, *Pseudomonas*, and *Pasteurella* when bite wounds are present. The importance of anaerobes, especially in bite-wound osteomyelitis, has been emphasized by Muir and Johnson, who reported a 64 percent incidence of anaerobic bacteria isolated from such cases.[3] Such isolates include *Actinomyces*, *Clostridium*, *Peptostrepto-*

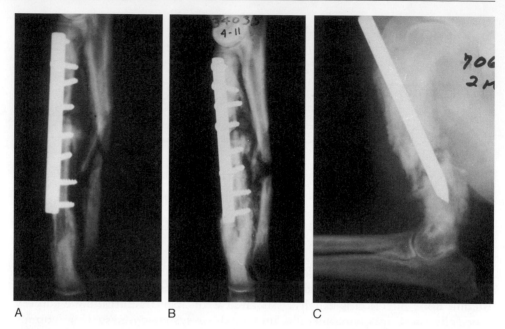

FIGURE 5–1. Radiographic signs of osteomyelitis. (*A*) Postoperative film of revision by bone plate fixation of an infected nonunion fracture. Hazy nonbridging callus is seen at the distal edge of the fracture gap, and periosteal new bone is present distal to the plate. (*B*) Postoperative day 19. Note resorption of bone under the center of the plate, increased periosteal new bone distally, and sclerosis of the ulna. The ulnar fragment is a sequestrum. The plate is loose as indicated by bone resorption around the distal screws. (*C*) Two months after intramedullary (IM) pin fixation this humerus shows classical signs of chronic infection and nonunion characterized by extensive mature periosteal bone formation.

coccus, *Bacteroides*, and *Fusobacterium*. About 50 percent of infections are caused by a single organism; others are caused by multiple organisms.

ROUTES OF INFECTION

The routes of infection, in order of occurrence, are as follows:

1.   Direct contamination from open fractures, surgical intervention in treatment of a fracture, and puncture wounds. The highest percentage of infected fractures follow either open fracture repair or open repair of closed fractures. The presence of a metallic implant is usually involved.

2.   Direct extension from infected adjacent soft tissue.

3.   The bloodstream, from such conditions as vertebral osteomyelitis, discospondylitis (*Brucella*, *Nocardia*, *Staphylococcus*), and bacterial endocarditis.[4] This source of osteomyelitis by comparison is rare and will not be discussed here.

TISSUE CHANGES

Bone is normally as resistant to infection as any other tissue. Clinical infection is always a result of more than simple bacterial contamination and usually implies concurrent soft tissue injury (hence compromised bone vascularity), sequestration, implants, instability of fracture fragments, or alteration of local tissue defenses.[1] Indeed, 72 percent of open fractures and 39 percent of closed fractures have bacterial contamination at the time of surgery, but only a small percentage become clinically infected.[5] The role of metallic implants in bone infection has been elucidated in a variety of studies that have explained how these implants create low-grade inflammation by depressing host defenses, thus providing a nidus for infection. Infective bacteria produce a biofilm (glycocalyx) that promotes bacterial growth by protecting bacteria from phagocytosis and antibodies and causing adherence to implants or other foreign material.[1,6]

Infection in bone produces vascular congestion, edema, and an inflammatory exudate that spreads through the bone, killing osteocytes and marrow cells. Polymorphonuclear cells release proteolytic enzymes, causing tissue necrosis, drop in local pH, and demineralization of bone matrix and breakdown of trabeculae. Sometimes the involvement is confined to a localized area; in other cases, large areas are involved. Spread of infective exudate is easiest along the medullary canal; however, it also occurs beneath the periosteum and in the cortex via vascular channels. As the quantity of exudate increases, intraosseus pressure increases and further compromises blood flow. Areas of bone served by the involved vascular channels become anoxic and die.

With subsidence of the acute phase, pyogenic granulation tissue attacks and absorbs dead spongiosa and separates as sequestra those parts of the cortex that are necrotic. Pus accumulating in the subperiosteal space may separate periosteum from the outer cortex. The periosteum responds by laying down new bone in an attempt to bridge and surround the involved area, the so-called involucrum. This process is not unlike the classical formation of an abscess. The involucrum is usually fenestrated, leading to the eventual drainage of pus through multiple sinus tracts, which are accompanied by extensive scar tissue formation in the surrounding soft tissue and distortion and thinning of overlying skin. These events are made worse by fracture instability, since interfragmentary motion discourages vascularization of the bone. The opposing surfaces become more widely separated due to bone resorption, leading to further instability.

Timely and aggressive surgical or medical intervention can arrest infection, leading to its elimination, followed by gradual remodeling of the involucrum into cortical bone that may look surprisingly like the original one. This process of healing can be discussed by considering (1) changes in necrotic bone; (2) formation of new bone; and (3) changes in old, living bone.

Necrotic Bone

Dead bone is absorbed by the action of granulation tissue that develops about its surface. If the dead bone is cancellous, it may be removed entirely, leaving a cavity behind. Dead cortex in any appreciable amount is gradually detached. After sequestration, the bone is less readily attacked and more slowly absorbed due to the physical barrier imposed by the scar tissue walls of the cavity surrounding the sequestrum. Cortical sequestra may take years or even the lifetime of the animal to be completely absorbed. Some sequestra are never absorbed and will continue to cause drainage until they are surgically removed.

New Bone

New bone forms from primitive mesenchymal cells in the surviving portions of periosteum, endosteum, and cortex. Recurrence of infection may result in the formation of superimposed layers of involucrum.

Old, Living Bone

In osteomyelitis, surviving bone usually becomes osteoporotic during the active period of infection because of disuse atrophy and decalcification resulting from inflammatory hyperemia. After subsidence of infection and resumption of function of the part, bone density increases again.

CLINICAL APPROACH

History, signs, and radiographic findings are essential in making a diagnosis and in determining the extent of the lesion. Treatment is based on the principles of appropriate antimicrobial drugs, open wound drainage and lavage, fracture stabilization, sequestrectomy, and grafting of bone deficits.[1] The first step is to culture and determine the antibiotic sensitivity of the causative organisms. Culturing for anaerobes is particularly important in chronic infection and those associated with bite wounds. It is imperative that the culture be taken from the infected area and *not* from the draining sinus tracts. The latter are commonly contaminated with skin organisms. In acute cases, it is best to perform fine-needle aspiration from the infected area. In chronic cases, culture at the time of sequestrectomy is indicated. Fractures will heal in the presence of infection, although healing will be delayed.

Acute Infection

Treatment must be aggressive and appropriate to forestall chronic disease.

1.   Place the animal on systemic antibiotics, initially based on either hospital epidemiology (previous iatrogenic infections) or on the knowledge that most infections are caused by β-lactamase–producing staphylococci; thus, cefazolin, clindamycin, cloxacillin, or amoxicillin–clavulanate are indicated. Culture and sensitivity testing will indicate the best choice for long-term treatment, which should be continued for 4 to 6 weeks.

2.   Complete and careful debridement of wound if indicated.

3.   Establishing surgical drainage to the area if exudate is present. This may necessitate leaving the wound open after debridement or use of drains with or without suction or irrigation. Because of the difficulty of maintaining drains in animals, it is much safer and easier to manage the patient if the wounds are left entirely open, even if this means leaving the implants exposed.[7] In this method, the open wound can be covered with a wet to dry bandage that is changed daily until the defect has stopped draining exudate or is filled with healthy granulation tissue. In a healthy wound, granulation tissue will quickly cover a metallic implant. At this time, it may be indicated to fill the bone defect with an autogenous cancellous bone graft by simply elevating granulation tissue and packing the cancellous graft beneath it (see Chapter 3 for details of graft collection).

A technique commonly used in human beings involves primary closure of the wound over drains to allow irrigation and suction. The drains are placed into the wound bed and exit the skin at a distant site. The tubes are used to flush the wound bed with fluids containing the appropriate antibiotic based on culture and sensitivity results. The difficulties of managing such a system almost preclude its use in animals. Open drainage is much more successful in completely evacuating exudate and preventing chronic infection.

4. Evaluate and modify, if necessary, the internal fixation to ensure stability of the fracture.

Chronic Infection

Treatment usually involves:

1. Antimicrobial therapy as outlined above, and continuation for 5 to 7 weeks. Anaerobic infection is much more likely in chronic cases, and mitronidazole and clindamycin are the most useful drugs. Aminoglycosides and quinolones are the most useful drugs against gram-negative infections.

2. Removing sequestra if present. In most instances, it is advantageous to follow the same surgical approach used in open reduction of the fracture rather than following the sinus tract if there is one present. As a rule, it is not necessary to curette the area of the sinus tract or to use chemical or proteolytic enzymes following removal of sequestra that are walled off with granulation tissue. It is useful to remove sclerotic bone involved in the involucrum, as this may be necrotic bone that will form a secondary sequestrum. Remove bone only until point bleeding is seen from the cortex to avoid creating a large cavity. If a draining tract persists, it is most probable that all sequestra have not been removed and a second or even a third attempt may be in order. A common site for sequestra is beneath a bone plate, and this may require removal of the plate to remove the sequestrum.

3. Critically evaluate fracture stability. If the fracture is healed and implants are present, they are removed. If implants are secure and stabilizing the fracture, they should be left in place until the fracture is healed. If instability is present and implants are loose, they should be removed and replaced by suitable fixation. Use of the external fixator or plates and screws is preferred over intramedullary pins. Once the fracture is healed, removal of implants is generally required to completely clear the infection due to the persistence of bacteria around the implant.

There is an exception to the rule that dead bone should be removed as soon as it is separated. This occurs when the sequestrum comprises the whole thickness of the shaft of a long bone. If these large fragments are removed at the time of the original surgery—shortly after injury or within a few weeks—the surrounding tube of periosteum may collapse and the subperiosteal hematoma may be obliterated. There is no longer a continuous hematoma between the fragments, and the fracture cannot unite. In such a case, it is better to defer sequestrectomy for several months until the surrounding involucrum of subperiosteal bone has been laid down, thereby ensuring continuity of the shaft. Bone grafting with autogenous cancellous bone is usually indicated after removal of sequestrum of this magnitude.

4. Leave the wound open and treat as described above for acute infection.[7]

Case Studies

CASE 1 ■ Figure 5–2 depicts acute bone infection. In *A*, a cocker spaniel struck by a car 5 days previously presented with an open draining area with bone protruding on the medial surface and a temperature of 104.5°F. The immediate objectives in treatment were to flush the area with Ringer's solution, apply rigid fixation, and place the animal on systemic antibiotics. The area was prepared for surgery, including a flushing of the area. In *B* and *C*, fixation was

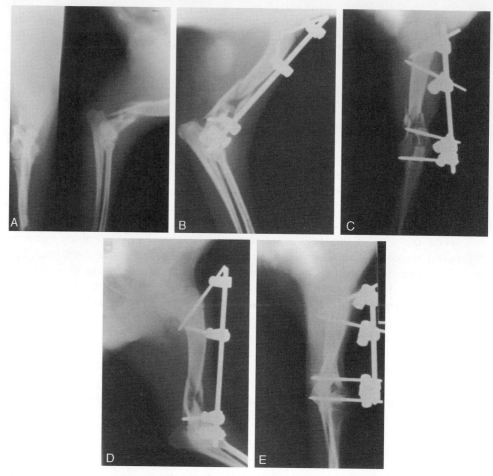

FIGURE 5–2. (*A*) Radiographic views of a distal humeral fracture, 5 days' duration, with an open suppurating wound. The dog's temperature was 104.5°F. (*B, C*) Lateral and craniocaudal views of the unilateral external fixator consisting of 2/2 pins applied for fixation. The draining area was treated as an open wound. It closed in about 2 weeks. (*D, E*) Lateral and craniocaudal views at 9 weeks; clinical union was present, and the splint was removed.

accomplished by application of a unilateral external fixator, 2/2 pins. Because the distal bone segment was too short for placement of two pins proximal to the supracondylar foramen, the distal pin was placed in a transcondylar position. The proximal pin was inserted next, followed by application of the connecting bar and clamps, then the two center pins. This arrangement allowed full use of the leg during the healing period. The draining area was treated as an open wound, and it closed in about 2 weeks. Healing was uneventful. In *D* and *E*, clinical union was present at 9 weeks, and the external fixator was removed.

CASE 2 ■ Figure 5–3 depicts the history of a fractured femur, which was originally treated 5 months previously. Infection had been a constant problem from the time of surgery. Several draining tracts were present in the region of the popliteal lymph nodes, and a walled-off sequestrum was present (*A, B*). Culture and sensitivity testing indicated *Staphylococcus pyogenes*, which was

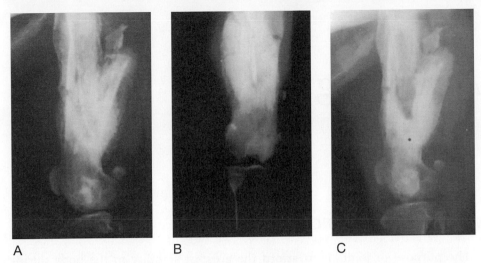

A   B   C

FIGURE 5–3. Fractured femur that had been treated 5 months previously; draining sinus tracts were present near the popliteal lymph nodes. (*A, B*) Lateral and craniocaudal views indicating a walled-off sequestra. (*C*) One large and two small sequestra were removed surgically using a lateral approach to the femur. The sinus tracts disappeared in 1 week.

sensitive to chloramphenicol, oxytetracycline, and chlortetracycline. In Figure 5–2C, one large and two small sequestra have been removed surgically by a lateral approach to the femur. The bone was well healed, and the infection was walled off in the local area. The animal was placed on systemic antibiotics, and the draining tract disappeared in 1 week.

References

1. Johnson KA: Osteomyelitis in dogs and cats. J Am Vet Med Assoc 205:1882–1887, 1994.
2. Love DN, Johnson KA: Antimicrobial sensitivity of staphylococci isolated from dogs. Aust Vet Pract 19:196–200, 1992.
3. Muir P, Johnson KA: Anaerobic bacteria isolated from osteomyelitis in dogs and cats. Vet Surg 21:463–466, 1992.
4. Smeak DP, Olmstead ML, Hohn RB: *Brucella canis* osteomyelitis in two dogs with total hip replacements. J Am Vet Med Assoc 191:986–989, 1987.
5. Stevenson S, Olmstead M, Kowalski J: Bacterial culturing for prediction of postoperative complications following open fracture repair in small animals. Vet Surg 15:99–102, 1986.
6. Smith MM, Vasseur PB, Saunders HM: Bacterial growth associated with metallic implants in dogs. J Am Vet Med Assoc 195:765–767, 1989.
7. Bardet JF, Hohn RB, Basinger BS: Open drainage and delayed autogenous cancellous bone grafting for treatment of chronic osteomyelitis in dogs and cats. J Am Vet Med Assoc 183: 312–317, 1983.

6

Arthrology

STRUCTURE AND FUNCTION OF JOINTS

The purpose of joints is to afford the greatest stability to the body during weight bearing and motion. Painless and full range of joint motion are needed for normal ambulation and performance of daily living chores. Interruption of normal joint mechanics leads to painful osteoarthritis and physical incapacity thereby reducing an individual's quality of life, and increasing the burden on others. This is an increasing problem in human and animal geriatric populations due to longer life spans. Proper diagnosis and management of joint disease depend on understanding the basic anatomy and physiology of the musculoskeletal system. Cures for stopping or reversing osteoarthrosis are on the horizon. The material presented in this chapter should guide clinicians in understanding and arriving at rational treatments for joint diseases.

Connective Tissues

The workhorse of the musculoskeletal system is connective tissue. Its components are outlined in Table 6–1 and are mentioned throughout the next two chapters. It is extremely important that their relationships be understood.

Classification of Joints

Joint classification[1,2] is summarized in the following way. Joint diseases of animals ordinarily involve diarthrodial joints.

FIBROUS JOINTS (SYNARTHROSES) ■ These joints have little motion.

1. Syndesmoses. These have considerable intervening connective tissue (e.g., the temporohyoid joint).
2. Sutures (e.g., the skull).
3. Gomphosis (e.g., the tooth socket).

CARTILAGINOUS JOINTS (AMPHIARTHROSES) ■ These joints have limited motion, which permits compression and stretching.

1. Hyaline cartilage (synchondrosis) (e.g., the costochondral junction, epiphyseal plate of the long bones of growing animals).
2. Fibrocartilage (amphiarthrosis) (e.g., the mandibular symphysis).

SYNOVIAL JOINTS (DIARTHROSES) ■ These joints allow the greatest amount of movement and are of primary concern to the orthopedic surgeon.

TABLE 6-1. COMPONENTS OF CONNECTIVE TISSUE IN JOINTS

Cell Types	Fibers (Proteins)	Matrix (Ground Substance)
Fibroblast	Elastin	Proteins
Chondrocyte	Reticulin	Mucopolysaccharides (proteoglycans),
Osteocyte	Collagen (hydroxyproline)	hyaluronic acid, chondroitin
Synoviocyte		sulfate, keratosulfate
Myocyte		Water

Components of Synovial Joints

All synovial joints have a joint cavity, joint capsule, synovial fluid, articular cartilage, and subchondral bone (Fig. 6–1). Some joints, in addition, have intra-articular ligaments, menisci, and fat pads.

The articular surface of bone is covered by hyaline cartilage. The bones are united by a joint capsule and ligaments. The joint capsule is composed of an inner synovial membrane that produces synovial fluid and an outer fibrous layer that aids joint stability. The range of motion in joints is limited by muscles, ligaments, joint capsule, and bone shapes.

Any mechanical system wears out with time, and animal joints are no exception. Wear and tear occur with aging but may be hastened or exaggerated by trauma, disease, and structural and biochemical changes in the articular cartilage. Lubrication—which decreases friction—is vital in keeping the "machine" in proper working condition. This lubrication can be affected by the nature and geometry of the articulating surfaces, the synovial membrane, the physical and chemical properties of the synovial fluid, the load on the joint, and the type of joint movement.

Synovial Membrane

The synovial membrane is highly vascular, blends with the periosteum as it reflects onto bone, and covers all structures within the joint except articular cartilage and menisci. The synovial lining may extend beyond the fibrous layer and may act as bursae under tendons and ligaments. Basically, the synoviocytes have two functions: phagocytosis and synovial fluid production.

Synovial Fluid

Synovial fluid is a dialysate of blood to which glycosaminoglycan (GAG) has been added by the synoviocytes. Its chief function is lubrication, which decreases friction, thereby decreasing wear and tear to articular cartilage. The synovial

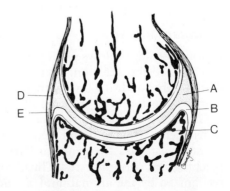

FIGURE 6-1. Schematic drawing of joint components. (*A*) Joint cavity with joint fluid. (*B*) Articular cartilage. (*C*) Subchondral bone. (*D*) Synovial lining. (*E*) Fibrous joint capsule.

TABLE 6–2.   CONDITIONS PREDISPOSING TO SECONDARY DEGENERATIVE JOINT DISEASE*

Congenital
1. Achondroplasia (generalized conformational defects of the limbs).
2. Localized conformational or postural defects (e.g., bowleggedness, straight hocks).
3. Chronic hemarthrosis with hemophilia.

Developmental
1. Osteochondritis dissecans.
2. Failure of ossification centers to fuse (e.g., ununited anconeal or possibly coronoid processes).
3. Abnormal development of joints (e.g., hip dysplasia, congenital elbow luxations).
4. Premature epiphyseal closure (e.g., radius curvus) resulting in carpal DJD from angular deformity and elbow DJD from joint incongruity, owing to asynchronous growth of the radius and ulna.
5. Miscellaneous conditions (patellar luxations).

Acquired
1. Damage to articular surfaces.
   a. Posttraumatic (e.g., fractures of articular surfaces, unusual shoulder stress seen in sled-pulling huskies).
   b. Sequelae to inflammatory joint disease (e.g., osteophytes seen secondary to instability from rheumatoid arthritis).
2. Damage to supporting structures of joints (e.g., tendons, ligaments, menisci).
3. Aseptic necrosis (e.g., Legg-Calvé-Perthes disease of the femoral head).
4. Neuropathies (e.g., abnormal range of motion resulting from abnormal pain and proprioception sense).

*From Pedersen NC: Canine joint disease. In 1978 Scientific Proceedings, 45th Annual Meeting of the American Animal Hospital Association, 1978, pp 359–366, with permission.

fluid also provides nutrition to the articular cartilage and maintains electrolyte and metabolite balance.

The chief GAG of synovial fluid is hyaluronic acid, which is highly polymerized and prevents serum proteins of high molecular weight from entering the fluid. Joint fluid proteins increase with inflammatory conditions either because of a decrease in this polymerized state of hyaluronic acid or as a result of an increase in the capillary permeability of the subsynovium. Both situations cause joint effusion. Corticosteroids are thought to interfere with production of hyaluronic acid.

Inflammatory joint conditions may be distinguished from noninflammatory conditions by analysis of joint fluid (see Table 6–2). In inflammatory conditions, the protein electrophoretic pattern of synovial fluid is altered, sugars are decreased, the cell population increases, and cell type ratios change. The polymerized state of hyaluronic acid can be estimated using the glacial acetic acid precipitate test.[3] The quality of GAG decreases rapidly in the presence of some infections and can slowly decrease in chronic osteoarthritis.

The viscosity of the synovial fluid is related to this mucoprotein; it is higher in small joints and at low rates of shear and use (walking, standing). A decrease in viscosity during more rapid joint movement causes less drag and, therefore, less friction of the joint surfaces. Cold temperatures may cause increased viscosity and, therefore, drag to joint surfaces. This partly explains the necessity for "warming up" prior to athletic pursuits.

Articular Cartilage

Joint cartilage allows gliding action of joints. It is the recipient of most blows and jolts to the skeleton. Its resilience buffers these blows, preventing erosion of the subchondral bone with subsequent shortening. The subchondral bone absorbs shock and in turn protects cartilage from damage.[4]

Grossly, normal adult articular cartilage is white, smooth, glistening, and translucent. It lacks blood vessels, lymphatic vessels, and nerve endings.[5] Nutrients must pass the synovial barrier and the cartilage matrix barrier before reaching the chondrocytes. Thus, a mechanical or chemical joint injury is not recognized by the animal until a synovial reaction occurs. Some agents used to

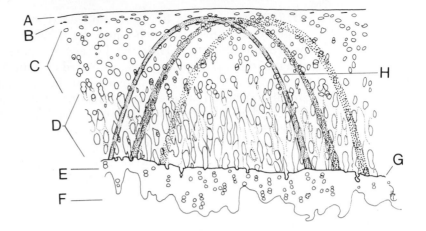

FIGURE 6–2. Schematic drawing of articular cartilage histology showing its layers and fibril arrangement. (*A*) Surface membrane. (*B*) Tangential zones. (*C*) Intermediate zones. (*D*) Radial zone. (*E*) Calcified zone. (*F*) Subchondral zone. (*G*) Tide mark. (*H*) Fibrils or "wickets."

treat synovial disease may be deleterious to the articular cartilage (e.g., corticosteroids in rheumatoid arthritis) but are not detected by cartilage cells owing to this lack of nerve endings in the cartilage. Because cartilage lacks blood vessels, the inflammatory repair process following trauma is impossible until deep lesions invade subchondral bone.[6]

The thickness of the articular cartilage is generally greater when:

1. The joints are larger.
2. The joints are under considerable functional pressure.
3. Friction is increased.
4. The joints are not very congruent.
5. The joints are greatly used.
6. The animals are younger.
7. The joints are exercised.[5]

Histologically, articular cartilage is composed of chondrocytes, fibers, and ground substance. Eighty percent of cartilage is water, 10 percent is collagen, and 10 percent is proteoglycan.[6]

There are four layers of articular cartilage, not including a surface membrane (lamina splendens), based on fiber orientation and shape of chondrocytes:

1. Tangential (surface layer).
2. Transitional (intermediate layer).
3. Radial (deep layer).
4. Calcified[5] (Fig. 6–2).

The chief nourishment for the cartilage comes from the synovial fluid, with 7 to 10 percent coming from the blood vessels of the subchondral bone.[7]

CELLS ■ Chondrocytes in mature cartilage are sparse but are metabolically quite active despite their appearance on light microscopy. The intermediate-zone cells are active in synthesizing protein and other components of matrix, as well as collagen. In immature cartilage, mitoses occur in the surface zone (resulting in growth of the cartilaginous mass during adolescence) and in the basilar layers (accounting for growth of the bony epiphysis). At skeletal maturity, however, mitoses are absent under normal conditions and cartilage cells are incapable of division. There is evidence that under certain situations, such as cartilage laceration and osteoarthritis, the chondrocyte can reinitiate cell synthesis and multiple division of a single cell (clone).[6]

FIBERS ■   Collagen fibers are imbedded in matrix. They are not normally visible by light microscopy because the refractive index is the same as that of the ground substance.[2] They may be seen by phase-contrast microscopy or electron microscopy.[5] Freyberg has postulated that the fibers form hoops or wickets[8] (Fig. 6–2). The surface arrangement of the cartilage fibrils provides a slightly irregular surface that prevents adhesions of opposing articular surfaces when lubricated by synovial fluid.[2] This superficial layer of tightly packed fibers resists shear forces during joint movement.[9] When pressure is applied at the surface, the fibrils expand laterally while the thickness decreases. When the pressure is released, the fibrils rebound as a result of their elasticity.[8] This elasticity decreases with continuous compression or with age. The resiliency of cartilage also depends on the fibrils being supported by matrix proteoglycans.[9] The intermediate layer has the greatest shock-absorbing capacity because of the high content of bound water.[9]

If the superficial layers of fibers are lost through erosion (trauma), the matrix comes into closer contact with joint enzymes, leading to further degradation. This layer can then be considered like the integument as a first line of defense for the rest of the cartilage.

MATRIX ■   The matrix or ground substance of articular cartilage is composed of bound water and proteoglycans. Subunits of proteoglycans are called glycosaminoglycans, such as chondroitin 6-sulfate, chondroitin 4-sulfate, and keratosulfate. These macromolecules are stiffly extended in space as a result of their strong negative charges, repelling one another. They are hydrophilic and bind to the collagen fibers, thereby creating a barrier to absorption of substances from synovial fluid. Only substances having a low molecular weight permeate normal articular cartilage. The barrier to outward flow of organic components is thought to be the factor for its resiliency and resistance to deformation of the articular cartilage.[6]

The health of cartilage matrix may be measured by using metachromatic histochemical stains such as toluidine blue O or safranin O. Loss of metachromasia (and thus chondroitin sulfate) is characteristic of degenerating cartilage and is directly proportional to the severity of the disease. Staining is thus an excellent research tool.

Significant softening of the articular cartilage has been seen in dogs undergoing experimental stifle immobilization for 11 weeks.[10] Rabbit knees immobilized for 6 days underwent extensive loss of metachromatic staining.[11] Mobilization, therefore, is critical to the health of articular cartilage.

Diseases, injuries, or toxic agents affecting matrix or fibers result in changes that can be permanent, painful, and crippling. Understanding these mechanisms may elucidate a cure or reversal of these changes.

Healing of the Articular Cartilage

In normal situations, mitotic figures are not seen in the articular cartilage of adult animals. However, in lacerations to the articular cartilage or in osteoarthrosis, the chondrocyte can reinitiate DNA synthesis and cell division possibly by release of biological suppression of the replicatory apparatus.[6]

If lacerations in adult animals are confined to the upper layers of the avascular articular cartilage, no inflammation or effective healing can occur. Mitotic activity does occur but ceases 1 week after initial injury. In rabbits, these superficial lacerations neither healed nor progressed to more serious disorders within

1 year of injury. When lesions were deep and invaded the subchondral vascular bone, reparative granulation tissue invaded the defect, which then changed to fibrocartilage by metaplasia. The end result, years after injury, is a discolored, roughened pit surrounded by smooth hyaline cartilage.[6] Allowing this vascularity to reach the surface is the theoretical reason for curetting or drilling a defect that results from osteochondritis dissecans. Continuous passive motion[12,13] (where the animal is placed in a confining apparatus with the affected limb attached to a machine that moves the leg at preselected rates and ranges of motion for 2 to 4 weeks) has shed new light on articular cartilage healing. However, it remains to be seen if there are practical applications in veterinary medicine.

CARTILAGE AND JOINT ABNORMALITIES

Pain, deformity, and limb malfunction can result from improper joint physiology. Many acute joint conditions progress to chronic osteoarthrosis. The aim of the orthopedist is to minimize or stop these changes. In chronic osteoarthrosis, the objective is to minimize patient discomfort and improve limb function.

Definitions

ARTHRITIS ■ The simple definition of arthritis is inflammation of a joint. Many chronic orthopedic conditions in veterinary medicine do not have any long-lasting appreciable inflammatory component of the synovial lining. Therefore, the term "arthritis" is a misnomer but so ingrained in the general population that this term will unfortunately persist.

ARTHROSIS ■ The term arthrosis refers to a noninflammatory degenerative joint condition characterized by a lack of inflammation in the synovial lining and the presence of normal or near-normal synovial fluid.

OSTEOARTHRITIS (OSTEOARTHROSIS) ■ The common arthritis seen in veterinary medicine is a slowly progressive cartilage degeneration with osteophyte production usually caused by trauma or microtrauma (abnormal wear). There is very little inflammation of the synovial lining (and therefore few changes in the synovial fluid) compared with the more inflammatory joint diseases. The synovial response is the basis for classifying joint disease. Because it is degenerative and not inflammatory, a more proper term is osteoarthrosis, or degenerative joint disease (DJD).

Classification of Joint Disease

Joint diseases are classified in the following way[14]:

Noninflammatory Joint Disease
1. Degenerative joint disease (DJD), osteoarthritis, osteoarthrosis
   a. Primary
   b. Secondary
2. Traumatic
3. Neoplastic

Inflammatory Joint Disease
1. Infectious
2. Noninfectious
   a. Immunological
      (1). Erosive
      (2). Nonerosive

Noninflammatory Joint Disease

Osteoarthrosis

PRIMARY DEGENERATIVE JOINT DISEASE ■ Primary DJD is a degeneration of cartilage in elderly individuals occurring for no known reason other than the wear and tear that comes with aging. Mankin, however, points out that aged cartilage does not show the same changes as osteoarthrotic cartilage.[15] Consequently, contradictions in various histochemical and biochemical data exist because of the types of abnormal cartilage that are analyzed and not identified as to source.

Most people older than 40 years of age have some degree of degeneration in the hip, knee, or interphalangeal joints of the fingers (Heberden's nodes). Much interest in this phenomenon has been generated in human medicine. Animals are useful as research models for osteoarthrosis. Bentley has stated that a suitable model is valuable in facilitating further study of the pathogenesis of the disease and the effects of various treatments upon it.[16] The ideal model for DJD should start with the loss of cartilage matrix and should progress to fissuring, fibrillation, erosion of cartilage, subchondral sclerosis, osteophyte production, and mild synovial inflammation.

SECONDARY DEGENERATIVE JOINT DISEASE ■ Secondary DJD develops secondarily from known conditions that affect the joint and supporting structures. This is perhaps the most common type observed in small animals. Those conditions predisposing animals to secondary DJD are outlined by Pedersen[14] and appear in Table 6–2.

Degeneration of the Articular Cartilage

Bentley[16] states that the cartilage breakdown starts when compression or shear stresses cause cell damage, releasing cathepsin, which in turn induces loss of proteoglycans and water. This decreases cartilage resiliency and leaves collagen exposed so that fissuring (fibrillation) occurs. Additional chondrocyte damage then occurs, and additional cathepsin is released ad infinitum (Fig. 6–3).

Other investigators hypothesize that excessive wear occurs in this damaged cartilage with normal physical stresses and that the degradation products released into the joint space produce secondary synovitis and sometimes inflammation (hence, pain and effusion in acute flare-ups of a chronic situation). There are attempts at repair in the forms of granulation tissue, chondrocyte proliferation, clones, increased proteoglycan production, and osteophytes. However, with degradative enzymes, lack of orientation in regenerating tissue, and abnormal stress caused by these unstable joints, physiological repair attempts are usually negligible. Two instances, however, have been reported that may show some reversibility of osteoarthrosis.[17]

In a case of hip osteoarthrosis, devitalized tissue was removed and a metal device interposed between the acetabulum and femoral head. Imperfect hyaline

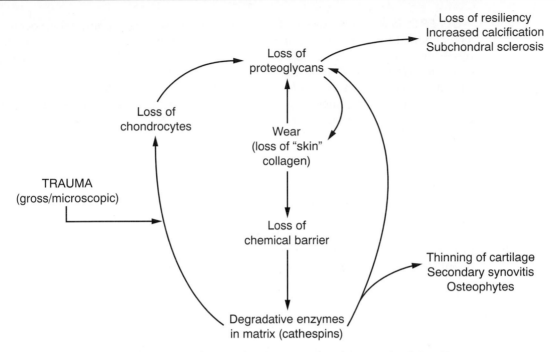

FIGURE 6-3. The vicious cycle of progressive degenerative joint disease.

articular cartilage formed under the prosthesis. The implication is that the prosthesis protected the reparative granulation tissue from mechanical abrasion.

In another case of osteoarthrosis of the hip, wedge osteotomies of the femur with reangulation of the femoral head were performed. Subsequently, radiographs showed regression of the osteoarthrosis.[17] Wilson stated that there was an increase in the joint space and more reformation of cartilage.[18]

CHANGES IN BONE

Two changes in bone occur in the presence of osteoarthrosis: the production of marginal osteophytes and the appearance of subchondral sclerosis.

OSTEOPHYTES ■   Marginal osteophytes may protrude into the joint or may develop within capsular structures or ligamentous attachments to joint margins. Their shape is determined by mechanical forces and the surface contour from which they protrude.[15] McDevitt and colleagues showed this to begin histologically 7 days after experimental rupture of the cranial cruciate ligament in dogs.[19] At first, there was an accumulation of fibroblast-like cells at the synovial membrane–articular cartilage junction, which by 4 weeks had changed to woven bone with a few chondrocytes. By 8 weeks, trabecular patterns were seen in the early osteophyte along with resorption of the femoral cortex underneath, allowing some communication of bone marrow from each area. By 16 weeks after the rupture, the osteophytes consisted of trabecular bone covered by thick cartilage. By 48 weeks, the trabeculae and marrow of the osteophyte and distal femur were confluent. Some investigators have proposed that hyperplasia of the cartilage margin is invaded by vascular granulation tissue with subsequent bone formation.[20] The reason for these osteophytes is unclear, and the theories are contradictory.[8,20–22]

SCLEROSIS ■   Under areas of cartilage erosion, sclerosis (eburnation) occurs. The denuded bone becomes polished and grossly resembles ivory or marble and represents advanced cartilage destruction. Turek believes that an early stage of this condition results from endochondral ossification of the lower layers of cartilage, which histologically are detected by double "tidemarks" (wavy hematoxylin-staining lines demarcating the interface between calcified and non-calcified hyaline cartilage).[22]

Changes in Synovial Membrane

The synovial membrane in degenerative joint disease generally appears normal. The surface may show some hyperplasia, but very little inflammatory response, except in certain forms of hip osteoarthritis in humans and large animals. With some partial cruciate ligament tears, however, we have noticed a red, proliferative synovial lining consistent with Griffen and Vasseur's suggestion that immune mechanisms may play a role in the development of spontaneous cruciate ligament rupture.[23]

Changes in Cartilage

Early gross changes in articular cartilage consist of a localized soft or velvety area that changes to a yellow to dull white color with pits, and with depressions and linear grooves becoming apparent. In advanced disease, the cartilage may be soft and spongy. In areas where subchondral bone is exposed and subjected to wear, a highly polished eburnated surface may be present. In joints with apposing articular surfaces, "kissing" or mirror-image lesions develop. Osteophytes develop at joint margins where the synovium reflects off the chondral-perichondral junction. Osteophytes sometimes form in an area not covered by synovium. Bone spurs that form outside joints where tendons insert are termed enthesiophytes.

HISTOLOGICAL ■   Collins has defined the histological progression of osteoarthrosis as follows[24]:

1. Loss of surface cartilage layers.
2. Diffuse increase in numbers of cells.
3. Moderate decrease in metachromatic staining, indicating loss of proteoglycans. In experimental sectioning of the cranial cruciate ligament in dogs, McDevitt[19] and associates found this loss 16 weeks after the rupture.
4. Ingrowth of subchondral vessels through the tidemark (the wavy hematoxylin-stained line demarcating the interface between calcified and noncalcified hyaline cartilage).
5. Vertical clefts beginning at the surface (flaking).
6. "Fibrillation" when clefts extend to the calcified zone.
7. Further loss of metachromatic staining.
8. Cloning or clumping of chondrocytes.
9. Focal areas of erosion down to the subchondral bone, leaving exposed sclerotic bone.
10. Subchondral cyst formation.
11. Patches of new cartilage seen over eroded areas and osteophytes.

The stages just enumerated are not always present and do not always occur in the order given. In some cases extensive erosions and eburnation occur without marginal osteophytes, whereas in other cases many osteophytes may be seen without appreciable change in the articular cartilage—such as in many spontaneous cruciate ligament ruptures in dogs. Dogs infrequently have subchondral cyst formation.

BIOCHEMICAL ■ In osteoarthrotic cartilage, collagen is renewed with a different type of collagen that is larger in diameter than the type found in skin and bone. The synthesis of protein and glycosaminoglycans is markedly increased—although the total quantity found is decreased—and is proportional to the disease severity in mild or moderate cases. In severe cases, there is a failure of this reparative process. This irreversibility suggests that treatment should be instituted at a relatively early stage of the disorder while there is still a capability of providing cells and matrix for repair of minimal to moderate defects.[25] Lacerations and chemical lesions do not show this reparative reaction. It may be feasible to treat lesions of cartilage with agents that decrease enzymatic degradation or with materials that could enhance repair (salicylates, uridine diphosphates).[25]

The interchange between the terms "osteoarthrosis" and "degenerative joint disease" are somewhat confusing at times. Human orthopedists frequently stress the decreased thickness of articular cartilage (with decreased joint space and sclerosis seen upon radiography), while small animal clinicians usually are referring to marginal osteophytes. Often with cruciate rupture, severe osteophytosis may occur and yet the articular surfaces look fairly normal rather than yellow, pitted, or eburnated. This joint performs better than when the cartilage is lost. Joint replacement in humans is considered with the surface articular cartilage is gone. Judging the severity of the arthritis based solely on osteophytes may be incorrect.

Clinical Signs

Osteoarthrosis in Humans

Because subjective patient descriptions are lacking in veterinary medicine, the clinical signs and symptoms of osteoarthrosis in people will be reviewed.[26]

PAIN ■ The prominent sign is pain that occurs upon use of the part and that is relieved by rest. The pain is usually described as aching and poorly localized. With more advanced cases, pain may occur with minimal activity or even at rest. At times, it may awaken a person after tossing and turning during sleep owing to loss of joint "splinting," which limits painful motion during the waking hours. Pain may be exacerbated by changes in the weather, such as temperature, humidity, and barometric pressure.

The origin of this pain may arise from several areas:

1. Elevation of normally sensitive periosteum due to marginal osteophytes.
2. Pressure on exposed subchondral bone.
3. Trabecular microfracture.
4. Pinching or abrasion of synovial villi.
5. Mild synovitis.
6. Capsular inflammation.

According to Gardner, pain in capsules and ligaments is stimulated by twisting or stretching.[27] There are pain fibers in the capsule and ligaments but few in the synovium. However, there are pain fibers in the adventitia of blood vessels supplying these areas. Gardner theorizes that increased sensitivity during weather changes is due to reflex blood flow to the area of joints; in addition, the pain may be referred from one area of the limb to another as a result of reflex spasms of the flexor muscles.

Pain is often nonexistent in osteoarthrosis. In one study, only 30 percent of people with radiographic or pathological evidence of osteoarthrosis had any symptoms.[26] Generally, when there were symptoms, there was little correlation between degree of pathology and severity of pain.

STIFFNESS ■ Stiffness upon arising from a resting position is common and usually lasts less than 15 minutes. The stiffness is due to a change in the elasticity of periarticular structures. Loss of joint range of motion (ROM) may be due to joint surface incongruity, muscle spasm and contracture, capsular contraction, or mechanical block from osteophytes or joint mice.

CREPITATION ■ Upon palpation, the human joint may show localized tenderness. Pain elicited by passive motion may be prominent. Joint crepitation (grating, crackling) from erosion or incongruity may be palpated; however, normal joint cracking or snapping is believed to be a slipping of tendons or ligaments over a bony prominence when the joint is flexed. The examiner may note loss of ROM. Bony ankylosis (fusion) of joints is very uncommon with osteoarthrosis. The joint may be swollen because of synovial reaction, increased joint fluid, or the presence of osteophytes. While not a true crepitus, the noise that is made when knuckles can be "cracked" is due to a negative resting pressure (-4 mm Hg) that becomes more negative (over -117 mm Hg) with distraction forces. This causes gas to go out of solution, resulting in a "crack."[28]

OBESITY ■ It is still unresolved whether obesity is a contributing causative factor in osteoarthrosis.[26] Logically, it appears that a heavier weight would mechanically abrade a damaged joint more quickly. In mice with a genetic predisposition for primary degenerative joint disease, obesity did not alter the course of the disease. Epidemiological studies in humans, however, indicate that osteoarthrosis is more common in obese, rather than nonobese, individuals. In one study[29] of 105 obese (50 kg or more) patients with chronic musculoskeletal pain, significant weight reduction was achieved by surgery on the stomach. Eighty-nine percent of patients had complete relief of pain in one or more joints. Two patients regained their weight and their pain as well.

OSTEOARTHROSIS IN DOGS

Most of our experience with osteoarthrosis deals with the dog; the cat rarely has osteoarthrosis except after obvious injury. Hip dysplasia has been diagnosed sporadically in cats.[30] In the dog or cat osteoarthrosis is usually not idiopathic or primary. It is usually secondary to trauma, unstable joints, malalignment or conformation defects, or congenital conditions such as osteochondritis dissecans and hip dysplasia. Exceptions may occur in very old or obese dogs. The clinician should try to discover the cause of the arthrosis in order to intervene in situations where treatment may decrease the amount of discomfort and future osteoarthrosis an animal will have.

PAIN ■ A discussion of pain is noteworthy, since our clients usually complain that their pet is in pain, or they may ask whether the animal is in pain when known osteoarthrosis exists. First of all, many dogs, as with some people, are stoic and do not let their pain bother them. Since they cannot tell us they are in pain and even though they may not cry or yelp, it is difficult to advise an owner whether an osteoarthrotic animal is experiencing pain, especially since we know that human patients with osteoarthrosis are commonly without pain.

An example of stoicism in a dog occurs in the event of fresh fractures. Many times, a dog will allow gentle palpation, radiographic positioning, and body movement without wincing, cringing, gasping, crying, yelping, or biting. Is this dog in pain? The answer is believed to be yes.

Another finding is that excitement or nervousness may override the dog's sensitivity to pain. For example, a client may say, "He limps all day except when he goes out chasing rabbits"; or lameness may disappear as the pet approaches the veterinary environment.

The most prominent sign of limb pain with osteoarthrosis is lameness. Limping or unusual gait can occur with other conditions, such as shortened limb (without pain), mechanical dysfunction (i.e., patellar ectopia, contracture of the infraspinatus muscle), a stiff leg (usually from previous fracture), neurological problems, or neuromuscular weakness. After examination of the limb, shortening or mechanical problems can be eliminated. Limping, then, is usually caused by pain. This is contradictory to a client's comment that the limping dog "doesn't seem to be in any pain." Clients fail to understand that dogs are more tolerant and less vocal than humans.

Other signs of pain—besides crying out, yelping, sensitivity upon palpation, and favoring a limb—include loss of tolerance to exercise and reluctance to play, jump on furniture, or go up and down stairs. When rear legs are involved, the dog may "bunny hop," take short, mincing steps, sit with the painful leg cocked to the side rather than underneath the body, or show pacing, irritability (especially with children), and personality change. When the owner or veterinarian has judged that the dog has a "shoulder" or "hip" lameness, the clinician must keep an open mind. In our experience, locating the source of pain based upon gait observation is difficult. The astute clinician should not make preconceived diagnoses based upon other opinions.

Pain elicited upon palpation is variable. Many dogs with known osteoarthrosis of a joint will not react to palpation. Identifying the area where pain has been elicited can be challenging at times. It is difficult to isolate and move one joint without moving other tissues or without pressing on a sensitive area during the manipulation. For example, a young dog has panosteitis of the radius or ulna, the area may be grasped tightly while the shoulder joint is examined. When the dog cringes, the examiner is thinking about the shoulder joint and forgets that the elbow is extended and the forearm tissues are compressed.

The osteoarthrotic dog is similar to humans in regard to the pain worsening with cold, damp weather or a change in physical activity. This altered physical activity may include taking longer walks or runs than usual; slipping on ice and stretching contracted tendons, joint capsules, and other parts; or climbing stairs that have not been part of the daily routine. Although pain may be increased, it usually does not persist for more than a week or two. If it does, the clinician should be alerted to further problems (e.g., a ruptured cranial cruciate ligament with hip dysplasia, fracture of osteophytes, further progression of pathology—such as meniscal damage occurring with chronic cruciate ligament disease). However, some chronically osteoarthrotic dogs progress to the stage where lameness or pain is continual.

The fact that in humans the radiographic signs may not correlate with the severity of the symptoms may help the veterinary clinician understand why a dog with severe osteoarthrosis of the hips may act totally normal without clinical signs, or why the dog may be more lame on the less arthritic hip, as shown by radiography.

A few comments concerning the theorized origin of pain from osteoarthrosis are in order. If osteophytes stretch sensitive periosteum, does debridement of these proliferations alone help the patient? Experimental data are lacking. If reflex muscle spasms from osteoarthrosis accentuate pain in people, can this be one of the benefits of pectinotomy for hip dysplasia in dogs? In cranial cruciate ligament rupture or partial rupture, the synovium is frequently reddened and corrugated. Can synovectomy in dogs relieve pain by eliminating hypertrophied synovial villi that can become pinched or contain immune complexes?

STIFFNESS ■ Upon arising from a resting state, an arthritic dog experiences stiffness. As with people, in earlier stages, this stiffness disappears as dogs "warm out of it." As time goes by, this stiffness may become continual as fibrosis and decreased joint ROM occur. Decreased ROM is not as common or as great as in people, probably because of increased use a dog would have compared with a person, whose pain threshold is probably lower.

CREPITATION ■ Crepitation is palpated on dogs with severe osteoarthrosis. The examiner must be careful at times in determining the source of crepitation since, if great, it can resound throughout the limb. If the stifle is palpated and crepitation originates from the hip, the examiner may get the impression that the stifle is the origin of the crepitation. Sutures beneath the skin from previous surgery may also give a feeling of crepitation; however, this sensation will be of a quality different from the kind that comes from bone rubbing on bone.

OBESITY ■ The question of whether obesity contributes to the development of osteoarthrosis is pertinent in veterinary medicine. Most arthritic dogs that we see are overweight. Common sense tells us that extra stress on the joint contributes to abrading and degenerating cartilage more quickly. For instance, hypernourished puppies with hip dysplasia potential have shown more degenerative joint disease than those whose diets were restricted;[31] however, this does not indicate that the diet was the cause of hip dysplasia. In cases of ruptured cruciate ligaments, our clinical impression is that larger dogs develop osteophytes more quickly than smaller dogs. This may also be related to the fact that smaller dogs may "carry" or favor the leg, thus resulting in less damage from weight bearing. In some cases, dogs with chronic pain from osteoarthrosis seem to improve with weight reduction alone.

AGE ■ Osteoarthrosis rarely is seen (radiographically or pathologically) in very immature animals, as compared with adults, except for cartilage diseases such as Legg-Calvé-Perthes or osteochondrosis. For example, a mature, large dog with cruciate disease would begin to develop osteophytes within 7 to 10 days after the rupture. Although the literature is sparse concerning natural rupture in young dogs, a few cases have been seen in which young dogs with chronic lameness (i.e., 2 months or more) associated with cruciate disease do not have remarkable cartilage change.

Treatment

The best treatment for osteoarthrosis is prevention. When a known disease condition is present in which a potential for osteoarthrosis exists, the clinician should advise corrective measures or environmental changes to lessen the problem (e.g., surgery for cruciate ligament rupture, diet for overweight dogs with hip dysplasia, and slinging for early Legg-Calvé-Perthes disease of the femoral head). It is interesting to note that Murray states that excessive athletic activity in children is likely an important cause (especially in males) of subsequent degenerative joint disease of the hip.[32] This contradicts those veterinarians and owners who believe that young dogs with hip dysplasia or with a potential for hip dysplasia should be heavily exercised to develop muscle mass and prevent or minimize osteoarthrosis.

OBJECTIVES

The objectives of treatment for osteoarthrosis in animals are to relieve pain, to maintain function and range of motion (unless undertaking arthrodesis), and to maintain or regain normal activity.

NONSURGICAL METHODS

REST ■   During flare-ups of osteoarthrosis, mild inflammation exists as debris is being absorbed and removed by the synovium. Weight-bearing activities tend to aggravate and prolong this inflammation. Rest includes short leashed walks, and the elimination of running and jumping. Total disuse, however, may lead to excessive muscle atrophy and joint stiffness. In most animals, total limb inactivity is unusual. If inactivity seems to be a problem, gentle passive ROM exercises may be warranted. When the animal is overusing a joint affected by early osteoarthrosis or in cases of early traumatic arthroses, coaptation splints, casts, or slings for 2 to 3 weeks may be useful.

HEAT ■   Heat is very beneficial in relieving muscle spasm and pain. This may be accomplished by soaking a facecloth or towel in fairly warm water and applying it around the joint for 10 minutes, two to three times per day. Therapeutic ultrasound is an effective method of applying heat in animals. The dose range depends on the depth of penetration desired and ranges from 5 to 10 watts (total dose) twice daily for 5 to 10 days. In acute joint injuries, however, cold rather than heat is indicated to decrease pain, swelling, and hematoma formation.

EXERCISE ■   Our usual recommendation concerning degree of exercise is rest during acute flare-ups and moderate self-regulated activity during remission. Encouraging an animal to overexert behind a bike or car or on an exercise treadmill is not advised. A dog will often not "feel" (until later) its limitations when excited to please an owner, chase a rabbit, or follow another dog in a race. Swimming is an excellent exercise for osteoarthrosis of joints since non–weight-bearing ROM exercise decreases joint capsule adhesions. If the animal has an athletic function (hunting, performance), permanent reduction of strenuous activity may have to be instituted to achieve a good quality of life for the pet.

MEDICATION ■   Most medications do nothing to reverse osteoarthrosis. By eliminating the animal's own defense mechanism (pain), overexertion and aggravation of joint degeneration are possible. Therefore, any pain-killing drugs administered should be accompanied by rest. Medication should be used only if needed as determined by the animal's discomfort or decreased function, not by radiographs. The use of medication may also eliminate the owner's concern about pain and may thus delay diagnosis and proper management of some orthopedic conditions (e.g., osteochondritis dissecans of the elbow and shoulder and cruciate ligament instability). Buffered aspirin (5 grains twice a day for a 25- to 40-pound dog) or aspirin with Maalox is the first drug of choice, since it is effective, free from most side effects, inexpensive and readily available in the home. If vomiting occurs, feeding prior to aspirin administration is often helpful.

The mechanisms of aspirin and aspirin-like drugs (acetaminophen, phenylbutazone, meclofenamic acid) are not totally known. The most recent tenable theory is that these agents inhibit the synthesis of prostaglandins, which are important mediators of inflammation. Aspirin has been shown to have a protective effect against the degeneration of articular cartilage,[33,34] while others state that aspirin and other nonsteroidal anti-inflammatory drugs (NSAIDs) may decrease proteoglycan synthesis.[34] Other substances such as phenylbutazone, selenium, vitamin E, orgotein, and meclofenamic acid have been used with varying success. Meclofenamic acid (Arquel, Ft. Dodge, Inc., Ft. Dodge, IA) has been used successfully in dogs at a dose of 0.5 to 1 mg/lb daily or every other day. It is now available in pill form but the owner should be cautioned that an occasional dog may develop a hemorrhagic diarrhea necessitating stoppage or dose modification. Other NSAIDs used in humans are often toxic in dogs (acetaminophen, indomethacin, ibuprofen) and should not be used.

Corticosteroids are frequently used by clinical veterinarians to treat lameness. Although short-term use is tolerated, long-term systemic use has undesirable systemic mineralocorticoid effects. Intra-articular corticosteroids repeatedly given to rabbits have been shown to decrease synthesis of proteoglycans and therefore hasten a type of cartilage destruction resembling chondromalacia.[6] This condition may lead to a Charcot-like joint[33] (see Neurectomy section, below). Corticosteroids, if used, should be given only occasionally and accompanied by rest for 2 to 3 weeks. In general, a continuing regimen of corticosteroids for arthritis should be used only as a last resort. Fortunately, cats infrequently need chronic pain medication. They are, however, more resistant to the various side effects of exogenous corticosteroids than are dogs and humans.[35] As with other animals, the reduction in pain caused by medications should be accompanied by rest.

The recent use of polysulfated glycosaminoglycans (PSGAG) (Adequan, Luitpold Pharmaceuticals, Inc., Shirley, NY) by practitioners has yielded many positive anecdotal results for treating arthritic syndromes. It is believed to be chondroprotective and possibly anti-inflammatory. However, controlled clinical and research studies utilizing animals and in vitro methods have had conflicting results. When given prior to the onset of arthritis after experimental meniscectomy in dogs,[36] PSGAG protected the articular cartilage from degenerative change compared to controls. While it stimulated production of proteoglycan in human cell cultures of chondrocytes,[37] it decreased proteoglycan production explant cell cultures derived from equine osteoarthritic cartilage.[38] In dogs with clinical signs of hip dysplasia, there was no statistical difference in clinical improvement with three different intramuscular doses and the placebo control.[39] To date this drug has not been approved for dogs and cats. The only known adverse effect in dogs is inhibition of coagulation test profiles, and it should be used with caution in dogs with bleeding disorders, or those being treated with drugs known to affect coagulation (e.g., aspirin). At this time, it appears PSGAG may be more beneficial in prophylaxis than in the treatment of advanced osteoarthrosis.[40]

Newer medications for osteoarthrosis in people aim to decrease joint stiffness. Stiffness is due to new collagen formation in joint capsules that has unstable intermolecular covalent bonds. In normal mature collagen, these bonds are not reducible biochemically, but new or pathological collagen can lose its strength completely when broken down by drugs such as penicillamine. Its practical use in animals is unknown. Other medications are aimed at increasing proteogly-cans (e.g., uridine diphosphate in rabbits[25]), decreasing its degradation, replacing proteoglycans with synthetic analogs, or increasing the limited healing properties of articular cartilage. These drugs are on the horizon.

DIET ■ Although it has not been conclusively proven that obesity causes osteoarthrosis, common sense and positive clinical results lead us to recommend weight loss in overweight animals. Weight reduction alone has been very effective for some animals in reducing pain from osteoarthrosis.

SURGICAL METHODS

Surgery for osteoarthrosis should be considered where pain or function is not helped by reasonable conservative measures. Operations include debridement of osteophytes and joint surfaces, soft tissue or muscle release, arthrodesis (bony fusion of a joint), arthroplasty, osteotomy, pseudoarthrosis, neurectomy, and limb amputation.

DEBRIDEMENT ■ The removal of osteophytes may decrease the "tugging" on the joint capsule and therefore prevent pain, although the real efficacy is unknown. Regrowth of osteophytes may occur, especially if the inciting cause (e.g., instability) is not corrected. Removal of fractured osteophytes has also provided some pain relief in elbow, shoulder, and stifle joint osteoarthrosis. Debridement of joint mice, cartilage flaps, proliferative synovium, or degenerative ligaments is also performed. Debridement is often used in conjunction with other procedures. Smoothing joint surfaces may enhance joint congruency and improve stability and joint fluid lubrication.

MUSCLE RELEASE ■ A prime example of helping pain and function involves cutting the pectineus muscle or tendon in canine hip dysplasia. The exact effect is uncertain, but improvement may be due to destroying a painful spastic muscle, decreasing the forces between the painful femoral head and acetabulum, or reangulating an eroded area in the coxofemoral joint to allow weight bearing on a less damaged area of cartilage.

ARTHRODESIS ■ Fusion of the carpal and tarsal regions is a fairly common procedure in dogs and is effective in relieving instability and pain. The canine limb functions satisfactorily with these fusions. Shoulder, elbow, and stifle fusions are attempted less often; they have a slightly greater chance of fusion failure, and greater gait impairment results than with fusions in the more distal areas. When arthrodesis is performed properly, however, a remarkable degree of function is obtained. At times amputation results in a better ambulation function for the animal but is often unpalatable for the owners.

ARTHROPLASTY ■ Arthroplasty means any plastic or surgical reconstruction of a joint. A synovectomy may fall into this category.[41] It is helpful in synovial chondrometaplasia and early cases of rheumatoid arthritis as well. Total hip replacement is another example of an arthroplastic procedure. This is now a fairly common procedure in small animal referral centers. Other prosthetic joints are not commercially available at present.

OSTEOTOMY ■ In humans, wedge osteotomy on the proximal femur is an older, accepted treatment for coxofemoral arthritis. The reangulated femoral head is nailed or plated in a more varus precalculated position, which brings immediate relief of pain and can increase the joint space radiographically as some reformation of surface cartilage occurs.[18] Wilson stated that simply breaking the bones is what brings relief, possibly owing to a decongestive effect by altered venous drainage; mere trochanteric osteotomy without altering the femoral angle also gave immediate pain relief.[18] It was not clear whether reformation of cartilage is possible. With unicompartmental osteoarthrosis of the knee in people, tibial osteotomy is successfully used. In small animals, however, most osteoarthrosis involves the entire joint and is an impractical option.

Bentley produced osteoarthrosis in rabbits by injecting papain into coxofemoral joints.[16] He then studied the effects 3 and 6 months after osteotomy. Results showed an increased blood supply to the femoral head and acetabulum, increased bone formation in the femoral head, and increased marrow activity. These changes can cause the clearance of bone cysts and subchondral sclerosis. The subchondral marrow cells produce fibrocartilage, and, coupled with a more favorable redistribution of forces in the hip, a continuous surface layer is reformed.

Wedge osteotomy of the proximal femur of dysplastic dogs has been performed in North America after having been used with encouraging results in Switzerland.[42] Our experience is that, although dogs are helped clinically, osteoarthrosis is still progressive.[43] Pelvic osteotomy (see Chapter 15) is another example of an osteotomy usually used to prevent osteoarthrosis rather than to treat osteoarthrosis.

PSEUDOARTHROSIS ■   A good example of pseudoarthrosis is resection of the femoral head and neck in dogs and cats. It is a simple, effective technique for relieving pain in dogs and cats. With congenital luxation of the radial head in dogs' elbows, resection has resulted in good limb function. Pseudoarthrosis can also be useful for treating problems with the digits, if necessary.

NEURECTOMY ■   Sectioning a sensory nerve to relieve pain has been used in large animals but not in companion animals. The diffuse nerve supply to an area is one reason why neurectomy may fail in dogs. In humans lacking nerve supply to a joint (Charcot's joint, often caused by syphilis or diabetes), joint destruction is massive as a result of the absence of normal body responses in protecting a painful area.[22] Pursuing therapies along this line seems unwarranted.

AMPUTATION ■   A final treatment that should be avoided but considered is amputation of a limb or toe. In a few instances, however, such as a chronically infected, destroyed joint caused by a resistant organism, or where arthrodesis would result in a severe mechanical gait impairment, amputation may be in the patient's best interest.

In conclusion, treatment of osteoarthrosis should include a proper balance of client instruction, moderate medication, and surgery if applicable.

Traumatic Joint Disease

Obvious traumatic joint conditions involve dislocation (luxation), instability from ligamentous disruption, and fracture. They are categorized under acquired degenerative joint disease. There are some general guidelines for selecting a rational treatment.

Dislocation (Luxation)

Dislocations result in obvious mechanical dysfunction. Normal nourishment and lubrication of the articular cartilage are lacking, and weight bearing on incongruent surfaces leads to further traumatic injury to the cartilage surfaces. In some instances, open reduction is less traumatic than prolonged abortive attempts at closed reduction (e.g., an elbow that has been dislocated 5 or more days). Therefore, gentle closed reduction should be attempted as soon as possible before muscle spasticity prevents easy relocation or before the animal tries to bear weight too soon on an unstable joint. Most joints should be immobilized from 1 to 4 weeks after reduction, depending on the degree of instability remaining after reduction. A relocated elbow may not need any support, whereas a relocated hock may require 4 weeks of support. When the joint is so unstable that immobilization will not maintain reduction, then some form of internal stabilization may be needed, such as capsular or ligament repair, pinning across joints, and other techniques that assist the coaptational support.

Fracture

A fracture through a joint is obviously serious when it affects a major movable joint. The hip, stifle, and elbow joints are most frequently involved. The aim of repair is to reduce the fracture line perfectly in order to decrease incongruency and subsequent degree of osteoarthrosis. Another objective in surgery is to stabilize fractures well enough to allow early weight bearing, which helps decrease joint stiffness and maintain range of motion. In general, pins, wires, and screws should not be placed through articular cartilage unless absolutely necessary. If so, non–weight-bearing areas of cartilage should be selected if a choice is possible.

Instability

Instability from ligament rupture often involves the stifle joint. The ligament or its function should be repaired as soon as possible so that instability does not cause osteophytes, erosion, or possible discomfort from the resulting arthritis. Instability seen with congenital laxity, such as in hip dysplasia or patellar luxation, causes microtrauma of articular surfaces, deformity of bony contours, eventual erosion of cartilage surfaces, and osteoarthrosis. Simple "reefing" or imbrication of the joint capsule does not result in a permanent stability in these hips or patellas, in luxating patellas, or in cruciate rupture instability.

Thus, early repair of joint injuries is indicated to minimize the irreversible changes that may occur. Usually some osteoarthritis will form, and the surgeon attempts to minimize these changes so that the animal may lead a comfortable life. With cruciate ligament rupture, the client should be advised, however, that the joint will never be as normal as it was prior to injury, in spite of the best effort made. This may change the performance of a working dog. When performance has to be maximum (e.g., in police, tracking, or sled dogs), the dog's function in life may have to be changed. There have been cases, however, in which strenuous activities were resumed and the animal performed well.

Neoplastic Joint Disease

Neoplasms in joints are rare. From 1952 to 1978, there were only 29 cases in dogs and three in cats reported in the literature.[44] Primary tumors are termed synoviomas, synovial sarcomas, or giant cell tumors. These tumors are characterized by slow-growing swellings about a joint that occasionally cause pain upon joint movement. Initially upon radiography, only a soft tissue mass may be seen. There may be calcium deposits within the soft tissue. Later there is destruction of the adjacent cortical bone followed by cancellous bone destruction. The tumor may appear encapsulated, but often there are extensions into fascial planes and surrounding tissues, resulting in a high rate of recurrence following extirpation.[44]

Wide surgical resection is advisable. Postoperative radiation therapy results in the dogs are unknown. In humans, there is a decreased frequency of local recurrence following postoperative radiation. If recurrences appear, amputation may be the best course to follow.

Inflammatory Joint Disease

Inflammatory joint diseases caused by infection or immunological factors are not rare in pet practice, but they occur infrequently. These conditions are characterized by inflammation of the synovial membrane with resultant changes in the synovial fluid (Table 6–3).[14] Lameness and gait impairment are the signs seen most frequently. Systemic signs may include fever, lethargy, anorexia, and leukocytosis. In-depth discussion of systemic inflammatory joint disease is beyond the scope of this text and readers are referred to internal medicine textbooks for more detailed information.[45]

Infectious Disease

Arthritis

Joint infections are usually caused by bacteria that enter the joint either by way of penetrating wounds or by way of the bloodstream. Fortunately, these instances are rare, but when an infection occurs, it can be devastating to the joint. Our experience with pets (other than neonates) differs from that of other investigators[14] in that joint infections usually have been caused by external wounds (e.g., surgery, gunshot, abrasions, lacerations). The severity of joint destruction depends on the type of bacteria and the duration of infection. *Corynebacterium pyogenes* infection causes severe pannus formation (granulation) over cartilaginous surfaces, whereas *Clostridium* species can elaborate collagenase. *Streptococcus* and *Staphylococcus* produce kinases that activate plasminogen and result in plasmin, which removes chondroprotein from cartilage matrix. All these infections result in severe and widespread cartilage damage. Other bacteria may not produce destructive enzymes and widespread permanent damage may not occur.

SIGNS ■ Pain and lameness are consistent findings. The joint is swollen, warm, and tender upon palpation. If the soft tissue trauma is extensive, the former signs may be present without infection.

TABLE 6–3. SYNOVIAL FLUID CHANGES IN VARIOUS TYPES OF CANINE ARTHRITIS*

Condition	Nucleated Cells/cu mm	Differential	
		Mononuclear	Neutrophils
Normal	250–3000	94–100	0–6
Degenerative joint disease	1000–5000	88–100	0–12
Erosive arthritis (rheumatoid-like)	8000–38,000	20–80	20–80
Nonerosive arthritis (all types)	4400–371,000	5–85	15–95
Septic arthritis	40,000–267,000	1–10	90–99

*From Pedersen NC: Canine joint disease. In 1978 Scientific Proceedings, 45th Annual Meeting of the American Animal Hospital Association, 1978, p 365, with permission.

DIAGNOSIS ■ It is expedient to perform synovial fluid analysis and Wright's staining of the centrifuged exudate. This staining technique is more helpful than a Gram's stain in picking up the presence of bacteria. Culture and sensitivity of this fluid are mandatory, although synovial biopsy culture is better. Early radiographs may show capsular distension, and subchondral lysis may appear later. Bacteria readily attach to the synovium. Therefore, it may be well to massage and "pump" the joint prior to joint tap so that the bacteria may be liberated into the fluid.

TREATMENT ■ In acute joint infections, treatment should be undertaken immediately. The exudate should be evacuated (by aspiration or by arthrotomy), the synovium cultured, the fluid smeared on a slide, and Wright's stain applied. High levels of appropriate antibiotics, depending on the results of the smear, are given systemically. However, antibiotics given before the culture is taken may prevent bacterial growth of the culture. Antibiotics should be given before the culture and sensitivity results are reported because of the disaster that may result if protection had been withheld for the few days during which test results are being anticipated. Choice of antibiotics may be changed when the sensitivity results are known. Penicillin G in high doses (30,000 IU/lb twice a day) is good to start with. Ampicillin and the cephalosporins are also useful. These antibiotics should be continued from 2 to 4 weeks.

Early infections (within the first 24 to 48 hours) may respond to joint aspiration and systemic antibiotics without arthrotomy. Arthrotomy, however, allows debridement of necrotic material, removal of fibrin clots, which may serve as a nidus for infection, and subtotal synovectomy if joint motion is restricted by the thickened joint capsule encroaching on the articular cartilage. Local instillation of antibiotics is contraindicated for two reasons: Systemic antibiotics achieve adequate levels in the joint; and chemical synovitis may be created, thereby enhancing the inflammation.[46]

Initially, the joint should be supported by a soft splint or bandage to reduce pain and inflammation. When clinical signs regress, gentle ROM exercise and minimal weight bearing may be allowed. If the joint is destroyed, arthrodesis may be indicated after the infection clears.

Noninfectious Diseases

Immunological Joint Disease

Joint conditions believed to be the result of the immune mechanism can be divided into those that erode cartilage (rheumatoid arthritis) and those that do not (systemic lupus erythematosus). These conditions are becoming better known in veterinary medicine as the literature describing clinical cases and our diagnostic tools expand. Most of our knowledge comes from human medicine, where these diseases are common and potentially crippling or life threatening.

Erosive Inflammatory Disease

RHEUMATOID ARTHRITIS ■ Rheumatoid arthritis is defined as a severe, often progressive, polyarthritis of unknown etiology. It was first described in the dog in 1969,[47] and other cases have been described since.[45,48–49]

Pathogenesis ■ The exact pathogenesis is unknown but has been summarized as follows.[50] Endogenous IgG protein becomes altered for some unknown reason and stimulates IgG and IgM antibodies (called rheumatoid factors), which then combine to form immune complexes in the joint. These complexes activate the complement sequence, resulting in leukotaxis. Leukocytes phagocytize the immune complexes, thereby releasing lysosomal enzymes that alter the components of the joint. These enzymes contain collagenase; cathepsins, which disrupt basement membranes; and proteases, which can cleave glycoproteins.[51] The more prolonged the synovitis, the more prominent the joint damage.[52] This succession of events is the basis for using anti-inflammatory drugs. Surgical synovectomy[53] removes the immune complexes and can be effective in humans if it is performed early.

Signs and Symptoms ■   The clinical signs and course of the disease may vary, as they do in humans. Depression, fever, and anorexia may occur with or without lameness. Joint swelling may be subtle or obvious. Often, more than one joint may be affected. With severe and chronic involvement, cartilage erosion may be detected by palpating crepitation. Erosions may be explained by the proliferative granulation tissue arising from the synovium, which crosses the articular surface (pannus) or invades the subchondral bone at the synovial attachments. Erosions in cartilage not covered by pannus may be caused by granulation tissue arising from the epiphyseal marrow, which erodes the subchondral bone.[54] Joint instability of the carpus and tarsus may be apparent while the dog is ambulatory. Drawer movement from stretching or tearing the cruciate ligaments may be palpated. Toes may dislocate. Spontaneous exacerbations and remissions occur.

Diagnosis ■   The diagnosis of rheumatoid arthritis is not provable. In humans, there is no pathognomonic characteristic or test. The American Rheumatism Association has established 7 criteria (Table 6–4),[55] and a definitive diagnosis is made if a patient shows at least 4 of 7 characteristics. Subcutaneous nodules (criterion 5) have not been reported in the dog.

The rheumatoid factor test in humans yields false-positive and false-negative results. The latex particle rheumatoid factor test using human IgG as performed in clinical laboratories has given poor results in the dog.[56] In institutions using

TABLE 6–4.   DIAGNOSTIC CRITERIA FOR RHEUMATOID ARTHRITIS*

Criterion	Definition
1. Morning stiffness	Morning stiffness in and around the joints, lasting at least 1 hour before maximal improvement
2. Arthritis of 3 or more joint areas	At least 3 joint areas simultaneously have had soft tissue swelling or fluid (not bony overgrowth alone) observed by a physician. The 14 possible areas are right or left PIP, MCP, wrist, elbow, knee, ankle, and MTP joints
3. Arthritis of hand joints	At least 1 area swollen (as defined above) in a wrist, MCP, or PIP joint
4. Symmetric arthritis	Simultaneous involvement of the same joint areas (as defined in 2) on both sides of the body (bilateral involvement of PIPs, MCPs, or MTPs is acceptable without absolute symmetry)
5. Rheumatoid nodules	Subcutaneous nodules, over bony prominences, or extensor surfaces, or in juxtaarticular regions observed by a physician
6. Serum rheumatoid factor	Demonstration of abnormal amounts of serum rheumatoid factor by any method for which the result has been positive in <35% of normal control subjects
7. Radiographic changes	Radiographic changes typical of rheumatoid arthritis on posteroanterior hand and wrist radiographs, which must include erosions or unequivocal bony decalcification localized in or most marked adjacent to the involved joints (osteoarthritis changes alone do not qualify)

For classification purposes, a patient shall be said to have rheumatoid arthritis if he/she has satisfied at least 4 of these 7 criteria. Criteria 1 through 4 must have been present for at least 6 weeks. Patients with 2 clinical diagnoses are not excluded. Designation as classic, definite, or probable rheumatoid arthritis is not to be made.

*From Primer on the Rheumatic Diseases, 10th ed. Atlanta, American Rheumatism Association, The Arthritis Foundation, 1993.

canine antigen, if the titer is high and other clinical signs are compatible with rheumatoid arthritis, a presumptive diagnosis of rheumatoid arthritis can be made because there are not too many diseases that can cross react. A negative rheumatoid factor test, however, does not exclude the diagnosis. Synovial histopathology reveals lymphoid and plasma infiltrates and is very nonspecific.

Radiographic changes occurring in this disease can include soft tissue swelling, increased joint fluid, decreased joint space, and lytic areas in the subchondral bone and juxta-articular bone. Disuse osteoporosis appears at a later stage, and osteophytes form when instability occurs. The joint space decreases as cartilage becomes thinner, and it is seen especially in the carpal and tarsal joints.

In one report,[48] four of ten cases of rheumatoid arthritis occurred in the Shetland sheepdog. In our experience, the Shetland sheepdog and collie have been prone to this condition. Often, the presenting signs are breakdown of the ligaments and tendinous support of the carpus or tarsus. Minimal trauma (e.g., fighting or jumping out of a truck) may have made the owner suddenly aware of the lameness or joint angulation. The cartilage change seen on radiographs (i.e., lysis) or arthrotomy may be minimal. The inflammatory response may cause necrosis within bundles of collagen, leading to weakening and rupture of tendons and ligaments.[45,57]

Joint infections may be difficult to differentiate from rheumatoid arthritis. History and clinical course help to distinguish the two.

Other inflammatory diseases have joint fluid analyses as well as systemic signs similar to those characteristic of rheumatoid arthritis. In bacterial endocarditis, there may be a heart murmur, electrocardiographic changes, and little erosion of the cartilage. Systemic lupus erythematosus (SLE) may be difficult to distinguish from rheumatoid arthritis in the early stages. SLE does not tend to cause erosions of cartilage, and it can have a high antinuclear antibody (ANA) titer.

Other diseases that may mimic clinical signs of rheumatoid arthritis include traumatic arthritis and degenerative joint disease. History of sudden onset and the fact that only one joint may be involved help to distinguish these from rheumatoid arthritis. Usually, synovial fluid analysis is valuable. Shifting leg lameness is seen with hypertrophic pulmonary osteopathy (HPO); however, careful limb palpation for swelling and radiography can usually elucidate this disease. Panosteitis causes a shifting leg lameness in young dogs along with some systemic signs (fever, inappetence), but can be differentiated by age, presence of bone pain, and lack of joint swelling.

Treatment ■ Anti-inflammatory agents are used to block the production or action of the local mediators of the inflammatory response. Immunosuppressant drugs may be tried.[54] In general, it is wise to start treatment with the least toxic drug and to change therapy only when the maximum tolerated dose is ineffective.[58] In veterinary medicine, economics may play a considerable role. Salicylates (e.g., aspirin) are considered to be very effective in their anti-inflammatory and analgesic effects and are still considered the first form of therapy for humans.

The most common cause of aspirin failing to achieve therapeutic results in humans is administration of an inadequate dose.[57] The dose in dogs for rheumatoid arthritis is 25 to 35 mg/kg (5 grains/20 lb body weight) every 8 hours. Aspirin should be buffered and given with food to decrease gastric irritation. It is debatable whether salicylates retard the disappearance of cartilage,[59] whereas corticosteroids hasten it.[60] Corticosteroids (such as prednisolone 1 to 2 mg/lb acutely for 2 to 3 weeks and the dose tapered over 3 to 4 months to 0.1 mg/ lb every other day[45]) can be used as necessary if aspirin fails to decrease the active inflammation. Intra-articular injections of corticosteroids are seldom indicated. If the patient is not responsive to high levels of aspirin and is nonambulatory, the clinician may be forced to consider joint injections. However, multiple joint injections cause cartilage degeneration and cyst formation and thus should be used as a last resort.[6,61] Other drugs used with some success are the cytotoxic drugs (cyclophosphamide, azathioprine), and gold (sodium aurothiomalate).[45]

Other aspects of treatment consist of weight reduction, rest during flare-ups, mild exercise (swimming is excellent), synovectomy, and arthrodesis. Synovectomy and arthrodesis are practical only if one or two joints are involved.

Lyme Arthritis ■   Lyme arthritis is a relatively new disease caused by the spirochete *Borrelia burgdorferi*. It has been diagnosed mainly in northern California, the upper Midwest, and the Northeast. It can cause recurrent joint lameness, fever, inappetence, and lethargy. Less frequently associated signs include lymphadenopathy, central nervous system (CNS) disorders, and renal and cardiac disease. The diagnosis is presumptive and should be based on a history of tick exposure and clinical signs, which include the presence of inflammatory joint fluid. Serologic tests have a high proportion of false-positives and -negatives and are not generally helpful.[62] Treatment is usually successful with the administration of antibiotics (tetracyclines, penicillins) for 3 to 4 weeks.[45] The use of preventative vaccines is controversial at this time and is not recommended except where the disease is endemic.

NONEROSIVE INFLAMMATORY DISEASE ■   These joint conditions involve three categories of disease: SLE, those associated with chronic infectious processes, and idiopathic conditions. The symptoms can mimic rheumatoid arthritis, but erosions are rare and systemic involvement occurs. Lameness and weakness are common.

Systemic Lupus Erythematosus ■   The distinguishing feature of SLE is its serological abnormalities (LE cell or antinuclear antibody positive). In humans, glomerulonephritis caused by aggregation of immune complexes in the kidney may cause death. Aspirin may control the joint aspects of this disease, but not the kidney changes.[58] Therefore, prednisolone is recommended and may be combined with cytotoxic drugs such as cyclophosphamide or azathioprine.[63] Polymyositis has been reported in the dog.[64]

Arthritides with Concomitant Chronic Infectious Disease ■   The presenting symptomatology is the same as SLE, except that a disease process (dirofilariasis—chronic fungal or bacterial infections of the heart, ears, or genitourinary system) is concurrent. Reversal of inflammation has occurred upon resolution of the primary problem.[63] Rheumatic fever in humans (preceded by *Streptococcus* pharyngitis) may result in polyarthritis that is sterile, probably owing to circulating immune complexes.

OSTEOCHONDROSIS

Osteochondrosis is a disturbance of cell differentiation in metaphyseal growth plates and joint cartilage. If this condition results in a dissecting flap of articular cartilage with some inflammatory joint changes, it may then be termed "osteochondritis dissecans" (OCD). This condition is very common in many species. In the dog, medium, large, and giant breeds are affected. By understanding the origins of these lesions, the veterinarian can devise a rational treatment for this condition at various stages and degrees of severity. After a general discussion of osteochondrosis, each major joint will be covered later as to clinical signs, pertinent physical findings, radiographic diagnosis, treatment, and prognosis.

Pathology

Olsson[65] has characterized osteochondrosis as a generalized skeletal disturbance of endochondral ossification in which either parts of the physis (epiphyseal plate) or lower layers of the articular surface fail to mature into bone at a symmetrical rate. This results in focal areas of thickened cartilage that are prone to injury.

Bone growth (osteogenesis) in the metaphyseal area of the long bones occurs at the physis (growth plate) through endochondral ossification (bone formation following a cartilage precursor). The end of the bone—the epiphysis—must also grow. This occurs by endochondral ossification of the deeper layers of the surface articular cartilage. Osteochondrosis in the physeal area can result in an ununited anconeal process, retained cartilaginous cores at the distal ulna, and genu valgum (knock-knee). Osteochondrosis of the articular surface can lead to osteochondritis dissecans in several joints (shoulder, stifle, hock, elbow, and vertebral articular facets[70]) and, possibly, to a fragmented coronoid process and ununited medial epicondyle of the elbow.[65]

The form of osteochondrosis seen most frequently in the United States is OCD of the scapulohumeral joint. OCD and fragmented coronoid process (FCP) of the elbow are rapidly becoming a common concern, especially in the Labrador retriever and Rottweiler breeds. Ununited anconeal process (UAP), OCD of the talus (hock), and OCD of the stifle, are seen in lesser numbers. In Studdert's study[71] of 1247 Labrador retriever puppies in an Australian breeding colony for producing guide dogs, 15 percent had osteochondrosis of the elbow. In Grondalen's study of Rottweiler dogs in Norway,[72] 50 percent of 1423 screened radiographically for elbow arthrosis were positive. In our experience and that of others,[73,74] the cause of the arthrosis is some abnormality of the coronoid (fragmented or fissured) process and less commonly OCD of the humeral condyle.

Histopathology

Cordy and Wind[66] give a histological sequence for the various stages of osteochondrosis. They studied the "normal" histology of the humeral heads from 14 dogs of large breeds 3 to 18 months of age. The predilective site for OCD had thicker-than-normal subchondral trabeculae that contained calcified cartilage until the dogs were 8 months of age. Nonpredilective sites of the humeral head showed ossified cartilage remnants in the trabeculae, which remained only until the animal reached 5 months of age. In three of these "normal" control animals, however, there were tongues of unossified cartilage that extended into the subchondral bone region (Fig. 6–4A). The cartilage in the oldest of these three dogs contained necrotic chondrocytes. These three dogs probably had osteochondrosis, which might have progressed to the clinical lesions of OCD had they been allowed to live.

In the control animals, the "tidemark" (a wavy hematoxylin-stained line demarcating the junction of the calcified and noncalcified layers of cartilage) was

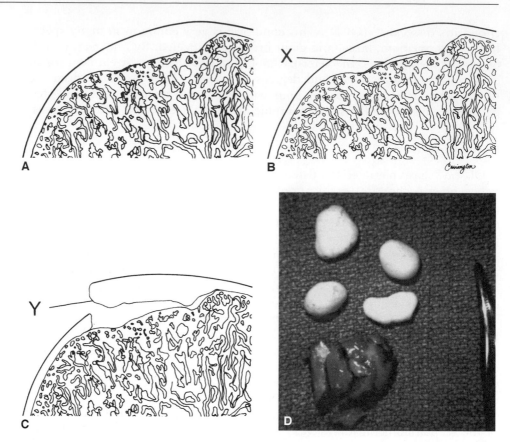

FIGURE 6–4. (*A*) Schematic diagram of thickened cartilage representative of osteochondrosis. (*B*) Osteochondrosis with a horizontal cleft that may heal or turn into osteochondritis dissecans. (X represents a crack in the calcified cartilage zone.) (*C*) Osteochondritis dissecans with flap formation. (Y represents the flap.) (*D*) Specimens from the radiograph shown in Figure 6–5E. Note the color difference between the fractured osteophyte and the four white joint mice.

faint in younger animals but dark-stained in those animals 6 to 7 months of age. In the predilective site, however, the tidemark was not prominent until the animals were 9 months old. The tidemark can be likened to a cementing substance. It may be that the predilective site has a weaker attachment (until the animal is 9 months of age) to the calcified cartilage zone than other areas of the humeral head.

A greater degree of asymptomatic pathology was seen in two other dogs.[66] Upon gross visualization of the smooth humeral head, a yellowish discoloration was seen bilaterally at the predilective sites. Histologically, there were debris-filled horizontal clefts along the tidemark region with thickened cartilage above it (Fig. 6–4B). This thickened cartilage superficial to the horizontal cleft contained some unorganized and necrotic chondrocytes.

When osteochondrosis progresses so that a vertical cleft breaks through the surface, the disease can then be termed osteochondritis dissecans. It is at this point that lameness may occur. According to Pedersen and Pool,[69] if the subchondral capillary bed is able to surround, bridge over, and bypass this area of chondromalacia, then endochondral ossification can occur without a clinical lesion developing. If the vertical cleft radiates and becomes more extensive than in one linear spot, the cartilage can then form a movable flap (Fig. 6–4C). These flaps, at this stage, are twice the normal cartilage thickness. Histologically, the surface appears normal, whereas the deep layers contain disorganized chondrocytes with some necrosis and calcification.[66] Bone was not found in these flaps except in 2 of 31 instances. In these cases, vascularized connective tissue extended to the flap from the underlying bone marrow of the bed. This vascularized cartilage then underwent endochondral ossification, thereby allowing bone to form within the flap. In our experience, OCD of the hock usually contains bone. The cartilage flap is usually attached to the synovial lining and therefore receives nourishment. It can later undergo endochondral ossification after detachment from the subchondral region.

The bed of the defect formed a saucer-shaped depression covered by a granular, grayish white material that histologically represented the calcified cartilage zone. Beneath this zone, there was a thin layer of new fibrous tissue or fibrocartilage. Deeper to this, trabecular bone was normal, and no necrosis, comminution, or eburnation was present, at least in the early stages of this condition.

After the flap forms (usually 5 to 7 months of age) it cannot heal back down to the bed of the lesion. It undergoes further dystrophic calcification and may either stay in place with gradual degeneration or become dislodged. Often, there is a "kiss" lesion on the articular surface touching the loosened piece. When free, these joint mice migrate to pockets within the joint or in tendon sheaths that communicate with the joint. These joint mice may be engulfed by synovium, or they may remain free within the joint. They may grow in size, since they are nourished by synovial fluid. Often they become rounded (Figs. 6–4D and 6–5E).

Pathogenesis

The pathogenesis of OCD can be considered as a thickened area of articular cartilage that is not cemented down well to the underlying subchondral bone. Some chondrocytes may die. A tangential force, such as the scapula hitting the humerus during running and jumping, can crack this weakened area horizontally; if the trauma is continued, it may crack vertically through the articular surface allowing synovial fluid to bathe the deep layers of degenerating cartilage, which in turn causes a synovitis. If there is no further stress (e.g., the stress of walking or running), the lesion may have a chance to heal. With further stress, the crack becomes circumferential, forming a nonhealing flap. The flap will continue to stimulate synovitis until removed. The cause of the thickened cartilage is unknown; however, a hereditary predilection is suspected. Feeding three times the recommended calcium intake has also produced osteochondrosis.[75]

Radiographic Appearance

Normal cartilage is not visible upon plain radiography unless significant dystrophic calcification or bone formation has occurred. Since OCD lesions consist of thicker cartilage than the surrounding cartilage, the lesion is observed as a flattening, "divot," or saucer in the bone. Each characteristic lesion will be described in the following sections.

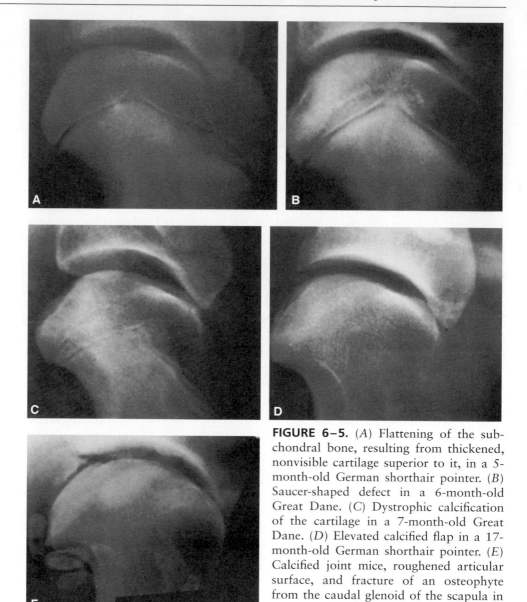

FIGURE 6–5. (*A*) Flattening of the subchondral bone, resulting from thickened, nonvisible cartilage superior to it, in a 5-month-old German shorthair pointer. (*B*) Saucer-shaped defect in a 6-month-old Great Dane. (*C*) Dystrophic calcification of the cartilage in a 7-month-old Great Dane. (*D*) Elevated calcified flap in a 17-month-old German shorthair pointer. (*E*) Calcified joint mice, roughened articular surface, and fracture of an osteophyte from the caudal glenoid of the scapula in a 2½-year-old Great Dane.

Treatment

When recognized early (4 to 6 months), some syndromes (OCD of the shoulder, hock, and stifle, retained cartilaginous cores) may be treated with rest and restricted diets. The latter consist of decreased caloric intake of a well-balanced cereal dog food, and cessation of calcium supplementation. Decreased activity may decrease shear forces and prevent flap formation. Once flap formation or separation has occurred, however, healing will not take place. Healing, or non-separation of the thickened cartilage, should occur by 6 months of age, and it has been our experience that dogs remaining lame after 6½ months of age have formed a nonhealing lesion and are surgical candidates at this point. Removal of the irritating flap or loose piece should be performed as soon as possible.

The first objective of surgery is to remove the flap or joint mouse that is irritating the synovium and gouging the opposite cartilaginous surfaces. A sec-

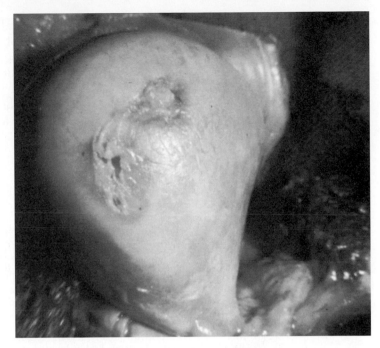

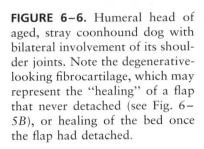

FIGURE 6–6. Humeral head of aged, stray coonhound dog with bilateral involvement of its shoulder joints. Note the degenerative-looking fibrocartilage, which may represent the "healing" of a flap that never detached (see Fig. 6–5B), or healing of the bed once the flap had detached.

ond objective is to remove any cartilage in the periphery of the bed that is not adherent to the underlying tissue. A third concern is whether the bed should be curetted. Curettage is sometimes recommended because granulation tissue from the bleeding subchondral bone invades the defect and fills it more quickly with fibrocartilage. This is especially true if the defect has dense sclerotic bone lining it. However, often a grayish material is already lining the defect (calcified cartilage layer) and may contribute to natural healing. Therefore, curettage may be unnecessary, and actually contraindicated. Another alternative is to use a Kirschner drill wire to drill a few holes in the defect (forage) to allow neovascularization without disturbing some of the cartilage elements already there.

Controlled experimentation using cases of natural disease is needed to provide guidance as to the proper therapy of the bed. Currently, we do not agree on recommending curettage of the bed.

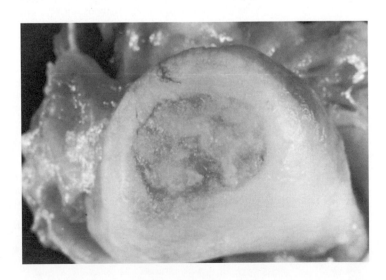

FIGURE 6–7. Humeral head of a 7-year-old Irish setter presented for forelimb amputation of an osteosarcoma of the radius. The dog had been lame all of its life. A rounded joint mouse 1 inch in diameter was also found.

The appearance of a humeral defect several years after natural flap detachment is shown in Figure 6–6. An example of an incompletely "healed" lesion (unoperated) is shown in Figure 6–7.

Panosteitis (Chapter 23) is a common condition of large young dogs and may coexist with osteochondrosis. Care must be taken to rule out this condition (moderate to severe lameness, pain on long-bone palpation, and characteristic radiographic lesions) as the source of pain to avoid operating on an osteochondrosis that has not formed a flap.

References

1. Evans HE, Christensen GC: Miller's Anatomy of the Dog. Philadelphia, WB Saunders Co, 1979, p 95.
2. Gardner E: Structure and function of joints. In Hollander JL (ed): Arthritis and Allied Conditions. Philadelphia, Lea & Febiger, 1972, pp 32–50.
3. Hollander JL: The Arthritis Handbook. West Point, PA, Merck, Sharp, & Dohme, Inc, 1974.
4. Radin EL, Rose RM: Role of subchondral bone in the initiation and progression of cartilage damage. Clin Orthop 213:34, 1986.
5. Jaffee HL: Structure of joints, bursal mucosae, tendon sheaths. In Metabolic Degenerative and Inflammatory Diseases of Bones and Joints. Philadelphia, Lea & Febiger, 1972, pp 80–104.
6. Mankin HJ: The reaction of articular cartilage to injury and osteoarthritis. N Engl J Med 291:1285–1292, 1974.
7. Moroudas A: Transport through articular cartilage and some physiological implications. In Ali SG, Elves MW, Leaback DH (eds): Proceedings of the Symposium on Normal and Osteoarthrotic Articular Cartilage. Middlesex, England, Institute of Orthopaedics, 1974, pp 33–40.
8. Freyberg RW; The joints. In Sodeman WA, Sodeman WA Jr (eds): Pathologic Physiology: Mechanisms of Disease. Philadelphia, WB Saunders Co, 1967, Chapter 32.
9. Johnson LC: Joint remodeling as a basis for osteoarthritis. J Am Vet Med Assoc 141:1237–1241, 1962.
10. Jurvelin J, Kiviranta I, Tammi M, Helminen JH: Softening of articular cartilage after immobilization of the knee joint. Clin Orthop Rel Res 207:246–252, 1986.
11. Troyer H: The effect of short term immobilization on the rabbit knee joint cartilage. Clin Orthop Rel Res 107:249–257, 1975.
12. Salter RB, Simmonds DF, Malcolm BW, et al: The biological effect of continuous passive motion on the healing of full-thickness defects in articular cartilage. J Bone Joint Surg 62-A:1232–1250, 1980.
13. Driscoll SW, Salter RB: The repair of major osteochondral defects in joint surfaces by neochondrogenesis with autogenous osteoperiosteal grafts stimulated by continuous passive motion. Clin Orthop Rel Res 206:131–140, 1986.
14. Pedersen NC: Canine joint disease. In 1978 Scientific Proceedings, 45th Annual Meeting of the American Animal Hospital Association, South Bend, IN, 1978, pp 359–366.
15. Mankin HJ: Discussion of pathogenesis of osteoarthrosis. In Ali SG, Elves MW, Leaback DH (eds): Proceedings of the Symposium on Normal and Osteoarthrotic Articular Cartilage. Middlesex, England, Institute of Orthopaedics, 1974, pp 301–317.
16. Bentley G: Experimental osteoarthrosis. In Ali SG, Elves MN, Leaback DH (eds): Proceedings of the Symposium on Normal and Osteoarthrotic Articular Cartilage. Middlesex, England, Institute of Orthopaedics, 1974, pp 259–284.
17. Sokoloff L: The pathology and pathogenesis of osteoarthritis. In Hollander JL (ed): Arthritis and Allied Conditions. Philadelphia, Lea & Febiger, 1972, pp 1009–1029.
18. Wilson JN: The place of surgery in the treatment of osteoarthritis. In Ali SG, Elves MN, Leaback DH (eds): Proceedings of the Symposium on Normal and Osteoarthrotic Articular Cartilage. Middlesex, England, Institute of Orthopaedics, 1974, pp 227–232.
19. McDevitt C, Gilbertson E, Muir H: An experimental model of osteoarthritis: Early morphological and biochemical changes. J Bone Surg 59:24–35, 1977.
20. Marshall JL: Periarticular osteophytes. Initiation and formation in the knee of the dog. Clin Orthop 62:34–47, 1969.
21. Brandt KD, Mankin HJ: Pathogenesis of osteoarthritis. In Sledge CB, Ruddy S, Harris ED, Kelley WN (eds): Arthritis Surgery. Philadelphia, WB Saunders Co, 1994, pp 450–468.
22. Turek SL: Orthopaedics—Principles and Their Application. Philadelphia, JB Lippincott Co, 1967.
23. Griffen DW, Vasseur PB: Synovial fluid analysis if dogs with cranial cruciate rupture. J Am Anim Hosp Assoc 28:277–281, 1992.
24. Collins DH: The Pathology of Articular and Spinal Diseases. London, Edward Arnold and Company, 1949.

25. Mankin HJ: The reaction of articular cartilage to injury and osteoarthritis. N Engl J Med 291:1335–1340, 1974.
26. Moskowitz RW: Symptoms and laboratory findings in osteoarthritis. In Hollander JL (ed): Arthritis and Allied Conditions. Philadelphia, Lea & Febiger, 1972, pp 1032–1053.
27. Gardner E: Structure and function of joints. In Hollander JL (ed): Arthritis and Allied Conditions. Philadelphia, Lea & Febiger, 1972, pp 32–50.
28. Simkin PA: Synovial physiology. In McCarthy DJ, Koopman WJ (eds): Arthritis and Allied Conditions, 12th ed. Philadelphia, Lea & Febiger, 1993, pp 199–211.
29. McGoey BV, Deitel M, Saplys RJF, et al: The effect of weight loss on musculoskeletal pain in the morbidly obese: J Bone Joint Surg (Br) 72-B:322–323, 1990.
30. Hayes HM, Wilson GP, Burt JK: Feline hip dysplasia. J Am Anim Hosp Assoc 15:447–449, 1979.
31. Olsson S, Hedhammer A, Kasstrom H: Hip dysplasia and osteochondrosis in the dog. In Proceedings of Voojaarsdagen 1978 (The Netherlands Small Animal Veterinary Association). Amsterdam, Royal Netherlands Veterinary Association, 1978, pp 70–72.
32. Murray RO: Aetiology of degenerative joint disease. A radiological re-assessment. In Ali SG, Elves MW, Leaback DH (eds): Normal and Osteoarthrotic Articular Cartilage. Middlesex, England, Institute of Orthopaedics, 1974, pp 125–130.
33. Short CR, Beadle RE: Pharmacology of antiarthritic drugs. Vet Clin North Am 8:401–418, 1978.
34. Clark DM: The biochemistry of degenerative joint disease and its treatment. Compend Cont Educ Pract Vet 13:275–281, 1991.
35. Scott DW: Feline dermatology, therapeutics. J Am Anim Hosp Assoc 16:434–456, 1980.
36. Hannan N, Ghosh P, Bellenger C, et al: Systemic administration of glycosaminoglycan polysulphate (Arteparon) provides partial protection of articular cartilage from damage produced by meniscectomy in the canine. J Orthop Res 5:47–59, 1987.
37. Huber ML, Bill RL: The use of polysulfated glycosaminoglycan in dogs. Compend Cont Educ Pract Vet 16:501–506, 1994.
38. Caron JP, Toppin DS, Block JA: Effect of polysulfated glycosaminoglycan on osteoarthritic equine articular cartilage in explant culture. Am J Vet Res 54:1116–1121. 1993.
39. de Haan JJ, Goring RL, Beale BS: Evaluation of polysulfated glycosaminoglycan for the treatment of hip dysplasia in dogs. Vet Surg 23:177–181, 1994.
40. Todhunter RJ, Lust G: Polysulfated glycosaminoglycan in the treatment of osteoarthritis. J Am Vet Med Assoc 204:1245–1250, 1994.
41. Bradney IW: Treatment of osteoarthritis of the femoro-tibial joint in the dog by synovectomy and debridement and repair of the anterior cruciate ligament. J Small Anim Pract 20:197, 1979.
42. Walker T, Prieur WD: Intertrochanter femoral osteotomy. Semin Vet Surg Med 2:117–130, 1987.
43. Braden TD: Personal communication. Unpublished data. Michigan State University, 1995.
44. Madewell MR, Pool R: Neoplasms of joints and related structures. Vet Clin North Am 20:511–521, 1978.
45. Bennett D, May C: Joint diseases of dogs and cats. In Ettinger SJ, Feldman EC (eds): Textbook of Veterinary Internal Medicine, 4th ed. Philadelphia, WB Saunders Co, 1995.
46. Van Pelt RW, Langham RF: Nonspecific polyarthritis secondary to primary systemic infection in calves. J Am Vet Med Assoc 149:505–511, 1966.
47. Tiu SK, Suter PF, Fischer CA, Dorfman HD: Rheumatoid arthritis in a dog. J Am Vet Med Assoc 154:495–502, 1969.
48. Newton CD, Lipowitz AJ, Halliwell RE, et al: Rheumatoid arthritis in dogs. J Am Vet Med Assoc 168:113–121, 1976.
49. Newton CD, Lipowitz AJ: Canine rheumatoid arthritis: A brief review. J Am Anim Hosp Assoc 11:595–599, 1975.
50. Ward PA, Zvaifler NJ: Complement-derived leukotactic factors in inflammatory synovial fluids of humans. J Clin Invest 50:606–616, 1971.
51. Robinson WD: The etiology of rheumatoid arthritis. In Hollander JL (ed): Arthritis and Allied Conditions. Philadelphia, Lea & Febiger, 1972, pp 297–301.
52. Anderson RJ: The diagnosis and management of rheumatoid synovitis. Orthop Clin North Am 6:629–639, 1975.
53. Sbarbaro J: Synovectomy in rheumatoid arthritis. In Hollander JL (ed): Arthritis and Allied Conditions. Philadelphia, Lea & Febiger, 1972, pp 623–629.
54. Pedersen NC, Pool RC, Castles JJ, Weisner K: Noninfectious canine arthritis: Rheumatoid arthritis. J Am Vet Med Assoc 169:295–303, 1976.
55. Primer on the Rheumatic Diseases, 10th ed. Atlanta, The Arthritis Foundation, 1993.
56. Lipowitz AJ, Newton CD: Laboratory parameters of rheumatoid arthritis of the dog: A review. J Am Anim Hosp Assoc 11:600–606, 1975.
57. Sokoloff L: The pathology of rheumatoid arthritis and allied disorders. In Hollander JL (ed): Arthritis and Allied Conditions. Philadelphia, Lea & Febiger, 1972, pp 1054–1070.
58. Mills JA: Nonsteroidal anti-inflammatory drugs. N Engl J Med 290:781–784, 1974.

59. Clark DM: Current concepts in the treatment of degenerative joint disease. Compend Cont Educ Pract Vet 13:1439–1446, 1991.
60. Roach JE, Tomblin W, Eysing EJ: Comparison of the effects of steroid, aspirin and sodium salicylate on articular cartilage. Clin Orthop 106:350–356, 1975.
61. Moskowitz RW, Davis W, Sammarco J, et al: Experimentally induced corticosteroid arthropathy. Arthritis Rheum 13:236–243, 1970.
62. Kazmierczak JJ, Sorhage FE: Current understanding of a *Borrelia burgdorferi* infection, with the emphasis on its prevention in dogs. J Am Vet Med Assoc 203:1524–1528, 1993.
63. Pederson WC, Weisner K, Castles JJ, et al: Noninfectious canine arthritis: The inflammatory nonerosive arthritides. J Am Vet Med Assoc 169:304–310, 1976.
64. Krum SH, Cardinet GH, Anderson BC, Holliday TA: Polymyositis and polyarthritis associated with systemic lupus erythematosus in the dog. J Am Vet Med Assoc 170:61–64, 1977.
65. Olsson SE: Osteochondrosis—a growing problem to dog breeders. Gaines Dog Research Progress. White Plains, NY, Gaines Dog Research Center, Summer 1976, pp 1–11.
66. Cordy DR, Wind AP: Transverse fracture of the proximal humeral articular cartilage in dogs (so-called osteochondritis dissecans). Pathol Vet (Basel) 6:424–436, 1969.
67. Johnson KA, Howlett CR, Pettit GD: Osteochondrosis in the hock joints in dogs. J Am Anim Hosp Assoc 16:103–113, 1980.
68. Olsson SE: Lameness in the dog: a review of lesions causing osteoarthrosis of the shoulder, elbow, hip, stifle and hock joints. Proceedings of the American Animal Hospital Association 42:363–370, 1975.
69. Pedersen NC, Pool R: Canine joint disease. Vet Clin North Am 8:465–493, 1978.
70. Hedhammar A, Wu FM, Krook L, et al: Overnutrition and skeletal disease: An experimental study in growing Great Dane dogs. Cornell Vet 64(Suppl 5):83–95, 1974.
71. Studdert VP, Lavelle RB, Beilharz RG, et al: Clinical features and heredity of osteochondrosis of the elbow in Labrador retrievers. J Small Anim Pract 32:557, 1991.
72. Grondalen J, Lingaas F: Arthrosis in the elbow joint of young rapidly growing dogs: A genetic investigation. J Small Anim Pract 32:460, 1991.
73. Grondalen J: Arthrosis with special reference to the elbow joint in young rapidly growing dogs. Part 2: Occurrence, clinical and radiographic findings. Nord Vet Med 31:69, 1979.
74. Grondalen J, Grondalen T: Arthrosis in the elbow joint of rapidly growing dogs. Part 5: A pathoanatomical investigation. Nord Vet Med 33:1, 1981.
75. Goedegebuure SA, Hazewinkle HA: Morphological findings in young dogs chronically fed a diet containing excess calcium. Vet Pathol 23:594–605, 1986.

7
Principles of Joint Surgery

The structure and function of joints, discussed in Chapter 6, should be well understood as a basis for surgery. An ever-increasing percentage of small-animal orthopedics cases have involved disorders of the joints, as stringent leash laws have limited the number of fractures seen in many urban practices. This chapter presents a few basic concepts necessary for success in arthroplastic procedures, and defines some terms that will be used in succeeding chapters.

In small animals, diseases of the joints should be repaired as soon as possible to avoid permanent changes. Strict asepsis must be adhered to in order to avoid devastating infection. Hemostasis is of utmost importance.

The objective of the orthopedic surgeon is to minimize the amount of uneven wear and abnormal stress across joint surfaces. This is accomplished by realigning joint fractures perfectly, removing loose bone (e.g., ununited anconeal process, fragmented coronoid process), correcting angular deformities, stabilizing instability (e.g., cruciates, patellar luxations), reducing dislocations, removing repetitive microtraumata (e.g., meniscal tears), reconstructing joints with diseases of cartilage (e.g., osteochondritis dissecans, Legg-Calvé Perthes disease), and arthrodesing nonreconstructible joints such as those with rheumatoid arthritis, severe osteoarthrosis, or chronic instability.

Correct diagnosis and understanding of the disease process are paramount in good patient care. All too often, the "grand old panacea" (cortisone or any pain medication) is given without diagnosing the problem correctly, sometimes at the expense of permanently crippling the animal. In other cases, when a correct diagnosis is made, eliminating the animal's signs may bring immediate relief to the owner and veterinarian; however, this may shorten the life span as the animal approaches old age and develops crippling arthritis as a result of misuse of the limb.

There are many treatments for any given disease, some directly contradictory. One has to bear in mind the client, the economic situation, the home care, the use and function of the animal, and the veterinarian's facilities and surgical abilities and ability to refer to specialists. The veterinarian has to adapt to those variables and may treat the same disease differently in different animals, depending on the circumstances.

Proper postoperative management is vital in achieving success. If the client is not advised on how to restrict the animal's activity for a certain length of time, how to take care of a splint (e.g., if a plaster of Paris cast gets wet), and how to look for complications, hours of the veterinarian's work may be wasted. If the patient or owner is uncooperative, longer hospitalization may be necessary. In all conditions in which osteoarthrosis is present or in which there is a potential for osteoarthrosis, the animal should be helped to reduce any excessive weight. To check for optimal weight, the owner should be advised to palpate and individualize each rib. When these ribs are palpable, and the abdominal area shows a discernible "waist," the animal has lost sufficient weight.

PRINCIPLES OF ARTHROTOMY

Surgical approaches to joints must be carefully planned to avoid damage to muscles, tendons, and major ligaments. Ideally, none of these structures would be incised, but in practice this is not always possible. It is very important, then, that these structures be properly sutured to maintain joint stability. Degenerative joint disease secondary to surgically induced instability of the joint is an unfortunate sequel to many otherwise successful procedures. Large ligaments and tendons should be detached, when necessary, by osteotomy of their bony origin or insertion rather than by incising and suturing. It is important to achieve adequate exposure for the proposed procedure; excessive retraction causes soft tissue trauma, and poor visualization of the joint usually results in an inadequate repair.

Incision into a joint often involves severing one or more fascial or fibrous tissue planes that function to stabilize the joint. These tissues are collectively known as the retinacula. The lateral retinaculum of the stifle, for instance, is composed of the fascia lata, the aponeurosis of the vastus lateralis and biceps femoris muscles, and the lateral patellar ligament. The fibrous joint capsule could also be considered part of the retinaculum. In some cases, these structures can be sutured collectively, and in some instances they need to be closed in layers to ensure normal function. The reader is referred to *An Atlas of Surgical Approaches to the Bones and Joints of the Dog and Cat*[1] for a discussion and illustration of specific approaches.

The actual incision into the joint capsule must be planned and executed to avoid damage to articular cartilage and to provide adequate tissue margins to allow suturing. Intraoperatively, damage to articular cartilage with retractors, knives, electrocautery, and other devices should be avoided. Frequent irrigation with saline or balanced electrolyte solution is valuable in maintaining superficial layers of articular cartilage in good condition. It is important to postoperative healing to maintain hemostasis to the extent possible and to remove large clots before closing the joint. Although the capsule is usually sutured, complete closure of the synovial layer is not necessary to prevent synovial fluid leakage. Like the peritoneum, the synovial membrane quickly seals itself by fibrin deposition and fibroplasia. Before a joint is closed, the joint space should be thoroughly irrigated to remove tissue debris and clotted blood.

Selection of suture material for joint capsule closure is the subject of a wide variety of opinions. Our general rules are as follows:

1.   When the closure can be made without tension and the capsule is not important in stabilizing the joint (such as shoulder osteochondritis dissicans [OCD] surgery or medial approach to the elbow for OCD), use continuous sutures of small gauge (sizes 2-0 to 4-0) absorbable material or an interrupted pattern with nonabsorbable materials. The synthetic absorbable materials such as polyglycolic acid (Dexon, Davis and Geck, Wayne, NJ) or polyglactin (Vicryl, Ethicon, Inc., Somerville, NJ) are more satisfactory than surgical gut, being initially stronger and more uniformly absorbed. The more slowly absorbed monofilament synthetic materials such as polydioxanone (PDS, Ethicon, Inc.,

Somerville, NJ) and polyglyconate (Maxon, Davis and Geck, Wayne, NJ) are also excellent materials for use in these applications.

2. If the capsule must be closed under tension or if it is being imbricated to add stability, use interrupted sutures of nonabsorbable material in sizes 3-0 to 1. The choice of material is not critical; however, monofilament materials such as nylon or polypropylene are not as prone to becoming infected as are the braided materials. Polydioxanone and polyglyconate sutures provide the long-lasting strength needed for healing of the capsule under tension as well as the advantage of ultimately being absorbed. This reduces the potential for long-lasting, suture-based infections to a very low level. For these reasons we are using these materials increasingly in joint surgery. It is important with any non-absorbable material that the suture not penetrate the synovial membrane in an area that would allow the suture to rub on articular cartilage. Such contact can cause erosion of the cartilage. Lembert and mattress patterns allow slight imbrication due to eversion, whereas the simple interrupted pattern allows edge-to-edge apposition. The cruciate interrupted pattern is excellent for holding the tension on the first throw of a knot and so is very useful with suture material that is "slippery" to tie under tension.

The question is often raised regarding the usefulness of debridement of osteophytes in the arthritic joint. Experimental work has indicated that this procedure probably has questionable value.[2] In experimental dogs, osteophytes returned to 60 percent of predebridement level within 24 to 28 weeks, and there was no measurable clinical difference between treated and untreated dogs. However, due to experimental conditions (i.e., minimal production of osteophytes after severance of the anterior cruciate ligament), the research cases had markedly fewer osteophytes than we typically see in clinical cases. Consequently, the results in this research protocol may not mimic clinical conditions. Therefore, we remove osteophytes when they mechanically interfere with joint motion, as commonly seen at the proximal trochlear sulcus of the stifle joint; however, partial synovectomy of hyperplastic synovial membrane is indicated to reduce inflammation within the joint. Osteophytes are also removed when they are rough and protrude into the overlying synovial lining.

LIGAMENTOUS INJURIES

A great deal of joint surgery in the dog and cat consists of treating various forms of ligamentous injury. We tend to think in terms of luxations or ruptured ligaments rather than in terms of sprain injury to ligaments. A brief review of the pathophysiology of sprain injury should help the clinician deal more confidently with these injuries.

Sprain

Although commonly used interchangeably, the terms sprain and strain have distinct definitions. A *strain* is an injury of the muscle-tendon unit, whereas a *sprain* is a ligamentous injury.

Ligaments are composed of longitudinally oriented bundles of collagen fibers that are so oriented as to have a much greater tensile strength in tension than in shear or torsion. Ligaments are very inelastic, however, and if tensile load exceeds the ligament's elasticity, the collagen fiber bundles will become per-

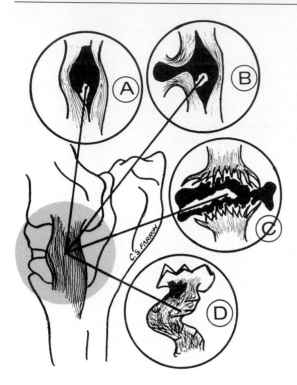

FIGURE 7–1. Sprain classification schemes generally focus on the qualitative aspects of the ligamentous injury. First-degree sprain injury involves minimal tearing of ligament and associated fibers, as well as a varying degree of internal hemorrhage (*A*). Second-degree sprain usually results in definite structural breakdown, as a result of partial tearing. Hemorrhage is both internal and periligamentous, with inflammatory edema being moderately extensive (*B*). Third-degree sprain is most severe and often involves complete rupture of the ligament body (*C*). Avulsion at the points of origin or insertion usually results in one or more small bone fragments, which may often be identified radiographically (*D*). (From Farrow CS: Sprain, strain, and contusion. Vet Clin North Am 8[2]:169–182, 1978, with permission.)

manently deranged at about 10 percent elongation. Damage to a ligament caused by external force is called a *sprain* (Fig. 7–1).

Sprains are conveniently categorized into three classes[3] (Table 7–1):

1. *First-degree* or *mild sprains* result from very short-lived application of moderate force. Relatively few collagen fibers are damaged, and minimal functional change results. Hematoma formation and edema occur in the parenchyma with rapid fibrin deposition. Invasion of the fibrin by fibroblasts results in rapid healing, with normal anatomy being restored and no functional deficit. Minimal or no treatment is needed.

2. *Second-degree* or *moderate sprains* (Fig. 7–2) are characterized by increased numbers of damaged collagen fibers, more extensive hematoma, and marked functional deficit. The ligament is grossly intact. Long-term restoration of normal function is unlikely without treatment.

3. *Third-degree* or *severe sprains* (Figs. 7–3 through 7–5) are characterized by actual interstitial disruption (partial or complete) or avulsion of the ligament from bone. Avulsion fractures of the ligamentous origin or insertion may also be present. Function is completely lost and vigorous treatment is needed to restore function. Spontaneous healing by fibroplasia is virtually certain to result in an unstable joint.

Treatment

First-Degree (Mild) Sprains.   Immediately following the injury, icing will reduce hemorrhage and minimize pain. Veterinarians rarely see the patient this early. Initial application of ice should be followed within a few hours by application of heat. External support is not necessary, although an elastic bandage may provide some comfort. Treatment is primarily directed at enforced rest for 7 to 10 days, followed by another 7 to 10 days of light exercise such as leash

TABLE 7–1.   CHARACTERISTIC FINDINGS IN *SPRAIN* INJURY IN THE DOG*

Disorder	Physical Findings	Roentgenological Findings
Chronic sprain	Regional soft tissue alterations, lameness, and variable degrees of limb deformity unaccompanied by signs of inflammation. There is almost always a history of prior trauma.	Regional soft tissue alterations often accompanied by signs of old bony trauma, osteoarthritis, and heterotopic bone formation.
Acute sprain Mild (first degree)	1. Minimal lameness. 2. Mild to moderate regional soft tissue swelling, which may be confined to the intracapsular location. 3. Tenderness on palpation. 4. Pain variable on manipulation.	1. Minimal regional soft tissue swelling; may be entirely absent. 2. No bony lesions. 3. No apparent instability; stress radiographs fail to identify spatial derangement.
Moderate (second degree)	1. Obvious lameness. 2. Obvious swelling. 3. Frank pain on palpation. 4. Pain readily elicited on minimal manipulation.	1. Prominent regional soft tissue swelling, usually both intra- and extracapsular in origin. 2. Bony lesions rarely present. 3. No apparent instability; stress radiographs may demonstrate spatial derangement (Fig. 7–2).
Severe (third degree)	1. Severe lameness often resulting in no weight bearing by the affected limb. 2. Gross swelling, which may extend well into the proximal metacarpus and the digits of the affected paw (Fig. 7–3). 3. Extreme pain on palpation or manipulation, frequently accompanied by crepitus or abnormal mobility.	1. Gross regional soft tissue swelling. 2. Bony lesions frequently present. Avulsion fractures are common and are often associated with subluxation. 3. Instability often apparent and readily demonstrable with stress radiographs (Figs. 7–4 and 7–5).

*From Farrow CS: Sprain, strain, and contusion. Vet Clin North Am 8(2):169–182, 1978.

walking or the freedom of a small kennel-run. Nonsteroidal anti-inflammatory drugs (NSAIDs) may be useful for a few days but may also encourage the animal to be overactive. By the end of the third week, most animals can be allowed unrestricted activity, although extremely vigorous exercise should be approached gradually.

Second-Degree (Moderate) Sprains.   More aggressive and definitive therapy is required in these injuries to ensure full return to function. It is extremely important to realize that 6 to 10 weeks may be required for initial healing and that full stability may not be achieved until 3 to 6 months after injury. If no instability can be demonstrated, the limb is splinted for 2 to 3 weeks, followed by 2 weeks in a firm elastic bandage if possible. Light activity is started at the removal of the splint and slowly increased toward normal between 6 and 8 weeks after injury, although maximal effort activities should be delayed until at least 12 weeks.

If instability can be demonstrated either by palpation or radiography, the best chance of success lies with early surgical repair (see the following section on surgical repair). Since the ligament is basically intact, the technique of suture imbrication or plication is employed to make the ligament taut in its functional position and to support it during the healing phase. The joint capsule and retinaculum can also be imbricated for additional support. The limb must be immobilized postoperatively with the affected joint at a functional angle in some manner that will protect the ligament from severe stress initially. However, it is important not to stress shield the ligament completely for too long; 4 to 6 weeks in the splint/cast is adequate. (See the discussion of splints and casts in Chapter 2 for more details.) Upon removal of the cast it is critical that the animal be

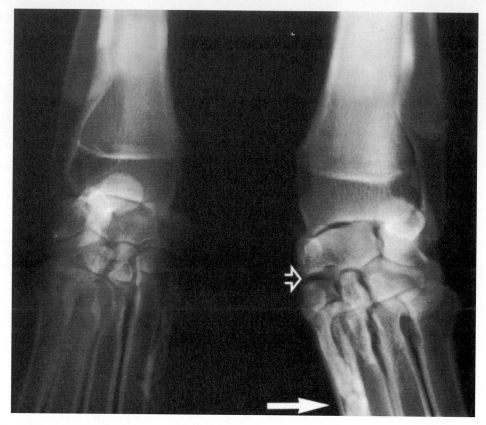

FIGURE 7–2. Second-degree sprain. The stressed radiograph (*closed arrow*) demonstrates slight instability on the medial site (*open arrow*) of the carpus, evidenced by excessive valgus deformity of the metacarpus. This view should be compared with a similar view of the contralateral limb to confirm the spatial derangement.

closely confined until 8 weeks postoperatively. Motion without undue stress will stimulate reorganization of collagen and produce more normal structure than will prolonged complete immobilization. An elastic padded bandage may be useful for the first 2 weeks after splint/cast removal.

Between 8 and 12 weeks after injury, a slowly progressive exercise program should be started. This may consist of short periods of leash walking or being turned loose in the yard for a few minutes. The activity level is gradually increased for another 4 to 6 weeks, at which point most patients will be able to return to near-normal activity.

Delayed surgery in the presence of instability is not as successful as early repair. The necessity of early surgical repair is directly related to the size and activity level of the patient. Small, sedentary animals may have a successful outcome when treated nonsurgically, whereas in the same type of situation a large, athletic dog would end up with a permanent instability and degenerative joint disease.

Third-Degree (Severe) Sprains. Suture repair (see Surgical Repair of Ligaments, below) of the torn ligament is the primary method of treatment for this class of injuries. The locking-loop (Kessler)[4] and pulley suture patterns[5] have proven most reliable. Monofilament nylon or polypropylene in size 0-4/0 is most commonly used. Shredding of the ligament (a crabmeat-like appearance) may

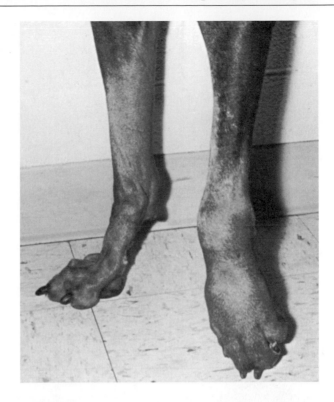

FIGURE 7–3. Third-degree sprain, showing marked swelling of the carpus and metacarpus and non–weight-bearing lameness.

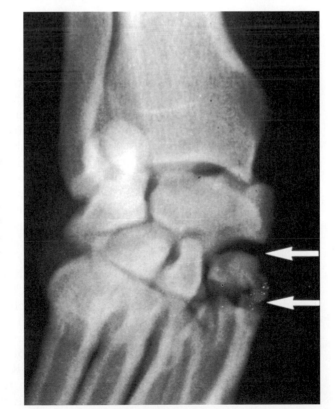

FIGURE 7–4. Third-degree sprain. Stressing the metacarpus in the lateral direction indicates severe valgus deformity due to complete rupture of ligaments at the midcarpal and carpometacarpal joints (*arrows*).

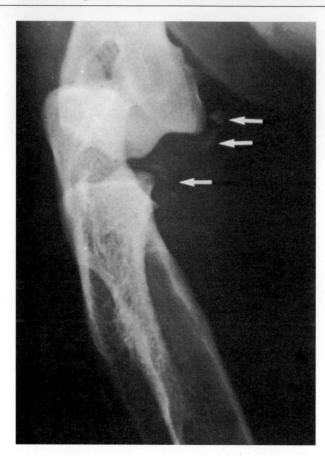

FIGURE 7–5. Third-degree sprain with avulsion of ligaments (*arrows*) on the medial aspect of the humeral condyle.

make it difficult to reappose the severed ends. In these cases, the ligament is augmented with strong suture material to support the joint while fibroplasia envelopes the suture and ligament. This fibrous tissue reorganizes in response to tension stress because of loosening or stretching of the suture and eventually can provide a functional substitute for the original ligament. Braided polyester sutures in size 0-2, monofilament nylon, or wire are materials that can be used. These sutures are usually anchored by means of bone screws or bony tunnels. It is important to make these anchor points of the ligament correspond to the normal origin or insertion point in order to allow a full and unrestricted range of motion. If a pedicle of nearby fascia or tendon can be harvested, it can be sutured to the remaining ligament to act as a source of fibroblasts and as a lattice for fibroplasia in the same manner that a bone graft functions.

If the ligament is avulsed close to a bony attachment, it can often be reattached with a screw and plastic spiked washer or a bone staple with a special insert. Likewise, it may be possible to anchor suture material in the ligament and then use the suture to pull the ligament into contact with the bone, following which the suture is tied around a screw or anchored through a bone tunnel.

Bony avulsions of ligaments can be reattached by small screws with or without spiked washers, multiple Kirschner wires driven through the fragment at divergent angles, tension band wire with or without a Kirschner wire, or stainless steel wire anchored through bone tunnels. Regardless of the method of fixation, reduction must be accurate in order to restore joint stability. If the joint is unstable following reduction, the ligament may need imbrication as described for second-degree injuries. Postoperative management is also as described for second-degree injuries.

Surgical Repair of Ligaments

Conservative treatment of many second- and most third-degree injuries with instability is discouraged because permanent joint laxity often results.[3] Ligamentous tissue shows little tendency to contract during healing, and very minor elongation, perhaps as little as 10 percent, causes loss of effective function and joint laxity. Additionally, scar tissue does not stand tension forces well and does not adequately substitute for ligamentous tissue.

Several basic methods are used in ligamentous reconstruction.

1. Stretched ligaments (second-degree injury) are imbricated by suturing (see Figs. 7–1 and 17–22G, H).

2. Torn ligaments are united by suturing as seen in Figures 7–6 and 7–7. Small, flat ligaments are repaired by incorporating sutures with the fibrous joint capsule and by use of the "prosthetic ligaments" (Fig. 17–22A, B) if necessary.

3. Avulsed ligaments are reattached as closely as possible to their original point of bony origin or insertion. If the ligament is pulled away from the bone cleanly, it can be reattached by a lag screw and plastic spiked washer (see Fig. 17–22D), or a suture placed in the ligament and then attached to either a bone screw (see Fig. 17–22F) or a tunnel through an adjacent bony prominence (see Fig. 19–12).

4. When bony avulsion of a ligament occurs, a lag screw with or without a plastic spiked washer is ideal if the fragment is large enough (see Fig. 17–

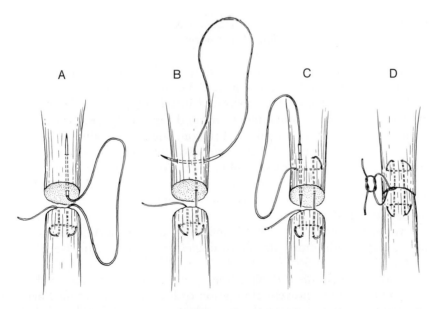

FIGURE 7–6. The locking loop tendon-ligament suture.[4] (A) The second half of the suture pattern is placed by entering the cut end with the suture needle and exiting the tendon at a distance from the cut end about equal to the width of the tendon. (B) A transverse bite is made superficial to the first bite. (C) The needle is passed deep to the transverse bite. The two corner loops surround and lock against a group of ligament-tendon fibers. (D) The suture is tied.

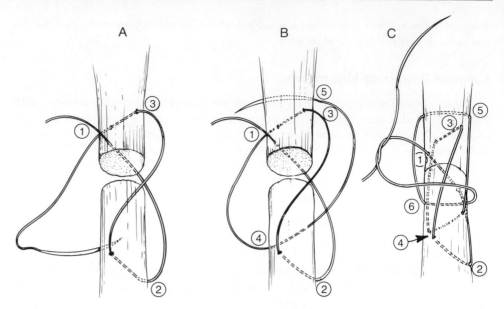

FIGURE 7–7. The pulley tendon-ligament suture. A monofilament material such as nylon or polypropylene must be used to obtain proper tightening of this suture. In theory, bites 1, 3, and 5 are rotated 120 degrees from each other. In practice, as much rotation as possible is obtained. (*A*) The first bite is made in a near-far pattern. (*B*) The second bite is mid-length between the near-far pattern; the third bite is made in the far-near pattern. (*C*) The suture is tied. (From Berg RJ, Egger EL: *In vitro* comparison of the three loop pulley and locking loop suture patterns for repair of canine weightbearing tendons and collateral ligaments. Vet Surg 15:107, 1986, with permission.)

19*A*, *B*). Smaller fragments can be attached with stainless steel wire (Fig. 17–19*C*) or with three diverging Kirschner wires drilled through the fragment (see Fig. 17–19*D*).

5.   Where the ligament is completely destroyed, as in shearing injuries of the carpus and tarsus, or in chronic injuries, the ligament must be prosthetically replaced. Such reconstruction is illustrated in Figures 19–4*C*, *D* and 13–24*B*, *C*. Large sizes of braided polyester suture and tape (Polydek, Tevdek-Deknatel Inc., Queens Village, NY; Mersilene, Ethicon, Inc., Somerville, NJ), sizes 0 to 2, have been commonly used for this purpose, but polyester arterial grafts may be stronger. Carbon and stainless steel filaments show promise as extra-articular ligamentous replacements because fibrous tissue infiltrates them well and can result in formation of a functional pseudoligament. However, carbon fibers have little initial strength.

6.   Any type of repair may be augmented by transposition of adjacent fascia to add strength and more fibroblastic elements for repair (see Figs. 17–22*I*, *J*, *K*).

Protection of the ligament during healing is necessary to prevent the sutures from tearing out and to prevent elongation of healing ligamentous fibers. None of the repair techniques available are able to withstand full weight-bearing stresses for several weeks. In some cases, internal support is supplied by prosthetic materials, as just described (see Fig. 17–22*A*). External skeletal fixators are often useful to support ligamentous repairs, particularly in the presence of open wounds (see Figs. 19–5 and 13–24*D*). Other cases are best supported by external casts and splints as detailed in Chapter 2. Casts and splints are generally maintained for 4 to 6 weeks, followed by 6 to 8 weeks of very gradual resumption of activity. Swimming is an ideal form of physiotherapy.

MUSCLE-TENDON INJURIES

Injuries of the muscle-tendon unit are termed *strains* (Fig. 7–8). Strains can be chronic and multiple or acute and singular in nature, can occur anywhere in the muscle-tendon unit, and can vary in their severity from mild to complete rupture (Table 7–2). Milder forms produce minimal changes in gait and are often overlooked except in animals such as the racing greyhound, in which a slight falling off of speed may be noted. The affected muscles can be located by deep palpation of muscle bellies and tendons. Digital pressure in these areas evinces pain in the patient.

The majority of strains resolve with conservative management consisting of rest and confinement for several days. Complete rupture of a muscle-tendon unit can occur in the muscle belly, in the musculotendinous junction, or in the tendon. Such injuries are usually characterized by an inability to actively flex or extend the associated joints and to support weight. Since the affected muscles undergo spasm and contract, such injuries in the large muscles require surgical repair and external coaptation until primary healing can occur. Techniques for suturing tendons and for aftercare closely follow those described above for ligaments (see Figs. 7–6 and 7–7). Deficits in muscle tissue heal by unorganized scar tissue and, if large enough, can seriously interfere with function. In such cases it may be possible to resect the scar tissue and reappose the muscle tissue. In other cases the muscle is so extensively replaced by scar tissue and so severely

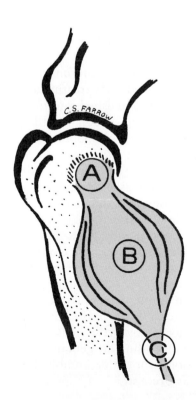

FIGURE 7–8. Strain injuries should always be considered in the context of *all* anatomical components associated with a muscle-tendon unit (MTU): origin or insertion (*A*), muscle belly (*B*), and muscle-tendon junction or tendon body (*C*). Injury to any part of the MTU is typically reflected by dysfunction of the unit as a whole. (From Farrow CS: Sprain, strain, and contusion. Vet Clin North Am 8[2]:169–182, 1978, with permission.)

TABLE 7–2. CHARACTERISTIC FINDINGS IN *STRAIN* INJURY IN THE DOG*

Disorder	Physical Findings	Roentgenological Findings
Chronic strain	Comparatively nonspecific; lameness often accompanied by localized muscle spasm. Often there is little patient response to palpation of the affected muscle-tendon unit.	A generalized decrease in regional muscle mass, which depends on both severity and longevity of the injury. Disuse osteoporosis may be present in advanced cases.
Acute strain	Comparatively specific lameness usually associated with signs of localized inflammation. The area of involvement is often painful to touch and manipulation.	Regional soft tissue swelling.
Mild (first degree)	Minimal lameness, which may be imperceptible to all but the owner.	Usually no radiographic abnormalities.
Moderate (second degree)	Easily perceived lameness, which appears to be the result of localized discomfort as opposed to frank, persistent pain.	Mild, often deceptively generalized regional soft tissue swelling, frequently associated with abnormality of associated fascial planes.
Severe (third degree)	Obvious lameness, which is often rapidly progressive. Pain is easily elicited.	Mild to moderate regional soft tissue swelling with distinct discrepancies of regional fascial planes.

*From Farrow CS: Sprain, strain, and contusion. Vet Clin North Am 8(2):169–182, 1978.

restricts motion of the affected joint(s) that the only recourse is to section the tendon, thus freeing the bone. Contracture of the infraspinatus muscle (see Chapter 9) is one of the more common clinical conditions of this nature.

OPEN WOUNDS OF JOINTS

An open wound into a major joint is a surgical emergency and requires vigorous and early treatment to prevent the inevitable contamination from becoming an established infection. Septic arthritis is a devastating injury, often totally destroying articular cartilage.

The animal should be sedated or lightly anesthetized to allow surgical debridement under aseptic conditions. The wound is covered by sterile lubricating jelly while surrounding hair is clipped, after which the jelly and embedded hairs can be washed away. The wound is enlarged to allow removal of intrasynovial foreign material, and devitalized tissue is excised. A culture and sensitivity sample is obtained.

The joint is flushed copiously with sterile Ringer's or saline solution before closure. Tissues are closed in layers with fine monofilament interrupted sutures, and any ligament damage is repaired at this time. Stabilization of the joint is important in preventing infection because better blood supply is maintained in stable tissues. Drain tubes in the joint are not necessary in most cases and probably do more harm than good. Daily drainage and Ringer's or saline lavage by arthrocentesis are preferable. Antibiotic therapy is initiated with ampicillin and gentamicin and changed if indicated from culture results. The joint should be immobilized for 7 to 10 days or longer if ligamentous damage is present.

IMMOBILIZATION OF JOINTS

Immobilization of major joints, especially of the elbow and stifle, is a double-edged sword. Although it can be very useful in protecting both boney and soft tissue during healing, it is also capable of producing undesirable side effects.

The most common side effect of joint immobilization is fibrosis and contracture of periarticular soft tissues, resulting in loss of range of motion. Articular cartilage is poorly nourished during periods of immobilization and will degenerate to a variable degree. Immobilization in rapidly growing animals, especially dogs of the large and giant breeds, often results in laxity of ligaments in the immobilized limb and in stretching (hence laxity) in the contralateral ligaments as a result of increased stress.

Despite these problems, the greater good is often done by immobilization of the joint following certain arthroplastic procedures. We specifically identify these situations and recommend appropriate immobilization devices in the procedures described in the applicable chapters. There is probably a tendency on the part of most veterinarians to overuse, rather than underuse, external immobilization following joint surgery. The theoretical ideal would be to never immobilize a joint because all the periarticular structures, muscles, tendons, and joint cartilage thrive better in the presence of motion. Therefore, we should examine each situation to see if immobilization can be omitted or at least minimized, rather than slavishly adhering to any specific regimen. Remember, our patients are four-footed and get along quite well on three legs. It is often possible to delay immobilization until the animal shows signs of recovering from the initial pain and swelling and begins to touch the foot tentatively to the ground. Such delay can shorten the period of immobilization by 2 to 10 days in most instances. Ideally, many conditions and/or postoperative management would be best handled by range-of-motion exercises without weight bearing. On the other hand, certain animals will overuse the limb and abuse the surgical repair, especially if the owners are not able to confine an active animal adequately. The intended athletic demands placed on the dog along with owner compliance will determine the balance of immobilization versus mobilization. Good judgment is necessary in evaluating these situations. See Chapter 2 for a discussion of casts, splints, and slings.

Transarticular Skeletal Fixation

The external fixator can be used to immobilize joints. It is particularly useful for open wounds, which make the use of casts and splints very difficult. In the case of multiple limb injuries, the pin splint provides rigid enough fixation to protect the joint, yet allows the animal to bear weight directly on the foot.

No standard patterns have evolved for the use of the external fixator in this matter. Two such applications are illustrated in Figures 19–5 and 13–24.

Arthrodesis

Surgical fusion of a joint to form a bony ankylosis is termed an *arthrodesis*. Spontaneous ankylosis rarely results in bony fusion of a joint in small animals; more often, it simply causes severe periarticular fibrosis and contracture. Arthrodesis and total loss of motion relieve pain originating in articular and periarticular tissues, whereas ankylosis often does not.

Arthrodesis is a salvage procedure and an alternative to amputation in many situations:

1. Irreparable fracture of the joint.
2. Chronically unstable joint.
3. Chronic severe degenerative joint disease from any cause.
4. Neurological injury causing partial paralysis of the limb, especially of the carpal and tarsal joints. For arthrodesis to succeed, there must be cutaneous sensation in the palmar-plantar foot region or self-mutilation may result.

Functioning of the limb after arthrodesis is never normal, but in most instances, it is adequate to allow a reasonably active life for a pet. The more proximal the fusion, the more pronounced the disability. Stifle and elbow fusion produce severe disability, and the animal would, in most cases, probably function better with an amputation. The shoulder is an exception to the basic rule because the scapula becomes more mobile on the trunk and so allows considerable movement to replace normal shoulder motion. Arthrodesis of the more distal tarsal and carpal joints, on the other hand, produces almost no visible change in gait. The hip joint is never fused, since excision of the femoral head and neck is a more useful procedure. Ensuring that the joint is fused in the proper angle is fundamental to success because the angle chosen is the primary means of producing correct leg length. Although a quadriped can make considerable compensation for lengthening or shortening of a single limb, function nevertheless suffers.

Surgical Principles of Arthrodesis

In order to achieve rigid and functional arthrodeses, the following principles should be observed:

1. The surgery should be performed only on a noninfected joint. Infection would lead to implant failure, loss of bone stock, and eventual loss of limb function.
2. Articular cartilage must be removed and subchondral bone exposed on what will be the contact surfaces at the fusion site (see Fig. 13–20A). Cartilage in noncontract areas can be left intact. Curettage, power-driven burrs, and power saws are all useful.
3. Contact surfaces may be cut flat to produce the proper joint angle and to increase the contact area, or they may be prepared by following the normal contours of the joint (see Fig. 19–20A, B). The former provides more stability against shear stress but creates more shortening and is difficult to accomplish without power bone saws. Following the normal contour is the much easier method if working with hand instruments such as curettes and rongeurs.
4. Proper angle at the joint is ensured by preoperative measurement of the opposite limb. Published ranges for each joint are only averages and may not fit any specific animal. Intraoperative use of a goniometer will allow the chosen angle to be duplicated. In the absence of a goniometer, a short piece of splint rod can be bent to the contour of the normal limb, sterilized, and used intraoperatively as a template. In some fusions such as that of the stifle (see Fig. 17–30), debridement of cartilage causes loss of limb length, which is fortuitous. During running movements, the contralateral limb flexes and "shortens" body height. The arthrodesed limb may become relatively too long, requiring abduction of the limb, or knuckling of the toes.

5.   Fixation of the bones must be rigid and long lasting, with compression of the contact surfaces preferred. Bone plates, lag screws, and tension band wire fixation techniques are most useful. When the fixation device is being attached to the bones, care must be taken to maintain the chosen angle and rotational alignment of the limb. Temporary Kirschner wires may be driven across the joint to help maintain normal relationships of the two bones (see Fig. 17–30C) while the permanent fixation device is applied.

6.   Bone grafting is useful to speed callus formation. Most commonly, autogenous cancellous bone is used to pack into and around the contact surfaces. See Chapter 3 for further discussion of bone grafting.

7.   External cast-splint support is needed for 6 to 8 weeks in certain cases, when the internal fixation device is not able to withstand weight-bearing loads before partial fusion has occurred.

PRINCIPLES OF JOINT FRACTURE TREATMENT

Intra-articular fractures are potentially devastating injuries that require prompt and aggressive surgical treatment. Open reduction and rigid internal fixation offer the best hope for uninterrupted function.

Failure to adequately stabilize joint fractures leads to malarticulation. Irregularities in the articular surface cause grinding of cartilage from the opposing surfaces. Liberation of intracellular proteoglycans is followed by inflammatory and degenerative changes within the joint, and varying degrees of degenerative joint disease (arthritis) follow. A certain amount of instability is also present as a result of malarticulation, which further adds to the degenerative joint disease.

Principles of Surgical Treatment

Treatment of specific fractures will be covered in succeeding chapters. There are several general principles that apply to all articular fractures that are discussed below.

Intra-articular Surgery

1.   Wide surgical exposure is needed. Consider osteotomy of ligamentous/tendinous attachments to allow generous exposure.

2.   In the presence of open wounds, it may be necessary to enter the joint through the wound, after appropriate debridement. If possible, however, enter through normal tissues.

3.   Make a general inspection of the joint to assess the damage and to correlate it with the radiographs. Identify all fracture lines and bony fragments.

4.   Remove cartilage chips without bone attachment and foreign bodies, and debride nonviable tissue.

5.   Save cartilage fragments that have subchondral bone attached.

6.   In reconstructing/reducing the fracture, handle cartilage gently. Use pointed reduction forceps, Schroeder vulsellum forceps, or Kirschner wires to hold pieces in reduction. Small gaps are better tolerated than "stair-step" defects.

7.   Size of fragments may dictate the fixation method. Some fragments are too small for anything but a small Kirschner wire. Where these are placed on gliding surfaces, they should be countersunk beneath the cartilage surface. Lag screw fixation is generally the most versatile and reliable method of fixation.

The interfragmentary compression produced generally is the most effective method of preventing shearing forces from disrupting the reduction. Very small screws, 1.5 to 2.0 mm, can be valuable for fixation of small fragments. In some cases it is possible to countersink the heads of these small screws sufficiently that they can be used on gliding surfaces. This is recommended only as a last resort, however, as late damage to the opposing cartilage surface is possible.

Use of plastic spiked washers (Synthes Ltd. [USA], Wayne, PA) can be useful in distributing the compression load of the screw head more evenly over small, thin fragments (Fig. 17–22D). When tension loads are the primary consideration, the pin/tension band wire technique may be useful, especially with small fragments. Lag screws are useful in large tension-stressed fragments if the screw can be positioned so that it is loaded only in the axial direction and is not subjected to bending loads (see Fig. 8–5B). Positioning of lag screws may be influenced by the type of fixation required when extra-articular fractures are present (see below).

8.   Know anatomy well. It is easy to misdirect a screw and not secure adequate fixation. The use of an aiming device (Synthes Ltd. [USA], Wayne, PA) can be very helpful. In some cases, it may be better to excise small fragments that cannot be adequately reduced and stabilized. For example, fractures of the distal one third of the patella are best treated by excision of the fragments and reattachment of the patellar ligament to the remaining patella.

Extra-articular Surgery

Many intra-articular fractures have an extra-articular component, such as the T-Y fractures of the distal humerus (see Fig. 10–20) and femur (see Fig. 16–29). Fixation of the extra-articular fracture should be completed at this time. Plates and external skeletal fixators are most widely applicable in these situations, although occasionally certain forms of pinning, especially with Rush pins, are applicable.

Cancellous Bone Grafting

Both intracapsular and extracapsular bone deficits may be present after reduction and fixation. Such defects can lead to loss of stability as a result of delayed bony bridging by callus formation. Autogenous cancellous bone grafts (see Chapter 3) will greatly speed callus formation. Do not place the graft where it is exposed to synovial fluid or where graft fragments could become free floating within the joint.

Repair of Soft Tissue Injuries

Ligamentous instability due to the fracture-producing trauma is the most common soft tissue problem. Appropriate reconstructive surgery should be done at this time because the instability is deleterious to the joint, and any additional insult to the fractured joint is definitely not needed at this point. Examine carefully for musculotendinous injuries, especially in gunshot fractures and those produced by sharp trauma.

Aftercare

Aftercare varies with the joint involved, the security of fixation achieved, and the size and activity level of the animal. The major question to be resolved is the necessity for cast or sling immobilization. Often, the fixation is less than adequate to allow weight bearing before some degree of fracture union is achieved.

As a general rule, immobilization of the elbow and stifle joints is best avoided. Both of these joints are susceptible to periarticular fibrosis and intra-articular cartilaginous degeneration, leading to loss of motion. If the fixation is so tenuous as to require external immobilization, try to delay applying the cast or splint for several days postoperatively until the animal starts to use the limb. Even the slight passive portion involved in non–weight-bearing activity gives the joint a chance to clear some of the hemarthrosis and inflammatory debris. Flexion bandages of the carpus and tarsus (see Figs. 2–30 through 2–32) are often effective in allowing some motion while preventing weight bearing. The shoulder and hip joints and the joints of the carpus and tarsus tolerate immobilization better and can be safely supported in the appropriate cast, splint, or sling. Generally 3 to 4 weeks of external support is sufficient to allow restricted activity throughout the rest of the healing period. Most animals can be returned to moderate levels of activity by 12 weeks postoperatively.

The determination of implant removal must be approached on a case-by-case basis. If bone plates have been used, they are often relatively short and end in the middiaphysis. This is a good situation for a pathological fracture to develop at the end of the plate after the animal returns to normal activity and is a good argument for plate removal at about 6 months. Screws can usually be left in place with no ill effects. Pin and tension band wire fixation, unless very carefully applied, may cause irritation of overlying soft tissues and will need to be removed as soon as practical. Twelve to 20 weeks is usually adequate to allow good healing in this situation.

References

1. Piermattei DL: An Atlas of Surgical Approaches to the Bones and Joints of the Dog and Cat, 3rd ed. Philadelphia, WB Saunders Co, 1993.
2. Nesbitt T: The effects of osteophyte debridement in osteoarthrosis. Presented at 17th Annual Meeting, American College of Veterinary Surgeons, San Diego, CA, February 18, 1982.
3. Farrow CS: Sprain, strain, and contusion. Vet Clin North Am 8:169, 1978.
4. Pennington DG: The locking loop tendon suture. Plast Reconstr Surg 63:648, 1979.
5. Berg RJ, Egger EL: *In vitro* comparison of the three loop pulley and locking loop suture patterns for repair of canine weightbearing tendons and collateral ligaments. Vet Surg 15:107, 1986.

PART II

FRACTURES AND ORTHOPEDIC CONDITIONS OF THE FORELIMB

8

Fractures of the Scapula

CLASSIFICATION

Fractures of the scapula are relatively uncommon and may be classified on the basis of the following anatomical locations.[1,2]

1. The body and spine.
2. The acromion process.
3. The neck.
4. The glenoid and supraglenoid tuberosity.

The most frequently encountered immediate complications are pulmonary contusions, rib fractures, pneumothorax, pleural effusions, foreleg paralysis, and injury to the suprascapular nerve.[3] The most common cause of scapular fracture is automobile trauma (68 percent), and 56 percent of cases have concurrent injury to other organ systems, including pulmonary trauma in 42 percent of vehicular trauma cases.[4] Long-standing complications include suprascapular neuropathy due to entrapment, and limitation of range of movement and osteoarthrosis in unreduced fractures of the neck or articular surface, particularly in large, athletic animals.

TREATMENT

Conservative Treatment

Most scapular body fractures are not grossly displaced because of the protection of the surrounding muscle mass and rib cage and can be treated closed unless there is loss of congruity of the articular surface or a distinct change in the angulation of the shoulder joint articulation, as will be true in most fractures of the neck. Healing is generally rapid due to the high proportion of well-vascularized cancellous bone, and stability of fixation is not critical except for articular fractures. Many fractures respond well to simple limitation of the animal's activity. In many instances, a modified Velpeau bandage adds greatly to the animal's comfort. The leg is flexed along the chest wall, padded, and bound to the body (see Fig. 2–29). The spica splint is also useful for stabilizing these fractures and reducing pain (see Fig. 2–23).

Internal Fixation

Open approach and internal fixation is indicated in fractures of the articular surface, the neck of the scapula, and most fractures of the acromion process.

Less commonly, some displaced body fractures are internally fixed, especially where athletic performance or cosmetic appearance are major concerns for the owner. The open approach varies considerably, depending on the area of involvement. Exposing the body simply requires elevating the spinati muscles from the spine and body, while exposure of the neck and glenoid cavity usually requires osteotomy of the acromion process, and in some cases osteotomy of the greater tubercle (Fig. 8–1).[5]

Acromion Process

This fracture includes the origin of the acromial part of the deltoid muscle, which pulls the fragment away from the spine if the fracture is complete, and results in a fibrous nonunion. Chronic soreness and lameness result. If the bone is large enough, pin and tension band wire is the most efficient fixation method (Fig. 8–2A). When the process and spine are too small to accommodate the K-wires (one K-wire is sufficient), a variety of interfragmentary wire patterns can be used (Fig. 8–2B, C). It is more important to ensure good stability of the fracture than perfect reduction.

Body and Spine

As previously stated, most fractures in this area can be conservatively treated, but if they are severely displaced recovery will be more rapid and certain with open reduction. The body usually folds outward in a tent-like configuration. In young dogs the body may fracture and the spine remain intact along the crest of the spine. Interfragmentary wire usually provides sufficient fixation once reduction is complete. Because the bone of the body is very thin it is best to place the wire in the thickened areas of the cranial and caudal border, and the crest or base of the spine (Fig. 8–3A). The wire diameter must not be too large or the wire will be so stiff that it will cut through the bone when tightened (20- to 22-gauge; [0.6- to 0.8-mm]) is sufficient.

When body fractures are multiple it is easier than multiple wiring to simply apply a plate along the base of the spine (Fig. 8–3B). This restores the basic alignment of the body and reduces the fragments to near normal position, where they do not require fixation. The use of the cuttable plate (VCP) referred to in Chapter 2 is extremely helpful here, and by stacking these plates they can be made sufficiently strong for most dogs.

Neck

The scapular body typically displaces distolateral to the neck fragment, and restricts outward rotation of the humerus. The scapular nerve can be damaged by direct impingement between the fragments, or can become trapped in callus in unreduced fractures. Although partial function of the shoulder remains in this situation, there is considerable cosmetic deformity due to atrophy of the spinati muscles.

A craniolateral approach with osteotomy of the acromion process is required for exposure (Fig. 8–1C).[5] Pin fixation is sufficient in simple transverse fractures (Fig. 8–4A, B). The pin from the supraglenoid tubercle into the scapular neck can also be inserted from the other direction, though with slightly less resultant stability. Occasionally the neck fracture is sufficiently oblique to allow fixation with lag screws. More commonly the obliquity is too short for screws only and a plate is required, as in Figure 8–4C. Right-angle or oblique-angle finger plates work well in this location, taking care to elevate the suprascapular nerve during placement. Two VCP plates, as shown in Figure 8–7C, are another option.

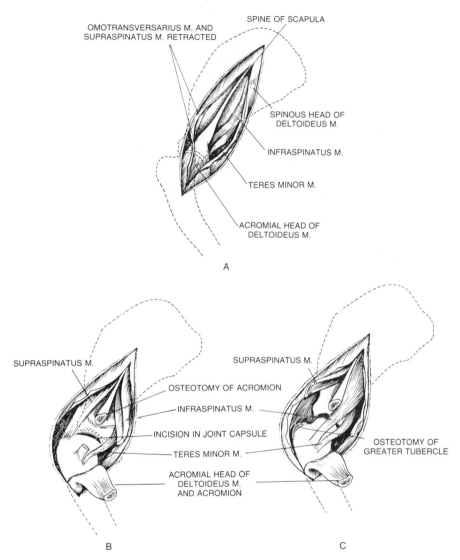

FIGURE 8–1. Open approaches to the scapula and shoulder joint. (*A*) Fractures of body and spine; the infraspinatus and supraspinatus muscles are reflected caudally and cranially, respectively, from the spine. (*B*) Fractures of neck; the acromion process is osteotomized so that the acromial head of the deltoid muscle can be reflected distally. The infraspinatus and supraspinatus muscles are reflected caudally and cranially, respectively. Their tendons of insertion may be severed for more exposure. The suprascapular nerve is located as it crosses the lateral surface of the neck just distal to the acromion process. In fractures involving the articular surface, the joint capsule is incised between the scapula and humerus for exposure. (*C*) In avulsion fractures of the supraglenoid tuberosity or in multiple neck fractures, the belly of the brachiocephalicus muscle is reflected cranially. The greater tuberosity of the humerus is osteotomized and insertion of the supraspinatus muscle is reflected proximally for exposure and working room.

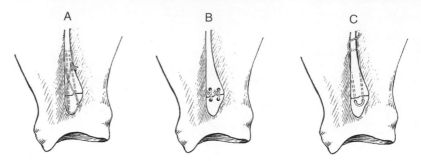

FIGURE 8–2. Fixation of fractured or osteotomized acromion process. (*A*) Tension band wire and Kirschner wires. (*B*) Simple interfragmentary wiring. (*C*) Interfragmentary wiring, applicable to animals too small for the technique in *A*.

An off-weight-bearing foreleg sling or Velpeau sling (see Figs. 2–30 and 2–29, respectively) is indicated for 2 weeks postoperatively, with exercise severely restricted the first month, and a gradual return to normal activity at 8 to 10 weeks. Use of the sling is especially indicated when pin fixation is used, or when the dog is very active and poorly controlled by the owner.

Articular

Treatment of articular fractures of the glenoid is difficult due to the small size of most bone fragments, and the relative difficulty of surgical exposure. Fractures of the cranial portion of the glenoid are most common, followed by the T-Y type.[4]

Supraglenoid Tubercle. Forming a separate center of ossification and the origin of the biceps brachii muscle, the tubercle (scapular tuberosity) is subject to avulsion from the tension of the biceps muscle in skeletally immature large-

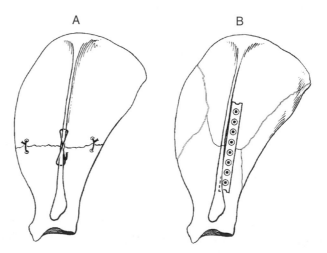

FIGURE 8–3. Fracture of the body of the scapula. (*A*) Simple fractures of the body and spine are amenable to interfragmentary wiring of the body and a tension band wire in the spine. Wires are placed to take advantage of the thicker bone of the cranial and caudal borders of the body and the crest of the spine. (*B*) Multiple fragment fractures are best fixed by a VCP plate (Synthes Ltd. [USA], Paoli, PA) with screws anchored at the junction of the spine and blade. The VCP plate shown here, or a semitubular plate, can be inverted to provide better contact with the bone.

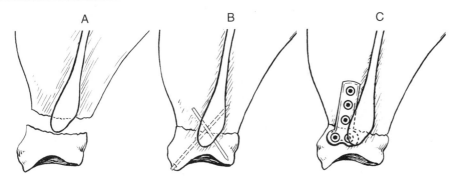

FIGURE 8–4. (*A*) Transverse fracture of the scapular neck. (*B*) Immobilization by insertion of two transfixation Kirschner wires. One wire was inserted at the acromion process and one in the scapular neck. (*C*) Immobilization by a small bone plate; the suprascapular nerve is elevated to insert the bone plate. The use of two VCP plates for a similar fracture is illustrated in Figure 8–7*C*.

breed dogs (Fig. 8–5*A*). Although the initial lameness is dramatic, this quickly disappears and many of these animals are not presented until the lameness is very chronic, with secondary degenerative joint diseases (DJD) present due to malunion or nonunion of this intra-articular fracture. Attempts to reduce the fracture are probably not worthwhile at this point, and biceps tenodesis (see Chapter 9) is indicated and quite successful if DJD is not advanced.

Recent fractures are best stabilized with either a lag screw or pin and tension band wire. As with all articular fractures, accurate reduction and stable fixation are necessary. Screw fixation is preferred, as less exposure is required and it can be applied from a cranial approach, while the pin and tension band wire usually require a craniolateral approach with osteotomy of the greater tubercle (Fig. 8–1*D*).[5] It is important that the screw be inserted into the scapular neck as parallel as possible to the biceps tendon in order to minimize bending loads on the screw (Fig. 8–5*B*). A cancellous thread screw will give the best security. Pin and tension band wire fixation requires that the wire span the suprascapular nerve, so care must be taken to protect the nerve during wire placement (Fig.

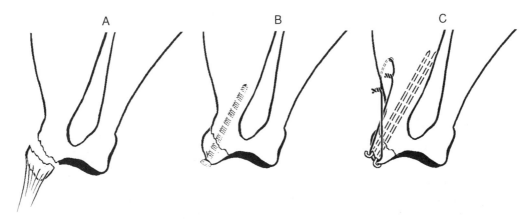

FIGURE 8–5. (*A*) Avulsion fracture of the supraglenoid (scapular) tuberosity. (*B*) Fixation with a lag screw, inserted as parallel to the tendon of the biceps brachii as possible. (*C*) Fixation with Kirschner wires and a tension band wire. The suprascapular nerve must be protected during placement of the tension wire.

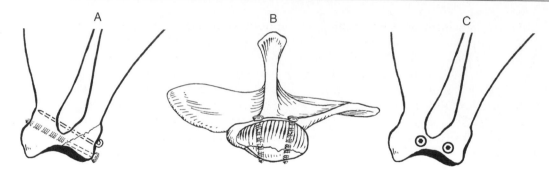

FIGURE 8–6. (A) Fracture of the caudoventral angle of the glenoid fixed with a Kirschner wire and lag screw. The K-wire is placed first. (B, C) Fracture of the medial rim of the glenoid fixed with two lag screws placed from the lateral side.

8–5C). An off-weight-bearing foreleg sling or Velpeau sling (see Figs. 2–30 and 2–29, respectively) is indicated for 2 weeks postoperatively, with exercise severely restricted the first month, and a gradual return to normal activity at 6 to 8 weeks.

Glenoid Rim. The most common fracture is of the caudoventral angle of the glenoid (Fig. 8–6A); similar fractures of the craniodorsal angle are less common. Fracture of the medial rim is also seen, as in Figure 8–6B, C. These fractures require lag screw fixation. Initial fixation with a K-wire is useful in order to get the reduction forceps out of the field for screw application. The K-wire is bent over at the protruding end to prevent pin migration and left in situ. The concavity of the glenoid cavity must be kept in mind when placing the screws to prevent their entering the joint.

An off-weight-bearing foreleg sling or Velpeau sling (see Figs. 2–30 and 2–29, respectively) is indicated for 2 to 3 weeks postoperatively, with exercise severely restricted the first 6 weeks, and a gradual return to normal activity at 10 to 12 weeks.

Glenoid and Neck; T-Y Fracture. As is typical in any fracture of this type, reconstruction of the joint is the first priority, followed by fixation of the neck. Methods of fixation are as described above for glenoid and neck fractures (Fig. 8–7).

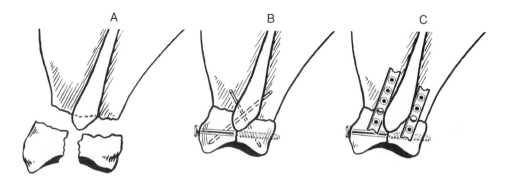

FIGURE 8–7. (A) Fracture of scapular neck and glenoid; T-Y fracture. (B) Immobilization by a cancellous screw and two transfixation Kirschner wires. (C) Fixation by a lag screw and two VCP plates (Synthes Ltd. [USA], Paoli, PA). Although there is only one screw on the glenoid fragment for each plate, this is sufficient stabilization for this fracture.

An off-weight-bearing foreleg sling or Velpeau sling (see Figs. 2–30 and 2–29, respectively) is indicated for 2 to 3 weeks postoperatively, with exercise severely restricted the first 6 weeks, and a gradual return to normal activity at 10 to 12 weeks. Use of the sling is especially indicated when pin fixation is used, or when the dog is very active and poorly controlled by the owner.

Prognosis for Intra-articular Fracture.   Long-term follow-up of 20 animals with articular fractures indicated that only 15 percent were free of clinical signs related to the fracture, with the remainder showing variable degrees of lameness. Thus, although prognosis for limb function is good, some degree of continued lameness is probable.[4]

References

1. Brinker WO: Fractures. In Canine Surgery, 2nd Archibald ed. Santa Barbara, American Veterinary Publications, Inc, 1974, pp 949–1048.
2. Piermattei DL: Fractures of the scapula. In Brinker WO, Hohn RB, Prieur WD (eds): Manual of Internal Fixation in Small Animals. New York, Springer-Verlag, 1984, pp 127–133.
3. Tomes PM, Paddleford RR, Krahwinkel DJ. Thoracic trauma in dogs and cats presented for limb fractures. J Am Vet Med Assoc 21:161–166, 1985.
4. Johnston SA: Articular fractures of the scapula in the dog: A clinical retrospective study of 26 cases. J Am Anim Hosp Assoc 29:157–164, 1993.
5. Piermattei DL: An Atlas of Surgical Approaches to the Bones and Joints of the Dog and Cat, 3rd ed. Philadelphia, WB Saunders Co, 1993, pp 92–101, 118–119.

9

The Shoulder Joint

Forelimb Lameness

Following a history and lameness examination as described in Chapter 1, it is usually possible to localize the source of lameness with some degree of accuracy. Following this comes the exercise of constructing a list of possible diagnoses and working through them until the correct cause is found. The following listing is not exhaustive, but includes the problems that are seen regularly.

FORELIMB LAMENESS IN LARGE-BREED, SKELETALLY IMMATURE DOGS

General/Multiple
- Trauma—fracture, luxation
- Panosteitis
- Hypertrophic osteodystrophy (HO)
- Cervical cord lesion—vertebral instability

Shoulder Region
- Osteochondritis dissecans (OCD) of humeral head

Elbow Region
- OCD of medial trochlear ridge
- Ununited anconeal process (UAP)
- Fragmentation of medial coronoid process (FCP)
- Avulsion and calcification of the flexor tendons of the medial epicondyle or ununited medial epicondyle (UME)
- Subluxation due to premature physeal closure

Carpal Region
- Subluxation/valgus or varus deformity due to premature physeal closure
- Valgus deformity due to retained cartilage cores in the ulna, or elbow conditions

FORELIMB LAMENESS IN LARGE-BREED, SKELETALLY MATURE DOGS

General/Multiple
- Trauma—fracture, luxation, muscle and nerve injuries
- Panosteitis
- Cervical cord lesion—disk, tumor, vertebral instability
- Brachial plexus tumor
- Bone cartilage or synovial tumor

- HO
- Synovial chondrometaplasia (SCM)

Shoulder Region
- OCD of humeral head
- Degenerative joint disease, primary or secondary
- Contracture of infraspinatus muscle
- Tenosynovitis of biceps brachii tendon
- Calcification of the supraspinatus
- Luxation

Elbow Region
- Degenerative joint disease
- FCP
- Calcification of the flexor tendons or UME
- Subluxation due to prior physeal injury or breed (chondrodystrophic) predisposition
- Subluxation due to premature physeal closure
- Luxation

Carpal Region
- Ligamentous instability/hyperextension
- Subluxation due to premature physeal closure
- Degenerative joint disease
- Inflammatory joint disease, with or without instability

FORELIMB LAMENESS IN SMALL-BREED, SKELETALLY IMMATURE DOGS

General/Multiple
- Trauma—fracture, luxation
- Atlantoaxial luxation

Shoulder Region
- Congenital luxation

Elbow Region
- Congenital luxation
- Subluxation due to premature physeal closure

Carpal Region
- Subluxation due to premature physeal closure

FORELIMB LAMENESS IN SMALL-BREED, SKELETALLY MATURE DOGS

General/Multiple
- Trauma—fracture, luxation, muscle and nerve injuries
- Cervical cord lesion—disk, tumor
- Brachial plexus tumor
- HO
- SCM

Shoulder Region
- Degenerative joint disease
- Medial luxation, nontraumatic

Elbow Region
- Degenerative joint disease

- Subluxation due to physeal injury

Carpal Region
- Degenerative joint disease

- Inflammatory joint disease

- Subluxation due to prior physeal injury

THE SHOULDER

Dorsal Luxation of the Scapula

Multiple ruptures of the serratus ventralis, trapezius, and rhomboideus muscle insertions on the cranial angle and dorsal border of the scapula allow the scapula to move dorsally on weight bearing. Onset of clinical lameness is usually acute and is often directly associated with jumps, falls, or bite wounds.

Considerable soft tissue swelling is evident several days after injury. Mobility of the scapula is easily demonstrated and is diagnostic. This uncommon problem is seen in both dogs and cats.

Surgical Technique

The objective of surgical repair is to attach the scapula to a suitable rib with heavy stainless steel wire and to reattach as many ruptured muscles as possible. An inverted L-shaped incision is made along the cranial and dorsal borders of the scapula. If any portions of the trapezius, serratus, or rhomboideus muscle insertions are intact, they are cut sufficiently to allow lateral retraction of the scapula so that its caudal angle and caudal borders can be visualized. Two holes are drilled from a medial to lateral direction through the caudal border of the scapula, close to the caudal angle (Fig. 9–1). Stainless steel wire of 20 to 22 gauge is carefully placed around an adjacent rib with the ends placed through the scapular holes, then pushed laterally through the muscles. The wire is twisted until dorsal movement of the scapula is minimized but still possible. All muscular insertions are sutured to the extent possible, and all tissues are closed in layers.

It is sometimes possible to eliminate the wire suture and simply attach muscle to the scapula through holes drilled near the cranial angle.

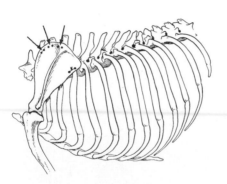

FIGURE 9–1. Dorsal luxation of the scapula. Heavy stainless steel wire is used to secure the caudal border of the scapula to an adjacent rib. Alternatively, holes are drilled through the cranial angle and vertebral border (*arrows*) to allow suturing to the serratus ventralis muscle.

AFTERCARE ■   The scapula is immobilized in either a Velpeau sling (see Fig. 2–29) or a spica splint (see Fig. 2–23) for 2 weeks. Exercise is gradually increased to normal in the 2 weeks after sling or splint removal.

Luxations of the Shoulder

Luxations of the shoulder are relatively uncommon in the dog. Obviously, traumatic luxations are seen in all breeds, but the toy poodle and sheltie show a particular propensity to develop medial luxations (Fig. 9–2) without any history of significant trauma. At the time of presentation, many of these animals have a history of lameness of several months' duration. Most luxations—perhaps 75 percent—are medial, and a large proportion of the remainder are lateral (see Fig. 9–4). Cranial and caudal luxations are rarely seen (see Figs. 9–6 and 9–8). Although the tendons of the parascapular muscles have long been thought of as the primary stabilizers of the shoulder joint, it was found experimentally that cutting the tendons that cross the shoulder joint resulted in minimal changes in joint motion, whereas cutting the joint capsule and glenohumeral ligaments caused marked alteration of joint motion.[1] This suggests that careful imbrication suturing of the capsule and associated ligaments should be an important part of any surgical repair.

The leg is usually carried with the elbow flexed and adducted and the lower limb abducted and supinated in the case of the medial luxation. With lateral luxation the position is similar except that the lower limb is adducted. On palpation, the relative positions of the acromial process and the greater tubercle are the keys to determining the position of the humeral head relative to the glenoid. These points should be palpated on the normal limb and then compared with the affected limb. Clinical signs and physical examination are usually diagnostic; but as with any skeletal injury, diagnosis should always be confirmed radiographically in order to eliminate the possibility of bone injuries such as

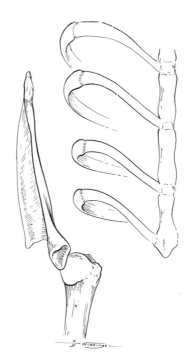

FIGURE 9–2. Medial luxation of the left shoulder (ventrodorsal view).

fractures. Stress radiography has been suggested as an objective method of measuring instability in this joint.[5] The presence of a severely eroded glenoid resulting from chronic luxation or the presence of a dysplastic glenoid or humeral head greatly reduces the probability of a successful reduction. Congenital luxations discovered later are usually irreducible because of severe malformations of both the glenoid and humeral head.

If an injury is seen within a few days following dislocation, and particularly if there is a known traumatic event, it is probably worthwhile to attempt closed reduction and immobilization of the limb for approximately 2 weeks. If the joint is relatively stable following reduction, there is a good chance that this type of treatment will be successful. If the joint remains unstable following reduction or if the luxation recurs while the leg is in the sling, surgical treatment is indicated.

Medial Luxation

Prosthetic ligaments and imbrication techniques have not been as successful as methods for transposing the biceps tendon. Medial transposition and tenodesis[2] of the biceps tendon create a stabilizing lateral force on the humeral head. If the glenoid is deformed, surgical stabilization will usually fail. Treatment in this situation is excision arthroplasty (see Fig. 9–11) or arthrodesis (see Fig. 9–12).

Surgical Technique

The shoulder joint is exposed by a craniomedial approach.[3] Typically, the subscapularis tendon of insertion is torn at its insertion on the lesser tubercle and has retracted a considerable distance making identification difficult. The tendon should be tagged with a suture when identified to assist in later suturing. If the joint capsule is not torn, it is opened carefully to inspect the joint. It is important to save as much capsule as possible for suturing. Careful assessment of the medial labrum of the glenoid and the lateral side of the humeral head is necessary. If the labrum is worn, successful stabilization is less likely. If there is significant chondromalacia of the humeral head articular cartilage owing to rubbing on the medial labrum, degenerative joint disease changes could limit long-term success even if the joint is stabilized. Arthrodesis or excision arthroplasty (see below) is probably indicated in these circumstances.

FIGURE 9–3. Surgical repair of medial luxation of the shoulder. (A) The left shoulder joint has been exposed by a craniomedial approach and the dislocation has been reduced.[3] The position for incision in the joint capsule is indicated. Elevation of the bone flap by means of an osteotome is being started. (B) Transposition of the tendon of the biceps muscle has been completed. It is trapped under the osteoperiosteal flap, which is then secured to the humerus with two Kirschner wires or a bone staple. The joint capsule is imbricated with mattress sutures of heavy absorbable material. (C) Another method of attachment is the use of a plastic spiked washer and bone screw (Synthes Ltd. [USA], Paoli, PA). The bone beneath the tendon is cut to form a shallow trough to encourage early attachment of the tendon. (D) The deep pectoral muscle has been advanced and sutured to the origin of the superficial pectoral muscle. The superficial pectoral muscle is advanced craniolaterad until it can be sutured to the fascia of the acromial head of the deltoideus muscle. The subscapularis muscle is attached to the proximal border of the deep pectoral muscle and to any humeral periosteum or fascia available.

If the articular surfaces are in good condition and the luxation is recent, it may be possible to stabilize the joint by suture of the joint capsule and the subscapularis tendon (Fig. 9–3B, D). If these tissues are friable, tenodesis of the biceps tendon is carried out.

Tenodesis of the biceps tendon to a medial position begins by transecting the transverse humeral ligament overlying the biceps tendon (Fig. 9–3A). The tendon is mobilized from the intertubercular groove after incising the joint capsule

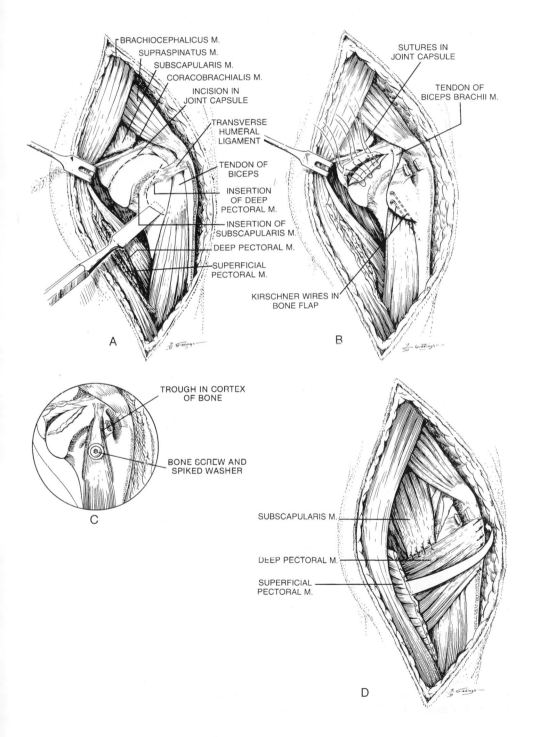

as needed. A crescent-shaped flap of bone is elevated from the lesser tubercle with an osteotome. This flap should hinge on the periosteum along its cranial edge. Bone, and sometimes articular cartilage, is curetted from underneath the flap to accommodate the tendon. The tendon is transposed caudally under the flap and held in place by Kirschner wires driven through the flap into the humerus (Fig. 9–3B). An alternative method of tenodesis is illustrated in Figure 9–3C. The tendon is bluntly split and a bone screw and spiked washer (Synthes Ltd. [USA], Paoli, PA) are used to fix the tendon to the bone in a shallow trough in the cortex. Removal of some cortical bone allows the tendon to heal to the bone more readily than if it were simply attached to the periosteal surface.

Joint capsule and medial glenohumeral ligament imbrication is accomplished by mattress or cruciate sutures of synthetic absorbable material. If the joint seems unstable when the humerus is externally rotated (thus turning the humeral head medially), a derotational suture to temporarily tether the humerus is helpful. Large-gauge nonabsorbable monofilament or braided polyester is anchored to the medial labrum of the glenoid by a bone tunnel or bone screw. A bone tunnel is then drilled through the greater tubercle in the region of the transverse humeral ligament. After passing the suture through the tunnel, it is tied moderately taut with the humerus *internally* rotated. Joint capsule and medial glenohumeral ligament imbrication is accomplished by mattress or Lembert suture patterns of absorbable material.

The deep pectoral muscle is sutured to the superficial pectoral muscle, and the subscapularis muscle is advanced as far cranially as possible and sutured to the deep pectoral muscle (Fig. 9–3D). The superficial pectoral muscle is pulled across the cranial border of the humerus and sutured to the acromial head of the deltoideus muscle. The effect of these transpositions is to tighten the muscles and to reinforce medial support of the joint. The remaining tissues are closed in layers.

AFTERCARE ■ The limb is supported in a foreleg (Velpeau) sling for 14 days (see Fig. 2–29). Exercise is restricted for 4 weeks. Passive flexion-extension exercise may be needed following removal of the sling, supplemented with swimming when possible.

PROGNOSIS ■ Hohn and colleagues[2] reported an overall 93 percent success rate (15 cases) for the tenodesis procedure applied to both medial and lateral luxations. Vasseur's group reported 40 percent (two cases) of their medial luxation cases had normal gaits, 20 percent (one case) had occasional limping, and 40 percent (two cases) had persistent limping following the tenodesis procedure.[4] If cases are carefully selected, and those with wearing of the glenoid or humeral head are eliminated, it is likely that these figures could be improved.

Lateral Luxation

Lateral luxations (Fig. 9–4) are more often seen in larger breeds of dogs and are usually traumatic in origin. They are more amenable to closed reduction when seen within a few days of injury. Fixation after closed reduction is by means of a spica splint (see Fig. 2–23) rather than a Velpeau sling, which tends to turn the humeral head laterally. For surgical treatment of irreducible or chronic luxations, biceps tenodesis can again be used to stabilize the joint.[2] By moving the tendon laterally, a "bow string" effect creates a medial force on the humeral head.

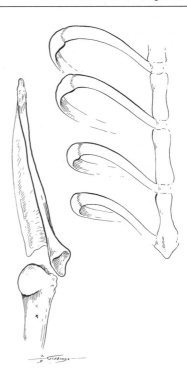

FIGURE 9–4. Lateral luxation of the left shoulder (ventrodorsal view).

Surgical Technique

A cranial approach to the shoulder is used with osteotomy of greater tubercle.[3] If the joint capsule is not torn, it is opened carefully to inspect the joint. All capsular material is saved for suturing. Careful assessment of the lateral labrum of the glenoid and the medial side of the humeral head is necessary. If the labrum is worn, successful stabilization is less likely. These changes are seen less with these luxations because of the more acute nature of most lateral luxations. If there is sufficient chondromalacia of the articular cartilage of the humeral head owing to rubbing on the lateral labrum, degenerative joint disease changes could limit long-term success even if the joint is stabilized. Arthrodesis or excision arthroplasty (see below) is probably indicated in these circumstances.

If the articular surfaces are in good condition and the luxation is recent, it may be possible to stabilize the joint by sutures through the lateral joint capsule (see Fig. 9–9). If this does not appear to be a viable option, tenodesis of the biceps tendon is carried out.

Tenodesis of the biceps tendon to a lateral position begins by transection of the transverse humeral ligament over the biceps tendon. The joint capsule is incised as needed to allow lateral transposition of the tendon (Fig. 9–5A). To transpose the tendon lateral to the remaining crest of the greater tubercle, it may be necessary to rongeur or curette a trough at the proximal end of the tubercular osteotomy site (Fig. 9–5B). The tendon is then held lateral to the tubercle by reattaching it to the humerus with Kirschner wires, pins and a tension band wire, or bone screws depending on tubercle size (Fig. 9–5C). Several sutures are placed between the biceps tendon and the deltoideus fascia. The joint capsule is imbricated with mattress or Lembert sutures. The superficial pectoral muscle is moved craniolaterally to allow attachment to the fascia of the deltoideus and biceps muscles.

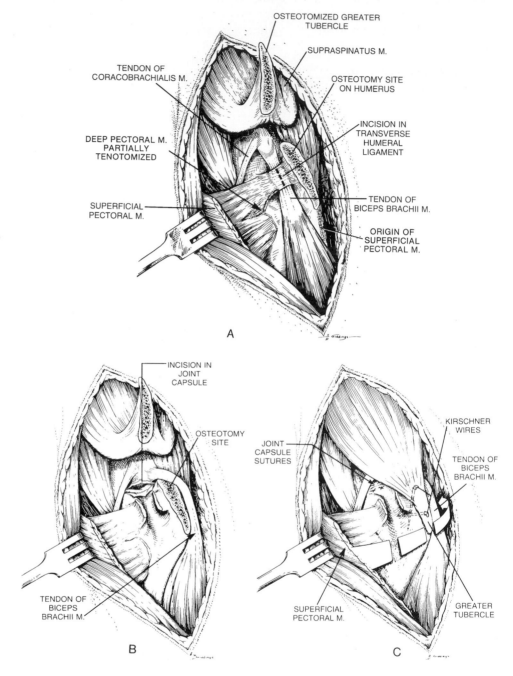

FIGURE 9–5. Surgical repair of lateral luxation of the shoulder. (*A*) The left shoulder has been exposed by a cranial approach.[3] The greater tubercle of the humerus has been osteotomized, and the incision is marked in the transverse humeral ligament. (*B*) The joint capsule has been incised to aid in moving the biceps tendon lateral to the greater tubercle osteotomy site. A small area of the proximal osteotomy site has been removed to ease positioning of the biceps tendon. (*C*) The greater tubercle is pinned back to its original site by two Kirschner wires or bone screws, thus trapping the biceps tendon laterally. The joint capsule is imbricated with mattress sutures, and the superficial pectoral muscle is attached to the fascia of the acromial head of the deltoideus and the biceps muscles.

AFTERCARE ■ A foreleg spica splint (see Fig. 2–23) is maintained for 14 days. Exercise is restricted for 4 weeks. Passive flexion-extension exercise may be needed following removal of the splint, supplemented with swimming when possible.

PROGNOSIS ■ In one series of six cases treated by lateral transposition of the biceps, five dogs had normal function and one limped occasionally at follow-up.[4]

Cranial Luxation

In our experience, cranial luxation, a relatively rare injury, is always the result of trauma. The biceps tendon can again be used for the stabilization of this infrequent luxation (Fig. 9–6). It is transposed cranially and thus is under increased tension and tends to hold the humeral head more tightly within the glenoid.

Surgical Technique

The shoulder is exposed by the cranial approach to the shoulder joint.[3] An incision is made in the transverse humeral ligament over the biceps tendon, and a trough is cut on the osteotomy surface on the crest and in the tubercle to accommodate the biceps tendon. If, as a result of tension, the tendon cannot be positioned within the osteotomy site on the humerus, sufficient bone is removed from the proximal osteotomy site to form a slight trough there (Fig. 9–7A). The tubercle is replaced and attached with Kirschner wires or pins and a tension band wire (Fig. 9–7B). Screw fixation should probably be avoided to prevent tendon injury. The joint capsule is imbricated with mattress or Lembert sutures.

AFTERCARE ■ The limb is supported in either a foreleg spica splint or Velpeau sling for 10 to 14 days (see Figs. 2–23 and 2–29). Exercise is restricted for 4 weeks. Passive flexion-extension exercise may be necessary after removal of the external fixation, and swimming is encouraged.

Caudal Luxation and Subluxation

Like cranial luxation, this injury occurs infrequently and may be either a self-induced or traumatic injury. Hyperextension of the joint is the probable cause.

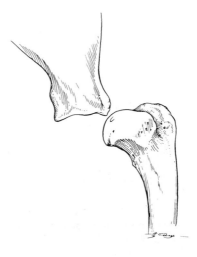

FIGURE 9–6. Cranial luxation of the left shoulder (mediolateral view).

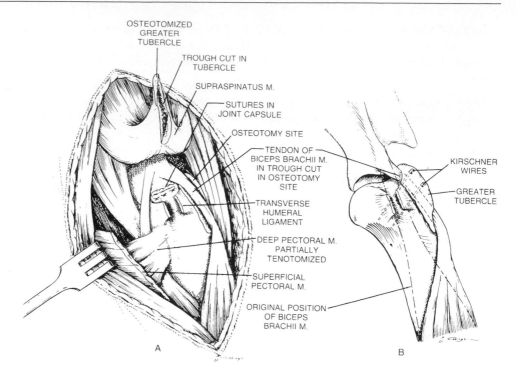

FIGURE 9–7. Surgical repair of cranial luxation of the shoulder. (A) The left shoulder has been exposed by a cranial approach.[3] The transverse humeral ligament has been cut, and the biceps tendon has been transposed cranially to lie in a trough created in the tubercular osteotomy site and in the tubercle itself. The joint capsule is imbricated with mattress sutures. (B) The tubercle is reattached to the osteotomy site with two Kirschner wires holding the biceps tendon in a position that pulls the humeral head into the glenoid.

The luxation may be total, as shown in Figure 9–8A, or subluxated. In the latter case, the joint space between the humeral head and the caudoventral rim of the glenoid is increased on extension-stress radiographs (Fig. 9–8B). Imbrication of the lateral and caudolateral joint capsule has worked well in these cases.

Surgical Technique

CAUDAL LUXATION ■ The shoulder joint is exposed by a craniolateral approach with osteotomy of the acromial process.[3] The joint capsule will be at least partially torn but may need to be opened farther to allow access to the joint. After inspection for intra-articular damage, the humeral head is reduced and the craniolateral and caudolateral joint capsule is imbricated with mattress or Lembert sutures of synthetic absorbable material (Fig. 9–9).

CAUDAL SUBLUXATION ■ The shoulder is exposed by a caudolateral approach.[3] The caudolateral joint capsule is imbricated with mattress or Lembert sutures of synthetic absorbable material (Fig. 9–10).

AFTERCARE ■ The limb is supported in a foreleg (Velpeau) sling for 14 days (see Fig. 2–29). Exercise is restricted for 4 weeks. Passive flexion-extension exercise may be needed following removal of the sling.

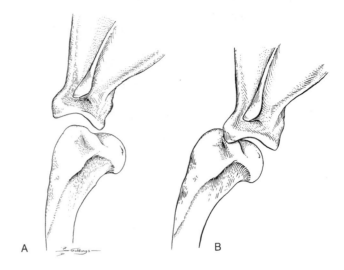

FIGURE 9–8. Caudal luxation and subluxation of the shoulder. (*A*) Caudal luxation of the left shoulder (lateromedial view). (*B*) Caudal subluxation of the left shoulder (lateromedial view). The joint space is increased caudally as extension stress is applied to the joint.

Excision Arthroplasty

In some cases, the glenohumeral joint cannot be reconstructed adequately. This is due most commonly to excessive wear of the medial labrum of the glenoid as a result of chronic medial luxation. Gunshot wounds on occasion damage the articular surfaces in such a way that nothing resembling normal joint function can result. The traditional method of treatment in these situations has been arthrodesis, which is technically demanding and requires bone-plating equipment in most cases.

An alternative salvage procedure is resection of the glenoid based on the method of Parkes.[6] This procedure has been modified by us to include partial excision of the humeral head in an attempt to provide a larger vascular surface. We postulate that this will result in a more rapid and proliferative fibroplasia and hence earlier stability of the pseudoarthrosis.

Surgical Technique

The joint is exposed by the approach to the craniolateral region of the shoulder by osteotomy of the acromial process.[3] The joint capsule is opened widely

FIGURE 9–9. Caudal luxation of the shoulder. The left shoulder has been exposed by a craniolateral approach with an osteotomy of the acromial process.[3] The infraspinatus and teres muscles have been freed by tenotomy. Mattress sutures of heavy-gauge absorbable suture have been used to imbricate the joint capsule as far cranially and caudally as possible, following the line of the rim of the glenoid.

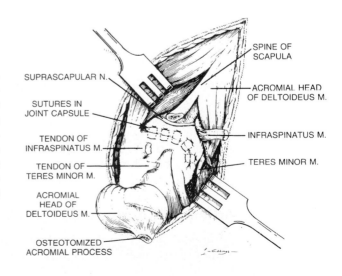

SPINE OF SCAPULA

SUPRASCAPULAR N.

ACROMIAL HEAD OF DELTOIDEUS M.

SUTURES IN JOINT CAPSULE

INFRASPINATUS M.

TENDON OF INFRASPINATUS M.

TERES MINOR M.

TENDON OF TERES MINOR M.

ACROMIAL HEAD OF DELTOIDEUS M.

OSTEOTOMIZED ACROMIAL PROCESS

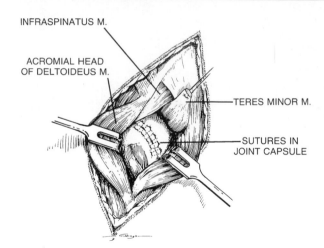

INFRASPINATUS M.

ACROMIAL HEAD
OF DELTOIDEUS M.

TERES MINOR M.

SUTURES IN
JOINT CAPSULE

FIGURE 9–10. Caudal subluxation of the shoulder. The left shoulder has been exposed by a caudolateral approach.[3] The caudolateral joint capsule has been imbricated with mattress sutures of heavy-gauge absorbable suture. The suture line follows the rim of the glenoid as far caudad as possible, taking care to avoid the caudal circumflex humeral artery.

and the tendon of the biceps muscle is detached from the supraglenoid tubercle (Fig. 9–11A). With care taken to protect the suprascapular nerve and caudal circumflex humeral artery, ostectomies are made in the glenoid and humeral head (Fig. 9–11B) with an osteotome or high-speed pneumatic surgical bur. The glenoid ostectomy is made obliquely to bevel the edge. The deep (medial) edge is longer than the superficial edge.

A notch is cut in the base of the spine of the scapula to allow the suprascapular nerve to be displaced proximally. The infraspinatus is reattached, but the teres minor muscle is pulled medially between the two ostectomy surfaces and sutured to the biceps tendon and medial joint capsule (Fig. 9–11C). Whatever joint capsule is available is then pulled into the "joint space" and sutured to the teres minor muscle and biceps tendon. The purpose of these maneuvers is to interpose soft tissue between the ostectomies and hasten formation of a fibrous false joint. It may be necessary to wire the acromial process to the scapular spine more proximally than normal in order to remove laxity in the deltoideus muscle created by the ostectomies, which shorten the distance between the acromial osteotomy site and the insertion of the muscle.

AFTERCARE ■ The limb is not immobilized postoperatively. Early, gentle use of the limb is encouraged by leash walking. More vigorous activity is forced starting 10 days postoperatively, and swimming is encouraged. Early activity stimulates the fibrosis necessary to create a false joint without any bony contact.

PROGNOSIS ■ It must be appreciated that this is a salvage procedure and that normal function of the limb is not to be expected. Moderate, pain-free exercise capability is the objective, and it usually is achieved. A slight limp and some atrophy of the shoulder girdle muscles are expected.

Thirteen cases have been reported in two series.[7,8] Good to excellent pain-free function was noted in each case. One case had bilateral surgery for chronic medial luxations of the shoulders, and, at 6 months postoperatively, the animal was using both limbs at all times and bore about 80 percent of normal weight on the limbs.

Arthrodesis of the Shoulder Joint

Surgical fusion of the shoulder joint results in remarkably little functional disability because of the extreme mobility of the scapula. This scapular motion

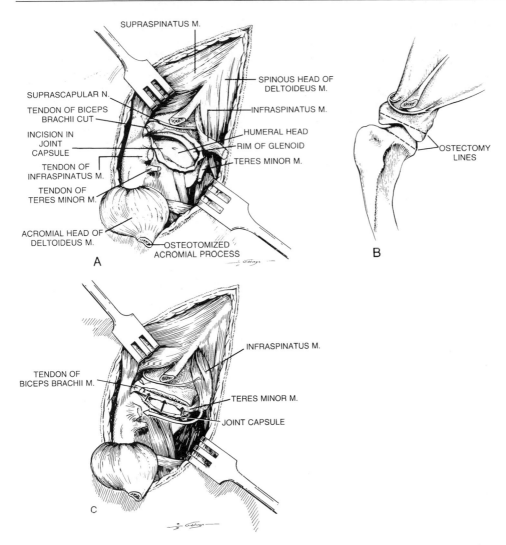

FIGURE 9–11. Resection of the glenoid and humeral head. (*A*) The left shoulder has been exposed by a craniolateral approach.[3] Tenotomies have been performed on the biceps, infraspinatus, and teres minor muscles. The joint capsule is cut close to the glenoid rim. The joint capsule that is left attached to the humeral head is preserved. (*B*) Positions of both ostectomy lines. (*C*) Both ostectomies have been completed. The teres minor muscle has been pulled medially where it has been sutured to the biceps tendon, which has previously been sutured to the fascia of the supraspinatus muscle. Accessible joint capsule from the humeral head is sutured to the teres minor. A small notch may be cut in the base of the spine of the scapula to allow the suprascapular nerve to be positioned more proximally if it is too near the ostectomy. The infraspinatus is reattached to its insertion, and the acromial process is wired to the spine more proximally than normal.

compensates for loss of motion in the shoulder joint. This is not to indicate that use of the limb is normal but that enough function remains for active use of the limb. In one study, the only gait abnormalities noted were limited circumduction and inability to advance the limb quickly when running.[5]

Common indications for arthrodesis of the shoulder are comminuted fractures of the glenoid, neck of the scapula, or head of the humerus. Additionally, chronic shoulder luxations often result in severe erosion of the glenoid and humeral head, making surgical repair impossible. Severe degenerative joint disease is a legitimate but uncommon indication. As with all arthrodeses, this is a mutilating operation and should be considered only as a last-resort salvage procedure. It is important that other joints of the limb be normal if this procedure is performed.

Surgical Technique

A combined craniolateral and cranial approach to the shoulder joint is performed with osteotomy of both the acromial process and the greater tubercle (Fig. 9–12A).[3] This widely exposes the joint and allows the joint capsule to be opened for debridement of cartilage on both articular surfaces.

The biceps tendon is detached at the supraglenoid tubercle, and the suprascapular nerve is protected during 20 osteotomies which parallel the lines shown in Figure 9–12B. Flat osteotomy surfaces eliminate shear stress at the bone surfaces, especially when compression is exerted. The greater tubercle of the humerus is osteotomized with rongeurs or saw to provide a gentle curve on a line from the spine of the scapula to the cranial aspect of the humerus. To temporarily immobilize the joint during plate application, a small intramedullary pin or Kirschner wire is driven from the cranial humeral cortex into the glenoid with the shoulder at a functional angle of about 105 degrees (Fig. 9–12C). An eight- to ten-hole plate is contoured to fit the cranial surface of the humerus and the dorsocranial junction of the spine with the body of the scapula. Some torsion of the plate will be necessary in order to make it fit the junction

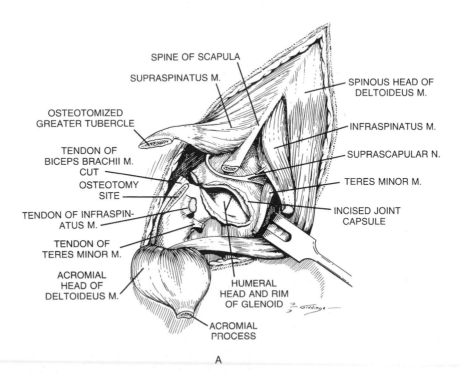

A

FIGURE 9–12. Arthrodesis of the shoulder joint. (A) The left shoulder has been exposed by a combined cranial and craniolateral approach.[3] The biceps tendon has been detached from the supraglenoid tubercle, and the joint capsule is opened. *Figure continues on following page*

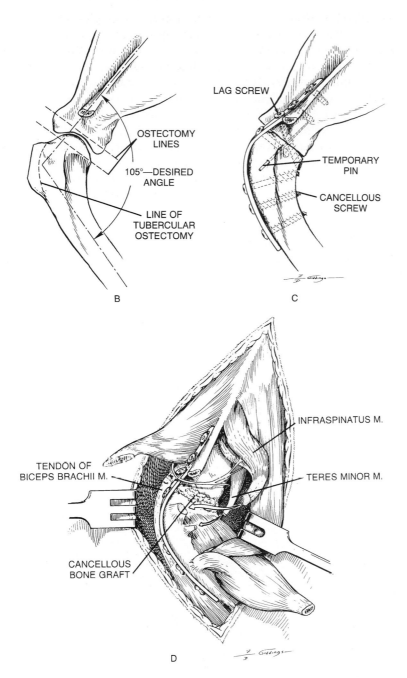

FIGURE 9–12. *Continued* (*B*) With the joint positioned at a functional angle of 105 to 110 degrees, ostectomies of the glenoid and humeral head are performed to remove articular cartilage and produce flat opposing surfaces. The greater tubercle is further ostectomized to provide a gentle curve from the humeral neck to the cranial cortex. (*C*) A small pin is driven across the joint to hold the bones at the correct angle while the plate is contoured and attached, after which the pin is removed. At least one screw must be a lag screw between the scapula and the humerus. (*D*) Bone graft obtained from the greater tubercle is placed around the opposed bones. The biceps tendon is sutured to the supraspinatus muscle fascia. The osteotomized portion of the tubercle attached to the supraspinatus muscle is pinned or screwed lateral to the plate, and the rest of the tissues are closed routinely.

of the spine and the body of the scapula. The reconstruction plate (Synthes Ltd. [USA], Paoli, PA) is especially suitable for this procedure because it is more easily contoured than conventional plates. The plate must either pass over the suprascapular nerve with sufficient room for the nerve or be placed underneath the nerve. In attaching the plate, thought must be given to placing at least one screw in lag fashion across the debrided bone surfaces to create compression. As shown in Figure 9–12C, the third screw hole was chosen.

One or two cancellous screws can be used to advantage in the humeral head. (Some types of plates do not accept cancellous screws except at the end holes.) The pin can be removed after the plate is attached. The bone removed from the greater tubercle during the contouring process is used as a bone graft in and around the joint (Fig. 9–12D). The biceps tendon is reattached to the fascia of the supraspinatus muscle or to the cortex of the humerus medial to the plate using a bone screw and spiked washer (see Fig. 9–15B, C). The osteotomized greater tubercle is attached to the humerus lateral to the plate with a screw or pins. The soft tissues are closed routinely in layers.

AFTERCARE ▪ The shoulder is immobilized in a spica splint for 4 weeks (see Fig. 2–23). Radiographic signs of fusion should be noted between 6 and 12 weeks postoperatively, at which time the splint is removed and the dog allowed to return to normal activity over a 4-week period. Barring complications, the plate is not removed.

Osteochondritis Dissecans of the Humeral Head

A general discussion of osteochondrosis dissecans (OCD) is found in Chapter 6. In the shoulder joint, the condition is manifested as a fragment of cartilage that becomes partially or fully detached from the caudocentral aspect of the humeral head, usually opposite the caudoventral rim of the glenoid. The cartilage flap usually remains attached to normal cartilage along the cranial edge of the flap; however, it may become free within the joint, in which case it usually becomes lodged in the caudoventral pouch or cul-de-sac of the joint capsule.

Free cartilage fragments within the joint can be resorbed, but some may remain viable and even grow in size, since they are nourished by synovial fluid. Others become attached to synovial membrane, where they can become vascularized and undergo partial ossification; they are then called *ossicles*. Those cartilage fragments that lodge in the caudal joint usually do not create clinical signs unless they grow in size sufficient to irritate the synovial membrane (see Fig. 6–2). Fragments that migrate to the bicipital tendon sheath often produce clinical lameness.[9]

Clinical Signs and History

Dogs of the large breeds are most commonly affected in a 2:1 to 3:1 male/female ratio. Various studies have reported bilateral involvement between 27 and 68 percent. Many dogs showing bilateral radiographic signs will be clinically lame in only one limb. It is worth noting that when an animal is markedly lame in one leg, it is difficult to assess lameness in the contralateral leg. It is likely that those animals diagnosed radiographically as bilateral in reality are showing only the signs of osteochondrosis in one shoulder and never develop a loose cartilage flap. This supposition is supported by a clinical series in which only 20 percent of the bilaterally affected animals needed bilateral surgical treatment.[10]

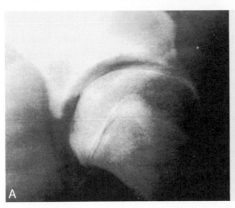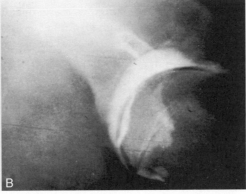

FIGURE 9–13. Osteochondritis dissecans of the humeral head. (*A*) A flattening of the subchondral bone of the caudal aspect of the humeral head can be appreciated here, but there is no visible indication of the presence or absence of a cartilage flap. This could simply be the manifestation of osteochondrosis. (*B*) This contrast arthrogram shows dye filling of the joint space and a filling defect that represents the cartilage flap.

Although most animals first show clinical signs between 4 and 8 months of age, some will present much later, at 2 to 3 years of age. In these cases, the owners have simply ignored, or did not notice, the early lameness. Lameness is often first noted after severe exercise, but it may be insidious in onset. Rarely is the dog three-legged lame. A shortening of the swing phase of gait leads to atrophy of the spinatus and deltoid muscles resulting in a more prominent acromial process. This is a constant finding if lameness has been present more than 2 to 3 weeks. The change of gait is most noticeable at a walk. Pain on palpation is variable and is more often noted on severe extension than flexion or rotation. Crepitus is also variable. Clinical signs are most notable after rest preceded by heavy exercise.

Radiology

OCD of the shoulder is usually detected by lateral radiographs of the shoulder. A flattening of the humeral head is usually seen if properly positioned (Fig. 9–13). Sedation is often necessary. Rarely, arthrograms may be needed if the flattening is inapparent (Fig. 9–13B). (See Chapter 1.) Usually 4 to 5 ml of diluted contrast is injected. The dye seeps under the flap (Fig. 9–13 B) and also travels to the bicipital tendon sheath, where it may outline joint mice.

Diagnosis

The diagnosis of OCD causing the lameness has to be based on clinical assessment of the history, radiographs, and physical examination. The lameness is usually of a mild to moderate severity. Often, pain may be elicited by palpation (flexion and extension). The radiographic lesion should be at least 4 mm wide. Other common rule-outs must be eliminated.

Treatment

Varying opinions have been expressed regarding surgical versus nonsurgical treatment of this condition. As experience has been gained, a more aggressive surgical approach has become evident. Although some animals do recover spontaneously, this can happen only if the flap breaks loose and is absorbed in the joint cavity. Furthermore, this process may take 9 to 12 months, and bilaterally affected animals are unlikely to recover to the point of clinical soundness. An additional little-appreciated danger is that the loose cartilage flap may survive within the joint, as described above. Large ossicles cause severe inflammatory changes and degenerative joint disease. We have retrieved such ossicles from 3- and 4-year-old dogs. If the flap never breaks free, a similar deterioration of the joint occurs. We have removed partially attached flaps in 3-year-old dogs.

Surgical treatment has yielded much more uniformly good results in our experience as well as others.[11,12] Not only is the final outcome more predictable but soundness is achieved within 1 to 2 months, and late degenerative changes are less probable. We recommend surgery if:

1.   Lameness has persisted more than 6 weeks.
2.   The animal is over 6½ months of age.
3.   The cartilage flap or joint mouse is confirmed radiographically.
4.   Pain is elicited from shoulder palpation, and no other radiographic lesion of the forelimb is found.

Osteochondroplasty of the Humeral Head

The aim of surgery is to remove cartilage flaps still attached and to remove all fragments of free cartilage from within the joint. Removal of the cartilage allows a fibrocartilage scar to fill the defect and seal the edges of the articular cartilage bordering the defect.

The choice of surgical approach is variable. The caudolateral approach[3] or variations of it have generally worked well for us if an assistant is present. A humeral head retractor (Scanlan Surgical Instruments, Inc., Englewood, CO) is useful for exposure of the lesion. If we work alone, the more generous exposure of the craniolateral approach with osteotomy of the acromial process[3] is preferable, lessening the need for retraction. However, this is a longer procedure and is associated with more postoperative morbidity (seroma/lameness).

The caudolateral approach provides adequate visualization of the lesion if the joint capsule is adequately retracted and if the leg is severely internally rotated (Fig. 9–14A). A scalpel blade or small curved osteotome is used to cut the cartilage flap free (Fig. 9–14B, C). Irregular and undermined loosened areas of cartilage at the periphery of the lesion should be trimmed and smoothed with a curette to create vertical walls. Curettage may or may not be done at this point, depending on surgeon preference. Curettage of the lesion floor should be very cautiously done to minimize removal of subchondral bone. There is often a film of unorganized material covering the lesion. This can be gently scraped to expose the bone. There may be merit in *forage*, which is a technique of drilling multiple holes in the bed of the lesion with a Kirschner wire. This creates vascular channels to the subchondral bone and hastens ingrowth of "repair" tissue in the defect. The caudal cul-de-sac of the joint cavity must always be explored for free fragments of cartilage. Exposure of this area is enhanced by a small Hohmann retractor and by flexing the shoulder and elbow (Fig. 9–14D). In chronic lesions, debridement of large caudal glenoid osteophytes may assist in removal of the flap and inspection of the lesion bed. The final step is forceful lavage of the joint to flush out small cartilage fragments. If cartilage fragments have been identified in the bicipital tendon sheath, they will have to be removed by a cranial approach, as they cannot be exposed from a caudolateral approach.[3]

Another surgical technique (lateral approach; Fig. 9–15) is to partially incise the caudal half of the acromial head of the deltoideus tendon to facilitate the

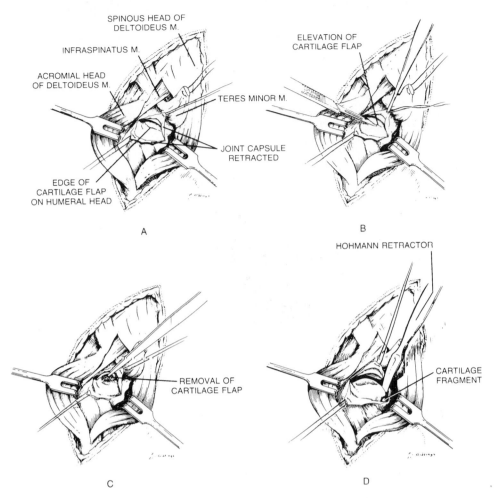

SPINOUS HEAD OF DELTOIDEUS M.

INFRASPINATUS M.

ACROMIAL HEAD OF DELTOIDEUS M.

TERES MINOR M.

JOINT CAPSULE RETRACTED

EDGE OF CARTILAGE FLAP ON HUMERAL HEAD

A

ELEVATION OF CARTILAGE FLAP

B

REMOVAL OF CARTILAGE FLAP

C

HOHMANN RETRACTOR

CARTILAGE FRAGMENT

D

FIGURE 9–14. Osteochondroplasty of the humeral head for osteochondritis dissecans. (*A*) The left shoulder has been exposed by a caudolateral approach.[3] The lateral edge of the cartilage flap is visible after retraction of the joint capsule by stay sutures. (*B*) The cartilage flap is elevated from the humeral head by sharp dissection. (*C*) When the flap has been sufficiently elevated, it can be cut free along its cranial border. (*D*) The caudal cul-de-sac of the joint capsule is retracted with a small Hohmann retractor to allow removal of any free cartilage fragments.

cranial incision into the joint capsule. The junction of the infraspinatus and teres minor is bluntly separated, followed by incision into the joint capsule (Fig. 9–15).

AFTERCARE ■ Seroma formation is more common with shoulder surgery than with virtually any other canine surgery. This is perhaps due to the extreme amount of sliding motion of the skin and subcutis in this region over the muscle fascia. The only prevention is enforced rest for the first 10 to 14 postoperative days. A Velpeau sling (see Fig. 2–29) may be indicated for some hyperactive animals. Small seromas clear spontaneously in 2 to 5 weeks; large ones are treated with hot packs. Needle aspiration is usually unnecessary, since the seroma disappears in 4 to 6 weeks regardless. Often, if drained, the fluid recurs.

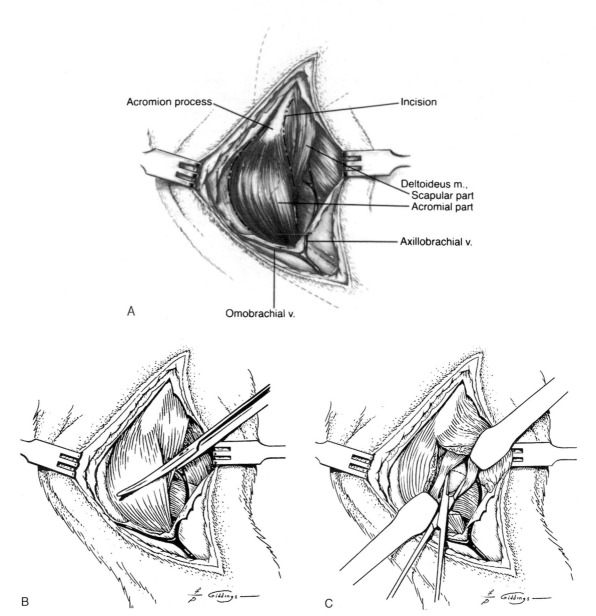

FIGURE 9–15. Lateral approach of the scapulohumeral joint. (*A*) A slightly curved skin incision is made from above the acromial process to the proximal fourth of the humerus. The deep fascia has been incised from the caudal edge of the acromial process to the junction of the omobrachial and axillobrachial veins distally. The junction between the acromial and spinous heads of the deltoideus muscle are developed. (*B*) The caudal half of the acromial deltoideus is incised 5 mm from its origin to gain increased exposure to the cranial joint. (*C*) After retraction of the deltoideus cranially, the junction between the infraspinatus and teres minor is separated. The teres minor is undermined off the joint capsule. The infraspinatus insertion and the deltoideus are retracted craniodorsally, while the teres minor is retracted caudoventrally. The joint capsule is incised as in Figure 9–14. (Part *A* from Piermattei DL: An Atlas of Surgical Approaches to the Bones and Joints of the Dog and Cat, 3rd ed. Philadelphia, WB Saunders Co, 1993, p 103, with permission.)

From 3 through 6 weeks postoperatively, very minimal activity (house confinement or leash) is suggested, followed by graduated exercise 2 to 3 months postoperatively.

Arthroscopy

Successful treatment of osteochondritis dissecans in 23 shoulder joints in 21 dogs has been reported by Person.[13] Force plate evaluation showed objective signs of improvement in gait in nine of 10 dogs seen postoperatively for follow-up. This method of treatment may well see much more application in the future but, at the present time, is not widely used.

PROGNOSIS ■ With shoulder OCD, the prognosis with surgery is excellent if treated before 12 months of age. The prognosis is still very good in older animals.

Calcification of the Supraspinatus Tendon

Calcification of the supraspinatus tendon of insertion is a newly reported[14] degenerative condition causing mild to moderate forelimb lameness in medium to large adult dogs. The etiology is unknown but is probably an overuse syndrome. It is often bilateral.

History and Clinical Features

Lameness is usually insidious in onset, producing chronic signs. Unlike osteoarthritic conditions, lameness worsens throughout the day with minimal or moderate activity. The presence of calcification radiographically is often asymptomatic and the clinician *must* eliminate other conditions before making the definitive diagnosis.

Physical Exam

Unfortunately, manipulations often do not produce pain. With few exceptions the calcium deposit is not large enough to palpate.

Radiographic Examination

Calcification is often seen upon careful scrutiny of a lateral view of the shoulder (Fig. 9–16). The condition is often bilateral radiographically but rarely produces bilateral lameness. Calcification is often subtle due to superimposition on the greater tubercle of the humerus. A tangential or "sky-line" view of the intertubercular region of the proximal humerus eliminates this superimposition and allows distinction between biceps tendon calcification. The cranioproximal-craniodistal (CP-CD) view is taken with the dog in sternal recumbency, with the radiographic cassette placed on top of the forearm with the elbow bent. The radiographic tube is positioned directly over the scapulohumeral joint (Fig. 9–17). Calcification occurs cranial and just medial to the greater tubercle of the humerus (Fig. 9–3). It may be smooth or irregular and have multiple "pockets." Calcification of the biceps tendon occurs more medial and caudal into the groove closer to the humeral head.

Diagnosis

Since the presence of calcification can be asymptomatic and since there is no particular physical exam finding, the diagnosis of the calcification causing lameness is only presumptive. Other conditions such as bicipital tendonitis and

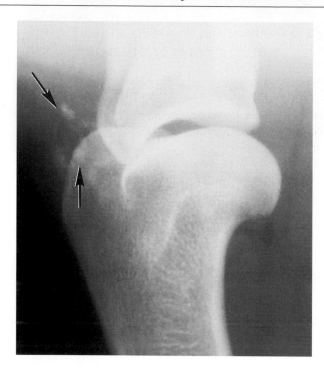

FIGURE 9–16. Calcification of the supraspinatus tendon. This calcification was asymptomatic in this 2-year-old Rottweiler. Its symptomatic calcified supraspinatus tendon on the opposite side was not as apparent radiographically. Note the numerous pockets of mineralized material located on and superficial to the greater tubercle of the humerus.

chronic congenital joint lesions must be ruled out (Figs. 9–18 and 9–19). When other conditions are found, a diagnostic quandary exists. Since the treatment is fairly simple, surgical treatment of both conditions at the same time may be undertaken. The amount of calcification is not relative to the amount of pain a dog may have.

Treatment

By longitudinally incising into the supraspinatus tendon, the calcium is evacuated. To accomplish this the dog is placed in dorsal recumbency with both

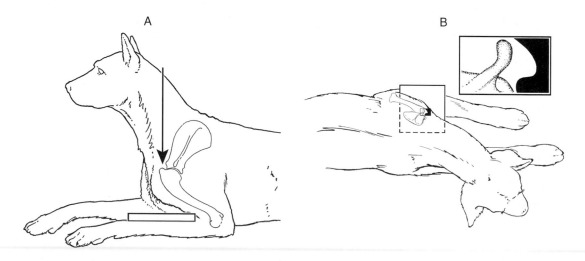

FIGURE 9–17. Positioning of dog for the CP-CD view. (*A*) With the dog in sternal recumbency, a radiographic cassette is placed on top of the flexed forearm. The radiographic tube is positioned directly over the point of the shoulder. (*B*) Dorsal view of how the greater tubercle is projected on the radiographic cassette. The dog's head is pulled to the side.

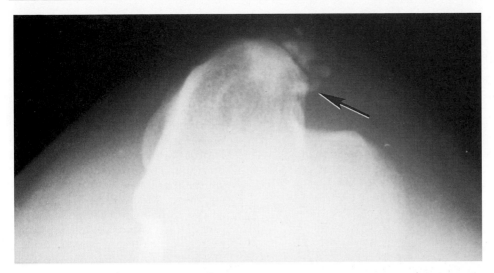

FIGURE 9–18. CP-CD view of the Rottweiler in Figure 9–16. The mineralization lies cranial and medial to the greater tubercle (*arrow*). The biceps tendon lies in the inter-tubercular groove situated under the arrow. The convex white area represents the greater tubercle while the concave area is the intertubercular groove.

forearms secured alongside the body wall. The radiographs are placed on a viewer to mimic the position of the dog to assist placement of the tendinous incision. A 6- to 7-cm cranial skin incision is followed by deeper dissection through the longitudinal fibers of the brachiocephalicus muscle (Fig. 9–20). The tendon of the supraspinatus is identified along with the proximal end of the humerus. Longitudinal incisions are made in relation to the humerus (Fig. 9–20B). Normal tendon is a yellowish white, while the tendon surrounding the

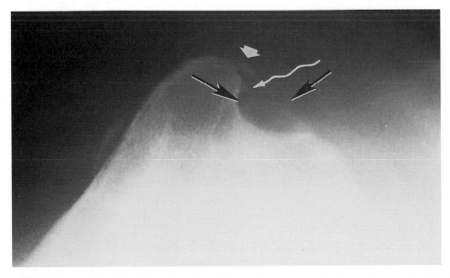

FIGURE 9–19. A CP-CD view of a shoulder arthrogram of a dog with severe foreleg lameness suspected of bicipital tendinitis along with calcification of the supraspinatus tendon. Note the calcified material on top of the greater tubercle (*white arrowhead*), osteophyte in the intertubercular groove (*curved arrow*), and dye outlining the normal biceps tendon in the intertubercular groove (*black arrows*).

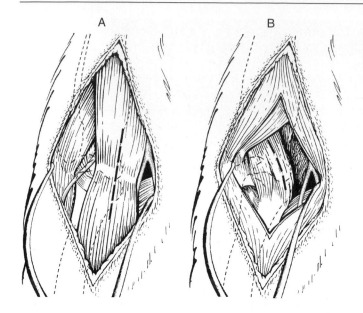

FIGURE 9–20. (*A*) A 6- to 7-cm skin incision is made over the point of the shoulder. A similar incision is made between muscle fibers of the brachiocephalicus muscle. (*B*) After retraction of the brachiocephalicus muscle, a blind longitudinal incision is made in the supraspinatus tendon depending on the location of the mineral seen on the radiograph. Pockets of mineral have a whiter appearance than the surrounding tissue. Multiple incisions may be needed to find all of the pockets. Closure consists of nonabsorbable sutures placed in the supraspinatus tendon, brachiocephalicus separation, and subcuticular and skin layers.

white calcium deposit is grayish white. The calcified material is very white and similar to what one sees when fenestrating a calcified disk. If multiple areas are seen radiographically, then multiple small incisions may be needed to evacuate the material. Closure is made in layers using absorbable or nonabsorbable flexion.

AFTERCARE ■ A flexion carpal bandage (see Fig. 2–30) is applied for 10 to 12 days to allow tendon healing followed by limited activity for another 2 to 3 weeks. While swimming is a good exercise for many orthopedic conditions, it may stress the supraspinatus and is not advised for several months.

PROGNOSIS ■ The prognosis, provided that this calcification was the cause of the lameness, is excellent. The dogs are usually better in 2 to 4 weeks and usually totally recovered in 6 to 8 weeks.

Tenosynovitis of Biceps Tendon

This disease process is a common cause of forelimb lameness in medium- to large-breed adult dogs. There is some predilection for animals that are not physically well conditioned.

Anatomy and Pathophysiology

After originating on the supraglenoid tubercle the tendon of the biceps brachii muscle passes distally through the intertubercular groove of the humerus, where it is stabilized by the transverse humeral ligament. The muscle inserts distally on the radius and ulna, and its main function is flexion of the elbow. It has little involvement in stabilizing the normal shoulder joint.[1] The tendon is surrounded by a synovial sheath that is an extension of the glenohumeral joint capsule. This sheath extends distally just beyond the transverse humeral ligament. There is no bursa associated with this tendon.

This injury is a *strain* injury to the tendon of the biceps brachii. These injuries are discussed in Chapter 7 in more detail. The mechanism of injury to the biceps tendon can either be direct or indirect trauma or simple overuse. Thus the pathological changes range from partial disruption of the tendon (grade 3 strain) to chronic inflammatory changes, including dystrophic calcification. Pathological changes also can be secondary to other diseases such as osteochondritis dissecans, where joint mice migrate to the synovial sheath and create an acute synovitis.[9] Thus it can be seen that the initial irritating source usually initially affects either the tendon or the synovial membrane individually, but soon the inflammatory process involves the opposite member. Proliferation of fibrous connective tissue and adhesions between the tendon and sheath limits motion and causes pain.[15]

History and Clinical Signs

An inciting traumatic incident may be recalled by the owner, but usually the onset of the disease is insidious, and many cases will be of several months' duration when presented. The lameness is subtle and intermittent and worsens with exercise. Since the pain is present only during gliding motion of the tendon, there is no hesitation to bear weight on the limb; therefore there is little change in the stance phase of gait.[15] The swing phase of locomotion is limited because the shoulder joint is guarded by limiting the amount of extension and flexion.[16–18]

Atrophy of the spinati muscle group is soon evident, but more distal muscles appear normal in size. Shoulder pain on manipulation is not a constant finding, especially in chronic cases. Pain is elicited by applying deep digital pressure over the tendon in the intertubercular groove region while simultaneously flexing the shoulder and extending the elbow. (See Fig. 1–5.)

Radiographic Findings

Tenosynovitis of the biceps tendon may stimulate a bony reaction on the supraglenoid tubercle (Fig. 9–21), calcification of the bicipital tendon, and osteophytes in the intertubercular groove (Fig. 9–22). The lateral and CP-CD or tangential radiographic views (Fig. 9–23) are helpful in defining these changes. Arthrography is often very helpful in diagnosing the condition.

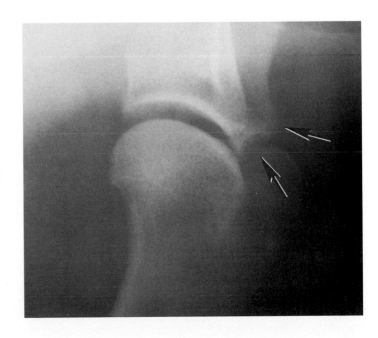

FIGURE 9–21. Reaction on the supraglenoid tuberosity in a 5-year-old mixed breed with a small rupture of the biceps tendon (*arrows*).

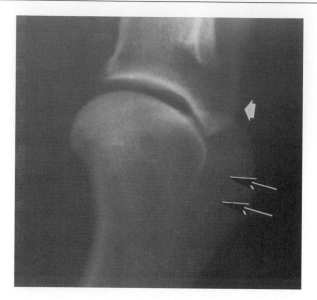

FIGURE 9–22. Osteophytes located in the intertubercular groove of a dog with chronic partial bicipital tendon rupture (*black arrows*). Note also a minor reaction on the suprascapular tuberosity (*white arrowhead*).

A normal arthrogram fills the tendon sheath, which is continuous with the scapulohumeral joint. The dye column should be continuous and has a lobulated appearance distally (Fig. 9–24). Abnormal findings include absence or decrease of dye filling the sheath (Fig. 9–25), leakage of dye from the sheath, and narrowing of the bicipital tendon.[16–18]

Diagnosis

The diagnosis of bicipital tenosynovitis is based on history, pain upon flexing the shoulder, and characteristic plain radiographs or arthrograms.[16–18] Not all cases will have all the characteristic signs, and at times the diagnosis is presumptive with definitive diagnosis only made after gross inspection or histopathology. Differential diagnoses include calcification of the supraspinatus,

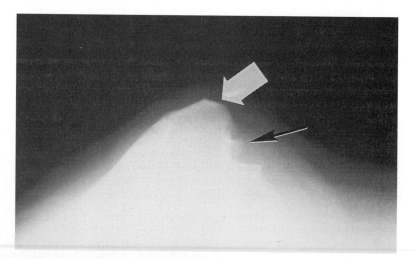

FIGURE 9–23. The CP-CD view is helpful in delineating the location of bony changes surrounding the proximal humerus. Note the greater tubercle (*white arrow*) and osteophyte (*black arrow*) in the medial aspect of the intertubercular groove. Compare with the calcification of the supraspinatus seen in Figures 9–18 and 9–19.

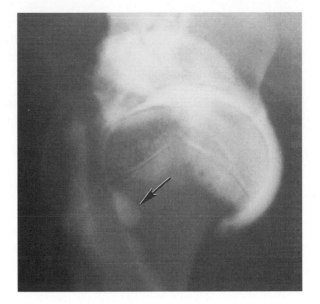

FIGURE 9–24. A normal shoulder arthrogram. Note the normal lobulations (*arrow*) surrounding the distal half of the bicipital tendon sheath and compare with Figure 9–25.

osteo- and chondrosarcomas of the proximal humerus, neurofibromas of the brachial plexus and spinal cord, and chronic elbow conditions related to osteochondrosis.

Treatment

In acute cases the treatment is aimed at reducing inflammation in the affected structures before the pathological changes become irreversible. Rest and anti-inflammatory nonsteroidal drug therapy (see Chapter 6) are often sufficient.

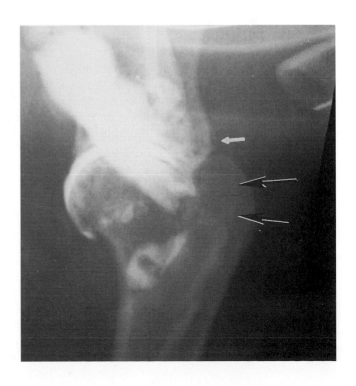

FIGURE 9–25. Shoulder arthrogram of a 6-year-old mixed breed dog with poor filling of the proximal (*black arrows*) and distal bicipital tendon sheath accompanying a bony reaction on the suprascapular tuberosity (*white arrow*) that was seen on plain radiographs. The biceps tendon was partially torn.

Strict confinement for 4 to 6 weeks is needed for resolution, and premature return to activity will almost ensure a chronic disease state. Systemic treatment with either nonsteroidal or corticosteroidal drugs has been unsuccessful in chronic cases in our hands. Intra-articular corticosteroid treatment can be successful in this disease if there are no mechanical causes, such as joint mice, and when the pathological changes are not well established. There is no way of knowing if this is the case initially, so treatment is always given on a trial basis unless the injury is relatively acute and uncomplicated.

Arthrocentesis must be done aseptically, and we prefer 1.5-inch, 22-gauge spinal needles, which cause less accidental damage to the articular cartilage. The joint is entered 1 cm from the acromial process, with the needle directed toward the glenoid and angled slightly cranially. Synovial fluid is aspirated and immediately observed for turbidity. If the fluid is off color or the viscosity markedly changed, a complete examination of the fluid is completed before injecting the joint with corticosteroid to prevent injection into a septic joint. If there are no contraindications, 20 to 40 mg of prednisolone acetate (Depo-Medrol, Upjohn Co., Kalamazoo, MI) is injected, which will fill the joint and go down the tendon sheath. Direct injection of corticosteroid into the tendon itself is contraindicated, as it is known to cause further tendon disruption. This is followed by strict confinement for 2 weeks and light activity the third week. If lameness is markedly improved but not eliminated, a second injection is given 3 weeks later. If this is not curative, the dog should have surgical treatment. Return of the lameness several months or years later is not uncommon, and many will respond again to corticosteroid injection.

Surgical treatment is recommended for dogs that do not respond to medical treatment or those in which a mechanical problem is found initially. The goal of surgical treatment is elimination of movement of the biceps tendon in the inflamed tendon sheath, and this is accomplished by tenodesis of the bicipital tendon.

Surgical Technique

The tendon is exposed by a cranial approach to the shoulder joint.[3] The transverse humeral ligament and joint capsule are opened to expose the tendon and the intertubercular groove, which often has osteophytes along each edge (Fig. 9–26A). Partial rupture of the tendon near its origin is not uncommon. Joint mice are sought and removed, and the tendon is transected near the supraglenoid tubercle. The tendon is reattached to the humerus distal to the groove by a bone screw and spiked washer (Synthes Ltd. [USA], Paoli, PA), as shown in Figure 9–26B, or more commonly the tendon can be pulled through a bone tunnel in the greater tubercle of the humerus and then sutured laterally to the supraspinatus muscle or the infraspinatus tendon (Fig. 9–26C). There is no loss of stability or mobility to the shoulder joint apparent from this procedure.[1] A section of the tendon should be saved for histopathological examination.

A simple procedure to reattach the biceps muscle after excision of the traumatized proximal tendon involves placement of a double Bunnell-Meyer suture pattern in the proximal biceps muscle. With the limb moderately extended, two parallel holes are made in the greater tubercle adjacent to the proximal end of the biceps. The ends of the suture material (No. 1 nonabsorbable suture material) are passed through these holes and tied laterally with the biceps relaxed (shoulder extended) (Fig. 9–26D).

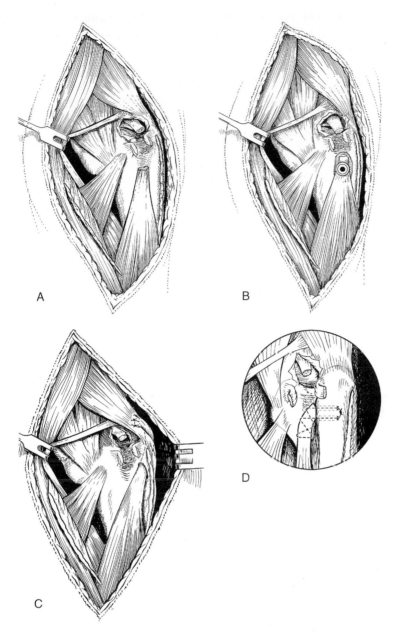

FIGURE 9–26. Tenodesis of the biceps brachii tendon. (*A*) The tendon is exposed by a craniolateral approach to the shoulder.[3] The tendon is cut near the supraglenoid tubercle and again distal to the intertubercular groove. (*B*) With the elbow flexed, the tendon is fixed to the humerus in a position that creates some tension on the muscle. After curettage of the periosteum, the tendon is bluntly split and attached to the humerus with a bone screw and an AO/ASIF plastic spiked washer (Synthes Ltd. [USA], Paoli, PA). (*C*) A second method of attaching the tendon is illustrated. The tendon is cut free from the tubercle but is not cut again distally as above. A hole is drilled laterally through the greater tubercle, and the tendon is brought through the bone tunnel and sutured to the insertion of the supraspinatus muscle. (*D*) Alternatively, a double Bunnell-Meyer suture pattern utilizing No. 1 nonabsorbable suture material has been placed in the proximal biceps muscle. Two parallel holes are made with an 0.045 Kirschner wire in the greater tubercle of the humerus adjacent to the proximal biceps muscle. The ends of the suture material are passed through the holes and tied laterally with the limb in extension.

AFTERCARE ■ The limb is supported in a Velpeau sling (Fig. 2–29) and the animal closely confined 3 weeks. Exercise is allowed to slowly increase to normal at 6 weeks postoperatively.

PROGNOSIS ■ About two thirds of the cases we have seen are treated medically, and approximately two thirds of these are cured by the treatment. The remainder of this group is divided between those that are treated again medically and those that do not respond and require surgical treatment. Those treated surgically early respond better than those that are operated on late. Normal gait and use of the leg return in 50 to 60 percent of the dogs, and the remainder stay variably lame, undoubtedly owing to chronic degenerative joint disease. Surgery is therefore recommended after one or less courses of corticosteroids. Medical management of this problem is discussed in Chapter 6. Surgical treatment of this problem in man is variably reported to be 50 to 94 percent successful.[19,20]

Rupture of the Tendon of the Biceps Brachii Muscle

The same forces that cause avulsion of the supraglenoid tubercle in young dogs cause rupture of the tendon of the biceps near its origin on the tubercle in the mature dog. Initially, there is pain and effusion in the cranial shoulder joint region. Although the animal will exhibit an obvious lameness on the affected limb, flexion of the elbow joint is not obviously impaired. It is not usually possible to palpate the area of rupture in the tendon digitally because of swelling of tissues. Partial rupture is not uncommonly a cause of bicipital tenosynovitis.

Arthrography in acute cases is essential for diagnosis.[17,18] The contrast media may not allow actual visualization of the ruptured tendon, but a filling defect tends to support the clinical diagnosis. Plain films may demonstrate a slight laxity in the joint, but this is not consistent. Chronic cases frequently show bony reaction on the supraglenoid tubercle.

Because repair of the tendon is difficult, and because there are no adverse effects from detaching the biceps tendon,[1] the treatment of choice is tenodesis (Fig. 9–26). This method is described in the section Tenosynovitis of Biceps Tendon (above).

Fibrotic Contracture of the Infraspinatus Muscle

This condition is an uncommon cause of shoulder lameness in hunting or working dogs. Electrophysiological and histological studies have indicated infraspinatus contracture to be a primary muscle disorder rather than a neuropathy. Affected muscle shows degeneration and atrophy with fibrous tissue replacement. The cause of this syndrome is hypothesized as an acute traumatic event that results in incomplete rupture of the infraspinatus muscle, leading to fibrotic contracture.[21] Although the trauma is usually self-induced, outside sources may also be the cause of injury such as a direct blow from a car or a horse kick.

Usually, there is a history of a sudden onset of lameness during a period of field exercise. Lameness and tenderness in the shoulder region gradually disappear within 10 to 14 days. Chronic lameness develops 3 to 4 weeks later. At this time, the animal elicits no pain but is completely unable to rotate (pronate) the shoulder joint internally. This results in a stance with the elbow adducted and the foot abducted (Fig. 9–27A). The lower limb swing in a lateral arc

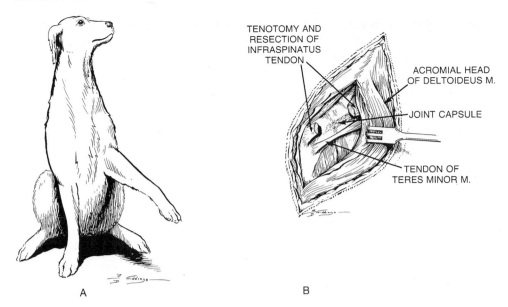

FIGURE 9–27. Fibrotic contracture of the infraspinatus muscle. (*A*) Typical sitting posture of a dog with infraspinatus contracture. The lower limb is permanently externally rotated and therefore shortened. (*B*) The left shoulder has been exposed by the craniolateral approach by tenotomy of the infraspinatus muscle.[3] The tendon is dissected free of the joint capsule until the shoulder moves freely; then about 1 cm of the tendon is excised.

(circumduction) as the foot is advanced during the stride. There is atrophy of the infraspinatus muscle on palpation; when the forelimb is forcibly pronated or adducted, the proximal border of the scapula becomes more prominent as it abducts from the thorax. Radiographs are usually normal. Although rare, the condition can be bilateral.

Treatment consists of tenotomy and excision of part of the tendon of insertion of the infraspinatus muscle on the greater tubercle of the humerus. The tendon is exposed by the approach to the craniolateral region of the shoulder joint.[3] The belly of the infraspinatus is inspected to confirm its fibrosis and contracture, following which the scarred tendon is undermined from the joint capsule and severed. If complete range of motion is not achieved, the joint capsule is also contracted and needs to be released (Fig. 9–27*B*). About 1 to 1.5 cm of tendon is excised. A distinct "pop" is often felt when the last of the adhesions is broken down. Full range of motion is immediately restored.

Aftercare/Prognosis

Dogs are leash walked immediately with no constraint of the limb. Normal activity is resumed in 10 to 14 days. These animals uniformly return to normal limb function.[22]

Fibrotic Contracture of the Supraspinatus Muscle

Although only a single case of this condition appears to have been reported,[23] we have seen it in conjunction with external trauma and in Doberman pinschers suspected of a spontaneous hemorrhage from von Willibrand's disease (platelet dysfunction). Clinical signs were identical to those described for infraspinatus contracture. Dogs respond well to sectioning of the tendon of insertion of the supraspinatus muscle. It would thus seem prudent to inspect both spinatus muscles for evidence of fibrosis and contracture before either tendon is sectioned.

References

1. Vasseur PB, Pool RR, Klein BS: Effects of tendon transfer on the canine scapulohumeral joint. Am J Vet Res 44:811, 1983.
2. Hohn RB, Rosen H, Bohning RH, Brown SG: Surgical stabilization of recurrent shoulder luxation. Vet Clin North Am 1:537, 1971.
3. Piermattei DL: An Atlas of Approaches to the Bones and Joints of the Dog and Cat, 3rd ed. Philadelphia, WB Saunders Co, 1993.
4. Vasseur PB: Clinical results of surgical correction of shoulder luxation in dogs. J Am Vet Med Assoc 182:503, 1983.
5. Fowler DJ, Presnell KR, Holmberg DL: Scapulohumeral arthrodesis: Results in seven dogs. J Am Anim Hosp Assoc 24:667, 1987.
6. Parkes L: Excision of the glenoid. Presented at 3rd Annual Meeting of Veterinary Orthopedic Society, Aspen, CO, 1976.
7. Breucker KA, Piermattei DL: Excision arthroplasty of the canine scapulohumeral joint: Report of three cases. Vet Comp Orthop Trauma 3:134, 1988.
8. Franczuski D, Parkes LJ: Glenoid excision as a treatment in chronic shoulder disabilities: Surgical technique and clinical results. J Am Anim Hosp Assoc 14:637, 1988.
9. LaHue TR, Brown SG, Roush JC, et al: Entrapment of joint mice in the bicipital tendon sheath as a sequela to osteochondritis dissecans of the proximal humerus in dogs: A report of six cases. J Am Anim Hosp Assoc 24:99, 1988.
10. Smith CW, Stowater JL: Osteochondritis dissecans of the canine shoulder joint: A review of 35 cases. J Am Anim Hosp Assoc 11:658, 1975.
11. Schrader SC: Joint diseases of the dog and cat. In Olmstead ML (ed): Small Animal Orthopedics. St Louis, Mosby, 1995, pp 437–469.
12. Birkeland R: Osteochondritis dissecans in the humeral head of the dog. Nord Vet Med 19:294, 1967.
13. Person M: Arthroscopic treatment of osteochondritis dissecans in the canine shoulder. Vet Surg 18:175, 1989.
14. Flo GL, Middleton D: Mineralization of the supraspinatus tendon in dogs. J Am Vet Med Assoc 197:95–97, 1990.
15. Lincoln JD, Potter K: Tenosynovitis of the biceps brachii tendon in dogs. J Am Anim Hosp Assoc 20:385, 1984.
16. Rivers B, Wallace L, Johnston GR: Biceps tenosynovitis in the dog: radiographic and sonographic findings. Vet Comp Orthop Trauma 5:51–57, 1992.
17. Barthez PY, Morgan JP: Bicipital tenosynovitis in the dog-evaluation with positive contrast arthrography. Vet Radiol Ultrasound 34:325–330, 1993.
18. Stobie D, Wallace LJ, Lipowitz AJ, et al: Chronic bicipital tenosynovitis in dogs: 29 cases 1985–1992. J Am Vet Med Assoc 207:201–207, 1995.
19. Becker DA, Cofield RH: Tenodesis of the long head of the biceps brachii for chronic bicipital tendinitis. J Bone Joint Surg 71-A:376, 1989.
20. Post M, Benca P: Primary tendinitis of the long head of the biceps. Clin Orthop Rel Res 246:117, 1989.
21. Pettit GD, Chatburn CC, Hegreberg GA, Meyers KM: Studies on the pathophysiology of infraspinatus muscle contracture in the dog. Vet Surg 7:8, 1978.
22. Bennett RA: Contracture of the infraspinatus muscle in dogs: A review of 12 cases. J Am Anim Hosp Assoc 22:481, 1986.
23. Bennett D, Campbell JR: Unusual soft tissue orthopaedic problems in the dog. J Small Anim Pract 20:27, 1979.

10

Fractures of the Humerus

The majority of fractures involving the humerus are in the middle and distal thirds.[1,2] In a study of 130 humeral fractures, 4 percent involved the proximal physis, 47 percent the shaft, 13 percent the supracondylar region, and 37 percent the distal articular surfaces.[3] Occasionally, fractures of this bone may be accompanied by foreleg paresis or paralysis resulting from radial nerve injury. Nerve injury may occur at the fracture site or in the brachial plexus (axillary nerve), or it may be due to avulsion of spinal nerves from the cord. Nerve impairment may be temporary or permanent; fortunately in most cases it is the former. Establishing the presence of withdrawal response by toe pinch, and sensorium by skin pricks, may be helpful in differentiation. Nerve conduction studies can be used to establish whether nerves are intact, but results are not reliable until about 7 days postinjury. In most cases, a patient with a humeral fracture carries the affected leg with the elbow dropped and with the paw resting on its dorsal surface because of pain and weakening of the extensor musculature. This mimics the appearance of loss of proprioception due to nerve injury, and response to the toe-pinch reflex may be obtunded due to pain, making early differentiation of nerve injury difficult.

FIXATION TECHNIQUES

Coaptation

There are very few fractures of the humerus that lend themselves to external fixation because of the difficulty of immobilizing the shoulder joint. The spica splint (see Fig. 2–23) is the only device that will stabilize the proximal fragment of a humeral fracture. Most diaphyseal fractures have considerable angular displacement of the distal segment due to muscular forces and these forces cannot be adequately neutralized by the spica splint. Greenstick or nondisplaced fractures in skeletally immature dogs are the major indications for this type fixation.

Intramedullary Pins and Wires

Steinmann pins have wide application in the humerus in the more stable fractures. These pins can be inserted either retrograde or normograde. The pins are most commonly driven distally into the medial condyle, which gives a very firm anchorage in the distal fragment (Fig. 10–1D). The pin must be small enough diameter to pass through the epicondylar crest into the epicondyle. This method is applicable to fractures at any level of the bone. A larger diameter pin, or multiple pins, can be anchored distally just proximal to the supratroch-

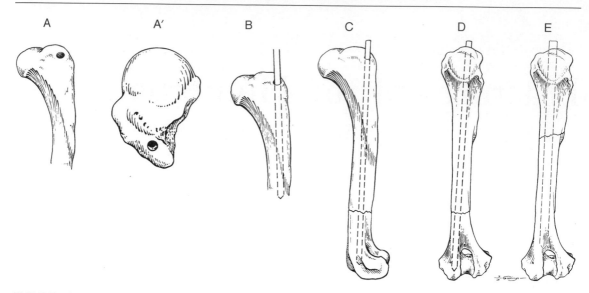

FIGURE 10–1. Internal fixation with an intramedullary pin. (*A, A'*) The Steinmann pin is inserted from the proximal end by entering the skin and bone in an oblique fashion just lateral to the ridge of the greater tuberosity of the humerus. (*B*) After the bony anchorage is secured in the outer cortex, the pin is directed distally in the marrow cavity. (*C, D*) Method 1: The pin is directed to pass along the medial cortex of the shaft and anchors well down in the medial condyle. Care must be taken that the pin is not too large to pass through the medial epicondylar area. If too large, it will break through into the elbow joint. (*E*) Method 2: A large diameter pin is directed centrodistad in the medullary canal, and is seated just proximal to the supratrochlear foramen.

lear foramen (Fig. 10–1*E*). The use of this type pin should be restricted to fractures proximal to the midshaft, as there is not firm anchorage of the pin in the distal fragment.

For *normograde* insertion, the Steinmann pin is driven from the proximal end by entering the bone on the lateral slope of the ridge of the greater tubercle near its base (Fig. 10–1*A, B*). Note that the pin enters near the base of the curve connecting the tubercle to the shaft. Initial drilling is done with the pin held perpendicular to the bone surface, and after bony anchorage is secured in the outer cortex, the pin is directed distally in the marrow cavity to pass along the caudomedial cortex of the shaft and anchors well down in the medial condyle, at least to the level of the epicondyle. The medial condyle forms a square corner with the caudomedial shaft that can be easily palpated to judge the depth of the pin (Fig. 10–1*C, D*). During insertion of the pin into the distal segment, the two segments are held firmly in the reduced position with one or two self-locking bone forceps. Allowing one segment to rotate on the other during insertion results in a loose-fitting pin. In order to ensure passage of the pin down into the medial condyle, the bone fragments are bowed slightly medially at the fracture site. For anchorage of the pin proximal to the supratrochlear foramen, it is allowed to follow the center of the medullary canal until resistance is felt, then driven slightly farther to secure bone anchorage without entering the foramen. These pins are all usually cut as close to the bone as possible, leaving just enough pin protruding to allow removal after fracture healing.

Retrograde insertion from the fracture site can be done by initially driving the pin either proximally or distally through the medial condyle. The pin is directed proximally toward the craniolateral cortex until it exits through the greater tubercle, after which it is withdrawn proximally until the distal pin tip is flush with the fracture. The fracture is reduced and the pin seated distally with either method as described above. If the medial condyle seating of the pin is chosen the pin can also be first driven distally until it exits from the condyle, after which the pin is retracted and the fracture reduced. The pin can now be seated by two methods:

1.   Drive the pin proximally through the greater tubercle, then pull it proximally until the distal end is within the medial condyle. The pin is cut proximally as described above. This method used in a supracondylar fracture is illustrated in Figure 10–24.

2.   Drive the pin proximally until it has just penetrated the greater tubercle, then cut the pin distally close to the bone of the condyle.

The chief indication for using a Steinmann intramedullary pin (IM) as the sole method of fixation is for transverse or short oblique type A fractures in small dogs and cats. The intramedullary pin may be used in combination with other methods of fixation in unstable fractures. Following an open approach, the fracture is first reduced, and the intramedullary pin is inserted in the proximal segment. The auxiliary fixation is applied next. The methods of auxiliary fixation are as follows:

1.   Cerclage wires, type A2 fracture (Fig. 10–2A).

2.   Hemicerclage wires, type A2 fracture (Fig. 10–2B).

3.   Interfragmentary wire inserted to secure the cortical fragments to each other and the intramedullary pin at the fracture site, type A3 fracture (Fig. 10–2C). This method does not establish complete rotational stability, as the cortex opposite the wire is still free to move unless the fragments interlock.

4.   Skewer pin and wire, type A fractures (Fig. 2–62G).

5.   Lag screw fixation, type A2 fracture (Fig. 10–2D). This is only possible in very large breeds.

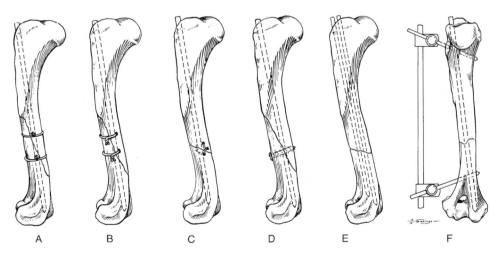

FIGURE 10–2. Intramedullary pin and auxilliary fixation. (A) Cerclage wires. (B) Hemicerclage wires. (C) An orthopedic wire secures cortical fragments to each other and the intramedullary pin at fracture site. (D) Lag screw fixation. (E) Use of two pins. (F) Unilateral external fixator, 1/1 pins.

A

B

C

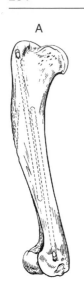
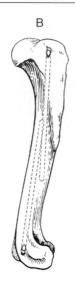
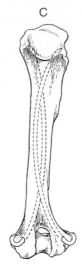

FIGURE 10–3. Rush pin sites in the humerus. (*A*) Proximal and distal sites on the lateral aspect. (*B*) Proximal and distal sites on the medial aspect. (*C*) Distal sites as seen from the caudal aspect.

6. Two or more intramedullary pins, type A3 fracture (Fig. 10–2*E*).
7. External fixator, type 1, 1/1 pins for stable type A fractures (Fig. 10–2*F*). The 2/2 pins configuration is used on unstable type B fractures.

Rush pin intramedullary fixation is useful in both proximal extra-articular type A and distal segment extra-articular type A1 fractures of the humerus because the ability to use double pins is effective in eliminating rotary motion. Pin entry sites are shown in Figure 10–3. Typically, a distal pin through the lateral epicondylar crest will have to be smaller in diameter than that in the medial side due to the small diameter of the bone of the lateral crest.

External Fixators

External skeletal fixation is applicable to all diaphyseal fractures as well as distal extra-articular type A fractures. Unilateral type 1 single- or double-bar fixators are used in shaft fractures (see Fig. 10–19), and a hybrid type 1-2 is very helpful for very proximal type B (see Fig. 10–13) or distal extra-articular type A2 and 3 fractures (see Fig. 10–27*B*).

The fixator may be used on most types of fractures; however, it is most commonly used on diaphyseal types B and C and open fractures. The splint is placed on the craniolateral surface of the bone to minimize muscle impingement. If the distal segment is short, the distal pin may be inserted in a transcondylar position (see Fig. 10–19). The distal (positive-thread-profile) pin is usually inserted first in the transcondylar position, in the same position as a transcondylar screw (see Fig. 10–28). The proximal pin is inserted next, followed next by application of the connecting bar and clamps, then by insertion of the center pins through the clamps. For the strongest buttress effect, particularly in dogs over 50 pounds (25 kg) with a diaphyseal type C3 fracture, a double connecting rod is advisable.

If the distal fragment is fragmented and strong buttressing is needed (type C3), the hybrid splint shown in Figure 10–27 can be used. This placement of pins allows full range of movement of the elbow joint during the healing period.

Fixators are also useful in combination with IM pins to control rotational and compressive shear forces (see Figs. 10–2*F* and 10–25*D*). The fixator can

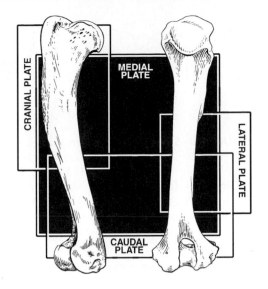

FIGURE 10–4. Various fracture zones on the humerus are indicated by the overlapping boxes. Suggested bone plate position is labeled within the boxes. There is considerable overlap of potential plate position for a specific fracture, thus the choice may be related to other factors such as patient size and bone shape, soft tissue injuries, or simply personal preference.

be removed as soon as callus formation is observed, usually 4 to 6 weeks, and the pin left in place until clinical union is achieved.

Bone Plates

Plates are indicated for all unstable type B and C diaphyseal fractures, as well as the more stable type A fractures in large breeds. Bone plates can be applied to every side of the humerus, depending on the fracture location (Fig. 10–4). In most cases where the fracture is proximal to the midshaft, the plate may be applied on the cranial surface to advantage (see Figs. 10–17C and 10–18). The lateral surface has two disadvantages: marked curvature of the bone and location of the radial nerve and brachialis muscle. The plate must be placed under these structures (see Fig. 10–17D). Fractures of the distal third, and fractures requiring a long plate (type C) are best handled with a medial plate.[4] Supracondylar fractures can be treated with a caudomedial plate (see Fig. 10–27A) or a caudal plate on the medial epicondylar crest (see Fig. 10–32G), sometimes supplemented with a plate on the lateral crest (see Fig. 10–32H). (See Fig. 2–74 for suggested plate sizes.) The choice between plates and external fixators is often arbitrary, following the preference of the surgeon.

Lag Screws

The interfragmentary compression afforded by lag screw fixation is essential for most type B and C intra-articular fractures (see Figs. 10–28, 10–29, 10–31, and 10–32). Because of the shear loads imposed on these screws with weight bearing, the use of a full threaded cortical screw as a lag screw (see Chapter 2) is preferred over partially threaded cancellous screws. The junction of the threaded and smooth shank in partially threaded screws is a stress raiser area and is prone to fatigue failure if this junction is near the fracture line. The dog's bone is dense enough in the condylar region that the cancellous thread is not important. (See Fig. 2–74 for suggested screw sizes.)

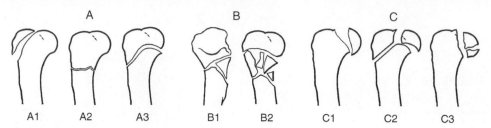

FIGURE 10–5. Proximal fractures of the humerus. (*A1*) Involving tuberosity, (*A2*) impacted metaphyseal, and (*A3*) nonimpacted metaphyseal. (*B1*) Metaphyseal wedge and (*B2*) metaphyseal complex. (*C1*) Simple, (*C2*) simple and metaphyseal, and (*C3*) multifragmentary. (From Unger M, Montavon PM, Heim UFA: Classification of fractures of the long bones in the dog and cat: Introduction and clinical application. Vet Comp Orthop Trauma 3:41–50, 1990, with permission.)

PROXIMAL FRACTURES

Fracture Type 11-A; Proximal, Extra-articular Simple (Fig. 10–5A)

Physeal fractures are uncommon injuries, comprising about 5 percent of humeral fractures, that occur in young animals prior to physeal closure.[3] They may be a result of direct or indirect force (avulsion). The proximal humerus has two epiphyses, the greater tubercle and the humeral head. These epiphyses may be confluent, with a bridge of cartilage between, or entirely independent from one another. Therefore, some fractures will involve both portions, as in Figures 10–6 and 10–7, while others involve either just the tubercle (Fig. 10–5A), or just the head (Fig. 10–5C). Impacted metaphyseal fractures (Fig. 10–5A) are quite rare.

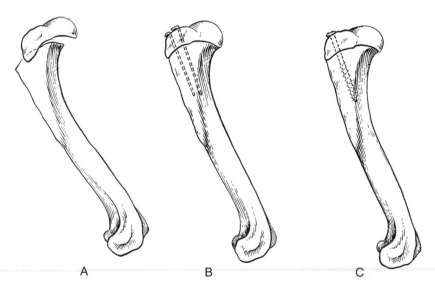

FIGURE 10–6. (*A*) Type A3 (Salter-Harris I) fracture of the proximal humeral physis and the apophysis of the greater tuberosity. (*B*) Fixation using transfixing Kirschner wires. (*C*) Fixation with a cancellous bone screw is reserved for animals that are close to maturity.

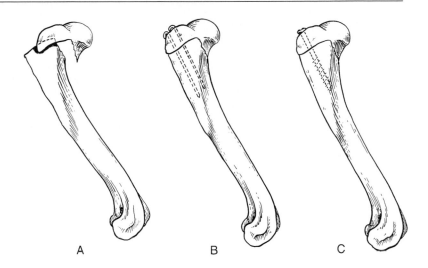

FIGURE 10–7. (*A*) Type A3 (Salter-Harris II) fracture of the proximal humeral physis and metaphysis. (*B*) Fixation using transfixing Kirschner wires. (*C*) Fixation with a cancellous bone screw is reserved for animals that are close to maturity.

Closed Reduction and Fixation

Usually closed reduction can be accomplished when the fracture leaves both epiphyses intact, particularly in cases of recent origin (Figs. 10–6 and 10–7). If the displacement of the fracture is 5 mm or less, immobilization may be accomplished by use of a modified Velpeau bandage encircling the chest and the affected leg with the joints flexed (see Fig. 2–29).[3] This area heals readily with minimal fixation and vigorous remodeling quickly restores normal alignment.

Open Reduction and Fixation

An open craniolateral approach to the shoulder joint and proximal humerus[5] and reduction can be performed if closed reduction cannot be accomplished. The fracture is reduced by levering. Internal fixation, which is necessary in most cases, is carried out by the insertion of one or more Steinmann pins or Kirschner wires in young animals with open growth plates. There is minimal chance of creating growth arrest with small smooth pins. Figures 10–6*B*, 10–7*B*, 10–8, 10–9*A*, and 10–10*A* show this technique. Due to the vigorous healing response of the physeal area, only minimal stability is needed. In animals at or near

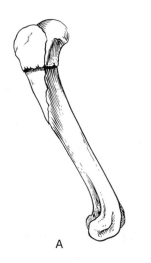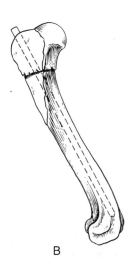

FIGURE 10–8. (*A*) Type A2 impacted fracture of the proximal humeral metaphysis. (*B*) The intramedullary pin is inserted closed, starting on the ridge of the greater tuberosity and proceeding distally into the medial aspect of the condyle.

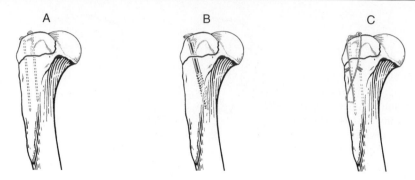

FIGURE 10–9. Type A1 fracture involving the apophyseal growth plate of the greater tuberosity of the humerus. (*A*) Fixation using transfixing Kirschner wires. (*B*) Fixation with a cancellous bone screw is reserved for animals that are close to maturity. (*C*) Fixation with Kirschner wires and tension band wire is also reserved for animals that are close to maturity.

skeletal maturity, a wider variety of fixation, to include lag screws and tension band wires, provide additional stability when needed (Figs. 10–9*B*, *C*, and 10–10*B*).

Fracture Type 11-B; Proximal, Extra-articular Multifragmentary (Fig. 10–5*B*)

Open reduction and internal fixation is always indicated in these fractures because the bone segment or callus may encroach on the joint or brachial plexus or change the functional angle of the shoulder joint and thus limit range of movement or alter function. As is typical of metaphyseal fractures they are quick to heal, but if they cannot be anatomically reconstructed (type B2) by interfragmentary compression, they present a challenge for fixation due to the shortness of the proximal fragment.

OPEN APPROACH ■   These fractures are exposed via the approach to the proximal shaft of the humerus (Fig. 10–11).[5]

Internal Fixation

Type B1 wedge fractures can usually be reduced and the fragment stabilized by lag screw or cerclage wire, which should be placed through a drill hole or notch in the bone to prevent migration. Fixation of the resulting two-piece

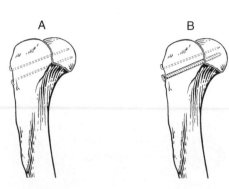

FIGURE 10–10. (*A*) Type C1 (Salter I) fracture of the proximal humeral physis fixed by double transfixing Kirschner wires. (*B*) Fixation by lag screw. The Kirschner wire is inserted first and maintains reduction while the screw is placed. Screw fixation is used only for animals that are close to maturity.

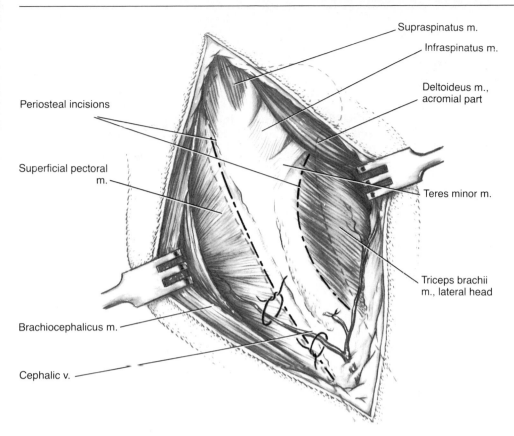

Supraspinatus m.

Infraspinatus m.

Deltoideus m.,
acromial part

Periosteal incisions

Superficial pectoral
m.

Teres minor m.

Brachiocephalicus m.

Triceps brachii
m., lateral head

Cephalic v.

FIGURE 10–11. Approach to the proximal shaft of the humerus. Because it is relatively superficial, this region is easily exposed. (From Piermattei DL: An Atlas of Surgical Approaches to the Bones and Joints of the Dog and Cat, 3rd ed. Philadelphia, WB Saunders Co, 1993, p 127, with permission.)

fracture is then done with a cranial plate or by pins and tension band wire, as in Figure 10–9C, except that long IM pins are used instead of the pictured K-wires.

Type B2 complex fractures require buttress or bridging fixation. This can be accomplished by a cranial straight or T-plate (Fig. 10–12), or by a hybrid external fixator (Fig. 10–13). Autogenous cancellous bone graft is packed into the unreduced fragment area if it is possible to do so without disturbing the fragments. A carpal flexion bandage (Fig. 2–30) is useful for the first 2 to 3 weeks postoperatively to protect the fixation.

DIAPHYSEAL FRACTURES

Fracture Type 12-A; Diaphyseal Simple or Incomplete
(Fig. 10–14A)

Considerable overriding resulting from spastic contraction of the brachial muscles can be seen with these fractures.[1,6] The distal segment is usually tilted cranially. Shaft fractures comprise approximately half of all humeral fractures.[3] Treatment recommendations are keyed to the Fracture Patient Scoring System detailed in Table 2–6.[7,8]

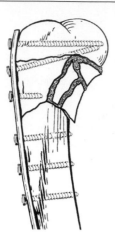

FIGURE 10–12. Type B2 fracture of the proximal humeral metaphysis stabilized by a buttress plate. The fragments are left as undisturbed as possible during the open reduction.

***OPEN APPROACHES*[5]** ■ Figure 10–15 shows the craniolateral open approach to the distal shaft of the humerus. This approach may be used to expose the proximal three fourths of the humerus when combined with the approach to the proximal shaft of the humerus. Figure 10–16 shows a medial open approach to the shaft of the humerus, useful for application of a long bone plate.

Closed Reduction and Fixation

Closed reduction is occasionally possible, particularly in cats and small dogs, when the fracture is of the transverse or short oblique type and can be readily palpated. Immobilization is most often done by intramedullary pinning, with a type 1 half pin external fixator added for supplemental fixation when needed for rotational stability (see Figs. 10–1 and 10–2). An external fixator can also be employed as primary fixation.

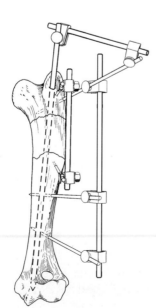

FIGURE 10–13. Type B2 fracture of the proximal humeral metaphysis shown in Figure 10–12, stabilized by two type IA external fixators, one of which is tied into a Steinmann intramedullary pin. The proximal fixation pin of the smaller fixator is driven deeply into the humeral head, in a manner similar to the proximal screws in Figure 10–12.

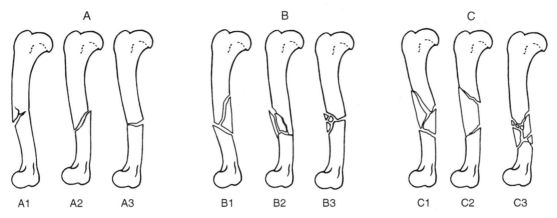

FIGURE 10–14. Diaphyseal fractures of the humerus. (*A1*) Incomplete, (*A2*) oblique, and (*A3*) transverse. (*B1*) One reducible wedge, (*B2*) reducible wedges, and (*B3*) nonreducible wedges. (*C1*) Reducible wedges, (*C2*) segmental, and (*C3*) nonreducible wedges. (From Unger M, Montavon PM, Heim UFA: Classification of fractures of the long bones in the dog and cat: Introduction and clinical application. Vet Comp Orthop Trauma 3:41–50, 1990, with permission.)

Internal Fixation

Potential methods of internal fixation are:

1. Intramedullary pin alone when the fracture patient score is 9 to 10 or more usually with supplemental fixation (see Fig. 10–2), when the fracture patient score is 8 to 9.

2. Type 1 external fixator alone or with supplemental fixation for fracture patient score of 7 to 8 or below. Four to six fixation pins and one connecting bar is used. There is the possibility of closed reduction and splint application, or of a limited open approach.

3. Bone plate, especially in large breeds, for any fracture score. The plate is applied as a neutralization plate in oblique fractures and as a tension band compression plate in transverse fractures.

Fracture Type 12-B; Diaphyseal Wedge (Fig. 10–14*B*)

These fractures all require open approach and internal fixation because they are all unstable in rotation and may be minimally stable relative to compression (weight bearing) loads.

Type B1, One Reducible Wedge

If the wedge can be reduced and fixed by cerclage or lag screw the fracture is then treatable as a simple type A fracture with any of the fixation methods detailed above, as long as the fracture patient score is 8 or above. Neutralization plate fixation of such a fracture is seen in Fig. 10–17.

Type B2, Several Reducible Wedges

Fracture patient score is typically in the 4 to 7 range and there is a choice of reconstruction or bridging osteosynthesis. Figure 10–18 depicts a reconstructive approach to a proximal shaft fracture, utilizing a neutralization plate. An external fixator and supplemental fixation of the fragments could also be used. Bridging osteosynthesis can be accomplished with either a bridging plate, or

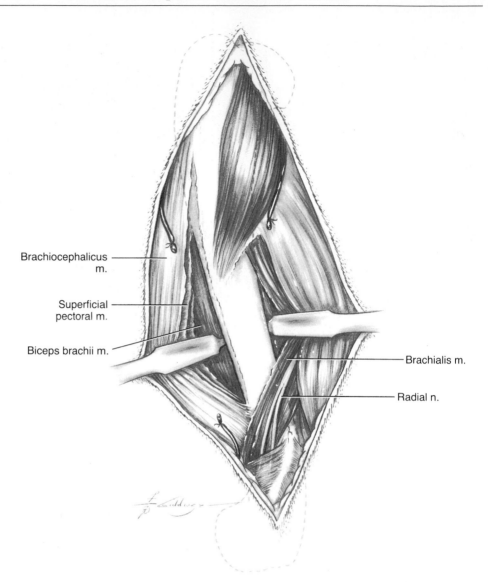

Brachiocephalicus m.

Superficial pectoral m.

Biceps brachii m.

Brachialis m.

Radial n.

FIGURE 10–15. Approach to the shaft of the humerus through a craniolateral incision. The triceps and brachialis muscles are retracted caudally, and the biceps, superficial pectoral, and brachiocephalicus muscles are retracted cranially. The radial nerve is protected by the brachialis muscle, which can also be retracted cranially to better expose the distal shaft (see Fig. 20–22). (From Piermattei DL: An Atlas of Surgical Approaches to the Bones and Joints of the Dog and Cat, 3rd ed. Philadelphia, WB Saunders Co, 1993, p 131, with permission.)

probably better with an external fixator, since a much more limited open approach can be utilized. The fixator would be applied as shown in Figure 10–19B.

Type B3, Nonreducible Wedges

With a fracture patient score in the 3 to 6 range, these fractures are treated by bridging osteosynthesis, as detailed above for B2 fractures. The interlocking nail is also applicable.[9]

FIGURE 10–16. Approach to the shaft of the humerus through a medial incision. The entire shaft of the bone can be exposed, and the relatively flat surface is advantageous for plate application. (From Piermattei DL: An Atlas of Surgical Approaches to the Bones and Joints of the Dog and Cat, 3rd ed. Philadelphia, WB Saunders Co, 1993, p 137, with permission.)

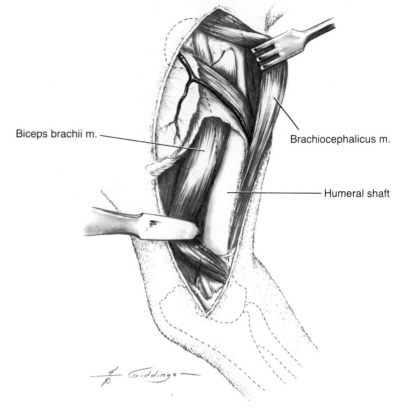

Biceps brachii m.

Brachiocephalicus m.

Humeral shaft

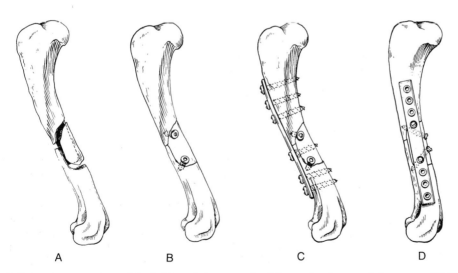

A   B   C   D

FIGURE 10–17. (*A*) Midshaft Type B1 one reducible wedge humeral fracture. (*B*) The wedge was first reduced with the proximal segment and fixed with a lag screw. The distal segment was next reduced and attached with a second lag screw. (*C*) Neutralization plate applied to cranial surface. (*D*) A neutralization plate may be applied to the lateral surface, although surgical exposure and contouring the plate may be more difficult.

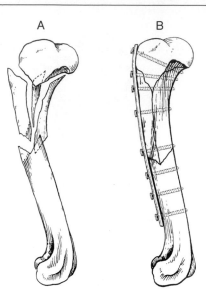

FIGURE 10–18. (A) Type C1 reducible wedges of the proximal humeral shaft. (B) Fixation by application of bone plate to cranial surface. Screws crossing the fracture line are inserted with a lag effect through the plate.

Fracture Type 12-C; Diaphyseal Complex (Fig. 10–14C)

These fractures all require open approach and internal fixation because they are all unstable both in rotation and compression (weight bearing) loads. Fracture patient scores range from 1 to 3.

Type C1 Reducible Wedge and C2 Segmental

Intramedullary pin fixation is rarely applicable to these fractures. The exception would be in a small-breed patient when the fracture lines are long enough to allow cerclage wire fixation. The more common options are:

1.   Reconstructive; interfragmentary compression by lag screws or cerclage wires and application of a neutralization plate or a type 1 external fixator.
2.   Bridging osteosynthesis; most commonly by a type 1 external fixator (Fig. 10–19), but a long bridging plate could be used.
3.   Bridging osteosynthesis by interlocking nail.

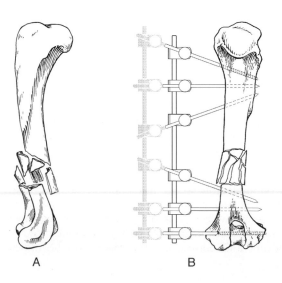

FIGURE 10–19. (A) Multiple fracture of the distal third of the humeral shaft. The reduction is done closed or by minimal open approach, and the fragments are not reduced. (B) Type IA external fixator with single or double (shaded) connecting bar. The distal pin is usually inserted first in the transcondylar position. The proximal pin is inserted next, followed by application of connecting bar and clamps, then the center pins. The double connecting bar is indicated in animals over about 40 pounds (18 kg) when there is no load sharing by the bone.

Type C3 Nonreducible Wedges

Bridging osteosynthesis is the only option available. This is usually accomplished by a type 1 external fixator (Fig. 10–19), but a long bridging plate or interlocking nail could be used.

DISTAL FRACTURES

Fracture Type 13A Distal, Extra-articular (Fig. 10–20A)

Distal humeral shaft and supracondylar fracture appear to be more frequent in cats than in dogs, where condylar fractures, type 13B, are more common.[10] In supracondylar humeral fractures, the fracture line may vary somewhat; however, it usually passes through the supratrochlear foramen.[1,3] In young animals, the injury may be a combination fracture and physeal separation (Salter-Harris type II injury). Even though the fracture may be reduced closed, an open approach is usually indicated for the application of internal fixation. Best results are obtained by using stable internal fixation, which allows movement of the joint during the convalescent period.

OPEN APPROACHES[5] ■   The skin incision may be medial (Fig. 10–21), lateral (Fig. 10–22), or both. In most instances, both the medial and lateral incisions are used. In some multiple type C2 or C3 fractures in this area, the transolecranon (caudal) approach may give the best visualization and working area (see Fig. 10–23).

Internal Fixation

TYPE A1, SIMPLE ■   The exact method of fixation may be dictated by the individual fracture. Following are several possibilities:

1.   Insert a double-pointed Steinmann pin retrograde through the shaft of the humerus along the medial cortex, reduce the fracture, and run the pin well into the medial aspect of the condyle (Fig. 10–24). This type of fixation will allow rotation at the fracture site unless the fracture is serrated and interlocking on reduction, and is best reserved for skeletally immature dogs where early callus formation is expected.

2.   Insert a double-pointed Steinmann pin as described above. In addition, insert another pin (usually of a smaller diameter) or K-wire from the lateral

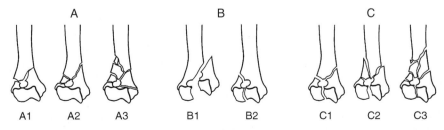

FIGURE 10–20. Distal fractures of the humerus. (*A1*) Simple, (*A2*) wedge, and (*A3*) complex. (*B1*) Lateral and (*B2*) medial. (*C1*) Simple, metaphyseal simple, (*C2*) simple, metaphyseal wedge, and (*C3*) simple, metaphyseal complex. (From Unger M, Montavon PM, Heim UFA: Classification of fractures of the long bones in the dog and cat: Introduction and clinical application. Vet Comp Orthop Trauma 3:41–50, 1990, with permission.)

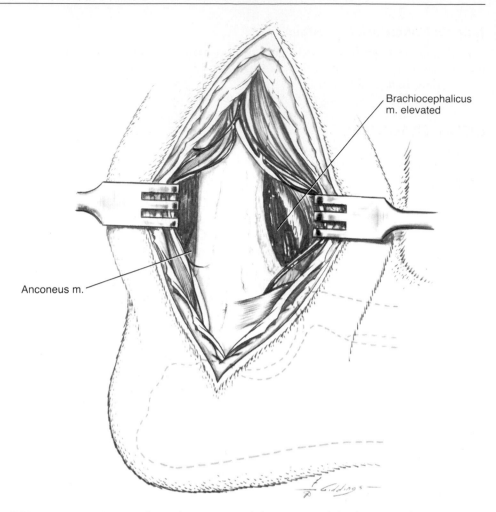

Brachiocephalicus m. elevated

Anconeus m.

FIGURE 10–21. Approach to the supracondylar region of the humerus from a medial incision. Cranial retraction of the median nerve and accompanying vessels and caudal retraction of the ulnar nerve and triceps muscle provides exposure of the medial aspect of the condyle and supracondylar region. (From Piermattei DL: An Atlas of Surgical Approaches to the Bones and Joints of the Dog and Cat, 3rd ed. Philadelphia, WB Saunders Co, 1993, p 145, with permission.)

epicondyle across the fracture to anchor in the medial cortex of the humeral shaft proximal to the fracture line (Fig. 10–25A).

3.   When the lateral fragment is slightly longer, insert a double-pointed Steinmann pin as in item 1 above. In addition, insert a lag screw through the lateral epicondylar crest and anchoring in the medial cortex of the humeral shaft (Fig. 10–25B). This will bring about compression at the fracture site and ensure rotational stability. When applicable, this is the preferred method.

4.   Insert a double-pointed Steinmann pin down into the medial condyle as described above. In addition, insert one or more cerclage wires if the fracture is of the oblique type (Fig. 10–25C).

5.   A Steinmann pin is inserted as above, and a two-pin type I external skeletal fixator is added for rotational stability (Fig. 10–25D). The distal fixation pin is inserted across the condyles in the same manner as a transcondylar

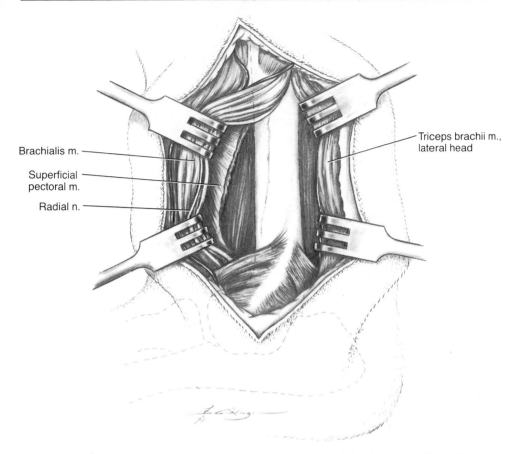

Brachialis m.

Superficial
pectoral m.

Radial n.

Triceps brachii m.,
lateral head

FIGURE 10–22. Approach to the supracondylar region of the humerus through a craniolateral incision. Caudal retraction of the triceps muscle combined with cranial retraction of the brachialis muscle and radial nerve are used to expose this region. (From Piermattei DL: An Atlas of Surgical Approaches to the Bones and Joints of the Dog and Cat, 3rd ed. Philadelphia, WB Saunders Co, 1993, p 141, with permission.)

FIGURE 10–23. Approach to the humeroulnar part of the elbow joint by osteotomy of the tuber olecrani. This approach allows reduction of both parts of the humeral condyle, and further elevation of the triceps muscle exposes the supracondylar region of the humerus.

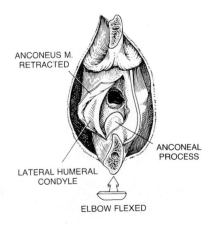

ANCONEUS M.
RETRACTED

ANCONEAL
PROCESS

LATERAL HUMERAL
CONDYLE

ELBOW FLEXED

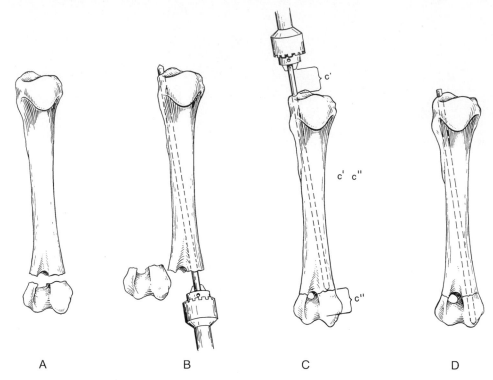

A   B   C   D

FIGURE 10–24. Placement of the intramedullary pin for a type A1 distal extra-articular fracture. (*A*) Fracture of the supracondylar type. (*B*) The fracture site is exposed from the medial side, and a double-pointed pin, started near the medial cortex, is inserted retrograde. (*C*) A pin chuck is attached at the proximal end at a distance (*c'*) that corresponds to the length of the condyle (*c''*). The fracture is reduced, and the elbow joint is extended prior to insertion. (*D*) Final position; if fracture segments do not interlock, rotation is possible at fracture site and supplemental fixation is indicated.

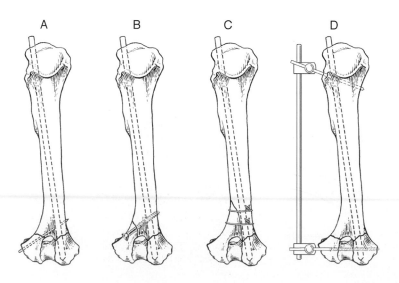

FIGURE 10–25. Intramedullary pin and auxiliary fixation for a supracondylar fraction. (*A*) An additional pin is inserted up the lateral epicondyle and penetrates the medial cortex. (*B*) A lag screw is inserted in addition to the pin. (*C*) Two cerclage wires are added for supplemental fixation. (*D*) Type I external fixator applied for rotational stability for this type A1 fracture.

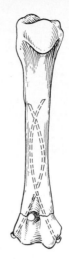

FIGURE 10–26. Two Rush pins give good stabilization.

screw. See the description of screw placement below in the section on distal partial articular fractures.

6.   Insert Rush pins at the medial and lateral epicondyles and drive them simultaneously into the shaft of the humerus (Fig. 10–26).

TYPE A2, WEDGE ■   The wedge is usually lateral, and if the fragment is large enough they can be fixed with the methods shown in Figure 10–25, utilizing an IM pin into the medial condyle and K-wires and/or lag screws to secure the wedge. A caudomedial bone plate (Fig. 10–27*A*) is more stable as it will better prevent rotation. The distal screws must be angled cranially into the condyle to prevent penetration into the supratrochlear foramen. If the wedge fragment cannot be captured by lag screw, double caudal plating can be applied (see Fig. 10–32*H*).

IM pins are not an option when the medial condyle is fragmented, and either a neutralization or buttress plate caudomedially as in Figure 10–27*A*, or a hybrid external fixator can be utilized (Fig. 10–27*B*).

TYPE A3 COMPLEX ■   A strong buttress effect is needed for these fractures, which can be supplied best with double caudal plating (see Fig. 10–32*H*) or the external fixator shown in Figure 10–27*B*.

Note that all methods of fixation allow movement of the joint during the convalescent period. Intramedullary pins are usually removed after the fracture reaches the stage of clinical union.

Fracture Type 13B Distal, Partial Articular (Fig. 10–20*B*)

Fractures of the lateral portion of the humeral condyle occur much more frequently than fractures of the medial portion.[3,10] The lateral portion is the major weight-bearing part, and its smaller lateral epicondylar crest makes it biomechanically weaker. There also appears to be a problem of incomplete ossification of the humeral condyle in cocker and Brittany spaniels in North America that predisposes them to humeral condylar fractures from minor trauma or normal activity.[11] Others have noted the tendency for condylar fractures caused by minor trauma,[10] but the cocker spaniel in Europe does not appear to be predisposed to these fractures.[12] Two distinct age groups are noted

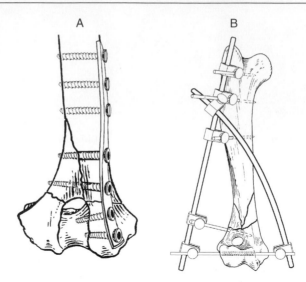

FIGURE 10–27. Distal extra-articular fractures of the humerus. (*A*) Type A2 wedge fracture stabilized by a caudomedially applied plate. Very little contouring of the plate is required. The wedge is lag screwed to the supracondylar region of the humerus and the condyle fracture line is compressed by using the load drill guide in the two distal plate holes. (*B*) Type A3 complex fracture stabilized by a hybrid type I-II external fixator. A minimal exposure open approach is used to partially reduce the fragments, and the transcondylar center-threaded fixation pin is placed first, followed by the most proximal half-pin. The remaining fixation pins are then inserted and a curved connecting bar is attached to one of the proximal half-pins and to the medial end of the transcondylar pin for rotational stability.

in this fracture type; those less than 4 months old (often toy or miniature breeds), and those older than 2 years.[10,12]

The procedure for reduction and fixation will vary, depending on the length of time since injury, the amount of swelling and edema, and the ease with which the fragments can be palpated. As a result of muscular pull, the prereduction radiograph will usually show the fractured lateral portion to be dislocated proximally and rotated laterally and cranially. The fractured medial epicondyle is usually rotated medially and caudally. Subluxation is present in the elbow joint. Recent fractures of the lateral and medial aspect of the humeral condyle are shown in Figures 10–28*A* and 10–29*A*. Within the first 36 to 48 hours after injury, there is usually minimal swelling, and the fragment can be palpated.

Reduction and Internal Fixation

The fractured leg may be placed in the Gordon extender (see Fig. 2–17) for 10 to 15 minutes to fatigue the muscles and overcome spastic contraction. The leg can be prepared and draped for surgery while still in the Gordon extender. By use of a lateral or medial approach (Fig. 10–30*A, B*), the fracture area is exposed.[5] The fracture is reduced, and a pointed reduction forceps or vulsellum forceps is applied across the epicondyles (Figs. 10–28*D* and 10–31*A*). On the side opposite the open approach this clamp will penetrate the skin, hence the need for a sharp pointed forceps. If additional rotational stability is desired, a transcondylar K-wire can be placed from epicondyle to epicondyle, as in Figure 10–31. Care must be taken to prevent this pin from entering the supratrochlear foramen.

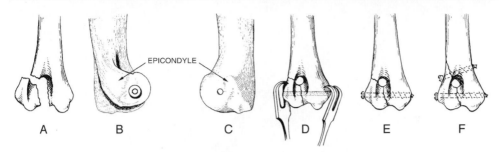

FIGURE 10–28. (*A*) Distal partial articular fracture of the lateral aspect of the humeral condyle. (*B*) Lateral view to show screw placement centered on the condyle. Note the proximocaudal position of the epicondyle relative to the screw. (*C*) Medial view to show the tip of the screw protruding distocranial to the epicondyle. (*D*) Reduction may be maintained during drilling of the screw hole by use of a vulsellum or pointed reduction forceps placed on the epicondyles. This leaves the area to accommodate transcondylar bone screw free for drilling. Also see Figure 10–31. (*E*) Bone screw insertion with lag effect. (*F*) Insertion of additional bone screw proximal to the supratrochlear foramen adds to stability and is important when the proximal fracture line does not provide any buttress effect to support the transcondylar screw.

The points of entry and exit of the transcondylar hole to be drilled are referenced to the epicondyles, and are halfway between the epicondyle and the articular surface of the condyle at an angle of about 45 degrees to the long axis of the humerus (Fig. 10–28*B, C*). It is necessary to bluntly separate the extensor or flexor tendons in order to get the drill sleeve anchored in these areas. The screw hole can also be started by a trocar-pointed pin, then enlarged with a drill of the appropriate size to accommodate the bone screw. Retrograde drilling of the fractured condyle can be accomplished by drilling from the fracture surface, then reducing the condyle and completing the drill hole as illustrated in Figure 10–31*B*.

Compression of the fracture site may be obtained by using a cancellous bone screw or a cortical bone screw inserted with a lag effect (see Fig. 2–65*E, F*); the latter is preferred because there is less chance of screw failure. In the very immature dog, minimal or no compression is advisable because of crushing of soft bone. In very small breeds drilling a glide hole for a full-threaded screw can remove a significant portion of the condyle, and in these cases a tap hole diameter drill is used through both cortices, and the only compression is that supplied by the bone clamp. Two or more small pins or K-wires placed in a diverging pattern may be substituted for the transcondylar screw in toy breeds that are less than 4 kg in weight.[13] Small vulsellum or pointed reduction forceps are used to obtain compression during the insertion procedure. This method is

FIGURE 10–29. (*A*) Recent type B2 fracture of the medial aspect of the humeral condyle. (*B*) Bone screw insertion with lag effect. (*C*) Insertion of additional bone screw proximal to the supratrochlear foramen adds to stability.

A   B   C

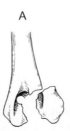 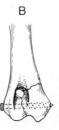 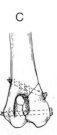

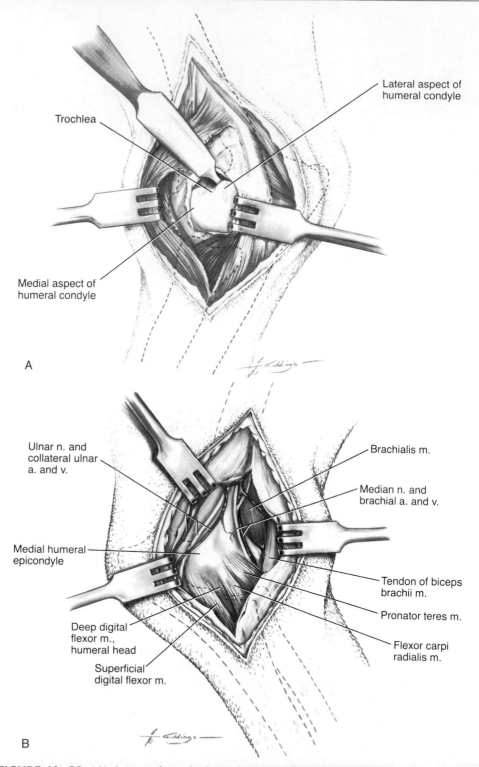

FIGURE 10–30. (*A*) Approach to the lateral aspect of the humeral condyle and epicondyle. The extensor carpi radialis muscle has been elevated and the joint capsule opened. (*B*) Approach to the medial humeral epicondyle. The medial and ulnar nerves must be protected during this approach. (From Piermattei DL: An Atlas of Surgical Approaches to the Bones and Joints of the Dog and Cat, 3rd ed. Philadelphia, WB Saunders Co, 1993, pp 149, 177, with permission.)

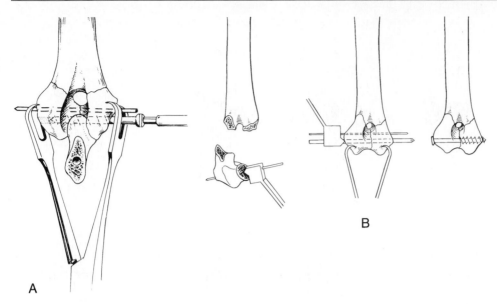

FIGURE 10–31. Methods of fixation for type C distal, complete articular fractures of the humerus. Reduction is usually maintained during the fixation procedure by use of a vulsellum forceps and transcondylar Kirschner wire. (A) The hole may be drilled and the screw inserted directly from the medial or lateral surface or (B) from the fracture surface. The Kirschner wire is usually removed after lag screw insertion.

definitely not recommended in larger breeds, and the availability of 1.5- and 2-mm screws lessens the need to use it even in small breeds. In some cases it is useful to utilize a K-wire through the lateral or medial epicondylar crest to supply additional rotational stability to the condyle, as shown in Figure 10–32A, B.

Additional fixation, preferably a second screw, is necessary in some cases, especially with lateral condylar fractures. Note that when the metaphyseal fracture line is relatively transverse (Figs. 10–28A, D, E and 10–29A, B) the bone can load-share weight-bearing forces with the fixation screw, and the screw is unlikely to fail. However, if the metaphyseal fracture line is less than 45 degrees to the long axis of the bone, no load sharing can occur and the screw is at jeopardy to fail in a few weeks (Figs. 10–28F and 10–29C). Since there is no callus formation in the intercondylar fracture area it is slow to regain normal strength through the Haversian remodeling process. Under these circumstances fixation of the metaphyseal fracture is important to prevent screw failure. A pin large enough in diameter to resist bending can be substituted for the screw if necessary.

For longer standing fractures of the lateral or medial region of the condyle, if the fragments cannot be accurately reduced or if the fracture is more than 3 to 4 days old, this procedure can be modified by performing a caudal approach with osteotomy of the tuber olecrani (Fig. 10–23) to expose the fracture site. When the patient is very young, a triceps tenotomy is advisable in preference to an osteotomy of the olecranon process. The additional exposure gained by these approaches simplifies reduction. Prognosis for good to excellent function following repair of lateral condylar fractures is reported to be 89 percent, and 87 percent for medial condylar fractures.[14]

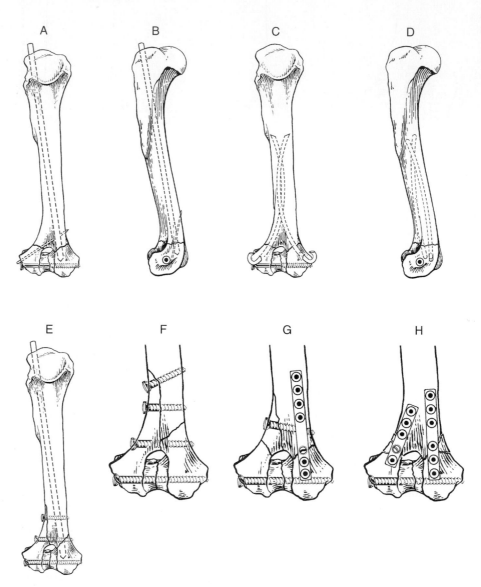

FIGURE 10–32. Fixation techniques for type C distal, complete articular fractures of the humerus. In all cases the transcondylar screw is placed first, followed by reduction of the supracondylar fracture line. (*A, B*) Type C1 fracture stabilized with a Steinmann intramedullary pin inserted in a retrograde fashion at the fracture site and seated in the medial aspect of the condyle. An additional pin, inserted just distal to the lateral epicondylar ridge and directed obliquely across the fracture through medial cortex of the shaft, gives good two-point fixation in these stable fractures. (*C, D*) Fixation of type C1 fracture using two Rush pins. (*E*) An intramedullary pin in combination with lag screws gives interfragmentary compression to all fragments when the fracture lines permit. (*F*) If the fracture lines are relatively long, they can all be stabilized using lag screws in a type C1 fracture. (*G*) Type C2 and C3 fractures are best fixed using two small bone plates placed caudally on both epicondylar crests. (*H*) Fixation of a type C1 fracture using one bone plate inserted caudally along the medial epicondylar crest, with a Kirschner wire in the lateral epicondylar crest for additional rotational stability.

Aftercare

It is important to maintain motion in the elbow joint postoperatively, so no external splintage is employed. Passive range-of-motion exercise is started as soon as it is tolerated. If the animal seems likely to damage the fixation, a carpal flexion bandage (see Fig. 2–30) will protect the fixation while still allowing motion of the elbow joint. The bone screw may be removed in the young growing animal (up to approximately 4 months of age), but it is usually left in place in those over this age unless otherwise indicated.

Fracture Type 13C Distal, Complete Articular
(Fig. 10–20C)

Bicondylar, or T-Y fractures occur most frequently in mature animals and usually result from trauma exerting torsional stress.[1,3] The spaniel breeds are particularly prone to this fracture. Spastic contractions of the muscles of the foreleg pull the ulna and radius proximally between the fractured medial and lateral portions of the condyle.

OPEN APPROACHES[5] ■ The caudal approach to the humeroulnar part of the elbow joint by osteotomy of the tuber olecrani usually gives the best visualization of the fracture area (Fig. 10–23). This approach gives good exposure of the caudal surface of the distal end of the humerus, including the condyle, trochlea, and anconeal process. Two other approaches that may be used are (1) approach to the elbow joint by osteotomy of the proximal ulnar diaphysis, and (2) approach to the supracondylar region of the humerus and caudal humeroulnar part of the elbow joint. In cats, two anatomical differences are to be noted when making surgical approaches in this area:

1. The median nerve passes through the supratrochlear foramen.
2. The ulnar nerve lies under the short portion of the medial head of the triceps muscle.

Reduction and Fixation

Perfect anatomical reduction of the fractured articular surfaces with uninterrupted rigid fixation and movement of the elbow is mandatory for the best functional results. This type of fracture is one of the most challenging to repair in veterinary medicine; any errors in reduction and fixation lead to decreased range of movement, abnormal wear, and degenerative joint changes.

After exposure of the fracture and following removal of the organizing clot and fibrin, the condyles are reduced and temporarily held by one or two vulsellum or pointed reduction forceps (Fig. 10–31). The addition of one or two transverse Kirschner wires proximally or cranially to the screw site increases rotational stability for drilling the condyle. The hole is drilled for insertion of the transcondylar bone screw. This hole may be drilled directly from the lateral or medial surface as described above for type B fractures, or from the fracture surface (Fig. 10–31B). Before the transcondylar hole is drilled, there should be perfect anatomical reduction of the articular cartilages of the humeral condyle along the fracture lines. The humeral condyles should be checked for good approximation at the intercondylar fracture site. Less than anatomical reduction may impinge the anconeal process, limit range of movement, and result in abnormal wear.

The transcondylar bone screw is then inserted with a lag effect. It now remains to fix the supracondylar fracture, and this is done in the same manner described above for type 13-A distal extra-articular fractures. The method is dictated by the fracture pattern, size of the animal, and the equipment available. The objective is rigid uninterrupted fixation that is capable of withstanding considerable abuse during the healing period. Documentation studies on T-Y fractures of the humerus indicate that less than adequate fixation in this area is the most frequent cause of failure.[14] Bone plate fixation gives the highest percentage of successful results, especially in type C2 and C3 fractures. In most cases, it is advantageous to carry out the reduction and fixation of the condyle first. In some cases, however, it may be advantageous to first reduce and fix one of the condyles to the humeral shaft and to then reduce the remaining condyle and insert the transcondylar bone screw. Figure 10–32 presents some suggested methods of fixation of the supracondylar fracture.

TYPE C1 FRACTURE ■   An intramedullary pin (Fig. 10–32A, B) is inserted in retrograde fashion at the fracture site and is then driven back into the medial epicondyle (Fig. 10–24). An additional pin is inserted just distal to the lateral epicondylar ridge and directed diagonally through the epicondylar crest, across the fracture, and through the medial cortex of the shaft. This gives good two-point fixation if the fracture is of the stable type. Alternatively, fixation can also be accomplished using two Rush pins (Fig. 10–32C, D), or by a caudomedial bone plate (Fig. 10–32G).

An intramedullary pin can also be used in combination with one or more lag screws when the wedge fragment is long enough to accept a lag screw proximally (Fig. 10–32E). This gives interfragmentary compression and is preferable to the use of a diagonal pin when applicable. If the arms of the Y fracture are relatively long, they may be attached using several lag screws (Fig. 10–32F).

TYPE C2 FRACTURE ■   A bone plate inserted caudally along the medial epicondylar crest and shaft (Fig. 10–32G) is applicable for most type C2 wedge fractures. This plate must be carefully positioned on the crest to avoid interference with the olecranon process within the supratrochlear foramen. Because the bone is almost perfectly straight in this region, very little contouring of the plate is necessary. The distal screws are quite long and well anchored in the medial condyle, but care should be taken to not penetrate the articular surface cranially. It is necessary to add lag screw or pin fixation to the wedge fragment. It is also possible in some cases to fix these fractures combining the methods shown in Figure 10–32A and E, with both a lag screw proximally and a pin distally in the wedge fragment, combined with an IM pin.

TYPE C3 FRACTURE ■   Double-plate fixation is the safest method of fixation in this situation (Fig. 10–32H). The medial plate can either be applied to the caudal surface of the epicondylar crest as shown here, or to the medial surface of the distal shaft and epicondylar crest. The difficulty with this position for the plate is that unless the most distal screws can be angled cranially into the condyle, they can only penetrate one cortex lest they enter the supratrochlear foramen.

Aftercare

It is important to maintain motion in the elbow joint postoperatively, so no external splintage is employed. Passive range-of-motion exercise is started as soon as it is tolerated. If the animal seems likely to damage the fixation, a carpal flexion bandage (Fig. 2–30) will protect the fixation while still allowing motion of the elbow joint. Exercise is limited during the healing period, and intramedullary pins are removed after healing. Other implants are left in place unless migration or soft tissue irritation is encountered. Prognosis is less than optomistic for type C fractures, only 52 percent attaining good to excellent results in one study.[14]

References

1. Brinker WO: Fractures. In Canine Surgery, 2nd Archibald ed. Santa Barbara, American Veterinary Publications, Inc, 1974, pp 949–1048.
2. Unger M, Montavon PM, Heim UFA: Classification of fractures of the long bones in the dog and cat: Introduction and clinical application. Vet Comp Orthop Trauma 3:41–50, 1990.
3. Bardet JF, Hohn RB, Olmstead ML: Fractures of the humerus in dogs and cats: A retrospective study of 130 cases. Vet Surg 12:73–77, 1983.
4. Harrari J, Roe SC, et al: Medial plating for the repair of middle and distal diaphyseal fractures of the humerus in dogs. Vet Surg 15:45–48, 1986.
5. Piermattei DL: An Atlas of Surgical Approaches to the Bones and Joints of the Dog and Cat, 3rd ed. Philadelphia, WB Saunders Co, 1993.
6. Kasa F, Kasa G: Fractures of the humerus. In Brinker WO, Hohn RB, Prieur WD (eds): Manual of Internal Fixation in Small Animals. New York, Springer-Verlag, 1984, pp 134–143.
7. Palmer RH, Hulse DA, Aron DN: A proposed fracture patient score system used to develop fracture treatment plans (abstract). Proc 20th Ann Conf Vet Orthop Soc, 1993.
8. Palmer RH: Decision making in fracture treatment: The fracture patient scoring system. Proc (Sm Anim) ACVS Vet Symposium, 1994, pp 388–390.
9. Durall I, Diaz MC, Morales I: Interlocking nail stabilisation of humeral fractures. Initial experience in seven clinical cases. Vet Comp Orthop Trauma 7:3–8, 1994.
10. Vannini R, Olmstead ML, Smeak DD: An epidemiological study of 151 distal humeral fractures in dogs and cats. J Am Anim Hosp Assoc 24:531–536, 1988.
11. Marcellin-Little DJ, DeYoung DJ, et al: Incomplete ossification of the humeral condyle in spaniels. Vet Surg 23:475–487, 1994.
12. Drape J: Etiology of distal humeral fractures in dogs: A retrospective study of 120 cases. Proc 18th Ann Conf Vet Orthop Soc, 1991.
13. Morshead D, Stambaugh JE: Kirschner wire fixation of lateral humeral condylar fractures in small dogs. Vet Surg 13:1–5, 1984.
14. Vannini R, Smeak DD, Olmstead ML: Evaluation of surgical repair of 135 distal humeral fractures in dogs and cats. J Am Anim Hosp Assoc 24:537–545, 1988.

11

The Elbow Joint

TRAUMATIC LUXATION OF THE ELBOW

Because of the bony anatomy of the region, virtually all elbow luxations are lateral (Fig. 11–1A, B). The large square caudodistal corner of the medial epicondyle of the humerus prevents the ulna from moving medially, whereas the rounded shape of the lateral epicondyle permits the anconeal process to clear the lateral epicondylar crest when the elbow is flexed more than 90 degrees. When medial luxations are seen, they are usually accompanied by severe ligamentous damage.

Clinical Signs

The general appearance of an animal with a lateral luxation is distinct, but similar to infraspinatus contracture shown in Figure 9–27. Palpation easily differentiates the condition, with the laterally displaced radius and ulna being quite prominent. The antebrachium and foot are abducted, and the elbow is flexed. There is usually marked pain and increased elbow width, and resistance to flexion and extension. Because of elbow flexion, the foot does not touch the ground when the animal is either standing or sitting.

Diagnosis

Although the basic diagnosis can be made by physical examination, radiographs in two planes are necessary to look for associated fractures and avulsion of ligaments.

Treatment

Closed Reduction

Virtually all lateral luxations can be reduced closed during the first few days after injury. Muscle contracture makes later reduction more difficult. The rarity of this condition and the lack of experience opportunities by clinicians contribute to reduction difficulties.

With the animal under general anesthesia, firm palpation is used to establish the position of the humeral condyles relative to the radius and ulna. In some cases, the anconeal process will still be inside (medial to) the lateral epicondylar crest. In such a situation, medial pressure is maintained on the olecranon while the elbow is flexed to 100 to 110 degrees. Medial pressure is then placed on the radial head to force it under the humeral capitulum to the reduced position.

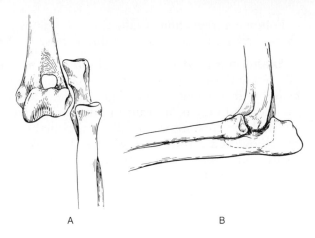

FIGURE 11–1. Lateral luxation of the elbow. (*A*) Craniocaudal view. (*B*) Lateromedial view. Note that in this case the anconeus is completely luxated.

A   B

The elbow is also abducted. If medial pressure on the radial head does not bring about reduction, additional pressure can be exerted by slightly extending the joint to lock the anconeal process inside the lateral epicondylar crest. The antebrachium should then be twisted inward (pronated) and adducted while abducting the elbow, causing the radial head to slip medially relative to the fixed fulcrum of the anconeus.

If the anconeus lies lateral to the lateral epicondyle, an additional step is required. With the elbow flexed to 100–110 degrees, the antebrachium is twisted inward (pronated) to force the anconeus inside the lateral condyle (Fig. 11–2*A*). The joint is extended slightly, then flexed while medial pressure on the radial head is continued. With pronation, the radial head can be forced under the capitulum (Fig. 11–2*B*).

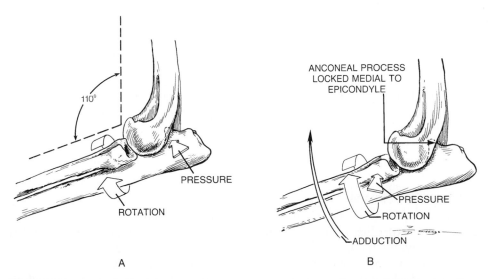

A   B

FIGURE 11–2. Closed reduction of lateral luxation of the elbow. (*A*) With the elbow flexed to 100 to 110 degrees, the antebrachium is twisted internally and the joint is slightly extended to lock the anconeal process inside the lateral epicondyle. (*B*) Continuous inward pressure is maintained on the radial head while the antebrachium is internally twisted. Gradual flexion and adduction of the antebrachium and abduction of the elbow forces the radial head medially, using the anconeal process as a fulcrum.

Following reduction, evaluation of ligamentous damage is necessary. Although most luxations can be reduced closed, a few will require open reduction.

Examination of Collateral Ligaments ■ The collateral ligaments of the elbow are illustrated in Figure 11–3A, B. These ligaments are intimately associated with the tendons of origin of the extensor (lateral) and flexor (medial) muscles and may be difficult to differentiate from these tendons at surgery.

The ligaments are evaluated by the method of Campbell.[1] After reduction, the elbow and carpus are both flexed to 90 degrees. Rotation of the paw laterally and medially causes similar rotation of the radius and ulna, which are constrained at the elbow by the collateral ligaments. If these ligaments are intact, lateral rotation of the paw is possible to about 45 degrees and medial rotation to about 70 degrees. If the lateral collateral is severed or avulsed, the paw can be rotated *medially* to about 140 degrees. If the medial ligament is damaged, the paw can be rotated *laterally* to about 90 degrees. In both cases, the paw rotation is about double the normal and can be compared with the opposite limb.

Excessive movement indicates damage to the collateral ligaments, and a decision must be made as to whether surgical treatment is indicated. If the joint is easily reluxated, the decision for surgical repair is simple to make. If the joint is reasonably stable despite the signs of ligament damage mentioned, the decision is more difficult. Immobilization will allow healing by fibrosis of periarticular soft tissues and may provide sufficient stability for smaller breeds, especially if they are not athletic or working animals. Conversely, surgical treatment is more often indicated in larger and more active animals.

Open Reduction

The elbow is exposed by a limited approach to the head of the radius and lateral compartments of the elbow joint.[2] This approach may be used up to 6 to 7 days following injury. Organized hematoma and shreds of ligament muscle and joint capsule are cleared from the joint. The procedure then continues as for a closed reduction. It may be necessary to use a smooth-surfaced instrument such as closed scissors blades or a bone lever to pry the radial head into the reduced position. Because of the inevitable damage to articular cartilage, this maneuver should be avoided if possible.

If reduction is still not possible, it may be necessary to extend the exposure by performing the caudal approach with osteotomy of the olecranon process.[2] It allows debridement of granulation and scar tissue in chronic cases. It also relieves the tension exerted by the triceps muscle and simplifies reduction. Following reduction, necessary repairs are performed as explained in the following discussion.

REPAIR OF LIGAMENTS ■ The surgical principles governing repair of ligamentous injuries are discussed in Chapter 7. Stretched ligaments are plicated (shortened), torn ligaments are sutured, and avulsed ligaments are reattached. Occasionally, ligaments are totally replaced or supplemented with various synthetic materials, although this is rarely necessary in the elbow.

Figure 11–4 illustrates repair of the lateral collateral ligaments. The elbow is approached laterally, with transection of the tendinous origin of the ulnaris lateralis[2] (Fig. 11–4A). The ligament is sutured or reattached to the bone (Fig. 11–4B). The adjacent extensor muscles are plicated with mattress sutures in the tendinous areas (Fig. 11–4C). Similar repairs are done medially if both ligaments are damaged. If the ligaments are torn near their distal insertions,

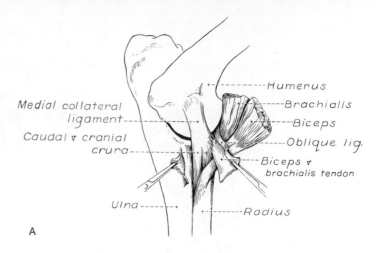

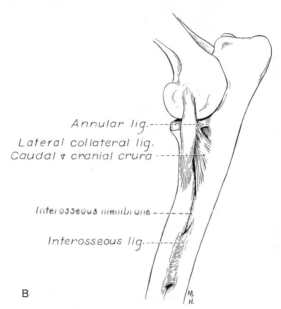

FIGURE 11–3. Collateral ligaments of the elbow. (*A*) Medial ligaments of the left elbow. (*B*) Lateral ligaments of the left elbow. (From Evans HE: Miller's Anatomy of the Dog, 3rd ed. Philadelphia, WB Saunders Co, 1993, with permission.)

they can be attached by suturing to the annular ligament. Damage in the midportion of the ligament is handled by suturing, using the locking loop suture described in Chapter 7.

Aftercare

CLOSED OR OPEN REDUCTION WITH NO LIGAMENT DAMAGE ■ The elbow is most stable when moderately extended to about the normal standing angle of 140 degrees. Because the elbow joint is very prone to lose range of motion as a result of periarticular fibrosis when completely immobilized, a soft splint (such as the modified Robert-Jones dressing, see Fig. 2–33) is useful. Five to 7 days is usually sufficient immobilization if exercise is restricted to the house or leash for 2 more weeks. Passive flexion-extension exercises are started immediately after removal of the dressing. This is facilitated by flexing the carpus while flexing the elbow.

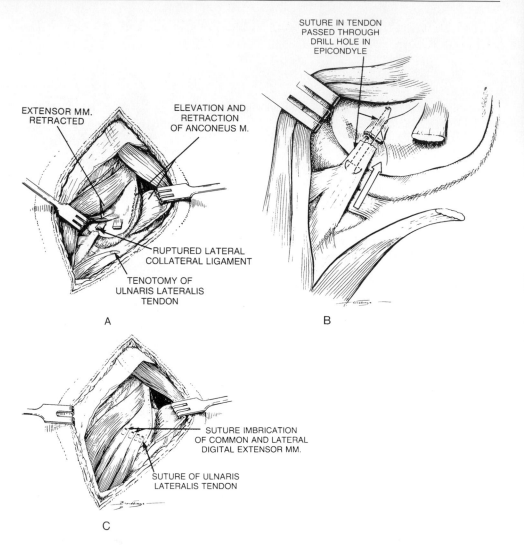

FIGURE 11–4. Surgical repair of lateral collateral ligaments of the elbow. (A) The left elbow has been exposed by a lateral approach with tenotomy of the ulnaris lateralis. Retraction of the other extensor muscles exposes the torn ligament. (B) The ligament has been torn close to the humerus. A locking loop suture has been placed in the ligament. One end of the suture is passed through a bone tunnel in the epicondyle to allow the ligament to be pulled to the bone. (C) The common and lateral digital extensors are imbricated with mattress sutures, and the ulnaris lateralis is sutured.

CLOSED REDUCTION WITH LIGAMENT DAMAGE ■ More rigid postoperative immobilization is needed in this situation despite the risk of joint stiffness. A spica splint (see Fig. 2–23) or Thomas splint (see Fig. 2–25) is maintained for 2 weeks. Passive flexion-extension exercise is important following splint removal. Exercise is restricted to the house or leash for 3 to 4 more weeks.

LIGAMENT DAMAGE SURGICALLY REPAIRED ■ Aftercare is similar to that above for ligament damage, except that the splint is maintained for 3 weeks.

DEVELOPMENTAL ABNORMALITIES AFFECTING THE ELBOW JOINT

Disturbed growth resulting from traumatic physeal closure of either the radius or ulna can produce subluxation of the elbow and is covered in Chapter 22.

Congenital elbow problems include luxation, asynchronous growth of the radius and ulna resulting in elbow incongruity, luxation of the radial head, and the presence of unstable and irritating cartilaginous bodies with or without bone.

Congenital Luxation

Congenital luxation of the elbow is occasionally seen in small breeds of dogs (terrier, Lhasa apso, pug, etc.). It can occur at birth or anytime up to 3 to 4 months of age. A proposed mechanism is aplasia of the medial collateral ligament leading to hypoplasia of the coronoid and anconeal processes and a shallow trochlear notch.[3] The proximal ulna is typically twisted laterally 45 to 90 degrees (Fig. 11–5A, B). When diagnosed early (7 to 10 weeks of age) and if closed reduction can be achieved, one or two temporary Kirschner wires driven from the olecranon to the humerus followed by a spica cast for 10 to 14 days has been successful in our hands. In older pups (12 to 16 weeks old), reduction usually requires an ulnar osteotomy distal to the semilunar notch. After the ulna is placed in the humeral trochlea, small Kirschner wires are driven across the joint (Fig. 11–6A) followed by spica coaptation until pin removal 2 to 3 weeks later. These dogs, if reduction is maintained, do surprisingly well (Fig. 11–6B). If reduction cannot be maintained, amputation or later arthrodesis are the only alternatives.

Elbow incongruity can be caused by physeal trauma or congenital factors. At times, the inciting cause is difficult to determine. Chondrodystrophied breeds are prone to asynchronous growth between the radius and ulna resulting in the ulna being too short relative to the radius (usual case) (Fig. 11–7A) or the radius being too short relative to the ulna (Fig. 11–8A). Traumatic physeal injuries resulting in elbow incongruity are covered elsewhere (see Chapter 22). In cases under consideration here, there is usually no known evidence of injury to the growth plate and the cause is unknown. Hereditary factors must be considered in the breeding animal.[4] Radiographs of the semilunar notch should be carefully inspected for a loose coronoid fragment, which we have occasionally observed when the radius is too short relative to the ulna.

Radiographic Findings

Mediolateral projections with the joint in approximately 90 degrees of flexion are most useful (Figs. 11–7A and 11–8A), although the craniocaudal view should also be examined. Varying degrees of degenerative changes will be seen, depending on the age of the animal. Ununited anconeal process may be seen concurrently in breeds such as the basset hound that are prone to this problem.

1. Normally the bottom of the semilunar notch lies on the same level as the radial head (Fig. 11–9A, B). With ulnar shortening, the coronoid process region lies below the radial head (Fig. 11–7A). In addition, the joint space surrounding the rounded humeral condyles may be pinched at the proximal anconeal process region, and widened distally at the coronoid region (Fig. 11–7A). With unusual

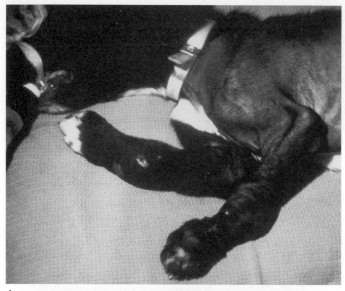

A

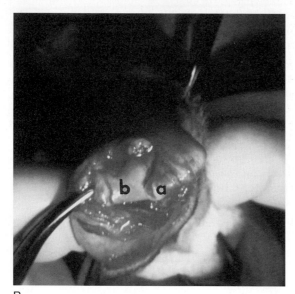

B

FIGURE 11–5. (A) Bilateral congenital luxation of the proximal ulna in a 9-week-old mixed-breed dog. Note the 90-degree or more internal rotation of the paw. Pressure sores of the cranial surface of the limb were present from abnormal weight bearing. (B) Intra-operative view demonstrating the 90 degrees or more of rotation of the anconeal process (*a*) and olecranon. The humeral trochlea is located at (*b*).

cases the radial head lies distal to the coronoid region due to radial shortening (Fig. 11–8A).

2. The usual surgical options involve lengthening the ulna (Fig. 11–7D) (when the ulna is too short relative to the radius), shortening the ulna (Fig. 11–8D) (when the radius is too short relative to the ulna), or lengthening the radius (see Fig. 22–15) (when the radius is too short). Lengthening the radius requires bone plate or external fixation, which is a more expensive procedure than altering the ulna, which is usually repaired with pins, or no internal fixation. See the discussion in Chapter 22 for further details.

Surgical Alternatives

The decision has to be made as to how much surgical limb shortening is acceptable in an already shortened limb. A crude method for ascertaining limb

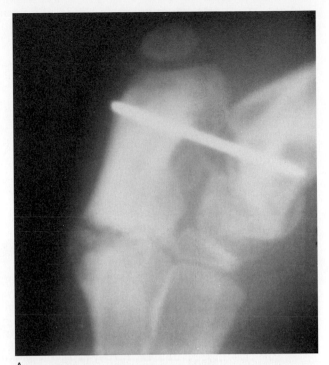

A

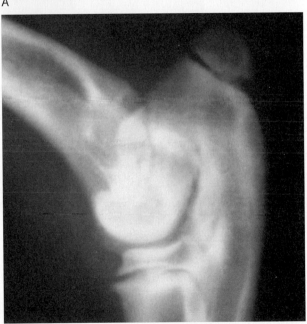

B

FIGURE 11–6. (A) Lateral radiograph 2½ weeks after surgery on the elbow of the dog in Figure 11–5A. (B) Lateral radiograph of the dog in Figure 11–5A taken 2½ months after bilateral elbow surgery. Note the elbow congruity. The puppy's forelimb function at this time was described by the owner as "normal."

length relative to the normal side during the physical examination is to align both olecranon regions parallel to each other and evaluate the relative position of the toe length. If the toes lie within a half inch of each other, then perhaps another half-inch shortening of the radius would be acceptable. If, however, the toe discrepancy is worse, and the radius is more than one fourth inch short at the elbow, then radial lengthening should be considered.

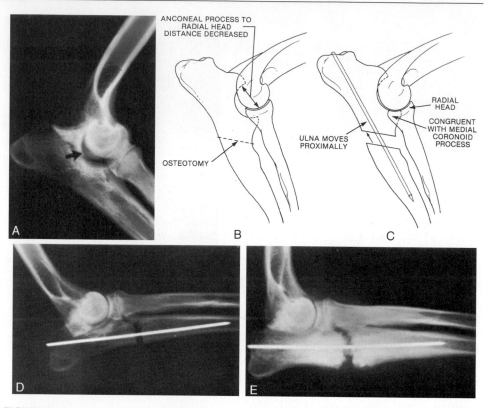

FIGURE 11–7. Incongruity of the elbow in the growing dog; the ulna is too short relative to the radius. (*A*) This mediolateral radiograph of elbow region illustrates that the trochlear notch (*arrow*) is not congruent with the radial head, resulting in subluxation of the humeroulnar joint. (*B*) Drawing illustrates the changes seen radiographically in *A*. Note the position and angle of the osteotomy. (*C*) Following osteotomy of the ulna the proximal ulna is free to move proximally due to muscular forces. (*D*) Postoperative radiograph of the case shown in *A*. Note the congruity of the trochlear notch of the ulna and the humeral condyles. A transverse osteotomy was performed here. (*E*) Three weeks postoperatively the ulnar gap is being bridged by callus, and the humeroulnar joint is congruent. Normal exercise can be resumed. (*B* and *C* from Gilson SD, Piermattei DL, Schwarz PD: Treatment of humeroulnar subluxation with a dynamic proximal ulnar osteotomy. A review of 13 cases. Vet Surg 18:114, 1989, with permission.)

When the ulna is too short, an ulnar lengthening osteotomy is performed, and the osteotomy site is wedged apart. The insertion of small nonthreaded intramedullary Kirschner wires provides some fixation (Fig. 11–7*B, C*) and yet allows muscular forces to reduce the proximal ulna upon weight bearing. This has a better chance of being truly anatomical compared to the surgeon's estimation of reduction. The intramedullary pin prevents the osteotomy site from "jackknifing," which could result in persistent lameness. Limb length is unaffected, and the surgical procedure is simple and effective.[5]

Alternatively, some surgeons prefer to perform the osteotomy in the distal third of the ulna, obviating pin insertion and removal. However, elbow joint exposure with visualization of the reduction is usually not performed. With either technique, active controlled limb use is encouraged postoperatively to allow muscular forces to provide final fine tuning of the reduction.

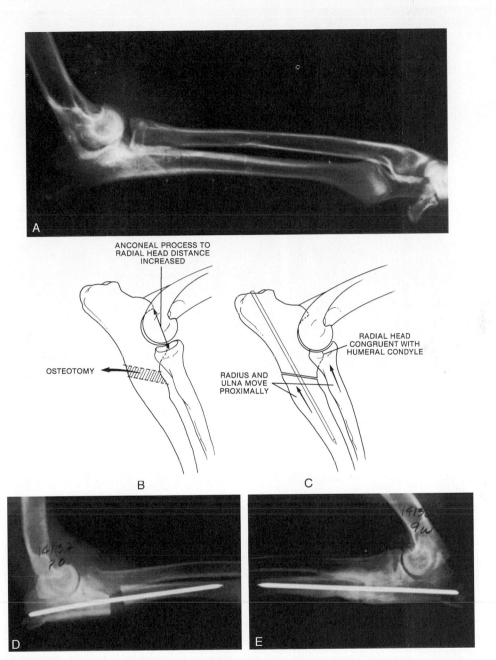

FIGURE 11–8. Incongruity of the elbow in the growing dog; the radius is too short relative to the ulna. (*A*) This mediolateral radiograph of elbow region illustrates a gap between the humeral condyle and the radial head, resulting in subluxation of the hu meroradial joint. (*B*) Illustrated here are the changes seen in *A* and the site for the ulnar osteotomy. (*C*) Following osteotomy, the radius and distal ulna are pulled into reduction by muscular forces. (*D*) In the postoperative radiograph the gap between the humeral condyle and the radial head has been partially reduced. An overly generous section was removed from the ulna. (*E*) At 9 weeks postoperatively the ulna has healed and the humeroradial joint is congruent. (*B* and *C* from Gilson SD, Piermattei DL, Schwarz PD: Treatment of humeroulnar subluxation with a dynamic proximal ulnar osteotomy. A review of 13 cases. Vet Surg 18:114, 1989, with permission.)

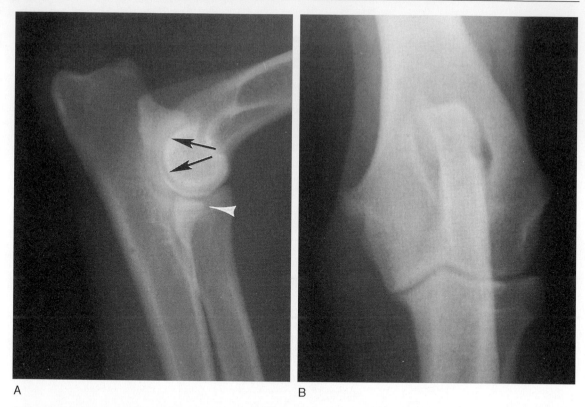

A   B

FIGURE 11–9. (A) Lateral radiograph of a normal elbow. Note the contour of the semilunar notch and its even joint space (*black arrows*). The rounded coronoid process (*white arrowhead*) lies on the same level as the radial head. (B) Cranial-caudal radiograph of a normal elbow.

Ulna Too Short

The ulna is exposed by a caudal approach to the proximal shaft of the ulna.[2] The joint capsule is incised on both sides of the ulna in the distal trochlear notch area to allow joint visualization. An oblique osteotomy of the ulna is performed distal to the trochlear notch (see Fig. 11–7B). This cut should be made with a Gigli wire saw or power saw, as an osteotome may split this hard bone. Typically the osteotomy will spontaneously gap apart as the osteotomy is completed, illustrating the dynamic muscular forces working on the proximal ulna. If such is not the case, a periosteal elevator is used to break down the interosseous membrane until the proximal ulna can be moved by forcing the osteotomy gap apart. A small nonthreaded intramedullary pin or Kirschner wire, $\frac{1}{8}$- to $\frac{3}{32}$-inch diameter (1.6 to 2.4 mm), is driven from the tuber olecrani across the osteotomy and seated into the midshaft region of the bone (Fig. 11–7C, D). The oblique osteotomy and the pin protect against angular displacement of the tuber olecrani from triceps muscle forces.

Radius Too Short

If the radius is too short in relation to the ulna, a similar approach is made to the proximal ulna. An ostectomy of the ulna distal to the trochlear notch is performed instead of a simple osteotomy (Fig. 11–8B, C). The width of the removed bone must be sufficient to allow the radius and distal ulna to move proximally until the radial head articulates normally with the lateral aspect of the humeral condyle. Some narrowing of the gap will be seen postoperatively (Fig. 11–8D). A pin is driven as in the previous case of ulnar shortening. If a radial lengthening is performed, stability must be rigid and is accomplished by plate fixation or by use of an external fixator (see Chapter 22).

AFTERCARE/PROGNOSIS ▪ With either type surgery it is important that early active weight bearing of the limb be achieved. A padded bandage is applied and nonsteroidal anti-inflammatory drugs (see discussion in Chapter 6) are administered to help achieve this by reducing pain and inflammation. Leash walking and limited free exercise are encouraged. Radiographic evaluation of healing should be pursued and the dog not returned to full activity until clinical union of the ulna is achieved (Figs. 11–7E and 11–8E). If a lengthening procedure of the radius (see Fig. 22–15) is performed, excessive activity could cause premature implant loosening in overly soft bone. Therefore, coaptation and very limited activity are recommended for several weeks.

The prognosis in these incongruent elbows depends on the severity of the incongruency, growth potential remaining after repair, and age at time of repair. If surgery is performed successfully at 6 to 7 months of age, the prognosis is very good. If surgery must be performed at a younger age due to severity, multiple surgeries may have to be done to achieve lasting congruency. If the incongruency is severe and surgery occurs later than 8 to 9 months of age, remodeling of the joint surfaces may be impossible and significant degenerative joint disease may ensue.

If surgery is done before degenerative joint disease is established, good results can be expected.[5]

Congenital Luxation of the Radial Head

This uncommon condition is seen in young chondrodystrophic breeds and sporadically in other breeds including the Akita.[6] The radial head migrates lateral relative to the humeral epicondyle along with ulnar shortening. Luxation may be partial or total, in which case the medial side of the radial head lies lateral to the non–weight-bearing aspect of the humeral epicondyle and is nonfunctional. Subluxation is common in chondrodystrophied breeds and at times may be relatively asymptomatic, while luxation can be very painful and result in severe elbow changes. This condition is often bilateral.

Clinical Signs

Beginning at 2 to 4 months of age, there is forelimb lameness, elbow swelling, valgus deformity of the carpus and varus deformity at the elbow (Fig. 11–10).

PHYSICAL EXAMINATION ▪ The limb deformities are noted, and crepitus may be palpated. The radial head lies more lateral than the humeral epicondyle (Fig. 11–11A, B).

RADIOGRAPHIC FINDINGS ▪ On the craniocaudal radiographic view, a subluxated radial head lies more lateral than normal, but still articulates somewhat with the weight-bearing surface of the humerus. A luxated radial head lies lateral, proximal, and caudal to the humeral weight-bearing surface (Fig. 11–11A–C). The ulna may be bowed.

PATHOGENESIS ▪ A proposed mechanism is ulnar physeal injury or improper intra-articular annular ligament formation, or hereditary factors.[4] The semilunar notch probably becomes a more important weight-bearing structure, as the radius becomes nonfunctional.

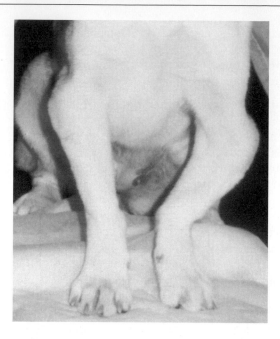

FIGURE 11–10. This 8-month-old Akita has severe radial head luxation and varus of the left elbow. The right radial head is also luxated.

TREATMENT ■ The radial articular surface becomes very deformed when luxated in very young puppies. Therefore, reduction should be achieved early. A corrective osteotomy with radial shortening, if done before 4½ months of age, will result in reluxation as asynchronous growth continues, thereby necessitating another surgical correction. Unfortunately, if performed after 5½ months of age, remodeling of the thinner articular cartilage is less likely. After osteotomy, the radial head is reduced and stabilized with pins (Fig. 11–12), or a plate. Postoperative care includes bandaging for 7 to 24 days, and severe activity restriction until radiographic evidence of bone healing (4 to 8 weeks).

Another procedure that can be performed in the 6- to 7-month old dog is a lengthening procedure of the ulna (see Fig. 11–7B). This allows reduction of the intact radius, which is then stabilized to the ulna utilizing screw fixation.[4]

A third option that we have used successfully in two cases involves amputating the radial head and neck (Fig. 11–13A–C). This is a simple, less costly procedure. However, stability of the elbow is less than if the humeral radial joint can be saved. Activity is restricted for 3 to 4 weeks.

Osteochondrosis of the Elbow

There are four conditions of the elbow presumed to be a result of osteochondrosis, which will be discussed in this chapter. They are: ununited anconeal process (UAP); osteochondritis dissecans (OCD) of the medial humeral condyle; ununited or fragmented coronoid process (FCP); and ununited medial epicondyle (UME), also known as calcification of the flexor tendons.

Ununited Anconeal Process

This condition is found primarily in large-breed dogs, especially German shepherds, basset hounds, and the St. Bernard. It is characterized by failure of the ossification center of the anconeus to fuse with the olecranon by 5 months of age. Instability or detachment of the process leads to inflammatory changes and eventual osteoarthrosis of the elbow joint. The condition can be bilateral.

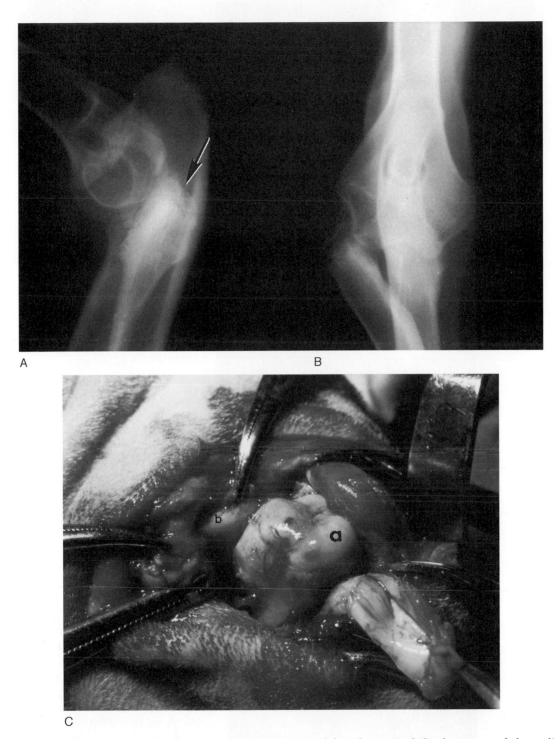

FIGURE 11–11. (A) Lateral radiograph demonstrates caudal and proximal displacement of the radial head (*arrow*) of a 4½-month-old German shepherd. (B) Cranial caudal radiograph of the dog in A demonstrates lateral displacement of the radial head. (C) Intraoperative photo of a deformed radial head (*a*) of a 3-month-old basset hound lying lateral and proximal to the articular weight-bearing surface of the humerus (*b*).

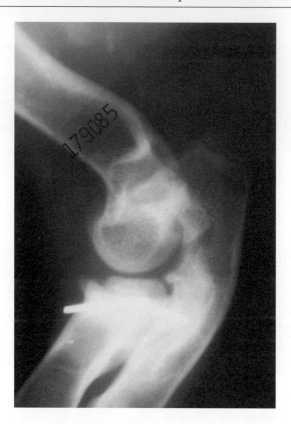

FIGURE 11–12. Healed corrective osteotomy of the proximal radius with pin fixation that was performed in this basset hound at 4 months of age.

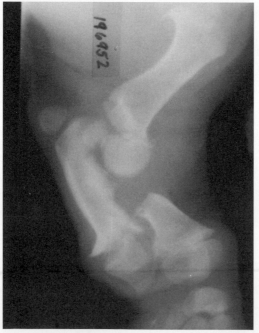

A

FIGURE 11–13. (*A*) Lateral elbow radiograph of a 3-month-old basset hound following amputation of the radial head for congenital luxation of the radial head. Note the radial head and metaphysis cranial to the foreleg that were removed and placed on the radiographic cassette. *Figure continued on opposite page.*

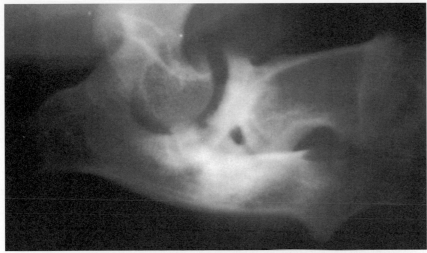

B

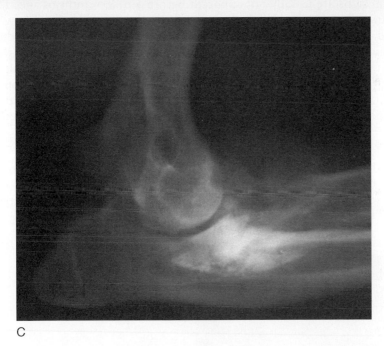

C

FIGURE 11–13. *Continued*   (*B*) Lateral elbow radiograph of the dog in *A* 4 months postoperatively. This dog had good function, but the opposite radial head was now luxated. Note regrowth of a "new" radial head. (*C*) Lateral elbow radiograph of a 9-year-old coon hound that underwent radial head amputation for radial head luxation 8½ years previously. The dog was still able to hunt and only became slightly lame after a strenuous hunt.

Hayes and associates[7] observed a positive association between risk and adult body weight; they suggested that in addition to familial genetics and hormonal factors, growth plate trauma associated with rapid or long periods of growth might be involved in the etiology. Olsson[8,9] has suggested that this condition is a manifestation of osteochondrosis, that is, a failure of endochondral ossification of the physeal cartilage.

The anconeal process has a separate ossification center in some of the larger breeds. It is not ossified and therefore visible radiographically until 12 to 13 weeks of age. It does not unite to the proximal ulna until 16 to 20 weeks of age in the German shepherd, and somewhat later in the St. Bernard and the basset hound. Therefore, the diagnosis of UAP should not be made until 5 months of age in the German shepherd, which is the breed most affected in the United States. We have seen spontaneous reattachment between 7 and 8 months of age in the other two breeds mentioned.

Wind[10] believes there is a growth disturbance of the proximal ulna resulting in an "elliptical" semilunar notch. It articulates poorly with the humerus, resulting in increased pressure against the anconeal process, thereby separating the thickened osteochondrotic physis. We have seen this obviously elliptical semilunar notch especially in the chondrodystrophied breeds.

Clinical Signs

Clinical signs are usually not apparent before 5 to 8 months of age. The signs consist initially of only a slight limp, with the lower limb and elbow slightly abducted. The swing phase of gait is limited by reduced motion at the elbow joint, which is virtually locked. The elbow circumducts laterally during the swing phase of gait. The dog stands and sits with the paw externally rotated, and the toes often seem widespread (Fig. 11–14). Crepitus on flexion-extension is more likely in older animals; joint effusion is also noticeable between the lateral epicondyle and the olecranon. This is best appreciated with the dog standing.

Diagnosis

Clinical signs, age, and breed form the basis for a provisional diagnosis; however, this must be radiographically confirmed. Both elbows should be examined. Acute flexion of the elbow moves the anconeus distal to the medial epicondyle and facilitates visualization (Figs. 11–15 and 11–16). Considerable arthritic

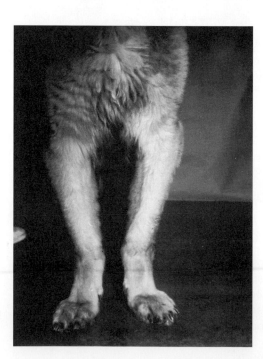

FIGURE 11–14. Typical stance of a dog affected with bilateral elbow osteochondroses. Note varus of the elbows and valgus of the carpi.

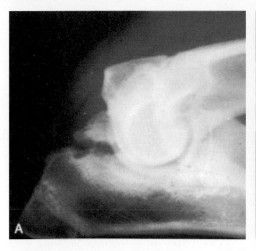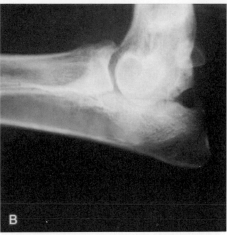

FIGURE 11–15. (*A*) Extreme flexion of the elbow permits good visualization of this ununited anconeal process in a 6-month-old dog. Note the wide lucent zone dividing the olecranon from the anconeal process (mediolateral view). (*B*) In this 24-month-old dog the anconeal process has become completely detached and is seen at the proximal extent of the joint. Signs of joint incongruency and secondary degenerative joint disease are evident (mediolateral view).

changes in the form of osteophytes may be visible throughout the joint and are best visualized from the craniocaudal view.

Treatment

SURGICAL EXCISION ■ Removal of the process is the most widely practiced method of treatment. Although it is unquestionably true that the joint is mildly unstable with the anconeus removed, it is much better to remove the source of inflammation and degenerative changes. In a series of 19 operations on 16 dogs, with an average follow-up of 19.5 months, good function was noted in most cases despite some loss of range of motion, crepitus, and arthritic changes.[11] Early removal—before marked arthrosis—produces the best results.

The elbow is exposed by a lateral approach to the caudal compartment of the elbow[2] (Fig. 11–17*A*). Considerable synovial hyperplasia may need to be resected in order to visualize the anconeus adequately. Usually, the process is still attached to the ulna by a fibrous union and must be sharply dissected to free it. This is usually done with a narrow osteotome or periosteal elevator (Fig. 11–17*B*). Grasping the process with a small pointed bone clamp or towel clamp aids in removing it from the joint. The anconeal process may be completely free within the joint, particularly in older dogs. In such cases, it may migrate to the

FIGURE 11–16. Ununited anconeal process (lateromedial view).

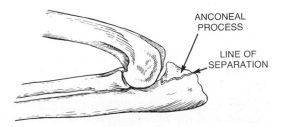

ANCONEAL
PROCESS

LINE OF
SEPARATION

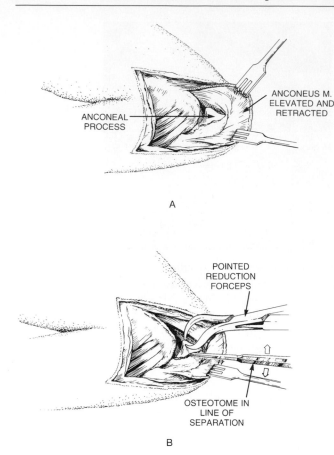

ANCONEAL
PROCESS

ANCONEUS M.
ELEVATED AND
RETRACTED

A

POINTED
REDUCTION
FORCEPS

OSTEOTOME IN
LINE OF
SEPARATION

B

FIGURE 11–17. Surgical removal of ununited anconeal process. (*A*) The left elbow has been exposed by an approach to the caudal compartment of the elbow joint.[2] With the anconeus muscle retracted, the anconeus is visualized. (*B*) A narrow osteotome is being used to free the anconeal process from the ulna. Grasping the process with a small pointed bone forceps aids in removing the process.

proximal portion of the joint. It usually is not well attached and can be removed quite easily.

Occasionally, the separation area is not readily observable. Approximately one third down the semilunar notch a small cartilage defect may be noted. Gentle probing may cause the nonunion area to "give way." The process removed is usually 25 to 30 percent larger than appreciated from the radiograph owing to its cartilaginous surfaces.

SCREW FIXATION ■   Repair of the ununited anconeal process by screw fixation has been advocated.[12,13] It is true that when a lag screw is properly placed, the process will heal. The difficulty in this approach lies in properly placing the screw. The primary consideration is that the process must be perfectly positioned or it will interfere with one of the humeral condyles on extension of the elbow. The wobble induced by such interference results in fatigue fracture of the screw. Screw fixation has the best chance of success in the animal that is presented early, between 5½ and 6 months of age. In this circumstance the process is still firmly attached to the ulna and has not moved. This will ensure that fixation of the process will be in an anatomically perfect position. The screw is placed from the caudal side of the ulna by first drilling a tap hole from the process caudally through the ulna, and then drilling a glide hole from the caudal ulnar side. This eliminates having the screw head in the joint as the original technique described.[12,13]

More recently, osteotomy of the proximal ulna has been used, which reduces pressure of the anconeal process on the humeral trochlea and allows the UAP to unite. Preliminary results by others look encouraging in selected cases.[14] We have seen this work in a few cases of UAP in conjunction with severe ulnar shortening in which release osteotomy was used to lengthen the ulna and improve congruity of the elbow.

AFTERCARE ■ Those animals with significant joint effusion tend to have slow soft-tissue healing. Immobilizing the joint in a modified Robert-Jones dressing (see Fig. 2–23) for 7 to 10 days aids significantly in preventing seromas and dehiscence.

Osteochondritis Dissecans of the Medial Humeral Trochlear Ridge

OCD affects the medial trochlear ridge of the humerus, sometimes bilaterally, in the same dog populations that are affected by OCD of the shoulder. Although retrievers, Bernese mountain dogs, and Rottweilers between the ages of 5 to 8 months are the most commonly affected, many other large breeds are affected as well. (A general discussion of osteochondrosis is found in Chapter 6.)

Clinical Signs

Affected dogs show a foreleg lameness or stiffness and stilted gait starting between the ages of 5 to 8 months. Occasionally, lameness is not obvious to an owner until later in life. Lameness is intensified by exercise and is often most prominent immediately after resting. Frequently, joint swelling can be palpated laterally between the lateral epicondyle of the humerus and the olecranon with the dog standing. There may be valgus of the carpus. Pain may be elicited by deep palpation over the medial collateral ligament or by stressing the ligament by flexing the carpus 90 degrees and rotating the foot laterally. Pain may also be evident on hyperflexion or extension of the joint. Crepitus is occasionally elicited in dogs over 1 year of age, when osteoarthrosis will be sufficiently advanced to produce palpable thickening.

Radiographic Signs

The radiographic diagnosis of OCD of the elbow joint has been well described by Olsson.[15] A triangular subchondral defect can be seen on the medial aspect of the humeral trochlea in the craniocaudal projection (Fig. 11–18A, B). Sclerosis of the medial condyle is often present near the lesion. Roughening of the medial epicondylar surface is an early sign. The lesion is radiographically visible by the age of 5 to 6 months. Later in the disease, osteophyte production is apparent in many areas of the joint. The lateral view also allows visualization of discontinuity of the medial trochlea (Fig. 11–18C). In dogs older than 9 to 10 months, osteophytes will be seen on the anconeus and radial head. Both elbows should be examined. Fragmented coronoid process (see below) is not uncommonly seen concurrently with osteochondritis.

On our experience with OCD of the elbow, the cartilage flap is traumatized and eroded away quicker than OCD of other joints. By 8 to 9 months of age, often only an oval area of "erosion" on the humerus is seen with or without joint mice observable (Fig. 11–18D). With FCP, there is usually a "kiss" lesion on the same area of the humeral condyle, but it is often narrower and longer than the OCD bed (Fig. 11–18E). Therefore, in dogs older than 10 months, it is very difficult to determine whether the damage to the humerus is attributable to an eroded OCD flap or trauma from an FCP. Therefore, statistics as to OCD occurrence with or without FCP may be misleading. In a recent study[16] using

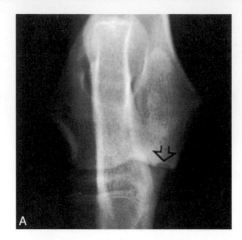

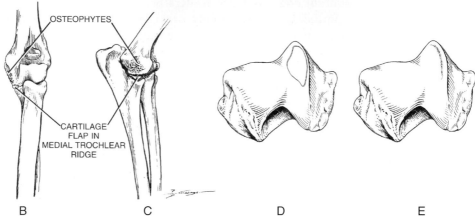

FIGURE 11–18. Osteochondritis dissecans of the medial humeral trochlear ridge. (*A*) A subchondral defect (*arrow*) is seen on this craniocaudal view of the right limb. (*B*) Similar changes are seen here in the trochlear ridge of the left limb, and, in addition, osteophytes are present on the medial epicondyle. (*C*) Although the cartilage flap is seen in this drawing, it is rarely seen radiographically owing to superimposition of the condyles, and its cartilaginous composition. (*D*) Typical bed of OCD lesion on medial humeral condyle. (*E*) Typical "kiss" lesion on medial humeral condyle caused by fragmented coronoid process in young dogs.

computerized study of elbows in 62 cases, only 2 of 64 elbows were believed to be OCD while 34 of 64 were diagnosed as fissured or FCP. In our experience at the surgery table we see many more cases of FCP than OCD, and occasionally the two together. Often we cannot tell, however, if OCD had accompanied the FCP as previously discussed. In the previously mentioned study,[16] 27 elbows underwent surgery with 2 OCDs found, 22 fragmented or fissured coronoids, 2 ununited medial epicondyles, and 1 undiagnosed arthritic joint.

Diagnosis

The specific diagnosis of OCD has to be made radiographically and while the dog is 5 to 9 months of age. Upon exploration, observation of a flap confirms the diagnosis. After 9 months of age, the triangular defect may fill in radiographically, and the flap may be gone upon exploration. The diagnosis is only presumptive at that point.

Treatment

Treatment consists of surgical excision of cartilage flaps and removal of loose cartilage from the joint. Good clinical results are obtained only if surgery is done before degenerative joint disease is well established. This means roughly that animals operated on after 9 months of age have a progressively poorer prognosis. In spite of surgery, further arthrosis will develop. Grondalen found that dogs with OCD had a better prognosis than FCP, which conflicts with Olsson's results.[17]

SURGICAL TECHNIQUE ■ The elbow is approached from the medial aspect.[2,18] This simple muscle-separating approach gives adequate exposure (Fig. 11–19A). Some prefer an osteotomy of the medial epicondyle (Fig. 11–19B). The epicondyle is fixed with a lag screw. Drilling for placement of the lag screw before osteotomy of the epicondyle ensures accurate replacement of the epicondyle and simplifies the drilling process. We have not found this technique necessary in the last several years.

Removal of the cartilage flap is easily accomplished with either approach because the usual location of the lesion is in the center of the surgical field (Fig. 11–19). Sharp excision frees partially attached flaps. Curettage should be just sufficient to clean the edges of the lesion. The joint should be thoroughly searched for free fragments of cartilage before the closure.

AFTERCARE ■ A light bandage is applied for 2 weeks with restricted activity advised for 4 weeks. Often the dogs are walking normally within a couple of days after surgery, even when done bilaterally.

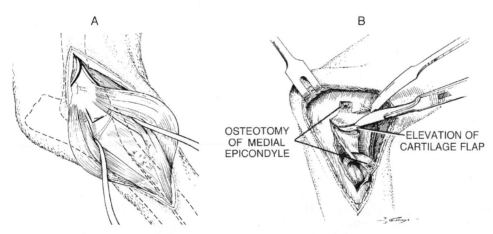

FIGURE 11–19. Surgical treatment of OCD of the medial humeral condyle. (A) The left elbow is exposed by a medial muscle-splitting procedure. After separating between the pronator teres and the flexor carpi radialis, the median nerve is undermined cranial and caudal to the pronator to facilitate retraction and avoidance while retracting with a Gelpi retractor. An L-shaped incision is made through the joint capsule and medial collateral ligament. Exposure is greatly assisted by applying a valgus stress to the elbow with the aid of a sandbag positioned laterally on the elbow. (B) The left elbow has been exposed by a medial approach with osteotomy of the epicondyle.[2] The pronator teres, flexor carpi radialis muscles, and medial collateral ligament are attached to the osteotomized bone. A cartilage flap is elevated with a scalpel.

Fragmented Medial Coronoid Process

The breeds of animals affected, clinical manifestations, and etiopathology of the FCP are similar to those found for OCD of the humeral trochlea. According to some,[15] OCD and FCP coexist 37 percent of the time. As explained in OCD of the elbow, the humeral lesion is often undefinable. It may represent the bed after the OCD flap has been eroded, or it may represent a "kiss" lesion from the FCP underneath it (Fig. 11–18D, E). Like OCD, this lesion is often considered to be part of the osteochondrosis complex,[19] but trauma[20] or growth discrepancies between the radius and ulna have been proposed as causes.

Wind found a developmental incongruity of the trochlear notch of the ulna that was associated with the development of UAP, FCP, and OCD of the medial humeral condyle.[10] In affected breeds a slightly elliptical trochlear notch with a decreased arc of curvature develops, which is too small for the humeral trochlea. This results in major points of contact in areas of the anconeal process and medial coronoid process and little or no contact in other areas of the trochlea. The incidence of FCP and OCD (which were not separated in this study) was 16 percent, and the incidence of FCP with UAP was 3 percent.[21]

In our experience, FCP is seen much more commonly at the surgery table than elbow OCD. The majority of FCP cases are bilateral radiographically, although clinically the dog may show unilateral or bilateral lameness. In some instances, one elbow may have an OCD lesion while the other may have an FCP or an FCP and OCD. Grondalen[22] has shown that, especially in the Rottweiler, there can be a "fissured" coronoid process, meaning that the process is not grossly loose, but usually has an observable line in the articular surface. This has paralleled our experience. Computed tomographic (CT) examination is especially helpful in assessing these cases for surgical decisions.

Surgical excision of loose cartilage or bony fragments before significant arthrosis develops affords a good prognosis, but later surgery in the presence of marked arthrosis is not as successful.[20] This is verified by our own experience. The fragmented coronoid process usually causes a "kissing" lesion on the medial aspect of the humeral condyle. This lesion is a cartilage abrasion and is difficult to distinguish from an old OCD lesion. The abrasion is usually 2 mm wide and extends practically the whole length of the articular surface of the medial condyle (see Fig. 11–18E).

Clinical Signs

There is little to clinically differentiate FCP from OCD of the elbow. Pain on flexion-extension of the elbow and lateral rotation of the paw is a little more consistent in FCP. In younger dogs, effusion is often present and detected as a bulge between the lateral epicondyle of the humerus and the olecranon process of the ulna. In dogs older than 10 to 11 months, joint effusion, crepitus, and general thickening resulting from osteophyte production are also more evident.

Radiographic Signs

Radiographic examination of the elbow is important despite the fact that radiographic signs of the FCP are often nonspecific. Excessive osteoarthrosis and superimposition of the radial head and coronoid process make identification of the FCP difficult. Usually the first radiographic sign seen is the appearance of an osteophyte on the anconeal process (Figs. 11–20A). This may be subtle at first and consists of a convex bony opacity on top of the normally dish-shaped convex anconeal process (Fig. 11–20B). This view and finding are

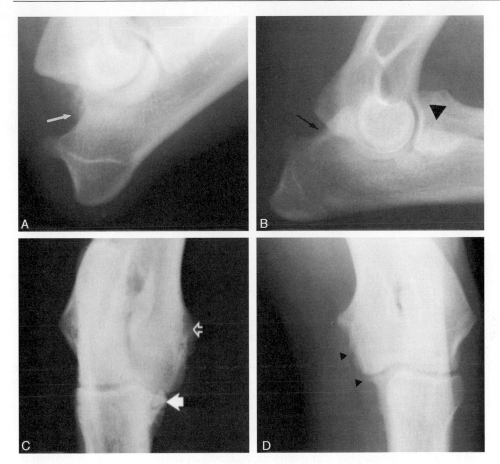

FIGURE 11–20. Fragmentation of the medial coronoid process. (A) Medial lateral view. Typical osteophytes on the dish-shaped anconeal process (*white arrow*). (B) Medial lateral view. Subtle osteophytes causing the anconeal process to lose its dish-shaped profile (*black arrow*). Note the vertical blunting of the coronoid process (*black arrowhead*). (C) Craniocaudal-lateromedial oblique view. Osteophytes are seen on the medial epicondyle (*open white arrow*), and the nondisplaced coronoid process is uncharacteristically well visualized (*solid arrow*). (D) The craniocaudal view of the dog seen in (B). Note the osteophytes on the medial epicondyle of the humerus and coronoid process (*black arrowheads*).

used for screening purposes for breeding dogs. On the craniocaudal view, osteophytes appear medially on the coronoid process (Fig. 11–20C, D) and the medial humeral condyle (Fig. 11–21A). There are occasional cases where the osteophytes are present on the coronoid but not obvious on the anconeal process (Fig. 11–20C). Therefore, three views are normally recommended for symptomatic dogs (lateral, flexed lateral, and craniocaudal). The second subtle radiographic finding is sometimes seen on the straight lateral view. The normal coronoid process has a beak-like projection cranially (Fig. 11–9A). However, with FCP there may be a squared or blunted cranial margin without the "beak" (Fig. 11–20B).

With chronicity, sclerosis of the proximal ulna surrounding the semilunar notch may be seen (8 to 10 months of age).

There is a normal sesamoid bone seen in some large dogs located just lateral to the radial head and should not be mistaken as a joint mouse (Fig. 11–21A).

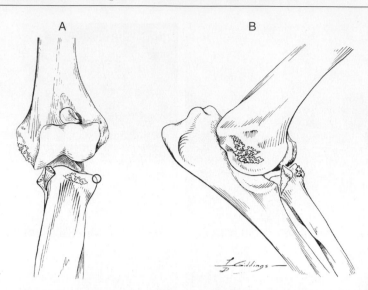

FIGURE 11–21. Fragmented coronoid process. (*A*) Osteophyte production is evident on the medial epicondyle and a displaced fragmented process is noted on this craniocaudal view. There is typically a faint erosion of the articular cartilage of the humeral condyle opposite the site of the fragmented process. The process may not be displaced in all cases. (*B*) In this mediolateral view, osteophytes are present on the radial head, but anconeal osteophytes are obscured by the humerus. The fragmented process can be seen here, but radiographically it is superimposed on the radial head. Note the normal sesamoid lateral to the radial head seen in some individual large breeds.

Although radiographic signs may be suggestive, definitive diagnosis often depends on arthrotomy. This should be undertaken immediately on any young large-breed animal that shows persistent lameness and radiographic signs of osteoarthritis or joint effusion, preferably between 6 and 8 months of age. We have seen some dogs, however, whose lameness did not begin until 2 to 3 years of age with minimal degenerative joint disease present. Perhaps it represents a fissured coronoid that recently breaks. These dogs have functioned well after surgery. Often these cases are bilateral and may be operated bilaterally. In affected Labrador retrievers, Studdert[23] cites a 90 percent occurrence of bilateral lesions.

Diagnosis

As mentioned earlier, FCP is usually not proven with conventional radiography. The diagnosis is presumptive based on the breed/age/joint swelling palpated laterally and radiographs demonstrating osteophytes without an OCD defect. A CT scan (see Chapter 1) may actually demonstrate the separate piece (Figs. 11–22 and 11–23), but is costly, often unnecessary (i.e., not needed for the surgical exploration), and unavailable to many practitioners. However, loose pieces seen on the CT exam and surgery may actually represent fractured osteophytes or joint mice from OCD, especially if not located in the typical locale of the FCP (between the radius and the coronoid). Therefore, making an absolute diagnosis based on surgical and CT findings may not be entirely accurate, especially in the dogs over 1 year old. This must be kept in mind in breeding and genetic studies.

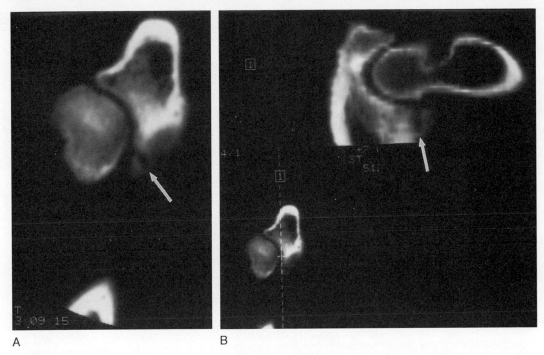

A   B

FIGURE 11–22. (*A*) A computed tomogram (CT) through the ulna and radius. Note the obvious black separation between the coronoid and its tip (*white arrow*). (*B*) Reformatted CT view in the plane of the dotted white lines in the lower left part of the picture. In the upper right, the black separation is seen (*white arrow*).

Surgical Technique

Exposure of the joint is identical to that for OCD, discussed above (Fig. 11–19*A, B*). Sharp adduction and internal rotation of the antebrachium are helpful in increasing exposure of the process. In most cases the process is loose enough to be readily apparent, but in some it is necessary to exert force on the process in order to find the cleavage plane. In fissured coronoids, an osteotome is used to break the top surface, and it usually breaks cleanly. A CT exam is especially helpful in these cases. Older dogs with secondary osteophytes present different problems. In these cases, the medial aspect of the process may be overgrown with osteophytes sufficiently to cover the cleavage plane and may give the process sufficient stability so that it is not easily moved. It is necessary to remove the osteophytes by rongeurs before the FCP can be appreciated.

Because of the possibility of slight malarticulation owing to discrepancies between the ulna and humeral condyle,[10,21] Olsson advised removal of the base of the medial coronoid so there is no possibility of contact with the condyle (SE Olsson, personal communication, 1988). The joint is carefully inspected for OCD lesions and then irrigated to remove cartilage fragments before closure.

AFTERCARE/PROGNOSIS ■ A soft bandage is applied for 2 weeks, with restricted activity for 4 weeks, followed by gradual return to full activity. The outlook for function is good if the FCP is removed before secondary degenerative joint disease (DJD) is well established. These animals will have recognizable signs of DJD later in life but usually function well, as the changes are not as severe as in untreated cases. This means that those animals operated on at

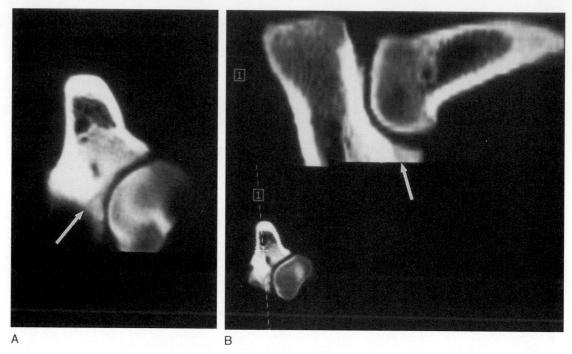

A   B

FIGURE 11–23. (*A*) Computed tomogram (CT) through the radius and ulna in a 9-month-old Rottweiler with a "fissured" or cracked coronoid (*white arrow*), which may not be apparent upon visual inspection. An osteotome is used to start the removal parallel to the cleavage plane denoted from the CT. (*B*) Reformatted CT view of the white dotted lines in the lower part of the picture. Note also a separate piece (fracture of an osteophyte) to the left of the dotted line. In the upper right, a dark abnormal coronoid process (*white arrow*) is seen, but no obvious "fracture" line.

7 to 9 months have the best outlook; the prognosis declines rapidly when surgery is delayed past 12 months and degenerative joint disease is extensive.

Ununited Medial Epicondyle

UME is an ill-defined uncommon elbow condition seen in several large breeds (especially the Labrador retriever) characterized by detached ossified bodies located either at the medial joint line or caudally just distal to the squared off medial epicondyle. In many cases they are located in both locations (Figs. 11–24 and 11–25C, D). Often they are seen in conjunction with other osteochondroses of the elbow. These pieces may actually grow to be 3 or 4 cm in length.

By themselves, they may cause lameness or be asymptomatic. There may be no history of trauma, or the lameness may result following nonviolent trauma

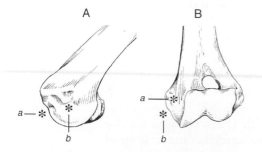

A   B

FIGURE 11–24. Schematic drawing of the two locations where loose pieces of bone (ununited medial epicondyle) are located. (*A*) Lateral distal humerus. (*B*) Craniocaudal view of the distal humerus. The asterisk at site *a* is the position of the fragment that detaches from the caudal distal medial epicondyle, while the asterisk at site *b* is the position of the fragment that detaches from the medial aspect of the medial epicondyle.

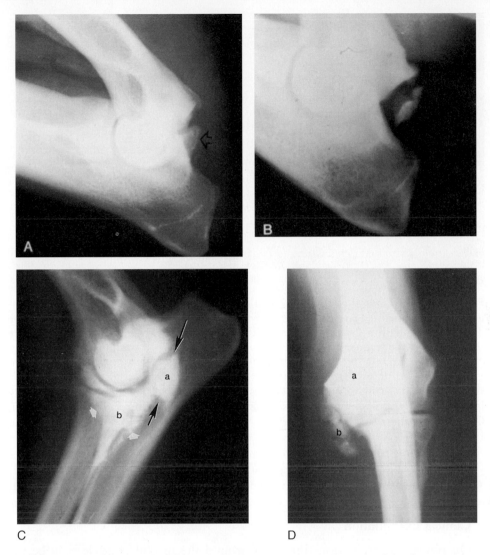

FIGURE 11–25. Ununited medial epicondyle (UME) or calcification of the flexor tendons arising from the caudal medial epicondyle. (*A*) A lateral view of UME located at the open arrowhead. (*B*) A lateral view of another dog with UME. (*C*) Lateral view of a large UME seen caudal as in site *a* (see Fig. 11–24) (*black arrows*). The mineralized densities at site *b* are not evident (*white arrowheads*). (*D*) Craniocaudal view of dog in (*C*). Note the densities in site *b* are obvious, but those in site *a* are obscured by the humerus. *Figure continued on following page*

such as hunting or playing with other dogs. Signs may begin at 4 to 5 months of age, or 5 years of age, or again may be an incidental finding. Others prefer to call this condition calcification of the flexor tendons of the medial epicondyle.[24] We believe, as do Olsson[9] and Bennett,[25] that it is a form of osteochondrosis wherein fragments of the cartilage avulse with tendons. With time, the cartilage changes to bone and enlarges, reaching a point at times where the bony pieces rub against the humerus or ulna, causing lameness (Fig. 11–25E, F).

The rationale in believing there is an underlying problem (i.e., osteochondrosis) other than trauma is that it is often bilateral, often without trauma in

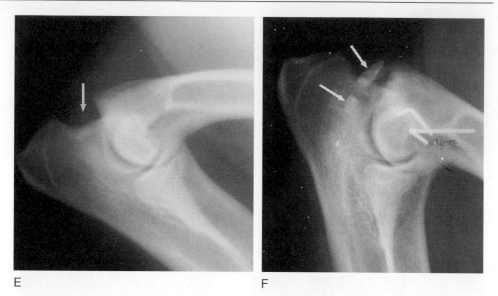

E   F

FIGURE 11–25. *Continued* (*E*) A 2-mm mineralized density (*arrow*) in a 14-month-old Labrador operated successfully for a fragmented coronoid. (*F*) Four years later, the dog presented with a 2-month lameness that resolved quickly after extirpation. Note the growth of the fragment seen in *E* (*arrows*).

the history, has been seen (all belonging to three different veterinarians!) in three littermates of English setters, and is seen especially in the Labrador retriever, German shepherd and English setter. We have seen a case in a 14-month-old Labrador retriever with FCP that was operated and did well for 4 years. Upon re-examination for a 2-month-old lameness, the 2-mm UME that was seen 4 years before had grown six to eight times in size (Fig. 11–25E, F). After excision, the lameness resolved within 3 weeks. Histological analyses of these pieces in the older dog is not helpful in elucidating its pathogenesis.

Clinical Examination

On physical examination, thickness around the medial condyle may be detected along with pain sometimes elicited by direct pressure.

Radiographic Findings

Two radiographic views (flexed lateral, craniocaudal) of the elbow must be studied carefully to determine the number and location of the fragments. These may only be found on the craniocaudal view spanning or just distal to the joint line. On the lateral view, they may be undetected due to superimposition of the humerus and radius. The fragments located on the distal caudal epicondyle may be seen on the flexed lateral view but not on the craniocaudal view—again due to superimposition (Fig. 11–25).

DIAGNOSIS ■ The diagnosis as to whether lameness is due to UME is problematic, since it may be asymptomatic and may coexist with OCD or FCP. However, in the mature dog, these fragments are just outside the articular surface and cause very little DJD. If DJD is present, other conditions (such as OCD and FCP) may be the real cause of lameness and should be explored.

TREATMENT ■ Surgical extirpation usually is rewarding if there is no other coexisting elbow condition. Lesion at site *a* is located in the fibrotic tissue surrounding the flexor carpi radialis, whereas lesion at site *b* is more caudal in the scarred origin of the deep and superficial flexors. The bony fragments are sharply dissected carefully avoiding horizontal transection of tendons. All fragments should be removed. If fragments are left, they may grow and result in return of lameness. If DJD is present, the elbow should be explored further. (See OCD/FCP sections.)

AFTERCARE/PROGNOSIS ■   The limb is bandaged for 10 to 14 days followed by another 2 weeks of restricted activity. If all fragments have been removed, and no other condition is present to cause the lameness, the prognosis is excellent.

ARTHRODESIS OF THE ELBOW

Arthrodesis of the elbow is an alternative to amputation for severely comminuted intra-articular fractures, chronic luxation or subluxation from a variety of causes, and severe osteoarthritis. High radial nerve palsy has also been suggested as an indication. Elbow arthrodesis, however, is a very disabling fusion and should be considered only when the owner refuses amputation. Amputation will provide better overall function than arthrodesis.

Strict attention to detail to establish proper joint angles and rigid internal fixation are necessary for success. Although a variety of fixation methods have been described, multiple-screw or bone plate fixation has yielded the best results in our experience. (See Chapter 7 for discussion of indications for and principles of arthrodesis.)

Surgical Technique

Bone Plate Fixation

The joint is exposed by a combined caudal approach with osteotomy of the olecranon process and the lateral approach to the elbow (Fig. 11–26A). A second ostectomy of the proximal ulna is performed to provide a smooth curve from the caudal humeral shaft to the caudal ulnar shaft with the joint at the functioning angle, usually 110 degrees (Fig. 11–26B). The lateral joint capsule is opened widely to allow the radius and ulna to be rotated medially and thus expose the interior of the joint. Articular cartilage is removed from all contact surfaces of the radial head, humeral condyles, and trochlear notch of the ulna. The humeral capitulum is flattened to fit against the radial head.

A temporary pin is driven across the joint to hold it at the selected angle, and an eight- to ten-hole bone plate is contoured to the caudal surfaces of the ulna and humerus (Fig. 11–26C). The proximal ulna may have to be further flattened slightly to allow good seating of the plate. One screw is placed as a lag screw through the plate and lateral epicondyle into the radial head. Ideally, a second lag screw is lagged through the plate and ulna into the medial epicondyle. The rest of the screws are inserted, and the temporary pin is removed.

Autogenous cancellous bone graft from the proximal humerus and the ulnar ostectomy is packed into and around the joint. The olecranon process is attached medial to the plate by a lag screw (Fig. 11–26D). The anconeus muscle is detached from the humerus and the ulnaris lateralis tendon sutured. The remaining tissues are closed in layers.

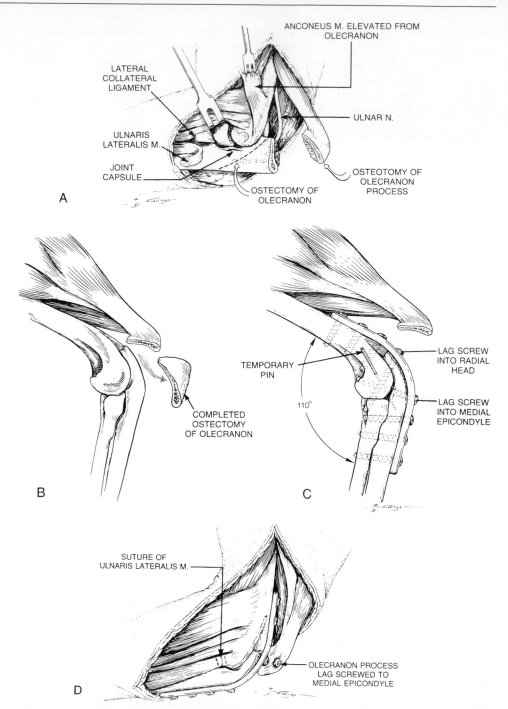

FIGURE 11–26. Arthrodesis of the elbow by bone plate fixation. (*A*) The left elbow has been exposed by a combined caudal approach with osteotomy of the olecranon process and a lateral approach.[2] The ulnaris lateralis and lateral collateral ligament have been sectioned and the joint capsule has been opened widely to allow for removal of joint cartilage. Ostectomy of the ulna is outlined here. (*B*) Ostectomy of the ulna is completed to form a smooth curve from the humerus to the ulna. (*C*) A temporary pin holds the joint at the selected angle, and the plate is contoured. A minimum of four plate holes for each bone is required. One screw is lagged through the plate and lateral epicondyle into the radial head and a second through the plate and ulna into the medial epicondyle. (*D*) The olecranon process is lag-screwed to the humerus medial to the plate, and the ulnaris lateralis tendon sutured. The anconeus muscle has been excised.

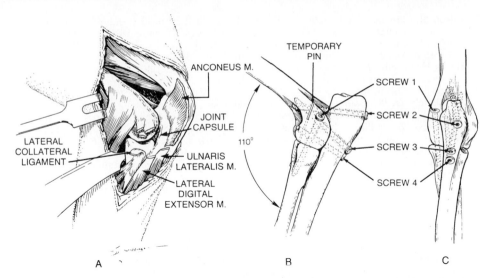

FIGURE 11–27. Elbow arthrodesis with lag screw fixation. (*A*) The left elbow has been exposed by a lateral approach. The ulnaris lateralis, lateral digital extensor, and lateral collateral ligament have been sectioned, allowing the joint capsule to be opened widely. Removal of articular cartilage follows. (*B*) A temporary pin fixes the joint at the desired angle, and the screws are placed in order. Screw Nos. 1, 2, and 3 are lag screws, and screw No. 4 is positional, threaded in both bones. (*C*) Caudal view of the screw placement.

Lag Screw Fixation

This technique to arthrodese the elbow requires less surgical exposure and operating time while eliminating the cost of a large bone plate. The joint is exposed by the lateral approach to the elbow.[2] Additional extensor muscles and the lateral collateral ligament are cut to widely expose the joint (Fig. 11–27A). Articular cartilage is debrided as detailed previously.

A temporary pin is placed across the joint to maintain the desired angle. Screw No. 1 is placed as a lag screw from the lateral epicondyle to the radial head (Fig. 11–27B, C). The second screw is lagged from the olecranon process into the humerus just proximal to the supratrochlear foramen. The third screw is lagged from the ulna into the medial epicondyle. Screw No. 4 is positional and threaded into the ulna and the center of the epicondyles. The temporary pin is removed. Autogenous cancellous bone graft from the proximal humerus is packed into and around the joint. Extensor and anconeus muscles are sutured, and the remaining tissues are closed in layers.

AFTERCARE ■ A spica splint is applied and maintained for 4 weeks (see Fig. 2–23). Exercise is restricted for 4 more weeks, at which time radiographic signs of fusion should be noted before exercise is gradually returned to normal.

References

1. Campbell JR: Luxation and ligamentous injuries of the elbow of the dog. Vet Clin North Am 1:429, 1971.
2. Piermattei DL: An Atlas of Approaches to the Bones of the Dog and Cat, 3rd ed. Philadelphia, WB Saunders Co, 1993.
3. Bingel SA, Riser WH: Congenital elbow luxation in the dog. J Small Anim Pract 18:445, 1977.
4. Guerevitch R, Hohn RB: Surgical management of lateral luxation and subluxation of the canine radial head. Vet Surg 9:49–57, 1980.

5. Gilson SD, Piermattei DL, Schwarz PD: Treatment of humeroulnar subluxation with a dynamic proximal ulnar osteotomy. A review of 13 cases. Vet Surg 18:114, 1989.
6. Flo GL, DeCamp CE: Surgical correction of congenital radial head luxations. Proceedings of the 1990 Veterinary Orthopedic Society annual meeting, Jackson Hole, WY, 1990.
7. Hayes HM, Selby LA, Wilson GP, Hohn RB: Epidemiologic observations of canine elbow disease (emphasis on dysplasia). J Am Anim Hosp Assoc 15:449, 1979.
8. Olsson SE: Osteochondrosis in the dog. In Kirk RW (ed): Current Veterinary Therapy VI. Philadelphia, WB Saunders Co, 1977, pp 880–886.
9. Olsson SE: Osteochondrosis—A growing problem to dog breeders. Gaines Dog Research Progress. White Plains, NY, Gaines Dog Research Center, Summer 1976, pp 1–11.
10. Wind AP: Elbow incongruity and developmental elbow diseases in the dog: Part I. J Am Anim Hosp Assoc 22:711, 1986.
11. Sinibaldi KR, Arnoczky SP: Surgical removal of the ununited anconeal process in the dog. J Am Anim Hosp Assoc 11:192, 1975.
12. Herron MR: Ununited anconeal process—a new approach to surgical repair. Mod Vet Pract 51:30, 1970.
13. Fox SM, Burbidge HM, Bray JC, Guerin SR: Ununited anconeal process: Lag screw fixation. J Am Anim Hosp Assoc 32:52–57, 1996.
14. Sjöstrom L, Kasström H, Kallberg M: Ununited anconeal process in the dog. Pathogenesis and treatment by osteotomy of the ulna. Vet Comp Orthop Trauma 8:170–199, 1995.
15. Olsson SE: The early diagnosis of fragmented coronoid process and osteochondritis dissecans of the canine elbow joint. J Am Anim Hosp Assoc 19:616, 1983.
16. Rosenstein DS, Stickle RS, Glo GL, et al: Computerized tomography of the canine elbow. Vet Rad Ultrasound (abstr) 35(4):244, 1994.
17. Grondalen J: Arthrosis in the elbow joint of rapidly growing dogs. Part 3. Ununited medial coronoid process of the ulna and osteochondritis dissecans of the humeral condyle. Surgical procedure for correction and postoperative investigation. Nord Vet Med 34:520, 1979.
18. Probst CW, Flo GL, McLoughlin MA, et al: A simple medial approach to the canine elbow for treatment of fragmented coronoid process and osteochondritis dissecans. J Am Anim Hosp Assoc 25:331, 1989.
19. Olsson SE: Osteochondrosis of the elbow joint in the dog: Its manifestations, indications for surgery, and surgical approach. Arch Am Coll Vet Surg 6:46, 1977.
20. Berzon JL, Quick CB: Fragmented coronoid process: Anatomical, clinical, and radiographic considerations with case analyses. J Am Anim Hosp Assoc 16:241, 1980.
21. Wind AP, Packard ME: Elbow incongruity and developmental elbow diseases in the dog: Part II. J Am Anim Hosp Assoc 22:725, 1986.
22. Grondalen J: Arthrosis in the elbow joint of young rapidly growing dogs. Part 5. A pathoanatomical investigation. Nord Vet Med 33:1–16, 1981.
23. Studdert VP, Lavelle RB, Beilharz RG, et al: Clinical features and heritability of osteochondrosis of the elbow in Labrador retrievers. J Small Anim Pract 32:557, 1991.
24. Zontine WJ, Weitkamp RA, Lippincott CL: Redefined type of elbow dysplasia involving calcified flexor tendons attached to the medial humeral epicondyle in three dogs. J Am Vet Med Assoc 194:1082, 1989.
25. Bennett D, May C: Joint diseases of dogs and cats. In Ettinger SJ, Feldman EC (eds): Textbook of Veterinary Internal Medicine, 4th ed. Philadelphia, WB Saunders Co, 1995.

12

Fractures of the Radius and Ulna

All the various types of fractures can be seen involving either or both the radius and ulna.[1-3] Distal to the proximal third of the radius these bones usually fracture as a unit, but proximal to this region independent fractures of both bones are commonly seen. The development of angulation and rotation at the fracture site, delayed union, and nonunion are not uncommon sequelae in distal third fractures, and measures to prevent them should be kept in mind constantly.

FIXATION TECHNIQUES

Coaptation

Stable type A1 and A2 (see Table 2–1) fractures of the diaphysis and distal radius/ulna (see Fig. 12–13A) respond to external fixation in a narrow range of cases. Lappin et al. reported a 75 percent serious complication rate in toy and miniature breeds, while medium-size dogs (10 to 65 pounds) less than 1 year of age responded well, with no serious complications.[4] Figure 12–1 illustrates the principle of location of fracture versus length of cast for applying coaptation fixation for these fractures. Reduction may be accomplished closed by a combination of traction, countertraction, and digital manipulation. In some instances, open reduction is preferable to closed manipulation, which may cause an undue amount of trauma to tissue in the fracture site. There is a tendency for the carpus to hyperextend, develop valgus deviation, and rotate outward postoperatively (owing to loss of tone in the flexor muscle group). The position of the foot on standing and walking while favoring the leg is also a factor. To prevent this unfavorable development when an external splint is used, the foot should be placed in a position of slight varus, flexion, and inward rotation. Ordinarily, this can be accomplished best with a molded cast.

Splinting

As the sole method of fixation, the use of a Mason metasplint, or similar coaptation splint (see Fig. 2–27) is limited to the more stable and more distal fractures (e.g., greenstick and certain intraperiosteal fractures) because it is impossible to immobilize the elbow joint adequately. Many splints have a tendency to loosen and need constant rechecking to make sure they are accomplishing the intended objective. For complete fractures, the position of slight varus, flexion, and inward rotation is difficult or impossible to obtain and maintain when

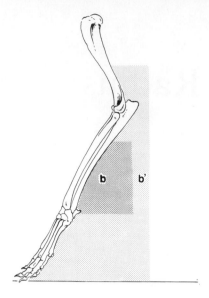

FIGURE 12–1. Stable fractures of the ulna and radius (*b*) may be immobilized with a cast extending to the midhumeral region (*b'*).

these splints are used. Thomas splints (see Fig. 2–25) can be satisfactorily used for diaphyseal fractures for those familiar with their application; however, the molded fiberglass cast is generally more satifactory.

Casts

In stable fractures, a plaster of Paris or fiberglass molded long leg cast (see Fig. 2–21) may be used as the sole method of fixation. If a cast is used on an unstable fracture, overriding frequently develops at the fracture site. Overpadding inside the cast allows for torsional movement at the fracture site and may result in delayed union, nonunion, or malunion. If the cast is applied when the leg is swollen, looseness and instability may result if the cast is not readjusted.

Intramedullary Pins and Wires

Because the radius is relatively straight, both ends are completely covered with articular cartilage, and the medullary canal is very narrow in the craniocaudal direction; thus the radius is not as amenable to intramedullary (IM) pin fixation as are the other long bones. In small dogs, the pin may be used to assist in holding end-to-end alignment in stable fractures. In general, the pin that is inserted is too small to approximate the marrow cavity in size. This type fixation must always be supplemented with coaptation. Attempts at intramedullary fixation, especially in small and toy breeds, are a common cause of delayed union and nonunion.[4,5] Intramedullary pinning is only practical in large breeds, and even here has the disadvantage of requiring supplemental coaptation. There are better methods of fixation available.

The method of insertion of an intramedullary pin in the radius in large-breed dogs is shown in Figure 12–2:

1.   The pin is started at the styloid process, then continues up through the marrow cavity, Rush pin style (Fig. 12–2A).

2.   The pin is inserted obliquely through the cranial cortex and medullary cavity of the distal segment into the proximal segment, Rush pin style.

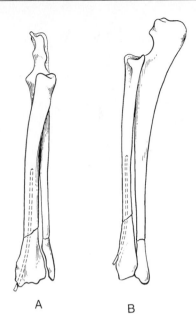

FIGURE 12–2. Insertion of intramedullary pins in radius. (*A*) A pin is started at the styloid process, continuing up through the marrow cavity in a Rush pin style. (*B*) Alternatively, the pin is inserted obliquely through the cranial cortex and marrow cavity of the distal segment into the marrow cavity of the proximal segment in a Rush pin style.

A   B

Intramedullary pinning of the ulna is easily accomplished from the tuber olecrani distally. The narrow diameter of the distal third of the bone limits the use of suitable size pins to the proximal two thirds of the ulna. Steinmann pinning of the ulna is generally indicated for additional support for a radial fracture fixation, the type A1 proximal extra-articular fracture (see Fig. 12–7) being the only ulnar diaphyseal fracture suitable to IM pinning as the primary fixation.

External Fixators

The fixator is adaptable to most shaft fractures of the radius and ulna. It is particularly indicated in open fractures, delayed unions, nonunions, and corrective osteotomies. The splint works particularly well with small dogs. In most instances, the pins are inserted on the medial or craniomedial border of the radius because the bone is more superficial in this location and the splint is in the position of least interference from cages, fences, and so forth.

All of the various configurations (unilateral and biplanar type I, bilateral type II, and trilateral type III) may be used. In the author's experience, however, the unilateral type I single bar is adequate in most all cases, is the simplest to apply, and has the fewest complications. This method requires the placement of all pins in the same plane (Fig. 12–3). A complex fracture of radius and ulna with single-bar type I fixator, 3/3 pins, is shown in Figure 12–17A, B, and a Type II fixator in 12–17C. Depending on the size of the animal and stability of the fracture, 2/2, 3/3, or 4/4 pins may be used. On some of the very fragmented fractures, a biplanar configuration type IA (one unilateral splint on medial surface and one on the cranial) may be indicated. This configuration is also useful for distal A2 fractures, as it allows placement of three fixation pins in the very short segment (see Fig. 12–22). A hybrid type II-III splint also has application in extremely short distal segments (see Fig. 12–23).

A very important advantage of the external fixator in radial fractures is the ability to employ the *biological osteosynthesis* concept by applying the splint with the fracture closed, or with a very limited open approach and reduction.

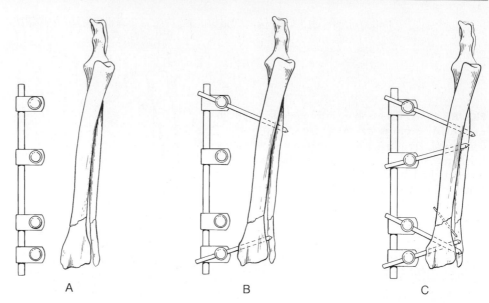

A   B   C

FIGURE 12–3. Applying a type IA unilateral external fixator with one connecting bar and all pins inserted in the same plane. (*A*) The fracture is openly reduced and held with locking forceps; a connecting bar with four single clamps is prepared. (*B*) The proximal and distal pins are inserted in the same plane; the connecting bar and outer clamps are attached. (*C*) Middle clamps are positioned; the two inside pins are inserted through holes in the middle clamps. The nuts on the clamps are securely tightened. In some cases, an additional obliquely directed Kirschner wire is inserted to give more stability at the fracture site. If the fracture pattern is a longer oblique, insertion of a lag screw is indicated.

Because of the limited musculature of the antebrachium, closed reduction is more feasible than in the humerus or femur. The animal is prepared and draped for surgery with the limb suspended as shown in Figure 2–12. Sterile towels or bandage material are wrapped around the suspending material a sufficient distance to prevent the chance of accidental contamination of the surgeon during reduction.

Although any type fixator can be used, the type II has special application during closed reduction. If the most proximal and distal fixation pins are inserted first, at 90 degrees to the bone, they become a visual indicator of the adequacy of reduction in the frontal plane, since they will be parallel to each other when angular deformity in this plane is reduced. Additionally, they can be employed to anchor a fracture distractor to aid in the reduction (Fig. 12–4A) if desired. If difficulty is encountered in reducing the fracture closed, it is often possible to make a small approach over the shaft of the ulna, and to then reduce the ulnar fracture under direct vision. If the ulnar fracture is simple, reducing it ensures that the radius is also adequately reduced. The other method is to employ a limited open approach to the radius to allow reduction under direct vision, but with minimal disruption of the fracture site, thus maintaining maximal vascularity of the fracture segments (Fig. 12–4B). The open approach also allows the use of auxiliary fixation such as K-wires (Fig. 12–3C), or lag screws (see Fig. 12–14), both of which can be inserted with minimal disruption of soft tissues.

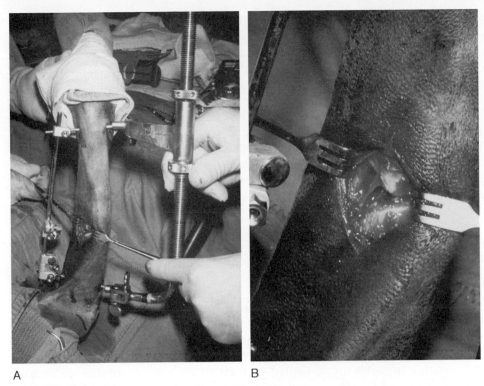

A   B

FIGURE 12–4. Application of a type IIA external fixator with a limited open approach to the radial diaphysis. (*A*) Fixation pins have been placed proximally and distally in the radius and the fracture reduced by means of the fracture distractor applied laterally to the fixation pins. The medial connecting bar is loosely positioned at this point. Note the varus angulation induced by the distractor; this can be adjusted when the lateral connecting bar is attached. (*B*) The adequacy of the reduction is verified by a small cutdown over the fracture site. If necessary, the ends can be levered into better contact, but the fracture hematoma is disturbed as little as possible.

Bone Plates

Plates are adaptable to most radial and ulnar shaft fractures.[1,3] For diaphyseal fractures the usual procedure is to only plate the radius. If the radius is well stabilized, fixation of the ulna is usually unnecessary. In large dogs, it is useful to use small plates on both the radius and ulna (see Fig. 12–16) in preference to one large plate on the radius. A large cranially placed plate may make it difficult to attain adequate soft tissue closure at the time of implantation, or it may interfere with movement of the extensor tendons. Round hole plates, DCPs, or semitubular plates may be used. The plate most frequently used is the DCP because it has the built-in potential of compression at the fracture site. A semi-tubular plate must be of sufficient size, and bending must be minimal in contouring it to fit the bone surface. For distal fractures, the T-plate allows placing two or three screws in a short segment (see Fig. 12–21A), and the cuttable plate (VCP) is also helpful in small breeds. See Figure 2–74 for suggested plate sizes.

Cranial placement of the plate has been the most widely used method for all diaphyseal fractures, because it is easily accessible and provides a broad and only slightly curved surface (Fig. 12–14B).[3] This surface serves well for fractures of the proximal and middle regions of the radius, but in the distal zone the plate is the source of some morbidity. Dissection and elevation of the extensor tendons from their synovial sheaths in the middle groove of the distal radius and the subsequent gliding of these tendons over the plate surface produce varying degrees of functional problems. Additionally, problems are sometimes encountered in closing the scant soft tissues over a distal plate. Most of these problems can be eliminated by medial plate placement for distal fractures (see Fig. 12–21B), and mechanical testing has shown this position to be equivalent in axial stiffness to cranially placed plates following distal osteotomy.[6] This despite the fact that the medial surface is narrower and the medial plate was therefore smaller (2.7 versus 3.5 mm) than the cranial plate. The smaller plate allows more screws to be placed per unit of plate length, and the medial position increases the possibility of incorporating a lag screw through the plate into an oblique fracture.

Postoperative swelling and pain are eased by use of a Robert-Jones dressing for 3 to 5 days (see Fig. 2–33).

Lag Screws

As primary fixation, lag screws are mainly used in distal articular fractures (see Figs. 12–24 and 12–25). Long oblique or spiral simple fractures of the radius and ulna may be stabilized with lag screws for holding alignment and exerting interfragmentary compression at the fracture site (see Fig. 12–14A). This fixation must be supplemented with either external coaptation or internal fixation. Internal fixation may consist of a bone plate (see Fig. 12–14B), an intramedullary pin in the ulna (see Fig. 12–14C), which may still need external splint support, or an external fixator (see Fig. 12–14D).

PROXIMAL FRACTURES

A major consideration in type B and C articular fractures is the pull of the triceps muscle on the tuber olecrani, with the tuber pivoting at the trochlear notch. Some form of tension band fixation is essential in these fractures to neutralize these muscle forces.

OPEN APPROACHES ■   Two open approaches can be used individually or combined to expose this region; the approach to the proximal shaft and trochlear notch of the ulna, and the approach to the head and proximal metaphysis of the radius (Fig. 12–5A, B).[7]

Fracture Type 21-A; Proximal, Extra-articular (Fig. 12–6A)

Type A1 Ulnar Fracture

This fracture is relatively rare because this region of the ulna is non–weight-bearing and not subjected to any indirect forces and so fractures can only be the result of direct trauma. Treatment is by external fixation by long leg cast (see Fig. 2–21), Thomas splint (see Fig. 2–25), or Velpeau sling (see Fig. 2–29). An IM pin could also be used, but is rarely necessary.

Monteggia Fracture[8]

This lesion is a fracture of the ulna and dislocation of the radial head, and is a special case injury that does not completley conform to the AO Vet fracture

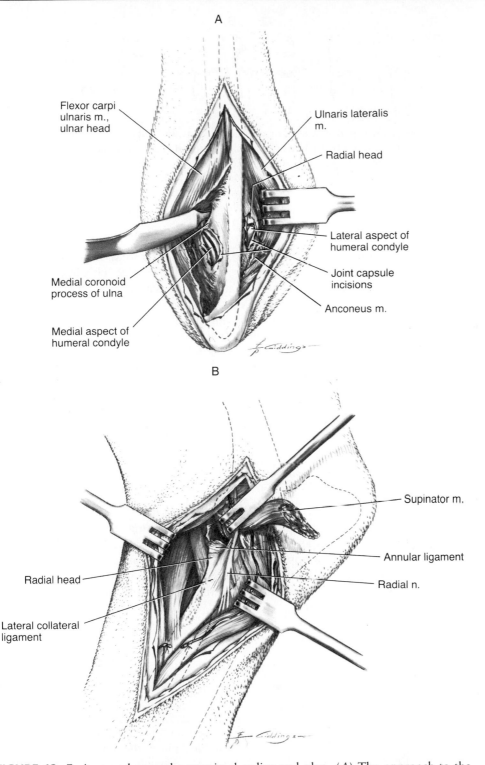

FIGURE 12–5. Approaches to the proximal radius and ulna. (*A*) The approach to the proximal shaft and trochlear notch of the ulna gives good visualization of the articular surface of the trochlear notch. (*B*) The radial nerve must be preserved during this lateral approach to the head and proximal metaphysis of the radius. (From Piermattei DL: An Atlas of Surgical Approaches to the Bones and Joints of the Dog and Cat, 3rd ed. Philadelphia, WB Saunders Co, 1993, pp 187, 195, with permission.)

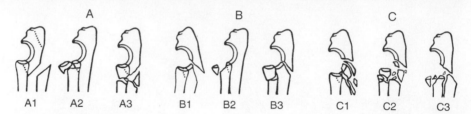

FIGURE 12–6. Proximal fractures of the radius and ulna. *(A1)* Ulnar, *(A2)* radial, and *(A3)* radial and ulnar. *(B1)* Ulnar, *(B2)* radial, and *(B3)* of one bone, the other extra-articular. *(C1)* One bone remains intact, *(C2)* of one bone, the other extra-articular, and *(C3)* radius and ulna. (From Unger M, Montavon PM, Heim UFA: Classification of fractures of the long bones in the dog and cat: Introduction and clinical application. Vet Comp Orthop Trauma 3:41–50, 1990, with permission.)

classification system. In a type I lesion, the luxated radial head is cranial in relation to the joint, and the bones are angulated cranially. This injury in dogs is usually a result of being struck by a car, while in cats it is usually a result of a fall. The proximal radioulnar joint can be intact (Fig. 12–7A), or the bones can become separated by rupture of the annular ligament of the radius and the caudal crus of the lateral collateral ligament (Fig. 12–8A). Type I is by far the most common type lesion. Type II lesions have a caudal dislocation of the radial head with caudal angulation, while in type III injuries the radial head is luxated in a lateral or craniolateral direction. Rarely seen are type IV lesions, with cranial luxation of the radial head and fracture of both the proximal radial and ulnar diaphyses.

REDUCTION AND FIXATION ■ If the fracture is relatively recent in origin, a closed reduction often can be accomplished by a combination of traction and countertraction along with caudal pressure on the radius to manipulate the radial head back into the reduced position.

Types I, II, and III; Proximal Radioulnar Joint Intact ■ Internal fixation may be accomplished by inserting a pin from the proximal end of the olecranon process into the shaft of the ulna (Fig. 12–7B). In some cases, it may be necessary to perform an open approach to the proximal ulna and trochlear notch to accomplish accurate reduction. The pin in the ulna may be inserted either from the proximal end or by use of the retrograde technique. If indicated, an

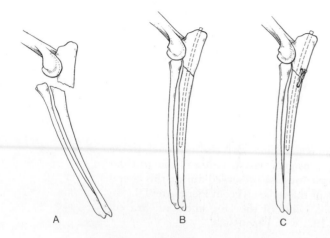

FIGURE 12–7. *(A)* Type A1 fracture of ulna with dislocation of the radial head (Monteggia fracture). The annular ligament is intact. *(B)* Immobilization by use of an intramedullary pin in the ulna and a coaptation splint. *(C)* The addition of an interfragmentary wire improves stability at the fracture site. This need not be a tension band wire.

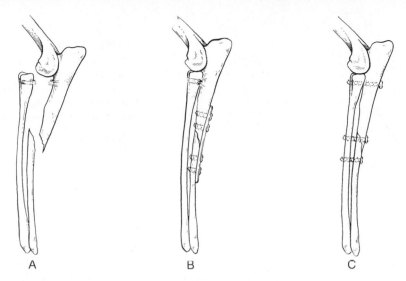

FIGURE 12–8. (A) Monteggia fracture with the annular ligament disrupted. (B) Repair by immobilizing the ulna with a bone plate and suturing the annular ligament. (C) Fixation by use of bone screws. The ulna is fixed to the radius. The proximal screw should be removed in 3 to 4 weeks to allow the return of some pronation-supination motion.

interfragmentary wire may be inserted in the ulna for additional stabilization and compression (Fig. 12–7C). If temporary additional external support is indicated, it may be in the form of a modified Robert-Jones dressing. Exercise is restricted during the healing period.

Types I, II, and III; Proximal Radioulnar Joint Luxated ■   Frequently, there is soft tissue (usually one or more of the extensor muscles) interposed between the two bones. An open approach may be necessary to accomplish reduction. The usual procedure is to repair the ulnar fracture (with a bone plate or intramedullary pin) and to then suture the annular and collateral ligaments to restore and maintain apposition of the radius and ulna (Fig. 12–8B). If suturing the annular ligament is not possible, apposition between the radius and ulna can be accomplished by the use of several bone screws (Fig. 12–8C). Ordinarily, this procedure is not used in the young growing animal because it interferes with normal shifting of the ulna on the radius in the growing process and may result in incongruency of the elbow joint and/or radius curvus. It should also be used with caution in cats because marked supination and pronation are a part of the normal function of the foreleg. If it is used out of necessity in either the dog or cat the screws should be removed 3 to 4 weeks postoperatively to allow return of normal motion between the radius and ulna.

Type IV ■   The radioulnar joint is typically intact in this injury. Reduction of the radial head luxation is followed by fixation of the radial fracture as is described below. Additional fixation of the ulna can be supplied by an IM pin if desired.

Type A2 Radial Fracture

The radial head is rarely fractured. It may or may not be accompanied by dislocation of the elbow joint. There is usually history of trauma. Separation at

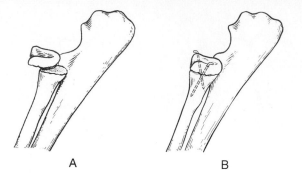

FIGURE 12–9. (*A*) Type A2 physeal fracture of the radial head. (*B*) Simple transfixation pinning with Kirschner wire. The wires enter the bone near the joint surface and proceed distally and diagonally into the opposite cortex.

the physeal plate always threatens to disturb growth. Premature closure of the physis and shortening of the radius are not uncommon sequelae (see Chapter 22). Anatomical reduction and fixation are indicated. Figure 12–9 shows an epiphyseal fracture-separation of the radial head. Open reduction and simple Kirschner wire fixation is used. Healing is rapid, and the wire may be removed in 2 to 3 weeks or left in place. A Robert-Jones dressing may be indicated for temporary additional support.

Type A3 Radial and Ulnar Fracture

Stabilization of the ulna by IM pin, IM pin and interfragmentary wire, or bone plating caudally (Fig. 12–10*F*) or laterally (Fig. 12–10*G*) may provide sufficient support for the radius. Additional radial fixation can be gained either by K-wire fixation or a small T or cuttable plate applied either cranially or laterally. A Robert-Jones dressing may be indicated for temporary additional support.

Fracture Type 21B; Proximal, Simple Articular (Fig. 12–6*B*)

Following fracture, the pull of the triceps brachii muscles pulls the tuber olecrani segment proximally, bending it toward the shaft of the humerus (Fig. 12–10*A*). For best results, this pull should be neutralized by use of the tension band principle. In general, the pin and tension band wire method is used on stable fractures, and a plate is used for unstable fractures (Fig. 12–10*B*, *C*, *E*–*G*). Although it seems reasonable to do, simple IM pin fixation of the ulna in these fractures never works well in any size animal. The medullary canal of the ulna is simply not large enough to accept a sufficiently large pin to resist the bending forces of the triceps muscle (Fig. 12–10*D*).

Type B1, Ulnar

Reduction and Fixation

The fracture site and the shaft of the ulna about 2 to 3 cm distal to it are exposed and the fracture is reduced. When the articular surface is involved, anatomical reduction is mandatory for restoration of good joint function. Two Kirschner drill wires are started in the proximal end near the caudal edge of the olecranon process and are driven distally into the shaft of the ulna. In small breeds it is advantageous to place the pins in the sagittal rather than the frontal plane. The pins are directed to engage the cranial cortex of the ulna distal to the trochlear notch in preference to going directly down the marrow cavity

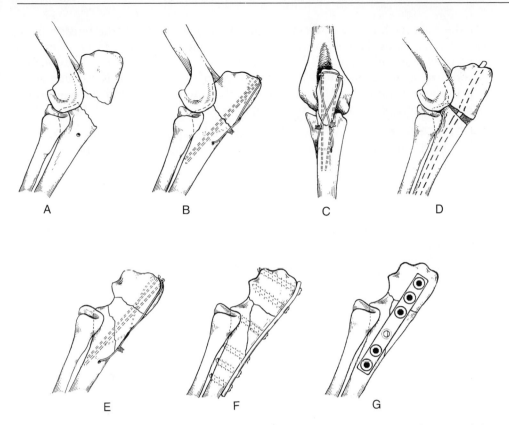

FIGURE 12–10. Fixation of olecranon fractures. (*A*) Type B1 transverse fracture of the olecranon process. (*B, C*) Fixation using two Kirschner wires and a figure-of-8 tension band wire works very well on simple fractures involving the articular surface. (*D*) Fixation with a smooth intramedullary pin alone is inadequate to resist the bending forces; as the proximal segment slides proximally due to pull of the triceps brachii muscle, a gap develops at the fracture site and delayed union or nonunion results. With a fracture in this location, pins or screws used alone as intramedullary fixation are subject to bending or fatigue fracture. (*E*) Type C1 fractures involving the articular surface must be anatomically reduced and may be stabilized using the tension band wire if the articular surface can be completely reconstructed on reduction. (*F*) In multifragmentary type C1 fractures (unstable fractures), the semitubular or dynamic compression plate (DCP) may be used as a tension band if the articular surface is intact after reduction. (*G*) In some multifragmentary fractures, it may be advantageous to place the plate on the lateral surface of the ulna, especially if the articular surface is not well reconstructed.

because this may not adequately prevent rotation (see Figs. 2–63 and 12–10*B, C*). A transverse hole is drilled through the ulna distal to the fracture line. A figure-of-8 wire connects the protruding pins on the proximal end with the hole that was drilled transversely in the distal segment. If the K-wires were inserted in the sagittal plane, the wire engages only the more caudal K-wire. It is important to place the wire through the triceps tendon, directly on the bone rather than over the surface of the tendon. The wire is twisted in both arms of the figure-of-8 to ensure that the entire wire is tight enough to resist the bending muscle forces, but not so tight that the articular side of the fracture is opened. The protruding portions of the pins are bent over caudally in hook fashion, cut off, and rotated 180 degrees cranially into the triceps tendon and driven against the bone with a nail set. This will minimize soft tissue irritation over the pins.

If the fracture line angles distally from the trochlear notch the tension band wire inserted as explained above can be quite long. The wire can be shortened if the proximal end is passed through a second drill hole in the tuber olecrani rather than around the pins. With this type of fixation, the Kirschner wires guard against rotation and shear forces at the fracture line, and the figure-of-8 wire transforms tension force into compression.

AFTERCARE ■   In most cases, no external support is required. Activity should be limited during the healing period. The pins and wire should be removed if there is any indication of irritation or loosening after the fracture is healed.

Type B2, Radial

Because these are articular fractures, simple K-wire fixation as described above for A2 fractures is not optimal. Lag screw or T-plate fixation is indicated. The plate is applied cranially or laterally, depending on the plane of the fracture line.

Type B3, One Bone Articular and One Bone Nonarticular

In the illustrated example the ulnar fracture is the articular fracture. The ulnar fracture is stabilized by the methods described above for type B1 fractures. The radial fracture is best treated by a short cranial plate, with at least four cortices engaged by plate screws in the proximal fragment. If the fractures were reversed, the radial fracture would be treated as in B2 above, and the ulnar fracture as in A1 above.

Fracture Type 21C; Multifragmentary Articular
(Fig. 12–6C)

These fractures are fortunately very rare, as they can present a real challenge to stabilize. Fixation is a combination of methods described above. If the fragments can be anatomically reduced, fixation is straightforward (Fig. 12–10E). If the trochlear notch portion of the fracture can be reconstructed, small plates can function as tension bands in larger breeds (Fig. 12–10F, G). If the ulnar articular portion cannot be reconstructed, the plate will not function as a tension band and will be subject to bending forces. In this situation a laterally applied plate is stronger than a caudal plate.

If plate application is not feasible, a hybrid external fixator can be employed (Fig. 12–11). Using an IM pin for one fixation pin provides some additional axial stability. This can be combined with plate fixation of the radius in type C2 and C3 fractures.

If fixation is less than totally stable, a carpal flexion bandage (see Fig. 2–30) is applied postoperatively for 2 to 3 weeks to prevent weight bearing while allowing passive motion of the elbow joint.

DIAPHYSEAL FRACTURES

A high percentage of the fractures involving the shaft of the radius and ulna occur in the middle and distal thirds with both bones involved.[1-4] However, these fractures occur at all levels and include all types; in a few cases, they may involve only the radius or ulna. The development of angulation, rotation, de-

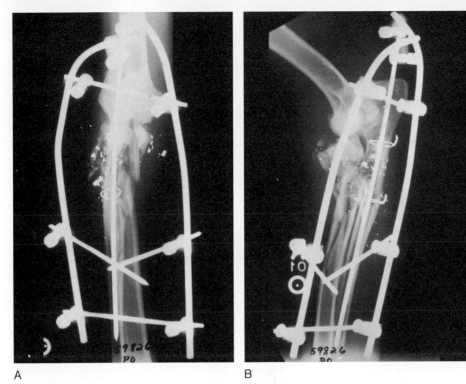

A   B

FIGURE 12–11. An extremely fragmented type A3 gunshot fracture. (A) An intramedullary pin in the ulna was used to restore angular alignment and the proximal end of this pin was tied into a type IIA external fixator by means of contoured connecting bars. (B) Note that the most proximal full fixation pin is placed in the ulna. No attempt was made to reduce the radial head; it was allowed to "float" against the humeral condyle and healed in a functional position.

layed union, and nonunion at the fracture site are not uncommon sequelae when the bones are handled improperly. Two of the more common mistakes are using fixation methods that allow rotation at the fracture site and removing the fixation device before the callus becomes sufficiently mature for weight bearing.

When applicable, treatment recommendations are keyed to the Fracture Patient Scoring System detailed in Table 2–6.[9,10]

OPEN APPROACHES[7] ■   The main indications for open approach are as follows:

1.   When reduction by closed methods is difficult or impossible.
2.   When there is difficulty in maintaining reduction in the process of applying fixation. (Viewing the fracture site during this process is most helpful.)
3.   When internal fixation is applied.

The choice of approach may vary, depending on the location of the fracture and the objective to be accomplished. The approach to the proximal radius is shown in Figure 12–5B. The diaphysis can be approached either laterally or medially, and in most instances, the latter is the preferred approach because the radius is subcutaneous in this area and can be exposed with a minimum of hemorrhage. Figure 12–12A illustrates this technique. The lateral approach might be chosen when there are medial skin wounds or where positioning the

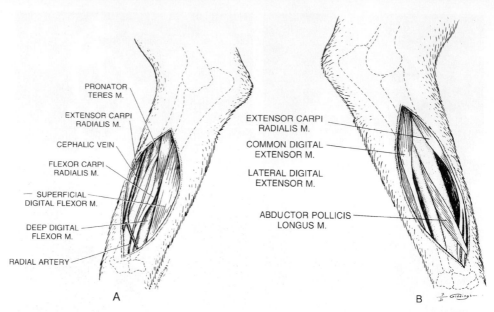

FIGURE 12–12. Approaches to the diaphysis of the radius and ulna. (*A*) The craniomedial approach provides good exposure without much muscle elevation. (*B*) The lateral approach is used when there is soft tissue injury to the medial side of the limb.

animal for access to other limbs makes it more convenient (Fig. 12–12*B*). The ulna is exposed by simple incision over the caudal border proximally (Fig. 12–5*A*), or in the diaphysis laterally.

Fracture Type 22-A; Diaphyseal, Radial Simple or Incomplete (Fig. 12–13*A*)

Type A1, Incomplete or of One Bone Only

Fracture Patient scores of 9 to 10 are typical for these fractures. If only the shaft of the *ulna* is fractured it can be treated by compression bandaging to reduce pain, and rest. Rarely, a short caudal splint (Fig. 2–27) might be applied.

If the *radius* is fractured, more aggressive treatment is indicated. Incomplete (greenstick) fractures respond to caudal splinting. Complete fractures can be handled either with a long leg cylinder cast (see Fig. 2–21) or Thomas splint (see Fig. 2–25). In a young animal, less than 6 months old, caudal splinting will usually suffice.

Type A2, Simple, Distal Zone and Type A3, Simple, Proximal Zone

Slightly more complex than type A1, Fracture Patient scores may range as low as 7, with 8 to 9 more common.

Closed Reduction and Fixation

Fixation by long leg cylinder cast is appropriate for relatively transverse fractures of the distal zone (stable relative to shortening, Fracture Patient score 9 to 10) in medium to large breeds, especially if under 1 year of age.[4] (See the discussion above in Fixation Techniques relative to cast fixation.)

A   B   C

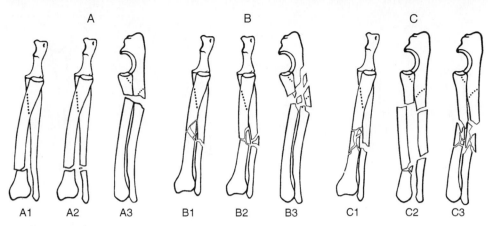

A1   A2   A3   B1   B2   B3   C1   C2   C3

FIGURE 12–13. Diaphyseal fractures of the radius and ulna. (*A1*) Incomplete or of one bone only, (*A2*) simple, distal zone, and (*A3*) simple, proximal zone. (*B1*) Simple, with ulnar fracture, (*B2*) distal zone, multifragmentary ulnar, and (*B3*) proximal zone, multifragmentary ulnar. (*C1*) With ulnar simple or wedge fracture, (*C2*) segmental radial, complex ulnar, and (*C3*) complex ulnar. (From Unger M, Montavon PM, Heim UFA: Classification of fractures of the long bones in the dog and cat: Introduction and clinical application. Vet Comp Orthop Trauma 3:41–50, 1990, with permission.)

Open Reduction and Fixation

Fractures that are not stable relative to shortening (Fracture Patient score 7 to 8), those in dogs older than 1 year, those in small and toy breeds, and proximal zone fractures are best treated by internal fixation. A variety of methods are applicable, the choice being personal preference or availability of equipment.

1. Type I external skeletal fixators are easily applied here (Fig. 12–3), often by closed, or minimal open, reduction as explained above in Fixation Techniques. Auxiliary fixation in the form of interfragmentary K-wires or lag screws can be used in oblique fractures (Figs. 12–3C and 12–14D). Proximal fractures with a very short proximal segment may require a type IB biplanar splint (see Fig. 12–22) with three pins in the proximal fragment.

2. Cranially placed compression or neutralization plates (Fig. 12–14B, E).

3. Intramedullary Rush type pins in large breeds for distal zone fractures (Fig. 12–2).

Fracture Type 22-B; Diaphyseal, Radial Wedge (Fig. 12–13*B*)

None of these fractures are amenable to coaptation fixation due to their instability. Fracture Patient scores will usually be in the 4 to 7 range, and occasionally as low as 3. The choice of fixation is limited to either bone plating or external skeletal fixators. The degree of fragmentation has little effect on the choice of fixation, since the radius is the weight-bearing bone.

Internal Fixation by Bone Plate

If the radial wedge is reducible, a reconstructive approach can be taken, with lag screw and neutralization plate fixation (Fig. 12–15). Cerclage wire fixation can be substituted for the lag screw(s) in some cases. Cranial application of the

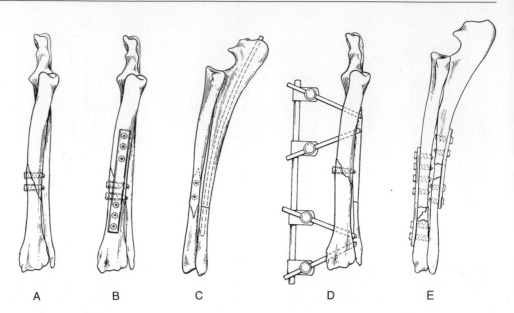

A　　　　B　　　　C　　　　D　　　　E

FIGURE 12–14. Fixation of type A simple fractures of the radius and ulna. (*A*) Long oblique or spiral fractures of the radius and ulna may be stabilized by lag screws to restore alignment and to exert interfragmentary compression at the fracture site. Additional stabilization may consist of a coaptation splint, (*B*) a neutralization plate, (*C*) an intramedullary pin in the ulna, or (*D*) a type I external fixator. (*E*) A proximal zone transverse fracture stabilized with a compression plate. Because the proximal segment is short and only two screws were used, additional stability was obtained by inserting an intramedullary pin in the ulna.

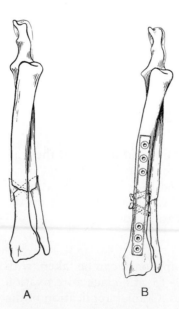

FIGURE 12–15. (*A*) Single radial wedge type B1 mid-shaft fracture. (*B*) Fixation with two lag screws and a neutralization plate on the cranial surface of the radius.

A　　　　B

radial plate is indicated. If the radial wedges are not reducible the plate is applied in compression, with autogenous cancellous bone graft added to the fragments. A long bridging plate on the ulna is useful for proximal zone radial fractures where only two screws (four cortices) are possible in the proximal fragment.

Internal Fixation by External Skeletal Fixator

Type I fixators are sufficient for those with higher Fracture Patient scores, while type II fixators are more certain for lower scores. Closed reduction or limited open reduction (*biological osteosynthesis*) is the best choice for application, as this will result in the least disruption of the vascular supply to the fragments. Proximal fractures with a very short proximal segment may require a type IB biplanar splint (see Fig. 12–22) with three pins in the proximal fragment.

Type 22-C; Diaphyseal, Radial Complex (Fig. 12–13C)

As stated above for wedge fractures, none of these injuries is amenable to coaptation. Fracture Patient scores will be 1 to 3 or 4.

Type C1, C3

Plate fixation in the bridging or buttress mode is applicable to these fractures (Fig. 12–16), and is supplemented with autogenous cancellous bone graft in the fragmented area, and in some cases involving large breeds the ulna is also plated.

Although bone plate fixation is feasible, these fractures heal more certainly and faster when a more biological approach is taken, with closed or limited open reduction and external skeletal fixation. Type IA external fixators (Fig. 12–17A) are sufficient for those patients with the highest Fracture Patient scores for this type fracture. A lower score is an indication for the type II fixator (Fig. 12–17C), or perhaps a type IB biplanar splint (see Fig. 12–22).

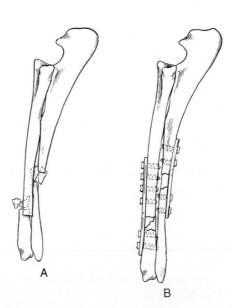

FIGURE 12–16. (*A*) Type B2 distal zone fracture of the radius and midshaft fracture of the ulna in a large St. Bernard dog. (*B*) Fixation using two bridging plates.

A

B

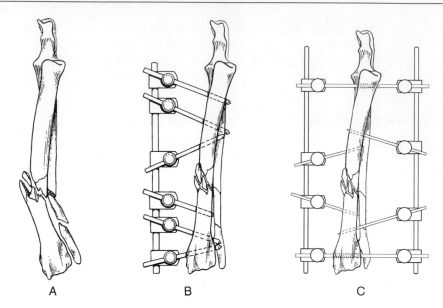

FIGURE 12–17. (*A*) Type C3 midshaft fracture of radius and ulna. (*B*) Fixation with a type IA external fixator, after closed reduction. (*C*) Somewhat more stability can be provided in large active breeds by this type IIB external fixator. Because of the cranial bow of the radius it is much easier to place half pins rather than full pins in the mid-portion of the splint.

Type C2

Segmental fractures are also treatable by either plates or external fixators. With dynamic compression plates both fracture lines can be compressed, as shown in Figure 2–71. The disadvantage with plate fixation can be the need for a very long plate if the middle bone fragment is long. External fixators of type IB or II are both applicable to this type fracture. A minimum of two fixation pins are required in each fragment.

DISTAL FRACTURES

Radial fractures of this region can be exposed by a cranial midline incision between the extensor tendons.[7] Ulnar fractures are virtually subcutaneous and are exposed by simple skin incision.

Fracture Type 23-A; Distal, Extra-articular (Fig. 12–18*A*)

Type A1 Ulnar

These fractures may occur in association with luxation or subluxation of the antebrachiocarpal joint (Fig. 12–19) or in isolation (Fig. 12–20). Because the ulnar collateral ligaments originate on the styloid process, it is essential to fix these fractures to help stabilize the joint, especially in large, active animals. Supplemental external fixation in the form of a short caudal splint (see Fig. 2–27) is necessary.

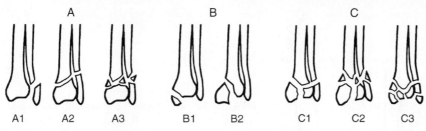

FIGURE 12–18. Distal fractures of the radius and ulna. (*A1*) Ulna, (*A2*) simple radial, and (*A3*) multifragmentary radial. (*B1*) Sagittal radial and (*B2*) frontal radial. (*C1*) Simple, metaphyseal simple, (*C2*) simple, metaphyseal multifragmentary, and (*C3*) multifragmentary. (From Unger M, Montavon PM, Heim UFA: Classification of fractures of the long bones in the dog and cat: Introduction and clinical application. Vet Comp Orthop Trauma 3:41–50, 1990, with permission.)

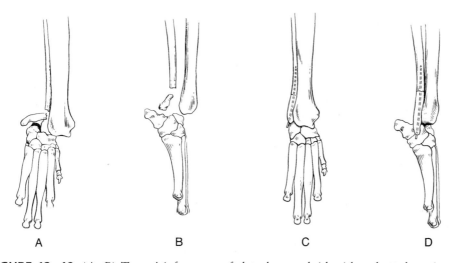

FIGURE 12–19. (*A, B*) Type A1 fracture of the ulnar styloid with palmar luxation of the antebrachiocarpal joint. (*C, D*) Intramedullary fixation of the styloid. If any ligaments and/or the joint capsule are ruptured, they are repaired and a coaptation splint is added.

FIGURE 12–20. (*A*) Type A1 fracture of the ulnar styloid. (*B, C*) Fixation with a Kirschner wire and tension band wire to secure the short distal fragment and collateral ligament. Add a coaptation splint for stability, if indicated.

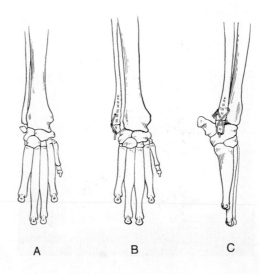

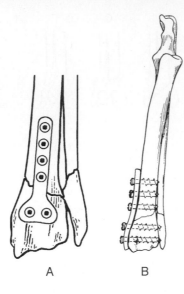

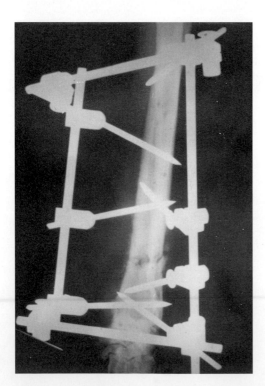

FIGURE 12–21. Type A2 simple distal radial fracture fixation. (*A*) A T plate on the dorsal surface allows two screws to be placed in the short distal segment. (*B*) Medial placement of the plate increases the area moment of inertia of the plate and the stiffness of fixation.

Type A2, Simple Radial and Type A3, Multifragmentary Radial

These injuries are common in small and toy breeds, usually the result of a jump or fall. Coaptation and intramedullary pinning are common causes of nonunion in these breeds.[4,5]

Closed Reduction and Fixation

Fixation by long leg cylinder cast is appropriate for relatively transverse fractures (stable relative to shortening, Fracture Patient score 9 to 10) *in medium*

FIGURE 12–22. Placing three fixation pins in a type A2 simple distal radial fracture with a short distal fragment is possible by means of the type IB two-plane external fixator.

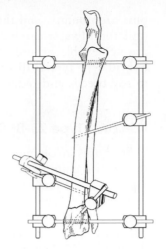

FIGURE 12–23. Fixation of this type A2 simple distal radial fracture with a very short distal fragment can be accomplished with a hybrid type I-II external fixator. In toy and miniature breeds the connecting bars and clamps are easily replaced by molded acrylic bars.

to large breeds, especially if under 1 year of age.[4] (See the discussion above in Fixation Techniques relative to cast fixation.)

Open Reduction and Fixation

BONE PLATES ■ The length of the distal fragment is the challenge for these fractures. A minimum of two screws (four cortices) are required in the bone, and three screws are ideal. For toy and miniature breeds, 1.5 to 2.0 mm screws and the mini T-plate or the cuttable plate are the best implants. The T-plate must be applied cranially (Fig. 12–21A), but the cuttable plate can be used medially (Fig. 12–21B), as discussed above in the section Fixation Techniques.

In medium-size breeds, a 2.7-mm T-plate is suitable, as is a standard 2.7-mm plate applied medially. In large breeds, a medial plate in 2.7- or 3.5-mm size is indicated.

EXTERNAL FIXATORS ■ Just as for plate fixation, the length of the distal fragment becomes the major consideration, and just as with plates, two fixation

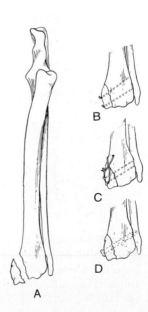

FIGURE 12–24. (A) Type B1 distal partial articular fracture of the styloid process of the radius. Progressively more stable fixation can be achieved by (B) two Kirschner wires, (C) addition of a tension band wire, or (D) a lag screw.

pins are minimal and three are ideal. If the fragment is long enough, a type IA unilateral fixator can be sufficient (Fig. 12–3). Three pins in the distal fragment are achievable by use of the type 1B biplanar splint (Fig. 12–22), or with a hybrid type type II/III splint (Fig. 12–23). Acrylic fixation rods work very well in toy breeds and reduce costs of the splint as well.

Fracture Type 23-B; Distal, Partial Articular (Fig. 12–18*B*)

Fractures involving the styloid process of the radius give rise to instability of the antebrachiocarpal joint. Open reduction and internal fixation are indicated. Figure 12–24 presents examples of some of the various methods of fixation of a *type B1* fracture. In this oblique fracture of the radial styloid process, fixation may be done with two Kirschner wires, a tension band wire, or a lag screw. The latter two methods provide better security than the simple K-wire fixation. Figure 12–25 depicts a *type B2* fracture combined with an A1 ulnar fracture. Since this fracture line is more directly in the weight-bearing surface of the radius, lag screw fixation is mandatory. In most cases, additional external support in the form of a short caudal splint (see Fig. 2–27) is indicated during the healing period (4 to 6 weeks).

Fracture Type 23-C; Distal, Complete Articular (Fig. 12–18*C*)

These injuries are rarely encountered,[2] which is fortunate, since they offer considerable challenge for adequate fixation, especially in toy or miniature breeds. *Type C1* and C2 fractures could be fixed by use of a medially placed plate (Fig. 12–21*B*) with one or more of the distal screws placed in lag fashion to stabilize the articular fracture. It is highly unlikely that *type C3* fractures could be adequately reduced and fixed to provide a functional articular sur-

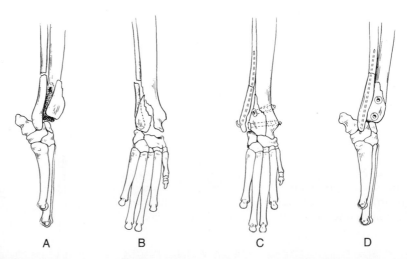

| A | B | C | D |

FIGURE 12–25. (*A, B*) Combined type B1 and B2 partial articular fracture of the distal radius and distal ulna. (*C, D*) Lag screw fixation of the distal radius with 4.0-mm cancellous screws and Kirschner wire intramedullary fixation of the ulna. A coaptation splint is usually indicated for additional stability for the first 4 to 6 weeks postoperatively.

face. Pancarpal arthrodesis is the most rational treatment of these injuries (see Chapter 13).

References

1. Brinker WO: Fractures. In Canine Surgery, 2nd Archibald ed. Santa Barbara, American Veterinary Publications, Inc, 1974, pp 949–1048.
2. Unger M, Montavon PM, Heim UFA: Classification of fractures of the long bones in the dog and cat: Introduction and clinical application. Vet Comp Orthop Trauma 3:41–50, 1990.
3. Harrison JW: Fractures of the radius and ulna. In Brinker WO, Hohn RB, Prieur WD (eds): Manual of Internal Fixation in Small Animals. New York, Springer-Verlag, 1984, pp 144–151.
4. Lappin MR, Aron DN, et al: Fractures of the radius and ulna in the dog. J Am Anim Hosp Assoc 19:643–650, 1983.
5. DeAngelis M, Olds RB, et al: Repair of fractures of the radius and ulna in small dogs. J Am Anim Hosp Assoc 9:436–441, 1973.
6. Wallace MK, Boudrieau RJ, et al: Mechanical evaluation of three methods of plating distal radial osteotomies. Vet Surg 21:99–106, 1992.
7. Piermattei DL: An Atlas of Surgical Approaches to the Bones and Joints of the Dog and Cat, 3rd ed. Philadelphia, WB Saunders Co, 1993.
8. Schwarz PD, Schrader SC: Ulnar fracture and dislocation of the proximal radial epiphysis (Monteggia lesion) in the dog and cat: A review of 28 cases. J Am Vet Med Assoc 185:190–194, 1984.
9. Palmer RH, Hulse DA, Aron DN: A proposed fracture patient score system used to develop fracture treatment plans (abstr). Proc 20th Ann Conf Vet Orthop Soc, 1993.
10. Palmer RH: Decision making in fracture treatment: The fracture patient scoring system. Proc (Sm Anim) ACVS Vet Symposium, 1994, pp 388–390

13

Fractures and Other Orthopedic Conditions of the Carpus, Metacarpus, and Phalanges

Injuries of the forepaw may consist of fractures, ligamentous injuries, and various combinations. The paw constitutes a complex and highly critical structure, and the larger and more athletic the animal, the more devastating are injuries in this area. The horseman's cliché of "no feet, no horse" can also be applied to the dog. There is a tendency to treat ligamentous injuries in this area very conservatively, with cast immobilization, and to hope for sufficient fibroplasia to stabilize the joint. Although this may be moderately successful in small and inactive breeds, it rarely restores full function in large breeds. Randomly oriented collagen in scar tissue cannot withstand tensile stress and soon breaks down, leaving the joint permanently unstable. Such instability soon leads to degenerative joint disease, as described in Chapter 7.

ANATOMY OF THE FOREPAW ■ The bony anatomy of the forepaw is depicted in Figure 13–1, and the ligamentous structures are shown in Figure 13–2. Distal to the radius, the terms *cranial* and *caudal* are replaced by *dorsal* and *palmar*. The six bones of the carpus are arranged in a proximal and distal row, with three joint levels: the antebrachiocarpal, the middle carpal, and the carpometacarpal. The middle carpal is often referred to as the intercarpal joint, but this term properly describes the joints between carpal bones of a given level. Ligaments of the carpus are generally short, none spanning all three joints, and most crossing only one joint level, connecting individual carpal bones. On the palmar side of the carpus, the joint capsule is well developed and blends with the palmar carpal fibrocartilage and ligaments. Note the dorsal sesamoids of the metacarpophalangeal and proximal interphalangeal joints; the former are often mistaken for fractures of the metacarpal bones.

SURGICAL APPROACHES AND TECHNIQUE ■ The carpal joints are most commonly opened on the dorsal aspect of the midline, elevating and retracting the carpal extensor tendons medially and the digital extensor tendons laterally (Fig. 13–3A).[1] The synovial capsule must be incised at each individual joint space because the synovium is adherent to each carpal bone. The palmar ligaments and carpal fibrocartilage can be exposed by an incision slightly medial

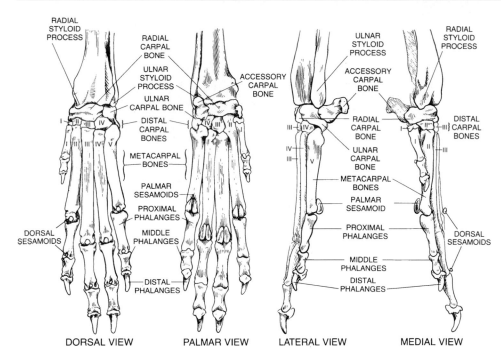

RADIAL STYLOID PROCESS
RADIAL CARPAL BONE
ULNAR STYLOID PROCESS
ULNAR CARPAL BONE
ACCESSORY CARPAL BONE
DISTAL CARPAL BONES
METACARPAL BONES
PALMAR SESAMOIDS
PROXIMAL PHALANGES
MIDDLE PHALANGES
DORSAL SESAMOIDS
DISTAL PHALANGES

ULNAR STYLOID PROCESS
ACCESSORY CARPAL BONE
RADIAL CARPAL BONE
ULNAR CARPAL BONE
METACARPAL BONES
PALMAR SESAMOID
PROXIMAL PHALANGES
MIDDLE PHALANGES
DISTAL PHALANGES

RADIAL STYLOID PROCESS
DISTAL CARPAL BONES
DORSAL SESAMOIDS

DORSAL VIEW   PALMAR VIEW   LATERAL VIEW   MEDIAL VIEW

FIGURE 13–1. Bones of the carpus, metacarpus, and phalanges.

to the midline. The flexor retinaculum is incised medial to the deep digital flexor tendon, which is then retracted laterally. From the dorsal aspect, metacarpal bones lie subcutaneously, covered only by digital extensor tendons and blood vessels (Fig. 13–3B).[1] Individual bones are exposed by incision of skin directly over the bone, with retraction of underlying vessels and tendons. Multiple bones are approached by parallel or a variety of S-, U-, or H-shaped skin incisions.

Surgery of the lower limbs can be done with a tourniquet, which is invaluable for decreasing oozing hemorrhage and so increasing visibility and decreasing operating time. Although pneumatic cuffs are the best way of creating the tourniquet more proximally in the limbs, distal tourniquets can be made more simply. Vetrap™ (3M Animal Care Products, St. Paul, MN) elastic bandage material has proven very satisfactory for this purpose, as illustrated in Figure 13–4. Although the bandage is best sterilized in ethylene oxide, it can be steam sterilized at minimal time and temperature, similar to the method of sterilizing rubber gloves (250°F for 12 minutes). Use of the tourniquet is limited to about 60 minutes, and has the disadvantage of producing more postoperative swelling. Application of casts or splints should be delayed 48 to 72 hours, with the lower limb supported in a Robert-Jones bandage (Fig. 2–33) during this time.

CLINICAL SIGNS AND DIAGNOSIS OF INJURY ■
Most carpal luxations and fractures occur as a result of a fall or jump, but automobile trauma is also common. Affected limbs are non–weight-bearing, have variable swelling and joint effusion in the carpal region, and may show gross instability of the carpus when ligaments are injured. The limb is commonly carried in abduction and flexed at the elbow and carpus.

Although clinical signs and palpation will usually be sufficient to localize the area of probable injury, radiographs are necessary to verify the diagnosis and to localize the damage. Stress radiographs will show the area of instability.

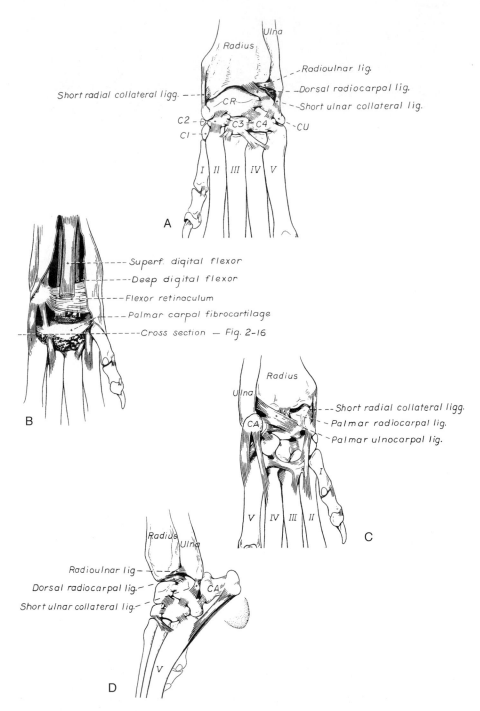

FIGURE 13–2. Ligaments of the carpus. (*A*) Ligaments of the left carpus, dorsal aspect. CR = radial carpal; CU = ulnar carpal; C1 to C4 = first, second, third, fourth carpals; I to V = metacarpals. (*B*) Superficial ligaments of the left carpus, palmar aspect. (*C*) Deep ligaments in the left carpus, palmar aspect. CA = accessory carpals; I to V = metacarpals. (*D*) Ligaments of the left carpus, lateral aspect. CA = accessory carpal; V = metacarpal V. (From Evans HE: Miller's Anatomy of the Dog, 3rd ed. Philadelphia, WB Saunders Co, 1993, with permission.)

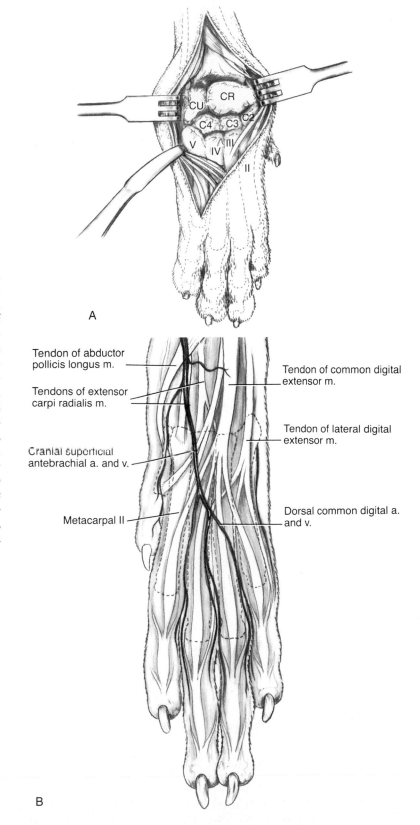

FIGURE 13–3. (*A*) Approach to the distal radius and carpus through a dorsal incision. (*B*) The most important of the vessels and tendons overlying the metacarpal bones are illustrated. Incisions to individual bones are made directly over the bones and these structures are retracted as needed. Multiple bones are approached by parallel, C- or H-shaped incisions. (From Piermattei DL: An Atlas of Surgical Approaches to the Bones and Joints of the Dog and Cat, 3rd ed. Philadelphia, WB Saunders Co, 1993, p. 205, 215, with permission.)

CR

CU

C4   C3   C2

V   IV   III

II

A

Tendon of abductor
pollicis longus m.

Tendons of extensor
carpi radialis m.

Cranial superficial
antebrachial a. and v.

Metacarpal II

Tendon of common digital
extensor m.

Tendon of lateral digital
extensor m.

Dorsal common digital a.
and v.

B

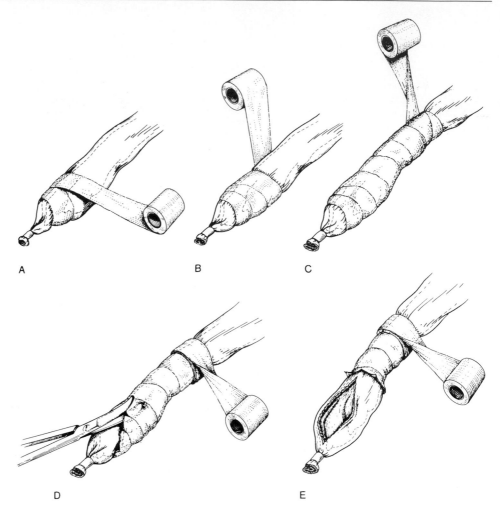

FIGURE 13–4. Application of a Vetrap (3M Animal Care Products, St. Paul, MN) tourniquet. (*A*) After the foot has been draped in sterile stockinet bandage, a roll of 2-inch sterile Vetrap is secured around the toes. (*B*) The Vetrap is wrapped very tightly as it is being wound proximally. (*C*) When well proximal to the surgical field, the elastic bandage is wrapped several times in one area while the bandage is twisted 180 degrees. This forms the tourniquet. (*D*, *E*) The stockinet and Vetrap are cut to expose the surgical field, in this case the phalanges.

Standard cranial and lateral or medial views, plus obliques, will identify ligamentous avulsions and fractures. Nonscreen film or fine-detail screens are essential.

THE CARPUS

Luxation of the Antebrachiocarpal Joint

Total luxation of the antebrachiocarpal joint is, fortunately, a rare injury (Fig. 13–5). Such total disruption of the ligamentous structure is disastrous. Panarthrodesis (see Figs. 13–22 and 13–23) is usually the only means of restoring

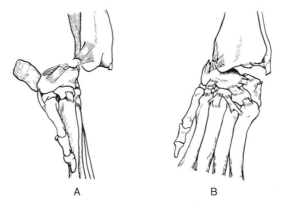

FIGURE 13–5. Luxation of the antebrachiocarpal joint. All the ligaments of the carpus are disrupted.

A   B

function. Fusion of the antebrachiocarpal joint only has not been successful in our hands.

Subluxation of the Antebrachiocarpal Joint

The most commonly injured ligaments at this joint level are the radial collaterals, resulting in medial instability and valgus (lateral) deformity of the foot (Fig. 13–6). Because the dog normally stands with the foot in valgus by a few degrees, the medial ligaments are always under tension. Injuries to the lateral ligaments are both less common and less serious because they are not subject to as much tension stress.

Surgical Technique

The long radial collateral ligament is important primarily when the joint is in extension. The short ligament limits and stabilizes mainly in flexion. Because

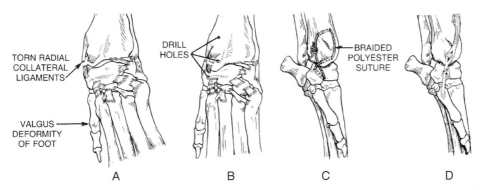

TORN RADIAL
COLLATERAL
LIGAMENTS

DRILL
HOLES

BRAIDED
POLYESTER
SUTURE

VALGUS
DEFORMITY
OF FOOT

A   B   C   D

FIGURE 13–6. Subluxation of the antebrachiocarpal joint resulting from tearing of the radial collateral ligaments. (*A*) Valgus deformity of the foot develops from medial instability. (*B, C*) Synthetic braided suture is threaded through bone tunnels placed in the radial carpal bone and radius to simulate both the long and short ligaments. An attempt is made to suture the ligaments, which have been omitted in these views for greater clarity. (*D*) The abductor pollicis longus muscle has been elevated and moved into a position overlying the torn ligaments. It is secured proximally to the radius with a bone screw and spiked washer (Synthes Ltd. [USA], Paoli, PA) through the split tendon, and sutured distally at the radial carpal bone to remnants of the ligament.

the carpus slides in a dorsopalmar direction during flexion and extension, the function of these ligaments is complex. An attempt is always made to suture the ligaments, but this is particularly difficult in the short ligament. The area is exposed by a medial incision directly over the area. The ligaments are found immediately deep to the antebrachial fascia and the tendon of the abductor pollicis longus. Bolstering a suture repair of the ligaments with synthetic material is usually advisable. Bone tunnels are drilled in the medial prominence of the radial carpal bone and in the radius (Fig. 13–6B, C). Braided polyester suture, size 0-2, is passed through these holes in a manner that simulates both the long and short ligaments. Although stainless steel wire is commonly advised for such application, its use is not recommended for situations in which it is subject to alternate stretching and relaxation. Monofilament wire will quickly fatigue and break under such conditions and should only be used when it is under a continuous tension stress. The suture is tightened until the joint is stable but still mobile, then tied. The knot can be oversewn with fine wire or lightly seared with electrocoagulation to prevent untying.

Earley was the first to report the use of autogenous tissue, such as the abductor pollicis longus or flexor carpi radialis muscle tendons, in replacing the radial collateral ligaments.[2] The tendons were placed through bone tunnels in a fashion similar to that used for the synthetic material. Additionally, the tendon of the abductor pollicis longus muscle can be directly attached to the sutured ligament, or the ligament replaced by securing the tendon to the bone and ligament. In Figure 13–6D the tendon has been secured to the radius by a small bone screw and plastic spiked washer (Synthes Ltd. [USA], Paoli, PA). Distally the tendon is sutured to remnants of the collateral ligament at its insertion on the radial carpal bone. The attachment procedure could be reversed, as the situation demands.

AFTERCARE ■ The carpus is immobilized in 10 to 15 degrees of flexion in a caudal splint (see Fig. 2–27) for 4 to 6 weeks. Strict confinement is continued through the eighth week, with a firm padded bandage in place after splint removal. A slowly progressive increase in exercise is then allowed, starting with leash walking, then short periods of free exercise. This program is slowly increased in intensity for another 4 to 6 weeks, at which point most patients are able to return to near normal activity.

Luxation of the Radial Carpal Bone

A relatively rare condition, luxation of the major bone of the carpus is possible following a jump or fall. The radial carpal bone pivots 90 degrees medially and dorsopalmar, coming to rest against the distopalmar rim of the radius (Fig. 13–7A, B). Severe lameness is always present with abduction of the limb and elbow flexion. Swelling is not remarkable, and the joint is not easily movable. Pain and crepitus are usually elicited by palpation, which easily reveals the displaced bone and a depression in its normal area.

Treatment

CLOSED REDUCTION ■ Surprisingly, the bone can often be reduced closed if seen soon after injury. Functional stability is unlikely to result in large breeds, however, because of damage to the radial collateral ligaments. Although splint fixation for a few weeks may well be justified in a toy or small breed, many patients will require surgical stabilization.

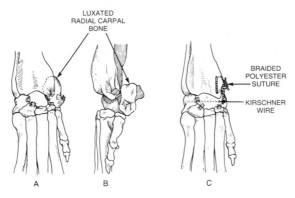

FIGURE 13–7. Luxation of the radial carpal bone. (*A*, *B*) Dorsal and medial views illustrating the palmaromedial luxation of the radial carpal bone. The bone is rotated 90 degrees medially and dorsopalmar. (*C*) The bone is reduced, and a Kirschner wire is driven through the bone into the ulnar carpal. Synthetic radial collateral ligaments stabilize the medial side of the joint.

OPEN REDUCTION AND FIXATION ■ The joint is exposed by a dorsal midline approach as described above. The following is a modification of the repair described by Punzet.[3] The lateromedial rotation is corrected first, and the bone is rotated in a palmodorsal direction to reduce it. A small pin or K-wire is placed from the medial nonarticulating surface of the bone into the ulnar carpal bone. The pin is cut short and countersunk into the articular cartilage. A synthetic radial collateral ligament is constructed as detailed previously (see Fig. 13–6). The remaining ligament is sutured if possible.

Aftercare ■ The carpus is immobilized in 10 to 15 degrees of flexion in a caudal splint (see Fig. 2–27) for 4 to 6 weeks. Strict confinement is continued through the eighth week, with a firm padded bandage in place after splint removal. A slowly progressive increase in exercise is then allowed, starting with leash walking, then short periods of free exercise. This program is slowly increased in intensity for another 4 to 6 weeks, at which point most patients are able to return to near normal activity.

Fracture of the Radial Carpal Bone

Fractures of this bone, which, with the radius, forms the antebrachiocarpal joint—the major joint of the carpus—are usually manifested as chips or slabs off the articular surfaces (Figs. 13–8 through 13–10). They are most often seen after injuries resulting from jumps or falls and in dogs undergoing heavy exertion such as sled dogs, field trial dogs, and other working breeds. Fragments are apparently created by a compressive force combined with shear. There is little tendency for these fragments to heal spontaneously, and the bony or cartilaginous fragments usually become joint mice, creating an acute inflammatory reaction in the joint, and leading to synovitis and degenerative joint disease. Lameness is severe but subsides somewhat in a few weeks. The dog may be sound when rested but becomes lame when exercised. Soft tissue thickening around the joint may become obvious after a few more weeks as a result of synovitis and arthritis.

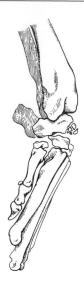

FIGURE 13–8. Comminuted dorsal slab fracture of the radial carpal bone. The fragments are excised in this type of injury.

Diagnosis requires a high index of suspicion because radiographs (nonscreen film or high-detail screens) must be made in oblique planes and in flexion and extension to verify the fracture. Sometimes, only a unilateral arthrosis is seen, but if the history supports a traumatic cause, this is sufficient justification for exploration of the joint.

Treatment

CLOSED REDUCTION ■ Undisplaced fragments may reattach if the joint is splinted for 4 weeks. The prognosis is uncertain, however, and many patients require surgery later.

OPEN REDUCTION AND FIXATION ■ Surgery may be performed with a tourniquet and most fractures can be exposed from a dorsal approach. Considerable synovial proliferation and inflammation may complicate the exposure. When the fragment is located, a decision is made to reattach or remove the fragment. To be reattached, the fragment must be large enough to handle; moreover, the fracture surfaces should not be severely eburnated, as may happen in a chronic fracture. If small screws are used, their heads must not interfere with any other structures (Figs. 13–9C, D and 13–10B, C). Miniscrews in 1.5 and 2.0 mm diameter are the most useful sizes. Kirschner wires countersunk below the level of the cartilage or bone are also used. (Fig. 13–9E, F). Fragments are often excised because they cannot be reattached due to chronicity and resulting eburnation (Fig. 13–11). In this situation, the desired result is an adequate fibrocartilage scar to fill in the defect.

Prognosis ■ The outlook for satisfactory function is usually good unless the bone is comminuted; this situation usually calls for arthrodesis (see Fig. 13–22).

Aftercare ■ A short molded palmar splint or short cast (see Figs. 2–27 and 2–22) is applied for 3 to 4 weeks following fixation of the fragments. Exercise is limited for 6 to 8 weeks, until there is radiographic evidence of healing. If the fragments are excised, the joint is rested in a similar splint for 10 days, after which light exercise is advisable through the fourth postoperative week.

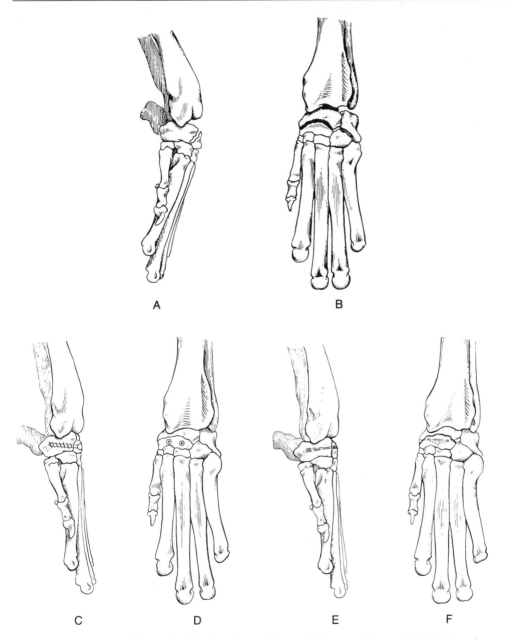

A   B

C   D   E   F

FIGURE 13–9. (*A, B*) Dorsal slab fracture of the radial carpal bone. (*C, D*) Two lag screws of 1.5- or 2-mm diameter are countersunk beneath the articular surface when the fragment is large enough. (*E, F*) Smaller fragments may be secured by two or more Kirschner wires countersunk beneath the surface of the articular cartilage or bone.

Fracture of the Accessory Carpal Bone

Fractures of the accessory carpal bone are seen most commonly in the racing greyhound but may be seen occasionally in most of the large breeds. Most fractures are self-induced avulsions (grade III sprains or strains; see Chapter 7), rather than caused by outside trauma. Johnson and co-workers have described these fractures and proposed the following classification system.[4,5]

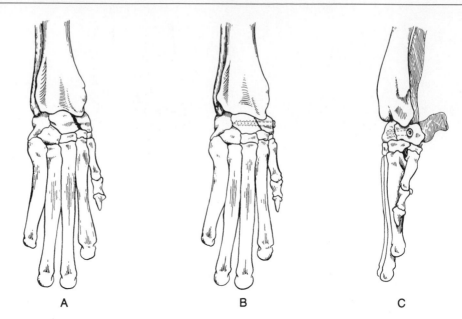

A   B   C

FIGURE 13–10. (*A*) Oblique fracture through the body of the radial carpal bone. (*B*, *C*) Lag screw fixation with a 2.7-, 3.5-, or 4.0-mm lag screw inserted from the medial surface of the bone. The screw is placed through the insertions of the radial collateral ligaments (see Fig. 13–2). In this position, the screw head will not interfere with joint motion.

Classification

Intra-articular Fractures

TYPE I, DISTAL BASILAR ■ Avulsion fracture of the distal margin of the articular surface at the origin of the accessoroulnar carpal ligaments (Fig. 13–12*A*).

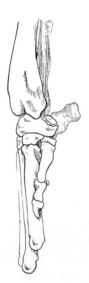

FIGURE 13–11. Fracture of the palmaromedial portion of the radial carpal bone (mediolateral view). Such fragments are simply excised because they are not on the main weight-bearing area of the bone.

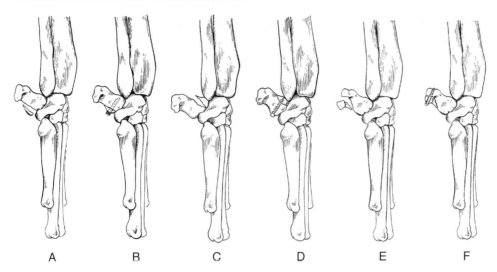

FIGURE 13–12. Fractures of the accessory carpal bone. (*A, B*) Type I distal-basilar fracture and fixation of the fracture with a 2-mm screw. (*C, D*) Type II proximal-basilar fracture and fixation with a 2-mm screw. (*E, F*) Type III distal-apical fracture and fixation with a 2-mm screw.

TYPE II, PROXIMAL BASILAR ■ Avulsion fracture of the proximal margin at the insertion of the ligaments to the radius, ulna, and radial carpal bone (Fig. 13–12C).

Extra-articular Fractures

TYPE III, DISTAL APICAL ■ Avulsion fracture of the distal margin of the palmar end of the bone at the origin of the two palmar accessorometacarpal ligaments (Fig. 13–12E).

TYPE IV, PROXIMAL APICAL ■ Avulsion fracture of the tendon of insertion of the flexor carpi ulnaris muscle at the proximal surface of the palmar end of the bone (see Fig. 13–14A).

Combined Intra-articular and Extra-articular Fractures

TYPE V, COMMINUTED FRACTURE OF THE BODY ■ May extend into the articular surface (see Fig. 13–15).

Type I fractures comprise 67 percent of the injuries in the racing greyhound and occur almost exclusively in the right limb, whereas type III injuries are the least common and occur mainly in the left limb.[5] Type II injuries rarely occur alone; they are usually seen concurrently with type I fractures. In other breeds, type IV and V fractures predominate.

Clinical Signs

In track injuries, the dog usually comes off the track mildly lame, but clinical signs may not be noted until the day following the injury when slight lameness and swelling are observed in the region of the accessory carpal bone. Clinical signs include swelling of the carpus, pain on digital pressure lateral to the accessory carpal bone, and pain on carpal flexion. Rest will lead to diminution of these signs, but a chronic low-grade lameness persists when exercise is resumed. There is very little tendency for complete healing to occur with conservative treatment such as external splinting or casting of the limb.

Treatment

Although simple excision of the fragment in type I injuries has been advocated, less than 50 percent of our animals so treated have ever returned to the track. With this technique, successful healing seems to depend on scar tissue reattachment of the distal ligaments to the bone. Failure to achieve this results in instability of the accessory carpal bone, leading to inflammation and degenerative joint disease. Because scar tissue does not have nearly the tensile strength of ligamentous tissue, it does not adequately replace the ligament in areas of high tensile stress. Screw fixation of type I, II, and III injuries has resulted in 91 percent of these dogs returning to training or racing, and 45 percent of those won one or more races.[6] Although these case numbers are small, nevertheless these results are encouraging and dramatically different from excisional treatment, and this approach is our preferred treatment (Figs. 13–12 and 13–13).

OPEN REDUCTION AND INTERNAL FIXATION, TYPE I ■ A palmarolateral approach is made.[1] The fragment is reduced and clamped with small, pointed reduction forceps, or Lewin forceps (Fig. 13–13A). Fixation is accomplished by a 2.0-mm screw (Fig. 13–13B) that is not placed as a lag screw due to the

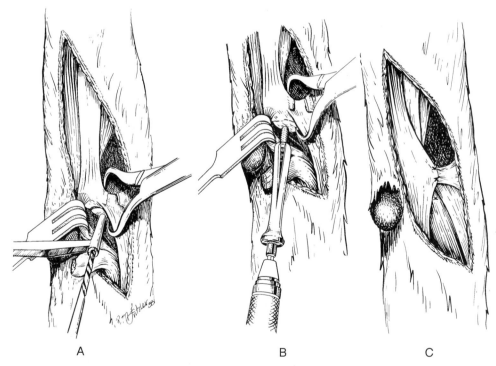

A   B   C

FIGURE 13–13. (A) Screw fixation of accessory carpal bone fracture. The accessoro-metacarpal IV ligament is retracted medially. The fragment is reduced and clamped with small, pointed, reduction forceps or Lewin forceps. A 1.5-mm drill is used to place a drill hole in the center of the fragment. If the drill is held parallel to the metacarpus, the angle will be correct to prevent entering the joint space. (B) The hole is measured and tapped, and a 2-mm screw driven with the clamp in place. This is not a lag screw; the clamp supplies compression. (C) The tendinous slip from the ulnaris lateralis tendon is sutured, followed by the antebrachial fascia, and then the skin.

difficulty of determining the depth of the glide hole required for lag effect and because drilling with a 2-mm bit to produce a glide hole probably poses an unnecessary risk of splitting the fragment. The bone clamp is used to supply compression. Closure of the approach includes suturing of the abductor digiti quinti muscle and the tendinous slip from the ulnaris lateralis tendon to the accessory carpal bone (Fig. 13–13C).

TREATMENT OF OTHER TYPES ■ Fractures seen most commonly in non-racing animals include the type IV proximal apical avulsion fracture of the free end of the bone (Fig. 13–14A) and type V body fracture with varying degrees of comminution of the bone (Fig. 13–15). The type IV avulsion is in the insertion of the flexor carpi ulnaris muscle and causes mild but persistent irritation until the fragment is removed (Fig. 13–14B–D).

Internal fixation of type V comminuted fractures by miniscrew fixation is feasible, but most limbs treated for this injury are cast in 20 degrees of flexion with surprisingly good healing and function if the fracture is entirely extra-articular. If there is an intra-articular component, an attempt should be made to do an internal fixation of that part of the fracture.

Aftercare ■ *Following screw fixation,* a molded palmar splint or short cast (see Figs. 2–27 and 2–22) is applied with the carpus flexed 20 degrees. The splint is maintained for 4 weeks. Complete confinement is enforced through the eighth postoperative week, followed by 4 weeks of gradually increasing activity. Regular training or activity is started by the 12th week. *Following excision of fragments,* the splint is maintained for 2 weeks, followed by an elastic bandage for 2 weeks. Exercise is restricted for 4 more weeks. Splinting of a comminuted

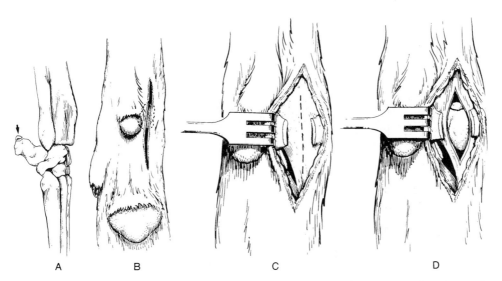

A   B   C   D

FIGURE 13–14. (A) Avulsion of part of the insertion of the flexor carpi ulnaris muscle on the free end of the right accessory carpal bone (type IV fracture). (B) Skin and antebrachial fascia incisions for removal of the fragment are slightly lateral to the bone. (C) The tendinous slip from the ulnaris lateralis muscle is incised over the free end of the bone and a midsagittal incision is made in the tendon of the flexor carpi ulnaris. (D) Careful dissection through the tendon will reveal the fracture fragment, which is then dissected free; care must be taken to avoid unnecessary trauma to the tendon. The tendon incision is closed with interrupted sutures, followed by the tendinous slip over the free end of the bone, the antebrachial fascia, and the skin.

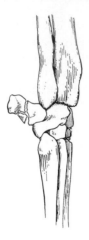

FIGURE 13–15. Comminuted nonarticular type V fracture of the accessory carpal bone. This fracture was splinted in 20 degrees of flexion and healed well.

fracture is maintained until radiographic signs of healing are obvious, usually in about 6 weeks. Full exercise should not be started until 3 or 4 weeks after splint removal.

Subluxation of the Accessory Carpal Bone

This injury is discussed in the section Hyperextension, below.

Fracture of the Ulnar and Numbered Carpal Bones

We have not observed fractures of the ulnar carpal bone. Fracture of the distal row of numbered bones is rare and usually is manifested as a small chip or slab on the dorsal surface (Fig. 13–16). Clinical signs of intermittent mild lameness and joint effusion are noted. Because these bones are smaller, radiographic diagnosis and reattachment of fragments are more difficult. Multiple oblique views are often necessary for visualization. Because these bones are all directly in contact with the synovium, adhesions form early between the fragments, or the damaged articular surface, and the synovial membrane. Most of

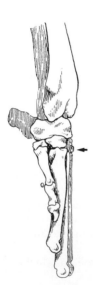

FIGURE 13–16. A small fracture on the dorsal surface of the third carpal bone. This fragment was excised.

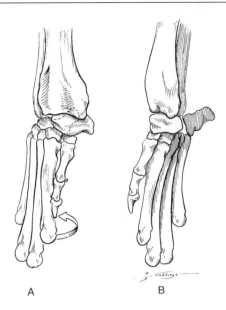

FIGURE 13-17. Middle carpal joint luxation, right limb. (*A*) This is actually a combined middle and antebrachiocarpal luxation because the ulnar carpal bone has remained with the distal carpals. The foot has supinated 60 degrees. Dorsal view. (*B*) Medial view showing supination of the foot.

A   B

these fractures are treated by excision of fragments and curettage of the damaged articular surface to ensure fibrocartilaginous scar formation. Small nondisplaced fragments may reattach and heal following 3 to 4 weeks of splinting of the carpus.

Middle Carpal Luxation

Complete disruption of the middle carpal joint is unusual but does occur, as illustrated in Figure 13–17. This was a combined antebrachiocarpal and middle carpal luxation because the ulnar carpal remained attached to the distal carpal bones in this 10-pound mixed terrier. In this case, the foot has twisted laterally (supination) about 60 degrees. A closed reduction was performed, and the lower limb was splinted for 6 weeks. Spontaneous ankylosis of the middle carpal joint adequately stabilized the carpus in this small animal. It is highly unlikely that adequate stability would occur in a larger animal that was treated conservatively in this manner. Hyperextension of the middle carpal joint would almost always develop, necessitating partial arthrodesis of the carpus (see Figs. 13–20 and 13–21). Because of the complexity of the injury, primary repair and stabilization of a complete luxation—though technically possible—are not very feasible.

Middle Carpal Subluxation

Subluxation of the middle carpal joint, with medial instability, is a much more common problem than complete luxation. Dorsomedial ligamentous disruption between the radial carpal and carpal 2 and occasionally between carpal 2 and metacarpal II results in valgus deformity of the foot (Fig. 13–18). Less easily appreciated is the fact that *the palmaromedial ligaments or carpal fibrocartilage is often damaged, with resultant hyperextension* (see discussion below). This hyperextension affects only the medial half of the carpus and therefore is not as dramatic as the examples shown below. The mediolateral projection stress radiographs mentioned below (Fig. 13–19) will need to be taken with slight

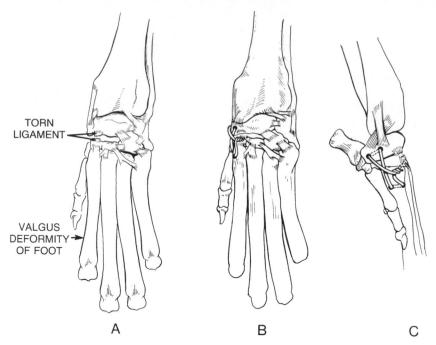

TORN
LIGAMENT

VALGUS
DEFORMITY
OF FOOT

A   B   C

FIGURE 13–18. Middle carpal joint subluxation with medial instability. Left limb, dorsal view. (*A*) Ligaments are torn between the radial carpal and carpal 2. (*B, C*) Bone tunnels are drilled in the palmaromedial process of the radial carpal bone and in the base of metacarpal II. Stainless steel wire of 20 to 22 gauge (0.8 to 0.6 mm) is threaded through the holes in figure-of-8 fashion and the wire tightened enough to eliminate the valgus instability.

internal rotation (pronation) of the paw to demonstrate hyperextension in this situation. If hyperextension is *not* present, the repair can proceed as described here. If hyperextension *is* present, the medial wire augmentation repair described here is performed, plus a partial arthrodesis of the medial half of the middle carpal and carpometacarpal joints (Fig. 13–20). The Kirschner wires seen in Figure 13–20 are placed in metacarpals II and III in this case.

Treatment

CLOSED REDUCTION AND EXTERNAL FIXATION ■ Conservative treatment can be considered for cats, toy, and small breeds when the observed laxity is minimal. A molded palmar splint or short cast (see Figs. 2–27 and 2–22) is applied with the carpus flexed 20 degrees. The splint is maintained for 4 weeks. Complete confinement is enforced through the eighth postoperative week, followed by 4 weeks of gradually increasing activity. Regular training or activity is started by the 12th week. Such treatment in larger breeds is reserved for type I and II sprain injury without laxity.

OPEN REDUCTION AND STABILIZATION ■ The dorsomedial instability is reduced by a synthetic monofilament wire because it is not possible to do a primary suture repair of the ligament. The incision for the dorsal approach to the carpus is positioned dorsomedially on the carpus. If a partial arthrodesis is to be performed concurrently, it is done first. (See the discussion below in the section Hyperextension for details.) The wire placement proceeds by exposure of the medial aspect of the joint. A bone tunnel is drilled through the palma-

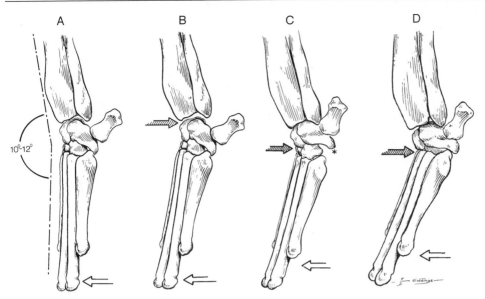

FIGURE 13–19. Stress radiographs for diagnosis of carpal hyperextension. Left limb, lateral views. (*A*) Lateral view of a normal carpus with the foot stressed (*open arrow*) to maximal extension of 10 to 12 degrees. Note the angular relationships of the proximal carpal bones to the radius and to the distal carpal bones. Note also the angular relationship between the carpal and metacarpal bones. (*B*) Lateral view of hyperextension at the antebrachiocarpal joint (*closed arrow*). The only difference from normal is the increased angle of exension. (*C*) Lateral view of hyperextension at the middle carpal joint (*closed arrow*). Note the gap between the palmar process of the ulnar carpal bone (*star*) and the base of metacarpal V. (*D*) Lateral view of hyperextension at the carpometacarpal level (*closed arrow*). The bases of the metacarpal bones appear to overlap the carpal bones.

romedial process of the radial carpal bone and through the base of metacarpal II (Fig. 13–18*B*, *C*). Stainless steel wire, 18 to 22 gauge (1 to 0.6 mm), is threaded through the holes in figure-of-8 fashion. The valgus deformity is reduced and the wire tightened until the instability is abolished. Care must be taken to turn the twisted end of the wire closely against the bone to minimize skin irritation. Closure of the skin completes the procedure.

Aftercare ■ The carpus is immobilized in 10 to 15 degrees of flexion in a caudal splint (see Fig. 2–27) for 4 to 6 weeks. Strict confinement is continued through the eighth week, with a firm padded bandage in place after splint removal. A slowly progressive increase in exercise is then allowed, starting with leash walking, then short periods of free exercise. This program is slowly increased in intensity for another 4 to 6 weeks, at which point most patients are able to return to near normal activity. If a partial arthrodesis was done, use the aftercare routine for that procedure described below.

Hyperextension of the Carpus

Among the most serious injuries to the canine carpus, hyperextension is also one of the more common, occurring in midsize and large breeds of dogs after falls and jumps. The structures responsible for maintaining the normal 10 to 12 degrees of carpal extension (Fig. 13–19*A*) are the palmar ligaments and

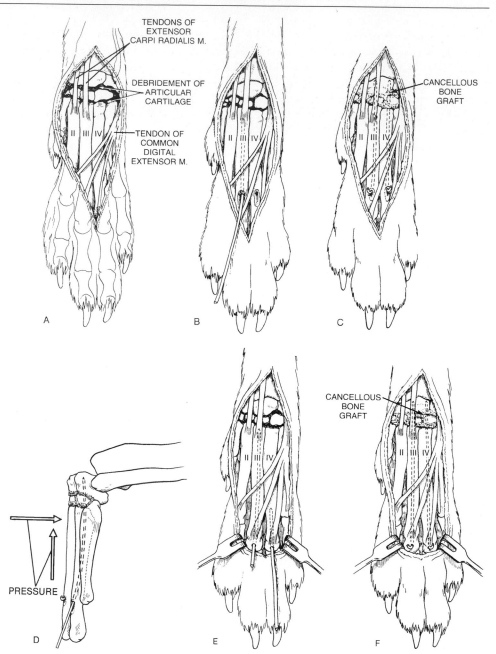

FIGURE 13–20. Partial arthrodesis of the carpus with pin fixation. (*A*) The carpus is exposed by a dorsal midline incision. The middle carpal, carpometacarpal, and inter-carpal joints are debrided of articular cartilage. (*B*) Slots are burred in the dorsal cortex of metacarpals III and IV in the distal third of the bones. Kirschner wire (0.045 or 0.062 inch) is introduced into the medullary canal in the manner of a Rush pin. (*C*) Both pins are seated (also See *D*), and the protruding end is bent into a hook shape and cut off. (*D*) Autogenous cancellous bone graft is placed in all the prepared joint spaces. The carpus is flexed 90 degrees, and palmar and proximal pressure on the metacarpal bones is applied to correctly position the carpal bones relative to the metacarpals. The Kirsch-ner wires are now driven into the proximal row of carpal bones as deeply as possible without penetrating the articular surface. (*E*) An alternative method of placing the Kirschner wires is to drive them from the metacarpophalangeal joints proximally. Two pins are placed and driven to the base of metacarpals III and IV. (*F*) Pins placed at the metacarpophalangeal joint are also bent to a hook shape and cut off.

palmar carpal fibrocartilage (see Fig. 13–2B–D). It is commonly held that hyperextension of the carpus is a result of tendon injury, but in fact the only tendon that bears on carpal stability in extension is the flexor carpi ulnaris, which inserts on the accessory carpal bone. Sectioning of this tendon results in very slight hyperextension at the antebrachiocarpal joint. Diagnosis of this problem is relatively easy because there will be either a laceration of the skin or, in the case of spontaneous rupture or avulsion (rare), palpable evidence of soft-tissue inflammation.

History and Clinical Signs

Invariably there is a history of injury caused by a fall or jump. If there is no history of injury and hyperextension has developed slowly, immune-mediated joint disease may be the cause (see Chapter 6). Surprisingly, minimal signs of pain and inflammation are associated with hyperextension injuries after a few days. Animals commonly will attempt weight bearing within 5 to 7 days. A seal-like or plantigrade stance is characteristic but variable in appearance. Some animals may be walking on their carpal pads, but others may show only 20 to 30 degrees of extension.

Diagnosis

In order to select the proper treatment, it is important to know at which joint level the injury has occurred. In our experience, the distribution of injuries has been as follows:

1. Antebrachiocarpal, 10 percent.
2. Middle carpal, 28 percent.
3. Carpometacarpal, 46 percent.
4. Combined middle and carpometacarpal, 16 percent.

A very rare injury, involving isolated subluxation of the base of the accessory carpal bone due to rupture of the accessoroulnar ligaments, with associated mild carpal hyperextension, has been reported.[7]

Definition of the joint level involved is possible only by radiographic examination. A medial or lateral exposure is made with the limb stressed to maximal carpal extension (see Fig. 13–19). A palmar intra-articular fracture of the radius is often seen when hyperextension is present at the antebrachiocarpal level (Fig. 13–19B). When the injury is at the middle carpal level the palmar process of the ulnar carpal bone becomes separated from the base of metacarpal V and the process is easily identified (Fig. 13–19C). The accessory carpal bone may show evidence of subluxation and proximal angulation. With carpometacarpal injury the proximal carpal bones override the distal row (Fig. 13–19D). Chronic antebrachiocarpal level injuries show wearing of the palmar edge of the distal radius due to the proximal carpal bones as they subluxate in a palmar direction. In chronic middle carpal instability, the radial and ulnar carpal bones can pivot in a distopalmar direction, their dorsodistal edges coming to rest on the base of the metacarpals, creating a wide gap between the craniodorsal surface of the radius and the radial carpal bone. In chronic injuries at all levels, varying degrees of bony proliferation will be present where the more proximal bones override the distal bones.

In the case of subluxation of the accessory carpal bone mentioned above, there was increased space in the accessoroulnar joint space in lateral radiographs taken in flexion. When the carpus was stressed in extension the accessory carpal bone and ulnar carpal bone shifted laterally, as visualized in dorsopalmar views.[7]

Treatment

Two basic types of arthrodesis are performed in the carpal region. Panarthrodesis involves surgical fusion of all three joint levels, the antebrachiocarpal, the middle carpal, and the carpometacarpal. Partial arthrodesis involves fusion of only the middle and distal joints. Panarthrodesis has been a widely practiced method of treating carpal hyperextension, regardless of the joint level involved.[8] This has been a satisfactory method of treatment, with 97 percent of owners reporting improvement in gait and 74 percent reporting normal use of the limb[8]; nevertheless, it destroys a normal joint (antebrachiocarpal) and requires the use of bone-plating equipment (see Figs. 13–22 and 13–23A, B) or external skeletal fixators (see Fig. 13–23C). Partial arthrodesis (fusion of the middle carpal and carpometacarpal joints only) is probably a better approach for those injuries that involve only the middle and distal joints (Figs. 13–20 and 13–21).[9] With this technique, flexion of the major joint of the carpus—the antebrachiocarpal joint—is maintained, and gait is affected little. Conversely, in chronic cases with

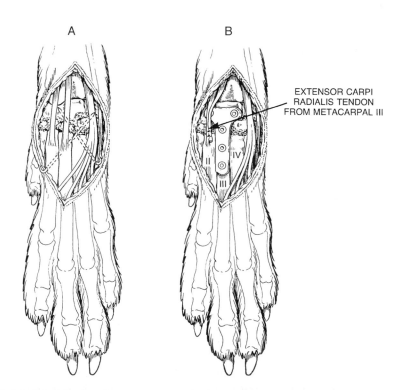

FIGURE 13–21. (A) An alternative transfixation method of pinning the middle carpal and carpometacarpal joints for partial carpal arthrodesis. The medial pin is driven from metacarpal II proximally into the ulnar carpal bone. The lateral pin is driven from the articular surface of the radial carpal bone (with the joint flexed) distally into metacarpal V, where it is then pulled distally until buried beneath the articular surface of the radial carpal bone. (B) Partial arthrodesis of the carpus using T-plate fixation. The plate is attached to the distal end of the radial carpal bone, the screws angling proximally. The first screw in the long end of the plate is placed in carpal 3, and the other two screws in the third metacarpal. The tendon of the extensor carpi radialis inserting on metacarpal III has been transposed to metacarpal II and is sutured there.

marked degenerative joint disease, panarthrodesis will yield better results. Conservative treatment by splinting in flexion or hyperextension seems to have little application, since virtually all animals will break down again following return to weight bearing. Patients with mild hyperextension at the antebrachiocarpal level and smaller animals are the best candidates for treatment by splintage. Arthrodesis can be performed later if necessary.

Partial Arthrodesis

Partial, or subtotal, arthrodesis involves surgical fusion of only the middle level and carpometacarpal joints. Subluxation of the accessory carpal bone need not be addressed. The function of the carpus remains essentially normal in this technique because there is little motion normally present in these joint levels. The antebrachiocarpal joint, which is responsible for virtually all flexion of the carpus, remains functional. The major indication for partial arthrodesis is hyperextension of the middle carpal and carpometacarpal joint levels, these cases comprising 90 percent of all hyperextension injuries of the carpus. Both joints are fused when either is injured because of the technical difficulty of fusing either individually. On occasion, instability will develop medially at either of these joints and will not respond to treatment (see Fig. 13–18); these cases could also be considered for partial arthrodesis.

PIN FIXATION METHOD ■ A dorsal midline approach to the carpus is made with the incision extending distally to the level of the metacarpophalangeal joints (see Fig. 13–20A). A tourniquet can be used. Preoperative preparations and draping are made to allow collection of a cancellous bone graft from the proximal humerus of the same limb (see Chapter 3). Articular cartilage of the middle carpal, intercarpal, and carpometacarpal joints is debrided with a curette or high speed bur. Care is taken to preserve the insertions of the extensor carpi radialis tendon on the proximal ends of metacarpals II and III. If the high-speed bur is available, slots are burred through the distal cortex of metacarpals III and IV at the level of the distal third of the shaft (see Fig. 13–20B). Kirschner wires (0.045 or 0.062 inch; 1.2 or 1.6 mm) are introduced through the slots into the medullary canal in the manner of a Rush pin and driven proximally into the base of the metacarpal bone. The cortical slots must be long enough to allow the pin to bend as it is introduced into the medullary canal. Failure of the pins to drive up the medullary canal easily means that the pins are too large in diameter or that the slot is too short. Autogenous cancellous graft is collected from the proximal humerus and packed into the debrided joint spaces. With the carpus held in extreme flexion to reduce the subluxation of the middle carpal or carpometacarpal level, pins are driven proximally into the radial carpal bone (see Fig. 13–20D). The pins must not penetrate the proximal articular cartilage of the radial carpal bone. The pins are backed out a few millimeters and then bent to form a hook at the distal end and cut off. The pins are then pushed or driven proximally to their original depth, after which the hook is rotated flat against the bone (see Fig. 13–20C).

If no power bur is available, it is difficult to cut slots in the metacarpal bones; two methods can be substituted in this situation:

1. The pins can be driven from the metacarpophalangeal joint proximally into the shaft of the bone similarly to pinning a metacarpal fracture (see Fig. 13–30). The pins should enter the bone slightly dorsal to the articular cartilage of the distal end of the metacarpal bone (Fig. 13–20E). After the pins are seated

in the radial carpal bone they are retracted a few millimeters, the distal ends are bent to form a hook, cut off, and driven back into their original depth. Finally the hook ends are rotated flat against the bone (see Fig. 13–20F).

2. Transfixation pins can be driven at an angle into the proximal carpal bones from metacarpals II and V (Fig. 13–21A) after reducing the joints as shown in Figure 13–20D. The medial pin must be driven from metacarpal 2 proximally into the ulnar carpal bone and the position of the tip of the pin verified to ensure it does not penetrate the articular surface, which will probably not be visible. The lateral pin is more easily driven from the articular surface of the radial carpal bone distally. The carpus is maximally flexed to allow the pin to be positioned under direct vision proximally in the radial carpal bone. After the pin exits metacarpal 5 distally the pin chuck is reversed and the pin pulled distally until it is below the articular surface of the radial carpal bone. An advantage of this method is that the exposure does not need to extend as far distally. The disadvantage is that the pins are more difficult to direct to insure that they penetrate the correct bones. A power drill is advisable, as it is easier to direct than a hand chuck.

BONE PLATE ■ A small T-plate can also be used for partial arthrodesis. The joint is exposed, prepared, and bone grafted as detailed previously for pin fixation. The plate is attached to the distodorsal surface of the radial carpal bone (see Fig. 13–21B) and is placed as far distally on the radial carpal bone as possible, in order to avoid interference with the dorsal rim of the radius. The two screws in the radial carpal bone are angled proximally to allow the plate to be properly positioned. The distal portion of the plate must lie over the third metacarpal bone, which necessitates cutting the tendon of insertion of the extensor carpi radialis. The tendon is sutured to the insertion of its paired tendon on metacarpal II. The two distal screws in the plate are placed in metacarpal III. The most proximal screw is either placed in carpal 3, as shown in Figure 13–21B, or in the base of metacarpal III.

Aftercare ■ If a tourniquet was used, a padded support bandage is applied for several days, and after swelling has subsided, a molded splint or short leg cylinder cast (see Figs. 2–27 and 2–22) is applied to the caudal surface of the limb. If no tourniquet was used the splint can be applied immediately if desired. This support is maintained until radiographic signs of fusion are noted, typically 6 to 8 weeks later. A gradual return to normal exercise is allowed over the next 4 weeks. If the pins were driven from the metacarpophalangeal joint, they should be removed before allowing exercise. Other implants are removed only if they migrate (pins) or loosen (plates).

Prognosis ■ Good results have been reported for this procedure.[9] At an average of 32 months postoperatively, 25 of 25 owners reported to be pleased or very pleased with the function of their animals. Some degree of hyperextension persisted in 11 percent of the cases, and degenerative joint disease was present in 15.5 percent of the cases. No cases required revision by panarthrodesis.

Panarthrodesis

Indications for panarthrodesis are primarily those that involve the antebrachiocarpal joint: polytrauma, such as fractures or multiple ligamentous injuries, degenerative joint disease, and hyperextension injuries at the antebrachiocarpal level. Arthrodesis for brachial plexus paralysis is not recommended because of the poor elbow function and self-mutilation of the foot that usually occur. It does not appear to be practical to fuse only the antebrachiocarpal level; therefore, when this level must be fused, the other two levels are also fused. Fusion of only the antebrachiocarpal joint is technically possible, but the stress placed on the metacarpal and carpometacarpal joints disposes them to increased laxity and degenerative changes. It should be remembered that because there is very little motion in the middle and distal joints of the carpus, fusion of the antebrachiocarpal level effectively destroys all motion in the carpus. Although function remains good, there is pronounced circumduction of the lower limb during the swing phase of gait.

Either bone plate or external skeletal fixation can be applied for stabilization of this fusion. Plate fixation was originally applied dorsally,[8] but this position is mechanically unsound, since the plate is not on the tension side of the carpus and is therefore subject to bending forces. The plate will loosen or break unless the carpus is supported in a cast or splint until fusion is radiographically verified. Dorsal plating has been used successfully in the cat, and in a case of hypoplasia of the carpal bone, where the radius was fused directly to the metacarpus.[10,11] A palmar position for the plate is obviously mechanically superior and has been found to be useful by Chambers and Bjorling.[12] This advantage may be negated by more difficult exposure (see below). External skeletal fixators can also be applied in a variety of configurations and are especially valuable in the presence of open injuries.

DORSAL PLATE TECHNIQUE ■ A dorsal midline approach from the level of the distal radius to the midmetacarpal level is used after a tourniquet ($\pm$) has been placed. Preparations are made to collect a cancellous bone graft from the proximal humerus of the same limb (see Chapter 3). Articular cartilage of the antebrachiocarpal, the middle carpal, the carpometacarpal, and the intercarpal joints is debrided with a curette or high-speed bur. The tendons of the extensor carpi radialis on metacarpals II and III can be sacrificed. After debridement of articular cartilage of all three joint levels (Fig. 13–22A), a seven-hole (minimum) compression plate is applied to the dorsal surface of the distal radius, bridging the carpus, and attaching distally to the third metacarpal (Fig. 13–22B). Plate and screw size vary with the size of the patient, with the width of the third metacarpal bone being the limiting factor. The screw diameter should not exeed 25 to 30 percent of the bone width or the bone could be seriously weakened. Suggestions for sizes are listed:

1. 3.5-mm screws/plates for large breeds over 60 pounds (27 kg).
2. 2.7-mm screws/plates for breeds from 20 to 25 pounds to 60 pounds (9 to 11 kg to 27 kg).
3. 2.0-mm screws/plates for breeds between 10 and 20 pounds (4.5 to 9 kg). Cuttable plates (Synthes; see discussion in Chapter 2) work well here. Two 1.5-mm-thick plates are stacked together to span the distance from the radius to the most proximal metacarpal screw. A single-thickness plate extends distally for two to three more screw holes. This simplifies skin closure and lessens the problem of late loosening of the most distal screw, as discussed below. Another option with this method is the use of 2.7-mm screws in the radius and radial carpal bone and 2.0-mm screws in the metacarpal.
4. 1.5-mm screws/plates for cats and toy breeds.[10] Two thicknesses of 1.0-mm-thick cuttable plates are used here. The 2.0-mm screws can be used in the radius and radial carpal bones and 1.5-mm screws in the metacarpal.

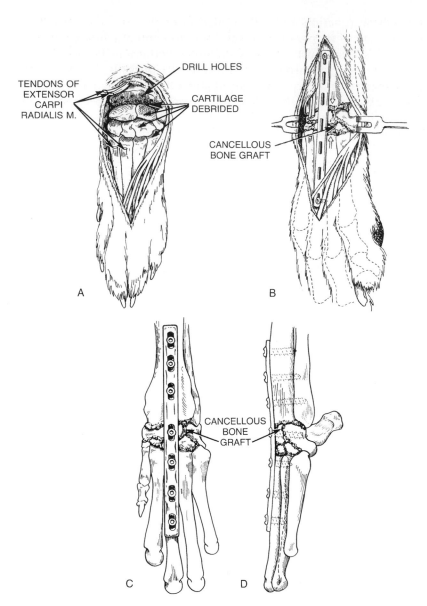

FIGURE 13–22. Panarthrodesis of the carpus with a dorsal plate. (*A*) The left carpus has been exposed by a dorsal midline incision, and the tendons of the extensor carpi radialis severed at metacarpals II and III. Removal of articular cartilage is eased by maximum flexion of the joint. Multiple drill holes penetrate the distal radius to aid in vascularization. (*B*) A seven- or eight-hole bone plate is contoured to provide 10 to 12 degrees of carpal extension (see *D*) and is attached distally to the third metacarpal and proximally to the radius. The abductor pollicis longus muscle must be cut to seat the plate on the radius proximally. The screws in this dynamic compression plate (Synthes Ltd. [USA], Paoli, PA) are placed in the load position to produce compression. It is important that the distal screw be placed first, in order to center the plate on metacarpal III. Autogenous cancellous bone graft is packed into the joint spaces. (*C*, *D*) The bone plate is completely attached, with three screws in the radius, three in the third metacarpal, and one in the radial carpal bone. Autogenous cancellous bone graft is used to pack the joint spaces and under the plate. Note that about 10 degrees of carpal extension have been maintained.

Three screws are placed in the distal radius, one in the radial carpal bone, and a minimum of three in the third metacarpal bone. The distal screw must be placed first in order to center the plate over metacarpal III and so ensure that the screws will be centered in this rather narrow bone. The self-compressing load position is used for the first two screws in the radius and metacarpal III in order to compress all the joint levels. Compression is not possible with cuttable plates. Plates are contoured to produce about 10 degrees of extension in the carpus (Fig. 13–22C, D). It is usually helpful to slightly flatten the flare of the distal radius to avoid having to double curve the plate. Autogenous cancellous bone from the proximal humerus is used to pack all the joint spaces and space beneath the plate. The extensor carpi radialis tendons are sutured to joint capsule in the area.

Aftercare ■ A short, molded palmar splint or cylinder cast (see Figs. 2–27 and 2–22) is maintained until radiographic signs of fusion are noted, usually 6 to 8 weeks. Exercise is gradually returned to normal over the following 4 weeks. If function of the limb is good, most plates will need to be removed in 6 to 12 months because of loosening or irritation. The metacarpal bones are flexible enough to bend slightly during weight bearing, and this may cause loosening of the distal screws due to the stiffness of the plate. Fatigue fractures of metacarpal III occur at the end of the plate on occasion. The plate should be removed and the foot splinted until bone healing is well advanced, usually about 4 weeks.

PALMAR PLATE TECHNIQUE ■ A palmaromedial approach to the distal radius and carpus is used to expose the area.[1] Preparations are also made to collect a cancellous bone graft from the proximal humerus of the same limb (see Chapter 3). Ligaments, palmar carpal fibrocartilage, and joint capsule are sharply dissected from the distal radius and carpal bones. Articular cartilage of all joint levels is removed by powered burs or curettes. This debridement is somewhat blind, since good visualization of the articular surfaces is difficult. Any bony prominences that prevent close contact of the plate and bone are removed in preparation for attaching an appropriate-size plate. The distal radius must be flattened quite aggressively to minimize contouring of the plate. Plate sizes are as discussed above and should be long enough to place at least three screws in the radius and in metacarpal III. The carpus is positioned in normal extension (10 to 12 degrees), and a Kirschner wire is drilled from the distal radius into the carpus to temporarily maintain the desired angle while the plate is contoured to fit the palmar surface of the distal radius and metacarpal III (Fig. 13–23A, B). The plate is attached first at the distal hole to ensure that the screw holes in metacarpal III will be centered in this narrow bone. The plate is then attached using the self-compressing load position for the first two screws in the radius and metacarpal III in order to compress all the joint levels. Cancellous bone graft is added to the joint surface areas and the Kirschner wire removed before closing the tissues in layers.

Aftercare ■ A padded support bandage is applied for several days, and after swelling has subsided, a molded splint (see Fig. 2–27) may be applied to the caudal surface of the limb. This splint is maintained until radiographic signs of fusion are noted, typically 6 to 8 weeks later. A gradual return to normal exercise is allowed over the next 4 weeks. If the animal can be closely confined, and if the use of a splint presents difficulties in treatment of soft tissue wounds, it is possible to dispense with use of the splint.

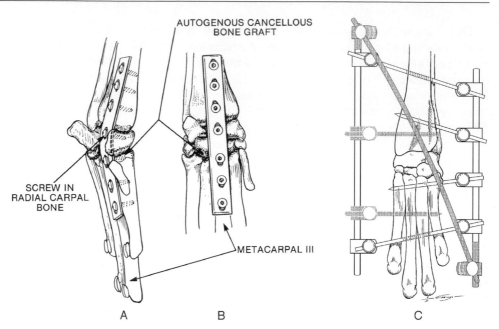

FIGURE 13–23. (*A, B*) Carpal panarthrodesis with a palmar plate.[12] A palmaromedial approach to the distal radius and carpus[1] is made to allow plate placement on the distal radius and metacarpal bone III. Autogenous cancellous bone graft is used in the prepared articular surfaces. Plate size for large-breed dogs is typically 2.7 to 3.5 mm. (*C*) A modified type IIB external fixator is applicable for panarthrodesis. Placement of the fixation pins is eased if the medial and lateral connecting bars are curved to match the normal extension angle of the carpus. The shaded fixation pins are used for maximum stiffness of the fixator, as is the shaded angular connecting bar, which is curved to arch dorsal to the paw.

EXTERNAL SKELETAL FIXATOR TECHNIQUE ■   There are occasions when it is desirable to perform panarthrodesis of the carpus in the face of actual or potential infection. Open comminuted fractures and severe shearing injuries are the most common indications. Early arthrodesis will help in management of the soft tissue injury by providing stabilization of the area, thus improving blood supply and optimizing the local defense reaction. Considerable time and expense are also saved. If bone plating equipment is not available, the external fixator represents an excellent method that is available to most practices.

The type IIB splint configuration shown in Figure 13–23C can be used to advantage to stabilize the joint after preparation of the joint surfaces, as described above. Curving of the connecting rods is helpful in establishing the proper angle of the carpus. Acrylic resin connecting bars are quite useful in this application, especially so in the small breeds. Type IIA splints can also be used, but it is quite difficult to get the intermediate pins aligned to the second bar (see discussion in Chapter 2). Autogenous cancellous bone graft (see Chapter 3) can be safely used in the presence of infection but should be withheld if there is frank suppuration. In this circumstance the graft will be washed out of the site by the exudate and therefore wasted. It is more useful to wait until healthy granulation has covered the area and then elevate the granulation tissue and insert the graft.

Aftercare ■   Bone healing in open injuries will probably be delayed, and the splint will have to be maintained for 10 to 12 weeks. Radiographic fusion in closed injuries will usually be attained by 8 weeks. If bone pins loosen before fusion is radiographically visible, the pins can be either replaced or removed and followed with a few more weeks of immobilization in a short leg cast (see Fig. 2–22).

Shearing Injury of the Carpus

This abrasion injury occurs when the dog's lower limb is run over by the tire of an automobile with its brakes locked attempting to avoid the animal. Soft tissues in contact with the pavement are simply ground away, often eroding skin, muscle, ligaments, and even bone. The medial carpal and metacarpal regions are most commonly affected, with the radial styloid process and radial collateral ligaments often completely destroyed (Fig. 13–24A). One or more carpal or metacarpal joints may be open, and varying amounts of debris are ground into all the tissues. The lateral side is less commonly involved and represents a less serious injury than a comparable injury on the medial side. Owing to the fact that the dog normally stands with a few degrees of valgus (lateral) deviation of the forepaw, ligamentous stability of the medial side of the carpus and metacarpus is much more critical than on the lateral aspect. Best results are obtained by treating these wounds in an open manner, with early aggressive stabilization of the joints and any accompanying fractures. Skin grafting is delayed and indicated only where granulation tissue does not adequately close the skin, a rare occurrence.

Early or delayed arthrodesis is indicated in those cases where it is not possible to restore reasonable joint function by ligamentous stabilization. Variables to be considered in choosing a plan of action are:

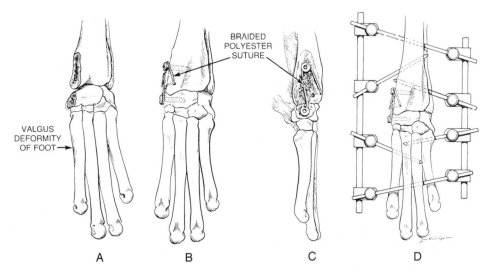

FIGURE 13–24. Shearing injury of the medial carpus. (*A*) The radial styloid process and medial aspect of the radial carpal bone and the associated collateral ligaments have been ground away. (*B, C*) Bone screws provide anchor points for the synthetic ligament of braided polyester suture. Placement of the screws and bone tunnel closely mimic the normal ligament. (*D*) In order to simplify open treatment of soft tissues, the joint is stabilized in 10 degrees of flexion with external skeletal fixation (Kirschner-Ehmer splint). The connecting rods are bent to allow the desired amount of extension.

1.   Assuming that the joint(s) can be stabilized, is there enough articular surface to allow good function? Loss of bone in the antebrachiocarpal articulation is critical. If the answer is no, arthrodesis is indicated.

2.   What will the owner accept as reasonable function? A large active breed presents problems different from those of a small and sedentary animal. In the former, aggressive ligamentous repair, augmentation, or replacement is necessary, while in the latter case it may be possible to obtain good results by very conservative methods. Stabilization of joints by scar tissue may well provide adequate support in the smaller and less active animals, but it rarely will support the tension loads of the medial side in large athletic individuals.

3.   How will support for the joints or fractured bones be provided? Regardless of which approach is taken to the ligamentous instability, the involved joints must be stabilized during the healing period. Because of the necessity for daily bandage changes for 2 to 3 weeks when treating these large open wounds, the use of conventional casts or splints is difficult. External skeletal fixation devices have greatly aided in solving this problem.

Treatment

RECONSTRUCTION ■   Initial debridement must be meticulous but not too aggressive, with emphasis on removal of obviously dead tissue and foreign matter from both soft tissue and joint spaces. Copious irrigation with saline or Ringer's solution is very important at this time. Addition of 10 percent povidone-iodine or 0.2 percent chlorhexidine is favored by some. After adequate debridement, it may be possible to partially close the wound by suturing skin. This can be helpful, but care must be taken to:

1.   Leave adequate open area for unimpeded wound drainage. Placement of Penrose or tube drains under the sutured skin is usually advisable for 2 to 5 days.

2.   Avoid closing skin under tension. Serious circulatory stasis develops owing to the tourniquet-like effect of excessive skin tension in the lower limbs.

3.   When in doubt about tissue viability, *do not suture skin*. Delayed primary closure can be done in a few days with no loss of healing time.

Several debridements over a number of days may be necessary to adequately remove all devitalized tissue because of the difficulty in determining viability of badly traumatized tissue. If there are portions of ligaments, joint capsule, or other tissues that can be sutured to support the joint and to close the synovial membrane, this should be done. Monofilament or synthetic absorbable suture is most trouble free relative to later sinus tracks.

Re-establishment of the radial collateral ligament complex is usually hampered by loss of bone, and small bone screws may be used to anchor a synthetic ligament. There is a tendency to use monofilament wire in this contaminated area, but heavy braided suture is a much more functional ligament and has resulted in very few problems related to suture sinus drainage tracks. Monofilament nylon fishing line of 40- to 60-pound test has also been successful. Two bone screws are positioned to mimic the normal ligaments as closely as possible (Fig. 13–24B, C). Precise placement of these bone screws for attachment of heavy braided polyester suture and adequate soft tissue debridement are necessary for successful treatment. The sutures are tied tightly enough to stabilize the joint, but motion without binding should still be possible. Washers can be used on the screws to prevent the suture from slipping over the head of the screw. Treatment of the open wound is simplified by use of transarticular type

IIB external fixator to stabilize the joint (Fig. 13–24D). Fixation is maintained until granulation tissue has covered the defect, usually 3 to 4 weeks. Sterile laparotomy sponges soaked in povidone-iodine or chlorhexidine solution are loosely bandaged to the limb for several days, and debridement is repeated daily or every other day until all dead tissue is removed. The wound must be kept moist and provision made for adequate drainage of exudate.[13] Moist gauze with copious absorbent padding covered by a moisture barrier such as polyvinyl sheet and dressing changes are used daily until healthy granulation covers the wound. Hydrocolloid, hydrogel, and polyethylene semiocclusive dressings have received considerable attention for treatment of full-thickness skin wounds. Hydrogel and polyethylene dressings were significantly better in all parameters tested in one study.[14] Once healthy granulation tissue is present, nonadherent dressings, either dry or with antibacterial ointments, and minimal absorbent padding are used in place of the moist dressings. Intervals between dressing changes can gradually be spread out as wound exudation lessens. The wound must be kept protected until it is well epithelialized, which may take up to 10 to 12 weeks.

Aftercare ■ When granulation tissue completely covers the wound, but not before 3 weeks postoperatively, the external fixator is removed. A firm elastic support bandage should be maintained for another 3 weeks with very restricted activity. Normal exercise is not allowed until weeks 8 to 12, depending on the stability achieved. Loosening of the bone screws and skin irritation from the screw heads are both indications for removing the screws. The screw in the radial carpal bone is particularly prone to loosening because of its motion. This should not be done before 3 to 4 months postoperatively if possible. Failure to adequately stabilize the joint will result in degenerative joint disease and poor function. In such a situation arthrodesis offers the best chance of restoring function. See the discussion above regarding arthrodesis.

Prognosis ■ A retrospective study of 98 shearing injuries by Beardsley and Schrader revealed some previously unknown facts regarding the outcome of these cases.[15] All were treated essentially as described above except that none received joint stabilization by means of external fixators; all were supported in some form of external coaptation. Healing time ranged from 2 to 9 weeks, depending on the size and depth of the wound and the amount of the wound that was able to be closed by suture. A mean of 1.7 surgical procedures were performed on each patient, and a mean of 5.5 rechecks were required after hospital discharge. Good to excellent outcome was attained in 91 percent of the dogs, defined as clinically normal or with only minimal functional abnormalities after healing of the injury. Only one case required skin grafting. As can be seen, these are expensive injuries due to the amount of care required, and those owners not prepared for this type care would be well advised to consider amputation as a primary treatment. It is our subjective opinion that support with external fixators simplifies treatment because owners can do more of it at home due to the absence of the coaptation splint, but we do not have data to suggest that it shortens the healing period or affects the final outcome.

ARTHRODESIS ■ Some injuries are too extensive to be successfully reconstructed. These are invariably those with extensive bone loss of the medial radial styloid process. If the bone loss extends laterally into the articular surface of the radius there may not be sufficient articular support for the radial carpal bone. Additionally, the ability to provide sufficient medial ligamentous support is questionable. In this situation, panarthrodesis of the carpus is the best method of maintaining limb function. Although it is possible to attempt reconstruction and then follow with arthrodesis if reconstruction fails, a great deal of time and expense can be wasted.

By the use of external skeletal fixation (Fig. 13–23C) the arthrodesis can be performed very early, before the wound is healed, with a high probability of successful fusion and a low chance of bone infection. The procedure can be delayed for a few days, until the debridement phase is complete and hopefully some granulation tissue has begun to appear. The carpus is supported during this phase entirely by the bandage, sometimes augmented by thermomoldable plastic splints or wire frames. If it seems necessary to use the external fixator immediately to support the joint, the fusion is done at the same time. The technique is performed basically as described above in the section Hyperextension. The major difference is in the manner of applying the autogenous cancellous bone graft, since there must be sufficient soft tissue available to cover the graft and allow its early vascularization. Exudation is another contraindication to early grafting, as the exudate may physically carry the graft fragments away. In this situation the joint debridement and fixation is completed as usual, but grafting is delayed until there is a healthy granulation tissue bed, without exudation. At that point the granulation tissue is carefully elevated from the joint surfaces sufficiently to allow the graft to be packed into the joint spaces. The area is kept covered by petrolatum-impregnated gauze sponges for several days, until granulation tissue again covers the area. Aftercare from this point onwards is as described above.

METACARPUS AND PHALANGES

Fractures of the Metacarpus

Fractures of the metacarpal bones occur in all three anatomical regions of the bone—the base (proximal end), the shaft, and the head (distal end).

Fracture of the Base

The medial (second) and lateral (fifth) bones are most commonly involved (Figs. 13–25A and 13–26A). Because these areas are points of ligamentous insertion, varying degrees of valgus (lateral) displacement of the foot are seen with fractures of the second metacarpal, and varus (medial) displacement with fifth metacarpal fractures. Some injury of the carpometacarpal ligaments may be noted, which may also result in hyperextension at the carpometacarpal level (see above).

CLOSED REDUCTION ■ Undisplaced fractures may be treated by external fixation, but there is usually some displacement of the fragment during healing and subsequent varus or valgus malunion. A very secure molded splint or short leg cast (see Figs. 2–27 and 2–22) must be used.

OPEN REDUCTION AND INTERNAL FIXATION ■ Fixation of displaced fractures is usually done by the tension band wire technique (Fig. 13–25B and Fig. 13–26B, C). Lag screws are also useful in some cases (Fig. 13–25C). Comminuted fractures in larger breeds may be handled with small plates, combined with lag screws and/or cerclage wires (Fig. 13–27).

Racing greyhounds are subject to stress fractures of the second metacarpal (and third metatarsal) of the right foot. These fractures are undisplaced and

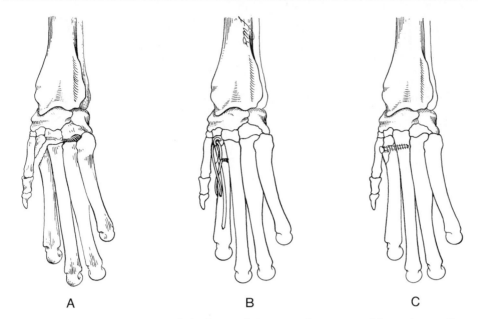

A   B   C

FIGURE 13–25. (*A*) Fracture of the base of the second metacarpal bone is usually associated with valgus (lateral) deviation of the foot. (*B*) Fixation with Kirschner wire and tension band wire. (*C*) Fixation with lag screw.

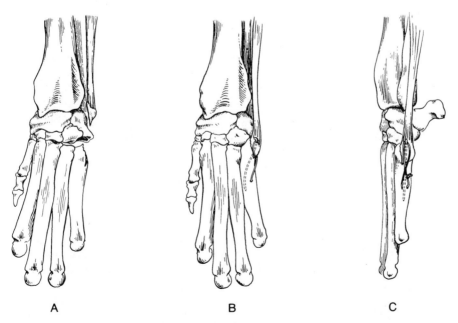

A   B   C

FIGURE 13–26. (*A*) Fracture of the base of the fifth metacarpal bone. The tendon of insertion of the ulnaris lateralis muscle causes the fragment to be displaced proximally. Some varus (medial) deviation of the foot may be present. (*B*, *C*) Fixation is by the tension band wire technique. The Kirschner wire is 0.045 inch in diameter, and the stainless steel wire is 22 gauge. This fracture could also be repaired with a lag screw.

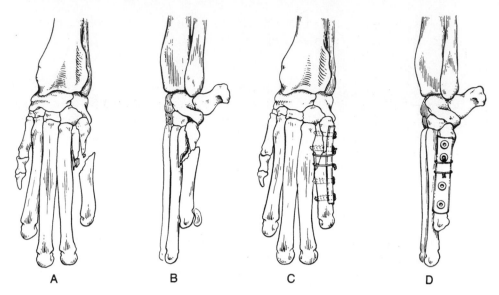

FIGURE 13–27. (*A, B*) Comminuted fracture of the proximal shaft and base of the fifth metacarpal bone. (*C, D*) A one-third tubular plate, 2.7-mm screws, and 22-gauge cerclage wire fixation. The two proximal screws were applied in lag fashion.

often show some callus formation (Fig. 13–28*A, B*). Fixation of acute injuries is by a palmar splint (Fig. 2–27), maintained for 4 weeks. Lag screw fixation with 2.0 mm miniscrews is indicated when there is no response to immobilization (Fig. 13–28*C*). Chronic injuries can be stimulated to start anew with a healing response by osteostixis.[16] Several 1.5- to 2.0-mm holes are drilled in the fracture area to stimulate a healing response, after which the foot is splinted for 4 weeks.

Aftercare ■   Primary fixation by casting or splinting will require the device to be worn for about 6 weeks, except in the case of the stress fracture, which requires only 4 weeks. If internal fixation is used, a molded palmar splint or

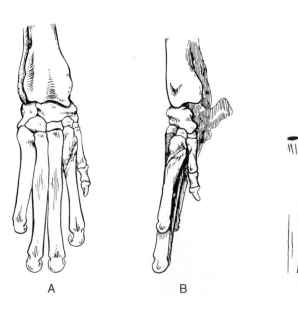

FIGURE 13–28. (*A, B*) Stress fracture of the second metacarpal bone, right forefoot. This fracture is specific in the racing greyhound. The fracture is usually incomplete and undisplaced and may extend into the articular surface of the base; unless it is seen very early, it will have some periosteal callus formation, which is usually palpable. (*C*) Fixation with 1.5- or 2.0-mm lag screws placed in a dorsal-palmaromedial direction.

short cast (see Figs. 2–27 and 2–22) is maintained for 3 to 4 weeks. Exercise is restricted for 3 to 4 weeks after splint removal.

Fracture of the Shaft

Fracture of one or even two metacarpals is not a serious injury, especially if the two middle bones are not involved. They heal quite readily in a simple palmar splint as a result of the splinting effect of the remaining bones. When three or all four bones (Fig. 13–29A) are broken, the situation is quite different, however, especially in the large and giant breeds. Here, simple splints often create a delayed union or malunion at best, with nonunion often resulting. This is a problem particularly when preformed spoon splints are used. Additionally, a valgus deformity and palmar bowing of the bones may occur because they are not adequately supported in the spoon splint (Fig. 13–29B, C).

CLOSED REDUCTION ■ When closed reduction and external fixation are used, a molded splint (see Fig. 2–27) or fiberglass short cast (see Fig. 2–22) is advisable. Because these devices are molded to the foot, the bony support is greatly improved. The splint or cast should be maintained until radiographic signs of healing are well advanced, which typically occurs within 4 to 8 weeks, varying with the age of the animal.

OPEN REDUCTION AND INTERNAL FIXATION ■ Internal fixation is indicated when two or more bones are involved, especially if they are the middle

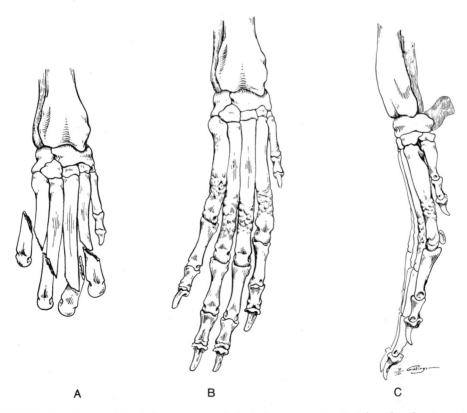

A   B   C

FIGURE 13–29. (A) Multiple metacarpal shaft fractures. (B, C) Closed reduction and inadequate external fixation resulted in valgus deformity and palmar bowing of the metacarpus.

bones. Other indications for internal fixation include severely fragmented or displaced fractures, nonunion, and malunion. Even simple single-bone fractures may warrant internal fixation for optimal functional results in large athletic breeds.

Intramedullary Pins ■ Kirschner wires, Steinmann pins, and Rush pins are all applicable to the metacarpal/metatarsal bones. They are indicated in transverse and oblique fractures that are not highly fragmented, often combined with cerclage wires in long oblique fractures. The pin should not fill the medullary canal too tightly because it will interfere with medullary blood supply and delay healing. K-wires of 0.045 to 0.062 inch (1.2 to 1.5 mm) generally suffice. In most cases it is best to think of the pin as merely an internal splint to maintain reduction of the bone and to rely on an external cast/splint to furnish a good deal of the immobilization needed for fracture healing.

A method of introducing the pins that does not damage or interfere with motion of the metacarpophalangeal joint will produce the best functional results and allow the external fixation to be removed as soon as there is sufficient callus to support the pin. One acceptable method is to introduce the pin from the distal end of the bone at the dorsal edge of the articular cartilage. Although this causes the pin to enter the bone at a slight angle, nevertheless, if the pin is not too large and stiff to bend slightly it should glide proximally in the medullary canal. The fracture is reduced and the pin driven into the proximal fragment until it is well seated in the base of the bone. The pin is then retracted 5 mm, a hook is bent and the end cut, and then the pin is driven back into the bone until the hook is close to the bone surface. In this manner, there is very little pin protruding from the bone to irritate the joint, yet the pin is easily removed (Fig. 13–30). This method is difficult in small breeds. Retrograde insertion (from the fracture site) is advocated by some, but it is difficult to avoid penetrating the distal articular surface with this method. If the bone is large enough to accept a ¹/₁₆-inch (1.5-mm) Rush pin (Osteo-Technology International Inc., Hunt Valley, MD), the hook will not have to be bent by the surgeon, and the pin can be inserted at some distance from the articular surface (Fig. 13–31C). Generally, a Rush pin will provide more rigid fixation than a straight intramedullary pin.

Aftercare ■ The metacarpophalangeal joint is kept in flexion in a splint or cast (see Figs. 2–27 and 2–22), and the pins are removed after healing. If the pins do penetrate articular cartilage, the splint should be maintained until healing is complete and the pins removed, before allowing active weight bearing. Rush pins do not generally require removal.

CERCLAGE WIRES ■ The general rules given in Chapter 1 apply to application of wires in the metacarpus or metatarsus. Useful wire sizes vary from 20 gauge to 24 gauge (0.8 to 0.4 mm). Of primary importance is that the cerclage wire must be tight or it will devascularize the underlying bone because of movement of the wire. An important difference in the metacarpus/metatarsus from their application in long bones is that on occasion cerclage wires are used as primary fixation. This is possible because external casts/splints are always used to support the internal fixation. More commonly, however, cerclage wires are combined with intramedullary pins (Fig. 13–31C).

LAG SCREWS ■ Interfragmentary fixation with lag screws, as with cerclage wire, is occasionally used as primary fixation in the metacarpus/metatarsus when supported with an external cast or splint. The advent of 1.5- and 2.0-

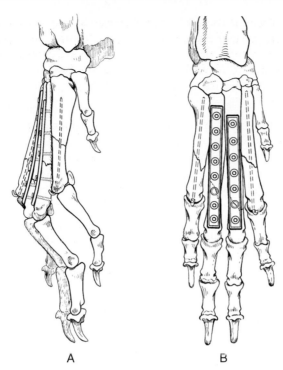

A   B

FIGURE 13–30. Combined bone plate and intramedullary fixation of multiple metacarpal fractures. Kirschner wires are inserted in the distal segment of metacarpals 2 and 5, staying as close as possible to the dorsoproximal edge of the metacarpophalangeal joint capsule. The fracture is reduced and the pins are driven proximally into the base of the bone. The pins are then bent to a hook shape and driven as close to the bone as possible to allow more extension of the toes and easier removal of the pins. Plate fixation is ideal for fixation of metacarpals 3 and 4, which are the major weight-carrying bones. Veterinary cuttable plates (Synthes Ltd. [USA], Paoli, PA) are the most adaptable plate for this application. Pinning of all four metacarpals is acceptable if plating is not possible. In either case the foot must be supported in coaptation for several weeks.

FIGURE 13–31. (A) Oblique shaft fracture of the fifth metacarpal in a racing greyhound. (B) Fixation by 2.7-mm lag screws. This method was chosen over pinning or cerclage wiring because there is less joint and soft tissue irritation. Primary bone union was achieved. (C) Cerclage wires and $\frac{1}{16}$-inch diameter Rush pin. The articular surface is not invaded.

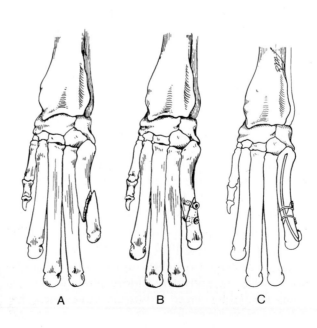

A   B   C

mm screws has increased the usefulness of this method in long oblique or spiral fractures. It is rarely possible to combine intramedullary pinning with lag screws because of the small size of the bones; thus screws are generally used alone (Fig. 13–31B) or in conjunction with bone plates (see Fig. 13–37C, D). The same general guidelines as discussed in Chapter 1 apply to the application of lag screws here.

BONE PLATES ■ Small plates are valuable in larger breeds for fixation of very unstable fractures (Fig. 13–30) and for nonunion fractures (Fig. 13–32). Because of their stability, external support does not have to be maintained as long as with other methods. Four weeks in a cast or splint is typically sufficient to allow limited active use of the limb. Plate and screw sizes typically range from 1.5 to 2.7 mm; both flat and semitubular style plates are useful. Cuttable plates (Synthes Ltd. [USA], Paoli, PA) have proven especially valuable in this application, as they allow placing of more screws in a given unit of length than conventional plates and their low profile minimizes soft tissue coverage problems. See Chapter 2 for a discussion of plating techniques.

Aftercare ■ In all cases of internal fixation, the foot should be supported in a molded splint or cast (see Figs. 2–22 and 2–27) until radiographic signs of bone healing are obvious. This typically ranges from 3 to 6 weeks. Bone plates are usually removed in 3 to 4 months, especially in athletic animals. Bone screws and cerclage wires can usually be left with no harmful effects. Intramedullary pins inserted from the distal joint area should be removed as soon as callus formation is well established. Rush pins can usually be left in place if desired.

Fracture of the Head

One of the most common injuries in this region is a fracture of the condyle. Such a fracture results in instability and luxation/subluxation of the metacarpophalangeal joint (Fig. 13–33) because the collateral ligaments of the joint originate on the condyle. The condylar fragment may be quite small (Fig. 13–33A), or it may involve half the head.

TREATMENT ■ Closed reduction and external casting usually result in an unstable joint, or the intra-articular alignment of the fragments may be poor, resulting in degenerative joint disease. Internal fixation offers the best chance for return to normal function, especially in the athletic animal. The approach is by incision of skin directly over the injury. Internal fixation may be done with wire (Fig. 13–33C, D) or by lag screws (Fig. 13–33D). Failure to repair these injuries may necessitate amputation at the metacarpophalangeal joint to restore function in the athletic animal, especially if the third or fourth bone is involved. For discussion of amputation, see below.

Aftercare ■ A molded palmar splint or cast is applied for 4 weeks, and exercise is limited for 6 to 8 weeks.

Fractures of the Phalanges

TREATMENT ■ Fractures of the head and base are handled in much the same way as described for metacarpal fractures, except that the fragments are often smaller and more difficult to secure (Fig. 13–34). As a result, amputation may need to be considered more often. Fractures of the shaft are most commonly treated by closed reduction and external fixation (Fig. 13–35), although

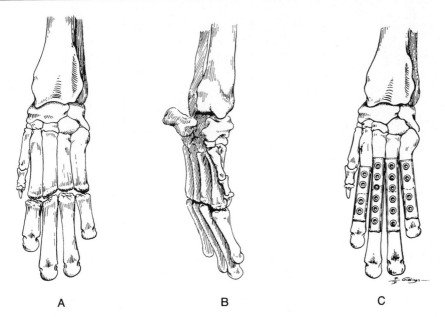

FIGURE 13–32. (*A, B*) Nonunion fracture of all metacarpals, 9 months' duration. (*C*) Multiple bone plate fixation. Size of plate will vary from a 1.5- to 2.7-mm screw size. Good healing was achieved using 2.7-mm plates and screws in this 80-pound (36-kg) dog.

internal fixation should be considered for a performance animal (Figs. 13–36 and 13–37). Surgical exposure is quite simple because the bone is immediately beneath the skin. As in the case of metacarpal fractures, both cerclage wires and lag screws are suitable as primary fixation when supplemented with external support.

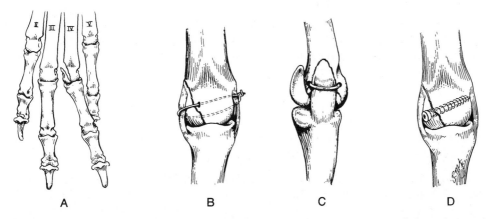

FIGURE 13–33. (*A*) Fracture of the medial condyle of the head of the fourth metacarpal bone. Valgus deformity of the toe results. (*B, C*) Wire fixation of fragments. To avoid having to drill a hole through the small fragment, two holes are drilled in the metacarpal bone and the wire (22 gauge in a 60-pound animal) passed through the holes and around the fragment. If the wire can be passed through the ligamentous tissue, it will have less tendency to slip off the fragment. (*D*) Lag screw fixation with 1.5- or 2.0-mm screws is ideal if the fragment is large enough.

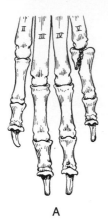
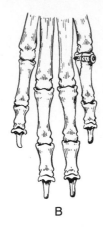

FIGURE 13–34. (A) Fracture of the base of the first phalanx. (B) Lag screw fixation using a 2.0- or 1.5-mm screw.

Aftercare ■ A molded plastic bivalve splint (see Fig. 2–28) is applied either as primary fixation or as support for internal fixation. Three to 6 weeks of splinting are usually needed for primary fixation, and 3 to 4 weeks are sufficient for support of internal fixation.

Fracture of the Proximal Sesamoids

Large-breed dogs are the primary victims of fractures of the proximal sesamoids of the metacarpophalangeal joint, although they are seen sporadically in all size dogs. This is a common injury of the racing greyhound, and the immature Rottweiler seems predisposed.[17] Excessive tension on the digital flexor tendons can cause the sesamoid bone, which is quite long and banana-shaped, to fracture near its midportion, although vascular compromise and bone necrosis has been proposed as a cause.[17] For convenience the sesamoids can be numbered from medial to lateral; because there are two sesamoids at each metacarpophalangeal joint, they are numbered from 1 to 8 (Fig. 13–38A). The sesamoids that are most commonly injured are the second and seventh (Fig. 13–38B, C). Either the forelimbs or hindlimbs can be involved. Sudden lameness occurs, accompanied by swelling, pain on palpation, and crepitus. This lameness rapidly subsides, and the animal shows lameness only on exercise. Tenderness on deep palpation over the bones remains. Bilateral injuries are not uncommon. High-detail screens or nonscreen radiographic techniques are helpful in diagnosing these fractures.

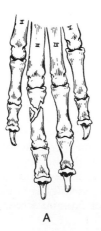
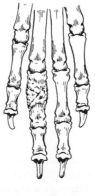

FIGURE 13–35. (A) Comminuted fracture of the first phalanx. (B) Four weeks after coaptation splintage. Although there is considerable callus at this stage, good alignment of the bone has been maintained.

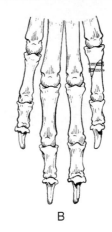
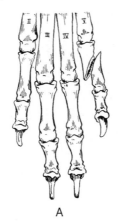

FIGURE 13–36. Because of the need for perfect reduction and rapid return to function, internal fixation with 1.5- or 2.0-mm lag screws was chosen. Such fixation must be protected by casting or splinting for several weeks.

TREATMENT ■ In the acute stage treatment may consist of splinting (see Fig. 2–28). Some fractures will heal sufficiently with splint fixation, but many will later require surgery for excision of the bone fragments. All chronic cases with persistent clinical signs should undergo operation. The bone is exposed by an incision just medial or lateral to the large central pad, directly over the joint.[1] The fragments are sharply dissected free of their ligamentous attachments. On occasion, only a small portion of the bone is fractured. If this piece is less than one third of the total bone, it is usual to leave the larger fragment and remove the smaller. When the fracture is in the midportion, both fragments are removed.

Aftercare ■ A snug bandage is maintained for 7 to 10 days postoperatively. Activity is restricted until 6 weeks postoperatively. A good prognosis can be given for surgically treated cases.

Fracture of the Dorsal Sesamoids

The dorsal sesamoid bones of the metacarpophalangeal bones (Fig. 13–1) are attached proximally to the common digital extensor and interosseous muscles,

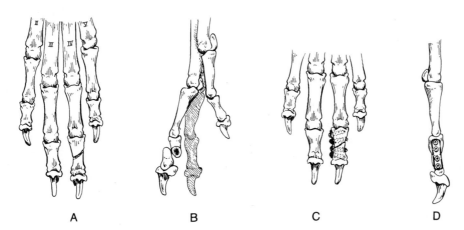

FIGURE 13–37. (*A, B*) Short oblique fracture of the second phalanx in a racing greyhound. (*C, D*) Because the fracture line was too short for a lag screw, a miniplate was used with 2.0-mm screws. An excellent functional result was obtained. The plate was left in place because it had not affected the dog's performance.

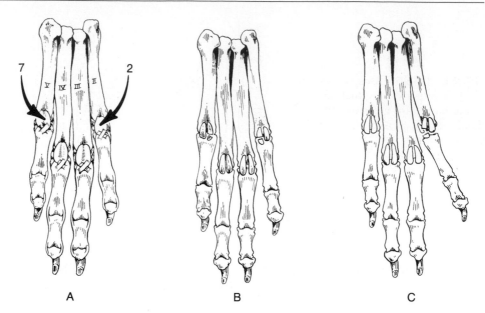

FIGURE 13–38. (A) Ligaments of the palmar sesamoids of the metacarpophalangeal joints. The sesamoids are numbered from medial to lateral. 1 to 8, with 2 and 7 being the most commonly injured. (B) Fractures of the distal third of sesamoid 7 and mid-portion of sesamoid 2. Only the small fragment of 7 is removed, whereas all of 2 is removed. (C) Fracture of sesamoid 2 with fracture of the base of the second metacarpal bone. The sesamoid is excised and the metacarpal fracture wired or lag-screwed as in Figure 13–33.

and distally via a ligament to the proximal phalanx. These small bones are rarely involved with any injury or pathological process, although they are commonly mistaken for chip fractures of the joint when seen radiographically. However, a dog has been seen in our practice that had a chronic lameness and exhibited pain and crepitus on flexion of the digits. Radiographic signs of enthesiophytes were present on the dorsal sesamoid bone and degenerative joint disease of the metacarpophalangeal joint were present. The lameness and clinical signs were relieved by surgical excision of the affected dorsal sesamoid.

Luxation of the Metacarpophalangeal and Interphalangeal Joints

Luxation or subluxation of the phalanges can occur at any joint level (Fig. 13–39), but the distal interphalangeal joint is the most commonly involved. These injuries are confined almost exclusively to racing greyhounds and working dogs. In greyhounds, the toe is usually luxated to the left side, that is, the inside of the track. In other breeds, the distribution is more random.

Clinical Signs

Lameness is usually absent to minimal at a walk when the animal is presented. Only when the dog is worked at faster gaits does it become evident that the dog is favoring a foot. Swelling, pain, and crepitus are not prominent, but the instability can be appreciated by careful palpation. The interphalangeal joints must be extended when palpating for stability to avoid rotational movement being mistaken for instability.

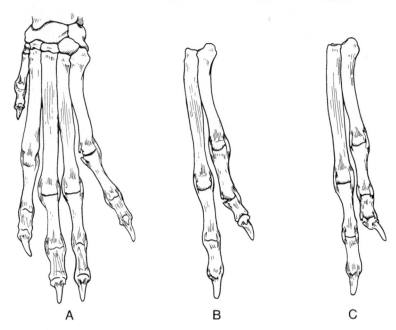

FIGURE 13–39. Luxation and subluxation of the phalanges. (*A*) Lateral subluxation of the metacarpophalangeal joint with rupture of the medial collateral ligaments. (*B*) Lateral subluxation of the proximal interphalangeal joint with rupture of the medial collateral ligaments. (*C*) Lateral subluxation of the distal interphalangeal joint with rupture of the medial collateral ligaments.

Diagnosis

Confirmation of the clinical diagnosis by radiographs is essential to rule out fractures and to allow identification of avulsions, which are treated as shown in Figure 13–33. Both total luxations and subluxations are seen.

Treatment

These are serious injuries for a running or working dog and should not be dismissed lightly. Aggressive surgical repair has yielded much better results than more conservative approaches, such as closed reduction and splintage. Many of these animals end up with instability of the joint and chronic degenerative changes in the joints that slow them markedly or leave them reluctant to traverse hard ground.

SUTURE RECONSTRUCTION ■ Surgical treatment by suture repair of collateral ligaments and joint capsule (Fig. 13–40) works best when performed within the first 10 days after injury, and the earlier the better. Fibroplasia of these structures makes accurate suturing more difficult after 10 days. Failure to stabilize the joint leaves only the alternatives of amputation (Figs. 13–41 and 13–42) or arthrodesis (Fig. 13–43). The interphalangeal joint is exposed through a dorsal incision (Fig. 13–40A). The torn joint capsule and collateral ligaments are visible beneath the skin. Three mattress sutures of 4-0 nonabsorbable monofilament or synthetic monofilament absorbable suture material are placed vertically to the tear in the capsule and collateral ligaments (Fig. 13–40B). These sutures are then encompassed within a single large purse-string mattress suture, as shown in Fig. 13–40C. Occasionally, the extensor tendon

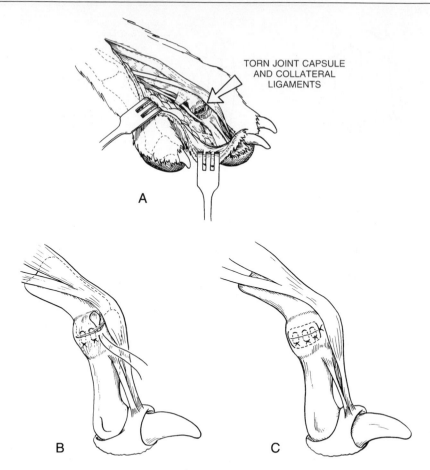

FIGURE 13–40. Suture repair of proximal interphalangeal subluxation. (*A*) The affected joint is exposed by a dorsal incision, with reflection of tissues on the side of the instability.[3] Tearing of joint capsule and collateral ligaments can be seen below the arrow. (*B*) Three main mattress sutures of 4-0 monofilament or synthetic absorbable material are placed across the torn capsule and collateral ligaments. (*C*) A purse-string–like suture encompasses the other sutures.

apparatus will be slightly luxated as a result of tearing of its retinaculum. A few sutures are placed in the edge of the tendon and joint capsule to stabilize it. After reduction of total luxations, usually only one side of the joint is unstable and that side is sutured. If both sides of the joint are loose after reduction, suture repair is performed bilaterally.

Aftercare ■ A molded plastic bivalve splint (see Fig. 2–28) is applied to the foot for 3 weeks. Following splint removal, exercise is severely limited for 1 week, after which activity is slowly resumed to normal 6 weeks postoperatively.

AMPUTATION OF TOE ■ Amputation of the second or fifth toe at any joint level is not too serious in most dogs, but in the middle toes the results are not as good because they are the main weight-bearing digits; the more distal the amputation, the better the prognosis. Although amputations usually give good results in working animals, the outcome in racing animals is more difficult to predict; some animals will run well and some will not. The surgical principles of toe amputation vary little with the joint level involved. The skin incision is

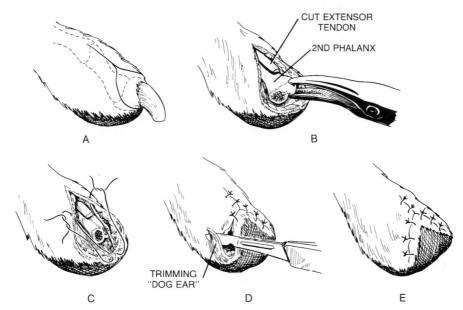

FIGURE 13–41. Amputation at the middle or distal interphalangeal joint. The procedure is drawn for the distal interphalangeal joint but does not differ in principle from a middle joint amputation. (*A*) The skin incision encircles the nail, sparing the digital pad, and continues proximally over the bones for a short distance. The incision shown would have to be extended proximally a short distance to expose the middle joint. (*B*) Soft tissue is sharply dissected away from the bone to be removed, and disarticulation is performed at the desired level. Rongeurs are used to remove the condylar portion of the remaining phalanx. (*C*) Skin sutures are placed to create a Y-shaped incision and to pull the pad over the cut end of the bone. (*D*) Excess skin is trimmed to allow smooth skin closure. (*E*) Skin suturing has been completed.

made to preserve the pad when amputation is at the interphalangeal level (Fig. 13–41*A*), but the toe pad is removed for a metacarpophalangeal amputation (Fig. 13–42*A*). The joint is disarticulated by sharp dissection, which also involves section of both the flexor and extensor tendons. It is desirable to remove the palmar sesamoids when amputation occurs at the metacarpophalangeal joint. The distal condyle of the proximal remaining bone is always removed. In the case of a distal interphalangeal amputation, the distal third of the middle phalanx is removed to provide more soft tissue between the skin and bone end (Fig. 13–41*B*). When amputating at the metacarpophalangeal level, the condyle is removed when metacarpal III or IV is involved, but bones II and V are beveled for a more cosmetic closure (Fig. 13–42*B*). Skin suturing may involve removal of skin dog ears to result in smooth skin closure (Fig. 13–41*D, E*).

Aftercare ■ A snug padded bandage is maintained for 10 days, and normal activity is not resumed until 3 weeks postoperatively.

ARTHRODESIS ■ Arthrodesis is a rational approach to metacarpophalangeal and proximal interphalangeal chronic instability in the racing animal. The most precise and predictable method of arthrodesis involves the use of miniplates or cuttable plates (Synthes Ltd. [USA], Paoli, PA) and 2.0- or 1.5-mm bone screws (Fig. 13–43*A*). Kirschner wires and a tension band wire are also applicable (Fig. 13–43*B*). Very little functional disability results from such a fusion, and joint pain is obviously banished.

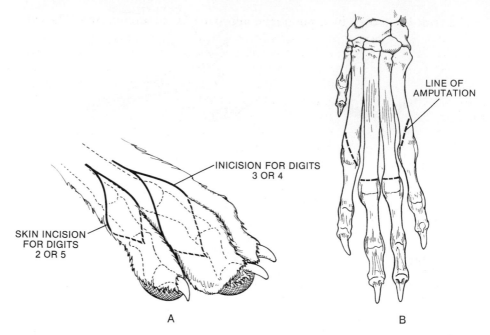

FIGURE 13–42. Amputation at the metacarpophalangeal (or metatarsophalangeal) joint. (A) Skin incisions are designed to remove the digital pad, and when sutured, they both create a straight line. (B) After disarticulating to remove the phalanges, the metacarpal bone is amputated at the indicated level. Beveling the medial and lateral bones improves the cosmetic appearance, especially on the lateral side.

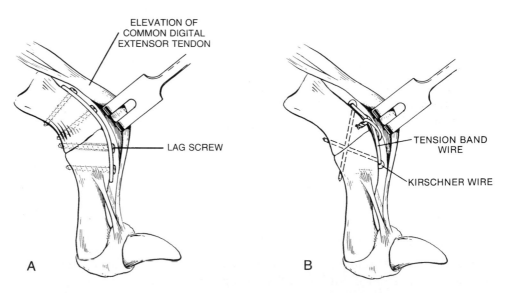

FIGURE 13–43. Arthrodesis of the proximal interphalangeal joint. Similar technique can be employed at the metacarpophalangeal (or metatarsophalangeal) joint. (A) An AO/ASIF straight Mini-Plate (Synthes Ltd. [USA], Paoli, PA) has been contoured over the dorsal surface of the proximal and middle phalangeal bones after removing articular cartilage at the joint. Mini L-Plates (AO/ASIF) can also be applied medially or laterally. Screws of 1.5- to 2.0-mm diameter are used to attach the plate. One screw has been lagged across the joint through the plate. (B) Kirschner wires and a tension band wire can also be used to stabilize this arthrodesis.

The joint is exposed by a middorsal approach as for amputation. The extensor tendon is reflected to one side by incising its retinaculum at the joint capsule. The joint is opened and articular cartilage removed by rongeurs or high-speed powered bur, conforming the surfaces to get good contact at the functional angle, which is judged by an adjacent toe. A four- or five-hole, straight mini-plate or cuttable plate (Synthes Ltd. [USA], Paoli, PA) is contoured to the dorsal surface of the bone and attached with 2.0- or 1.5-mm screws (Fig. 13–43A). An attempt is made to lag-screw across the joint with at least one screw. Bone grafting is not necessary. Alternatively, Kirschner wires can be driven across the joint and the joint compressed with a tension band wire (Fig. 13–43B).

Aftercare ■ A molded bivalve splint (see Fig. 2–28) is maintained for 6 weeks, at which time radiographic signs of healing should be seen. Exercise is slowly increased for 3 to 4 weeks before full activity is allowed.

References

1. Piermattei DL: An Atlas of Surgical Approaches to the Bones and Joints of the Dog and Cat, 3rd ed. Philadelphia, WB Saunders Co, 1993.
2. Earley T: Canine carpal ligament injuries. Vet Clin North Am 8:183, 1978.
3. Punzet G: Luxation of the os carpi radiale in the dog—pathogenesis, symptoms and treatment. J Small Anim Pract 15:751, 1974.
4. Johnson KA: Accessory carpal bone fractures in the racing Greyhound: Classification and pathology. Vet Surg 16:60, 1987.
5. Johnson KA, Piermattei DL, et al: Characteristics of accessory carpal bone fractures in 50 racing Greyhounds. Vet Comp Orthop Trauma 2:104, 1988.
6. Johnson KA, Dee JF, Piermattei DL: Screw fixation of accessory carpal bone fractures in racing Greyhounds: 12 cases (1981–1986). J Am Vet Med Assoc 194:1618–1625, 1989.
7. Lenehan TM, Tarvin GB: Carpal accessorioulnar joint fusion in a dog. J Am Vet Med Assoc 194:1598–1600, 1989.
8. Parker RB, Brown SG, Wind AP: Pancarpal arthrodesis in the dog: A review of forty-five cases. Vet Surg 10:35, 1981.
9. Willer RL, Johnson KA, et al: Partial carpal arthrodesis for third degree carpal sprains. A review of 45 carpi. Vet Surg 19:334–340, 1990.
10. Simpson D, Goldsmid S: Pancarpal arthrodesis in a cat: A case report and anatomical study. Vet Comp Orthop Trauma 7:45–50, 1994.
11. Kellar W, Chambers J: Antebrachial metacarpal arthrodesis for fusion of deranged carpal joints in two dogs. J Am Vet Med Assoc 195:1382–1384, 1989.
12. Chambers JN, Bjorling DE: Palmar surface plating for arthrodesis of the canine carpus. J Am Anim Hosp Assoc 18:875, 1982.
13. Swaim SF: Management and bandaging of soft tissue injuries of dog and cat feet. J Am Anim Hosp Assoc 21:329, 1985.
14. Morgan PW, Binnington AG, et al: The effect of occlusive and semi-occlusive dressings on the healing of acute full-thickness skin wounds on the forelimbs of dogs. Vet Surg 23:494–502, 1994.
15. Beardsley SL, Schrader SC: Treatment of dogs with wounds of the limbs caused by shearing forces: 98 cases (1975–1993). J Am Vet Med Assoc 207:1071–1075, 1995.
16. Specht TE, Colahan PT: Osteostixis for incomplete cortical fracture of the third metacarpal bone: Results in 11 horses. Vet Surg 19:34–40, 1990.
17. Cake MA, Read RA: Canine and human sesamoid disease. Vet Comp Orthop Trauma 8:70–75, 1995.

PART III

FRACTURES AND ORTHOPEDIC CONDITIONS OF THE HINDLIMB

- Cauda equina lesion
- Bone, cartilage, or synovial tumor
- Hypertrophic osteoarthropathy

Hip Region
- Degenerative joint disease, secondary to hip dysplasia
- Luxation

Stifle Region
- Degenerative joint disease, primary or secondary
- Rupture of cruciate and collateral ligaments, meniscal injury
- Patellar luxation
- Long digital extensor luxation

Tarsal Region
- Ligamentous instabilities/hyperextension
- Avulsion of the gastrocnemius tendon
- Luxation of the tendon of the superficial digital flexor muscle
- Degenerative joint disease, primary or secondary

HINDLIMB LAMENESS IN SMALL-BREED, SKELETALLY IMMATURE DOGS

General/Multiple
- Trauma—fracture, luxation

Hip Region
- Avascular necrosis/Legg-Calvé-Perthes disease

Stifle Region
- Patellar luxation

Tarsal Region
- Varus deformity due to premature physeal closure of distal tibia

HINDLIMB LAMENESS IN SMALL-BREED, SKELETALLY MATURE DOGS

General/Multiple
- Trauma—fracture, luxation, muscle and nerve injuries
- Spinal cord lesion—disk, tumor

Hip Region
- Degenerative joint disease, primary or secondary
- Luxation

Stifle Region
- Degenerative joint disease, primary or secondary
- Rupture of cruciate ligaments
- Patellar luxation
- Luxation of long digital extensor tendon

Tarsal Region
- Luxation of the tendon of the superficial digital flexor muscle
- Degenerative joint disease, primary or secondary
- Inflammatory joint disease

14

Fractures of the Pelvis

Fractures of the pelvis are relatively common, and in many veterinary practices they constitute 20 to 30 percent of all fractures. Most fractures are multiple in that three or more bones are involved. Rarely are they open or compound.

ANATOMY

Structurally, the pelvis roughly forms a rectangular box and is made up of the ossa coxae (ilium, ischium, and pubis), sacrum, and first coccygeal vertebra (Figs. 14–1 and 14–2). The structure is well covered with muscles and soft tissues. In fractures with minimal displacement, the muscles serve very effectively in supporting the bones. If there is gross displacement of the fracture segments, spastic contraction of the muscles increases the difficulty of surgical reduction and fixation.

FRACTURE CATEGORIES

Pelvic fractures can be grouped into six anatomical areas.[1]

SACROILIAC FRACTURE/LUXATION ■ Luxation of the sacroiliac joint, fracture of the sacral wing, or partial sacroiliac luxation with partial fracture of the sacral wing.

ILIAL WING FRACTURE ■ Fracture of the non–weight-bearing and nonarticular portion of the ilial wing.

ILIAL BODY FRACTURE ■ Ilial fracture between the sacroiliac joint and the acetabulum.

ACETABULAR FRACTURE ■ Any fracture involving the articular surface; may extend into the ilium or ischium.

ISCHIAL FRACTURE ■ Fracture of the ischial body, ramus, or fracture/avulsion of the tuber ischium.

PELVIC FLOOR FRACTURE ■ Fractures of the pelvic symphysis, pubic body or ramus, and ischial ramus.

HISTORY AND EXAMINATION

The patient's history usually includes traumatic injury and a sudden onset of symptoms. Because of the degree of trauma necessary to fracture the pelvis or

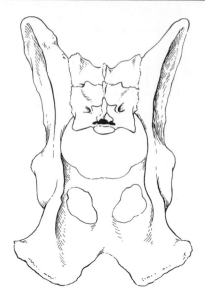

FIGURE 14–1. Pelvis, caudodorsal aspect.

cause a fracture-luxation, adjacent tissue and surrounding organ systems must be carefully evaluated. Fractures of the pelvis are always multiple in nature and, if displacement is present, at least three or more bones are assumed to be fractured. Dogs typically are weight bearing on three legs with unilateral injuries, but may also be weight bearing on all limbs with bilateral injuries. Inability to stand can be associated with neurological injury or extreme pain, which is seen most commonly with sacral injuries.

Examination should include:

1. Physical examination and evaluation of the entire body.

2. Special emphasis on some of the more common complicating injuries—traumatic lung syndrome, traumatic myocarditis, pneumothorax (chest radiographs are taken routinely), rupture of the bladder or urethra, fractures of the spine, fractures of the femoral head and neck, and neurological deficits.

3. Neurological examination of the rear limbs should be evaluated with the reservation that pain may obtund some reflexes such as proprioception and withdrawal. Include observation for voluntary leg movement while supporting the trunk, deep pain reflexes on all four toes of each foot, femoral nerve reflex (knee jerk), sciatic nerve reflex (withdrawal), as well as observations of the rectum and perineal reflex.

4. Palpation of the pelvic bones with emphasis on normal relationships between the bony prominences such as the tuber coxae and ischii, and the greater

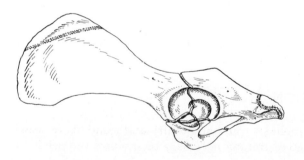

FIGURE 14–2. Left os coxae of young dog, lateral aspect, showing the acetabulum made up of the ilium, ischium, pubis and acetabular bones, and physis of ilium and ischium.

trochanter. Palpation is rarely adequate to form a good picture of the bone damage, and radiographs are always imperative. A digital rectal examination will provide information about pelvic canal compromise due to displaced bone fragments. Blood on the glove should lead to suspicion of rectal perforation/laceration, and inability to palpate the prostate in males would be suspicious of urethral avulsion.

5. Radiographs including ventrodorsal and lateral views. A lateral radiograph is taken with the affected side down, the lower hip flexed, and the upper hip extended. Tilting the pelvis to produce a slightly oblique view helps to separate the two sides. Extension of the hind legs for the ventrodorsal view can often be painful; the frog-leg position is adequate for initial evaluation. Complete radiographic examination may require anesthesia because of pain, and therefore may have to be postponed until the patient is stable. If surgical treatment is expected based on the initial films, more definitive views can be obtained when the patient is anesthetized for surgery.

PRINCIPLES OF TREATMENT

In regard to treatment, pelvic fracture patients may be divided into nonsurgical and surgical groups.[2,3]

Nonsurgical Group

Included in the nonsurgical group are patients with little or no displacement of the fracture segments, an intact acetabulum, and continuity of the pelvic ring remaining essentially intact. The pelvic musculature serves very effectively in immobilizing the fracture segments. Perfect anatomical alignment of fractures involving the bones of the pelvis (other than articular surfaces) is not necessary for healing or function. While posttreatment function may be adequate for most pets, the prognosis is much less certain for performance animals.

Management of the patient usually consists of cage rest, limitation of activity, and measures to ensure regular urination and defecation. To help prevent the development of decubital ulcers, a well-padded kennel is needed, particularly for those patients who are temporarily nonambulatory; many patients are able to stand up and move around within a day or two, or, in the case of multiple fractures, in a week or two. For large breeds, an enclosed space that can be covered with a thick layer of clean straw makes an excellent bedding that will carry urine away from the skin. Healing time for bones of the pelvis is approximately the same as for other bones in the body.

Surgical Group

Surgical intervention should be considered in animals with pelvic fractures characterized by one or more of the following[2,3]:

1. Marked decrease in the size of the pelvic canal.
2. Fracture of the acetabulum (displacement of articular surfaces).
3. Instability of the hip due to fracture of ilium, ischium, and pubis.
4. Unilateral or bilateral instability, particularly if accompanied by coxofemoral dislocation or other limb fractures.

Careful study of the radiographs can show the type and location of the fractures involved and can suggest the appropriate surgical approach. In some multiple fractures, it may be necessary to use a combination of approaches to expose the involved areas and to accomplish reduction and fixation. Most pelvic fractures are accompanied by extensive muscle trauma, hemorrhage, and soft tissue injury. Such conditions usually result in increased surgical risk. The condition of the patient may prohibit carrying out all of the surgery that may be indicated. Traumatic lung or myocardial syndromes may complicate anesthesia and delay surgery for 3 to 6 days. Reduction and fixation are accomplished much more easily and accurately if undertaken within the first 4 days of injury. Each day of delay adds to the injuries to major nerves and blood vessels and to the time required to obtain reduction of the bones. In some instances, a prolonged delay may limit or prevent surgical repair. The chief advantages of early reduction and fixation are minimal hospitalization time, early ambulation, and minimization of fracture disease.

The various means of fixation for pelvic fractures commonly include intramedullary pins, Kirschner wires, bone plates, bone screws, and interfragmentary wiring, or a combination of these techniques. Clinical experience indicates that the highest percentage of successful cases have been treated with bone plates and screws. For surgical treatment of pelvic fractures, *major emphasis is placed on the sacroiliac joint, ilium, and acetabulum.* If these three areas are properly reduced and fixed, the other areas (ischium, pubis) as a rule will be adequately reduced and stabilized, and, with very few exceptions, need no specific surgical treatment. In most cases, it is to the surgeon's advantage to proceed in the order of sacroiliac joint, ilium, and acetabulum if all three are involved. If the ilium and acetabulum are involved, reduction and fixation of the ilium first gives stability to the cranial portion of the acetabulum; thus, there is a stable segment to build on for reduction and fixation of the remaining portion.

SACROILIAC FRACTURE-LUXATION

In this condition, the ilium is usually displaced craniodorsally, with a portion of the sacral wing often remaining attached to it. Displacement is always accompanied by fractures of the pubis and ischium or by separation along the pelvic symphysis, making half of the os coxae unstable. Injury of the lumbosacral trunk in the form of sensory, voluntary motor, and reflex neurological abnormalities are common with these injuries. In two studies of pelvic fractures, 11 percent had peripheral nerve injury, and 41 percent of these were sacroiliac (SI) fracture-luxations.[1,4]

Minor luxations of the SI joint with little or no displacement may be treated conservatively with restricted activity. Indications for internal fixation chiefly include pain and instability. Inability to control adduction of the limb due to pain may present a problem in some cases. In many animals, this condition is accompanied by considerable discomfort and a prolonged period of favoring the involved rear limb, particularly when the lumbosacral nerve trunk is traumatized. Reduction and stabilization speed healing of the nerve trunk. Contralateral injuries may dictate stabilization of the SI joint in order to allow weight bearing to be shared between the hindlimbs and ease the load on the contralateral internal fixation. As a generalization, SI joint instability creates less problems in smaller breeds than large breeds and there is less need for internal fixation.

Open Approach and Reduction

The sacroiliac area may be exposed dorsally by the dorsolateral approach to the wing of the ilium and dorsal aspect of the sacrum (Fig. 14–3) or ventrally by the lateral approach to the ilium (Fig. 14–4).[5] Either approach may be used; the dorsal lends itself to fracture separations alone or in conjunction with ipsilateral acetabular fractures and to contralateral fractures of the os coxae; the ventrolateral approach lends itself to fracture separations alone or in conjunction with fractures of the ilium on the same side.

From the dorsal approach, the articular surface on the medial side of the ilium lies just ventral to the dorsal iliac spine in the caudal half of the wing (Figs. 14–5 and 14–6C). After location or visualization of the fracture separation surface on both the ilium and sacrum, reduction is accomplished by

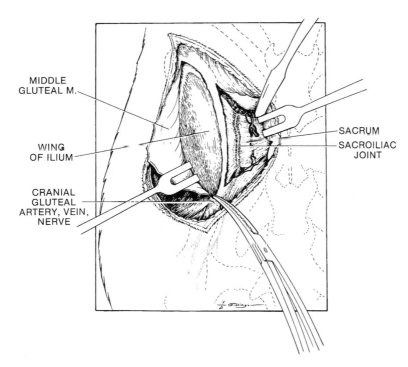

FIGURE 14–3. Dorsolateral approach for sacroiliac fracture-separations.[5] A skin incision is made over the crest of the ilium and extended caudally along the dorsal iliac spine. The middle gluteal muscle is incised at its origin just inside the cranial and dorsal borders of the wing and subperiosteally elevated from the ilium. As the caudal end of the straight portion of the dorsal iliac spine is approached during this elevation, a curved hemostat is used to run along the dorsal iliac spine to locate the caudal border of the sacrum. The cranial gluteal vessels and nerve pass from medial to lateral over the caudal iliac spine and enter the middle and deep gluteal muscles. The inserted hemostat helps to locate this area and also helps to avoid severing the cranial gluteal vessels and nerve. The hemostat is retained in place and the subperiosteal reflection stops just short of this area, thus avoiding injury to the gluteal vessels and nerve. In most cases, the tissue between the iliac crest and adjoining sacrum is separated and little additional cutting or blunt dissection is necessary to expose the opposing surfaces of the sacrum and wing of the ilium. Additional soft tissue is reflected off the dorsal surface of the sacrum to expose the sacroiliac joint. The hemostat remains in place during the entire procedure, including dissection, reduction, and fixation because it helps to protect the cranial gluteal vessels and nerve and serves as an aid in keeping anatomical landmarks in mind.

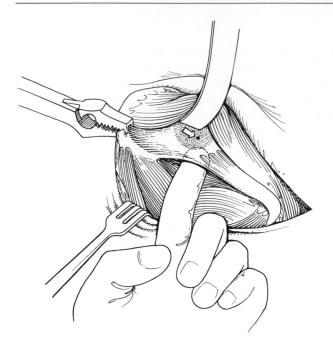

FIGURE 14–4. Ventrolateral approach for a sacroiliac fracture-separation is the same as the lateral approach for the ilium (see Fig. 14–9). In addition, the iliacus muscle is incised and subperiostally elevated along the ventromedial border of the iliac body as needed to allow insertion of one finger in the pelvic inlet.[9] The inserted finger is used to palpate the area of synchondrosis of the ilium and sacrum for reduction and screw placement. The Kern bone-holding forceps is used to move the ilium into reduction on the sacrum. The arrow and dot indicate the approximate location for inserting the lag screw through the ilium and into the body of the first sacral vertebrae. This is the same location for placement of the lag screw as in a dorsolateral approach.

grasping the edge of the iliac wing with a bone-holding forceps and moving it caudally into position. A countering cranial force on the sacrum by use of a hemostat is helpful in accomplishing reduction (Fig. 14–5). It is highly recommended that the surgeon visualize these areas on a cadaver specimen and to also be able to compare the anatomical positions of the ilium and sacrum with a bone specimen during surgery. Anatomical reduction is essential to allow for stable screw fixation.

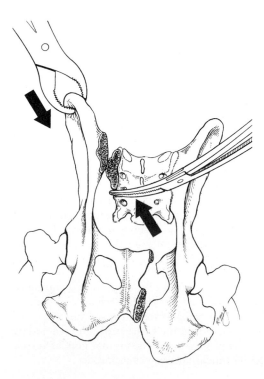

FIGURE 14–5. In a fracture-separation of the sacroiliac joint, the wing of the ilium lies in a craniodorsal position in relation to the sacrum. From a dorsolateral approach, reduction is usually accomplished by grasping the wing of the ilium with a bone-holding forceps and exerting a caudal and downward force. This is countered by a directly opposite force exerted on the sacrum by a curved hemostat or scissors.

Internal Fixation

Stabilization of the SI joint is accomplished by inserting a lag screw(s) (see Fig. 2–65) through the body of the ilium into the body of the sacrum. Two screws are stronger than a single screw of the same size, and two small screws are stronger than a single large screw.[6] Thus the ideal fixation would be two screws of the largest possible size.

Looking at the lateral surface of the ilium, the area for insertion of the screw through the ilial body and into the sacral body is indicated by the + mark on Figure 14–6C. This point is located by first dividing the length of the straight portion of the dorsal iliac crest into two equal parts. The craniocaudal location of + lies in the center of the caudal half. The dorsoventral location of + lies near the center of the ilial width in this area. The first screw goes into the sacral body (Fig. 14–6B). If a second screw is inserted, it is usually located just cranial and slightly dorsal to the first, and the length is just short of the neural canal (Fig. 14–6A). The ilial body hole should be glide hole diameter if full threaded screws are to be used. Screw length is measured on the dorsoventral view of the radiograph. A second screw is desirable, particularly where a portion of the sacrum is fractured or the first screw is not ideally placed in the body of the sacrum.

Drilling of the sacral body for the screw from the dorsal approach requires first visualizing the notch on the lateral surface of the sacrum (Fig. 14–6D). Pulling the wing ventrally and laterally aids in locating this area.[7,8] The tap hole into the sacral body should be drilled just caudal to this notch and cranial to the crescent-shaped auricular cartilage. The clear area on Figure 14–6D shows the area in which the screw can be inserted for maximum holding and that is free of important structures.[8] Although a perfectly placed central sacral body screw can penetrate the entire body, if there is any doubt about the location of the hole, drilling should proceed cautiously to a premeasured depth that will not take the drill into the neural canal. This hole is then tapped to receive the selected screw. The screw is advanced through the ilial hole and, when the tip appears on the medial side, the fracture is reduced and the screw is directed and inserted into the predrilled sacral hole.

From the ventrolateral approach, a finger is used to palpate the area of synchondrosis on the ilium and the ventral portion of the sacrum (Fig. 14–4).[9] A bone-holding forceps placed on the cranial ventral iliac spine is used to accomplish reduction. A Kirschner wire is inserted through the ilial body and into the sacrum for temporary stabilization until one or two lag screws are inserted through the wing into the sacrum. The sacrum must be drilled "blind," as it cannot be exposed for drilling as explained above. It is recommended that the surgeon visualize and palpate these areas as well as review the anatomical position of the ilium and sacrum on a bone specimen.

Note: Accurate reduction and placement of screws are at times challenging, especially if a week or more has elapsed since the injury. A common error involves screw placement in lumbar articular processes, the lumbosacral disk space, the seventh lumbar vertebra, or missing the sacrum entirely.

In some cases (e.g., in markedly overweight dogs, in impacted fractures involving a portion of the sacrum, and in some bilateral fractures), an additional stabilizing bolt will improve stability. This device passes transversely through the iliac wings and dorsal to the seventh lumbar vertebra (Fig. 14–6F). It can be either a partially threaded Steinmann pin, bent at the smooth end and with a nut placed on the threaded end, or a Hagie pin, which has a positive-thread-profile tip and a negative-profile thread at the other end to accept a nut.

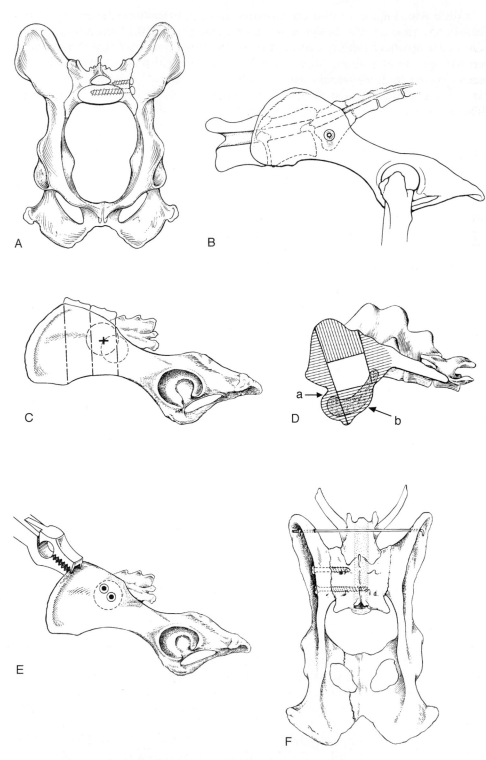

FIGURE 14–6. *See legend on opposite page*

Case Studies

CASE 1 ■ Figure 14–7A shows a mature St. Bernard with a unilateral fracture-separation of the sacroiliac joint and fractures of the ischium and pubis. On the fourth day after the trauma occurred, the animal still exhibited considerable pain on attempting to move and was unable to rise. Two cancellous bone screws were used for fixation of the SI joint (Fig. 14–7B). Reduction and fixation of the sacroiliac joint also aided in stabilization of the other fractures. The animal was able to stand and walk on the first postoperative day.

CASE 2 ■ Figure 14–8A depicts a large mixed-breed dog with bilateral sacroiliac luxations, a coxofemoral luxation, and fractures of the pubis and ischium. The animal was unable to rise and lay with its hindlimbs in the "spread-eagle" abducted position. Reduction and fixation were done using two cancellous bone screws on each side (Fig. 14–8B). It was necessary to stabilize the acetabulum before reduction of the hip joint could be maintained. An open approach was performed to reduce the hip joint and suture the joint capsule. The legs were hobbled together for 6 days (see Fig. 14–26) to protect against abnormal abduction.

ILIAL WING FRACTURE

Since these fractures involve neither a weight-bearing nor articular area, they are ordinarily not treated surgically. Cosmetic considerations might be an indication for internal fixation under some circumstances. Pins, interfragmentary wire, lag screws, or small plates could be employed. The dorsolateral approach (Fig. 14–3) is used for exposure.

FIGURE 14–6. Reduction and fixation. (A) Craniocaudal view of the pelvis showing proper position of the lag screw into the sacral body. Penetration is usually about 60 percent of the width of the sacral body. A second screw may be inserted for two-point fixation. (B) Schema of lateral view of pelvis with screw inserted into the body of the sacrum. (C) Lateral view of the ilium; + marks the spot for drilling and inserting the lag screw. Craniocaudally, the + is located in the center of the caudal half, and proximal-distally, it is located in the center of the ilial width. (D) The area of the lateral surface of the body of the sacrum available for proper screw placement is only slightly larger than 1 cm in the average-size dog, as denoted by the clear area in D. The cross-hatched area represents a thinner portion of the sacral wing, which can only accommodate short screws. This means that for many cases, there is only room for placement of one screw within the area of the sacral body. The notches (a) along the cranial border of the sacrum and the crescent-shaped auricular cartilage (b) are used as landmarks in locating the area for screw insertion into the sacral body. (E) After reduction, a Kirschner wire is inserted for temporary stabilization. The first lag screw is inserted through the ilium and into the sacral body. When a second screw is inserted, it is usually located slightly cranial and proximal. The depth for drilling this hole and length of the lag screw to be inserted are determined from the ventrodorsal radiograph. The drill hole and screw should stop just short of the neural canal. Two-point fixation is preferred in most cases. (F) If additional fixation is indicated for stabilization, a transilial bolt passing through the wings and over the dorsal surface of L7 may be inserted.

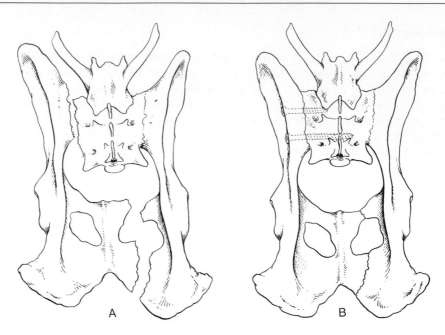

FIGURE 14–7. (*A*) Mature St. Bernard with a unilateral fracture-separation of the sacroiliac joint and fractures of the ischium and pubis. (*B*) Postoperative view showing two cancellous bone screws used for fixation.

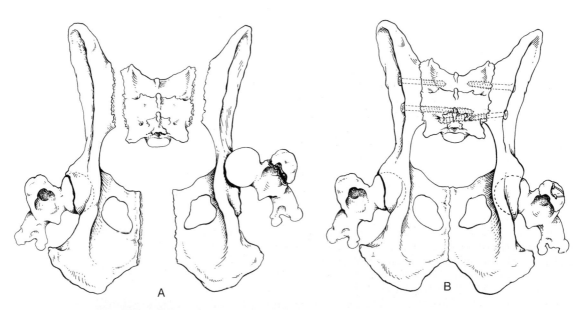

FIGURE 14–8. (*A*) Large dog with bilateral sacroiliac separations, a coxofemoral dislocation, and fractures of the pubis and ischium. (*B*) Postoperative view showing two cancellous bone screws on each side used for fixation. The acetabulum must be stabilized before reduction of the hip joint can be maintained. A dorsolateral approach was used to expose the hip joint; after reduction, the ruptured joint capsule was sutured in place.

ILIAL BODY FRACTURE

Most fractures of the ilial body are oblique in nature, and the caudal segment is depressed medially, resulting in a decreased size of the pelvic canal (see Fig. 14–10).[2,3] Some fractures are multiple, and most are accompanied by fractures of the ischium and pubis. Reduction and stable fixation of ilial body fractures aids in lining up and stabilizing fractures of the ischium and pubic bones (see Fig. 14–10C, D). If the body of the ischium is also fractured the hip joint will be quite unstable (see Fig. 14–11). Internal fixation of ilial body fractures is the most common surgical repair of the pelvis.

Open Approach and Reduction

Figure 14–9 shows an approach to the lateral surface of the ilium.[5] Reduction usually consists of a combination of levering, traction, and rotation. The caudal segment generally needs to be levered out from underneath (medial, or deep, to) the cranial segment. A bone-holding forceps on the greater trochanter (Fig. 14–10D) may be helpful in maneuvering and realigning the caudal segment. If the ischium is not fractured, a bone-holding forceps on the the ischiatic tuberosity, as shown for acetabular fracture reduction (see Fig. 14–14A), can also be used. Final reduction and fixation will vary according to the type fixation used. Application of a bone plate does not require total reduction initially, as explained below.

Internal Fixation

Many methods of fixation for fractures of the ilium have been presented and used. The highest percentage of successful cases, and ease of application, can be attributed to the use of bone plates. Plating of the ilium is very straightforward, requires a fairly small inventory of implants, and is an excellent place to

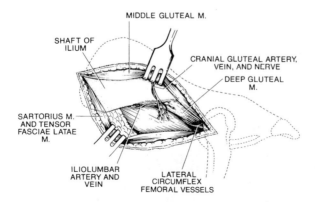

FIGURE 14–9. Approach to the lateral surface of the ilium.[5] Subperiosteal reflection upward of the middle and deep gluteal muscles exposes the ventral border and lateral surface of the body and wing of the ilium. The primary structures of importance encountered in this approach are the lateral circumflex femoral vessels (just cranial to the acetabulum), the cranial gluteal nerve (midway), and the iliolumbar vessels (located at the caudal iliac spine). The iliolumbar vessels are cut and ligated in carrying out the approach. The cranial gluteal vessels and nerve may be cut if necessary to obtain adequate exposure.

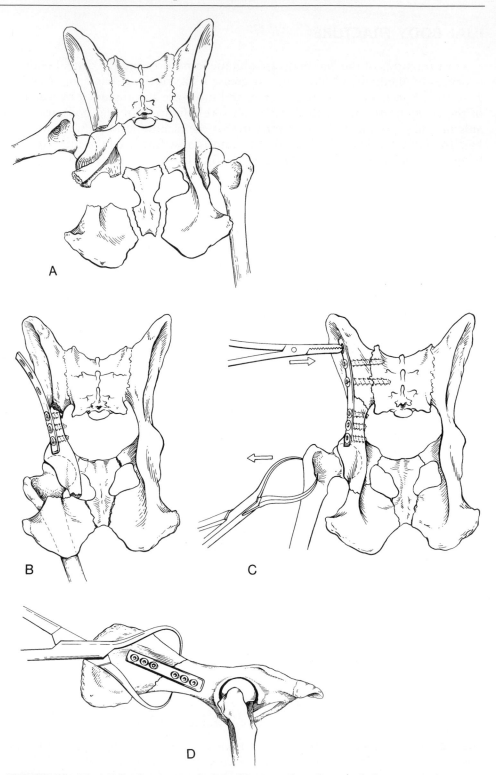

FIGURE 14–10. (*A*) Reduction and plate fixation of an iliac shaft fracture with accompanying fractures of the ischium and pubis. (*B*) A contoured plate is first attached to the caudal iliac segment. (*C*) Lateral traction by way of the trochanter major and medial pressure on the cranial end of the bone plate bring about reduction of all of the fractures. Cranial screws are then placed. (*D*) Bone-holding forceps maintains reduction while cranial screws are placed.

gain experience in bone plating before doing long-bone fractures. In certain cases (e.g., long oblique fractures and in relatively lean animals), the insertion of lag screws or pins and compression wire is very effective.

Bone Plates

There are two methods of plate application for ilial body fractures:

1. If the fracture can be adequately reduced, self-retaining bone forceps (e.g., compression, speed-lock, or Verbrugge forceps) are helpful in accomplishing and maintaining reduction while fixation is applied (Fig. 14–10D). A K-wire driven across the fracture line (see Fig. 14–12B, C) will help prevent sliding motion at the fracture line if there is difficulty maintaining stability with the forceps.

2. When the fracture can only be semireduced, the plate is first applied to the caudal segment (see Fig. 14–10B). Lateral traction is exerted on the trochanter major along with medial pressure on the cranial end of the plate prior to and during insertion of the bone screws into the cranial segment, which should proceed from caudal to cranial (see Fig. 14–10C). Driving the screws through the contoured plate (see below) acts to reduce the fracture.

The length and type of bone plate depends on the location of the fracture line, the limiting factor being the distance between the fracture line and the acetabulum. If there is room enough, a six-hole straight plate is applied as in Figure 14–10D. Anchoring one or more screws in the body of the sacrum greatly increases the holding power of the cranial screws. The cranial part of the wing of the ilium is thin, and screws may strip easily. Compression of the fracture line is desirable but seldom possible due to the obliquity of the fracture line. Two screws are sufficient in the caudal segment if the distance is short. If the distance is too short for two screws in a straight plate, T-plates, L-plates, or reconstruction plates (see Fig. 14–16B) may be necessary. The ilial plate must be bent slightly more concave than the normal curvature of the ilium, which is judged from the contralateral side on the dorsoventral radiograph. This is essential to help restore the normal size of the pelvic canal, which will always collapse slightly postoperatively due to the animal's tendency to lie on the operated side.

Figure 14–11 shows an oblique fracture of the ilium along with fractures of the ischium and pubis and sacroiliac luxation on the opposite side. If attention is directed toward reduction and fixation of the sacroiliac separation and the fractured ilium, the rest of the fractures will usually align in a satisfactory manner. The sacroiliac joint was treated first and stabilized with the use of two cancellous screws. This made reduction easier on the opposite side. The lateral approach was used to expose the ilium, which was fixed by the use of a bone plate. Note how the plate is contoured in a concave fashion to restore the pelvic canal to normal size and to realign the fractured ischium.

Lag Screws

Mechanical and case studies have shown that two or more lag screws (Fig. 14–12A) can be an effective method of stabilizing oblique fractures of the ilial body when the length of the fracture line is equal to two times the dorsoventral measurement of the ilium.[10,11] Shorter obliquities do not allow the screws to be placed at an effective angle to provide angular stability. The fracture is exposed by the lateral approach to the ilial body (Fig. 14–9).[5] The iliacus muscle is elevated from the ventral edge of the ilium and is retracted medially with a

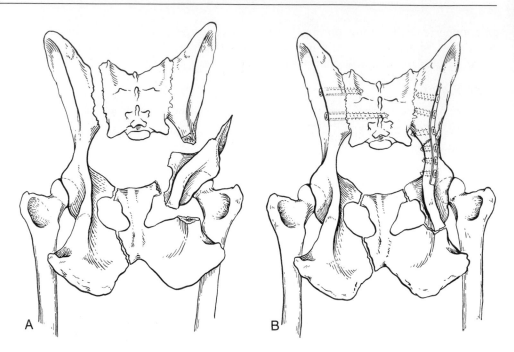

FIGURE 14–11. (A) Oblique fracture of the ilium, along with fractures of the ischium and pubis; sacroiliac separation on opposite side. (B) The sacroiliac is stabilized by two cancellous screws; a lateral approach exposes the ilium, which was fixed by use of a bone plate.

Hohmann retractor to allow drilling into the ilial body. If the animal is heavily muscled or obese it may be difficult to obtain the proper angle for the drilling. In this case, a smooth intramedullary (IM) pin can be used for drilling the screw hole, as the pin can be introduced into the exposed bone after passing it through soft tissues at the required angle. A cancellous screw can be used if the threads do not cross the fracture line; otherwise, a full threaded screw and glide hole are necessary. Self-tapping screws are advantageous, as it can be difficult to introduce a tap at the required angle. The ilial bone may also be soft enough to allow the use of a nontapping cortical thread screw without cutting threads in the bone with a tap.

Pins and Compression Wire

This technique (Fig. 14–12B, C) can be substituted for the screw technique, especially in smaller breeds, where screw size can be a problem. It is essential that a minimum of two pins be used to ensure angular stability and that the wire be tight enough to provide interfragmentary compression. The wire can be placed around the protruding ends of the pins or between two short screws in the ilium.

FRACTURES OF THE ACETABULUM

Conservative Treatment

Fractures of the acetabulum in skeletally immature animals that show no displacement on ventrodorsal and lateral radiographs may be treated conser-

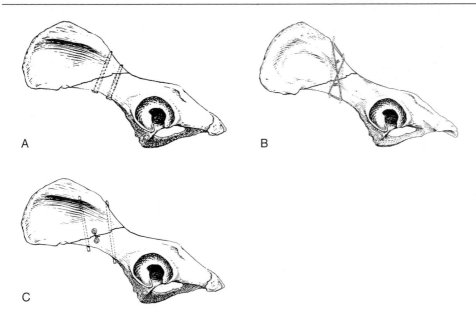

FIGURE 14–12. Ilial body fracture fixation methods. (*A*) Lag screw fixation is as stable as plate fixation, but is technically difficult in small breeds, in heavily muscled breeds, and in obese patients. (*B*) Two Kirschner wires and an interfragmentary wire to provide compression offer good stability and can be applied to small breeds. There is no specific advantage to crossing the wire in this application. (*C*) Another method of providing interfragmentary compression with Kirschner wire fixation is to place the compression wire between screws set on each side of the fracture line. Less dorsal muscle elevation is required as compared to *B*.

vatively, with marked restriction of activity indicated for 3 to 4 weeks. In most cases, it is advantageous to place the leg in a non–weight-bearing or Ehmer sling for a period of 10 to 14 days (see Figs. 2–31 and 2–32). Conservative treatment of apparently nondisplaced or non–weight-bearing area fractures in adult animals often yields disappointing results in the long run, with degenerative joint disease being the all-too-common sequela. Femoral head and neck excision arthroplasty or total hip replacement are indicated in this situation (see Chapter 15) if medical treatment is not successful.

Surgical Treatment

Open approach and internal fixation is indicated for those cases in which dislocation or instability of the fractured segments is present, and for any performance animal.[2,3,12] Crepitation is usually felt on movement of the hip joint. If these cases are untreated, pain and permanent lameness follow as a result of abnormal wear and ensuing degenerative joint disease. Another reason for surgical treatment is that the animal frequently lies on the affected side, which further displaces the fracture fragments. Early surgical intervention is needed to prevent chondromalacia of the femoral head due to abrasion from the acetabular fracture fragments.

If there is fragmentation of the fracture, the chances of successful internal fixation are reduced, especially if the fragments are too small to be stabilized, and when they involve the articular surface. This is often difficult to ascertain from preoperative radiographs. Therefore, the owner must often be given an uncertain prognosis preoperatively. Femoral head and neck excision arthroplasty is a reasonable primary treatment for irreducible acetabular fractures, and it is a good idea to discuss this preoperatively with the owner. If delayed total hip replacement is considered for long-term treatment, some reduction and stabilization is desirable to provide a reasonably intact acetabulum for later anchorage of the acetabular prosthesis.

Open Approach and Reduction

Figure 14–13 shows the approach to the craniodorsal and caudodorsal aspects to the hip joint with osteotomy of the greater trochanter.[5] The tendons of the obturator and gemellus muscles are only cut when access is needed to the most caudal part of the acetabulum.

The method of reduction varies with the type and location of the fracture. Acetabular fractures are often combined with ilial body fractures, and in such cases it is best to reduce and stabilize the ilial fracture first, as it then provides one stable fragment for the acetabular reduction (see Figs. 14–20 and 14–21). In many patients, reduction consists of a combination of traction, countertraction, levering, and rotation. The caudal segment is always angled ventrally and rotated due to the combined pull of the hamstring and external rotator muscles. Reduction is assisted by attaching a Kern or Lane bone forceps to the tuber ischii by means of a small cutdown over the tuber (Fig. 14–14A). In many cases, a bone hook moved down along the medial surface of the caudal segment is helpful in the reduction procedure (Fig. 14–14A). Rarely is the fracture stable after reduction. The fracture must be held in the reduced position while fixation is being applied. Use of a reduction forcep that straddles the trochanter major and anchors on the cranial and caudal rims of the acetabulum is helpful in maintaining reduction and compression in a stable fracture (Fig. 14–14B). If the fracture is oblique, the compression forceps is placed at right angles to the fracture line (Fig. 14–14C). Extreme care must be exercised to protect the sciatic nerve during reduction. Anatomical reduction is a must in acetabular frac-

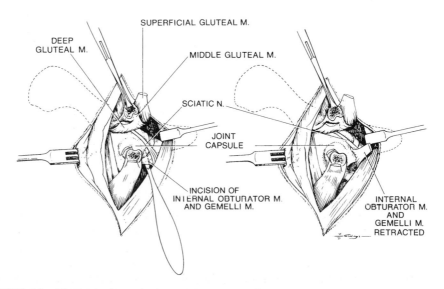

FIGURE 14–13. Dorsolateral approach to the hip joint with osteotomy of the greater trochanter.[5] Transection of the external rotator muscles close to the trochanter exposes the caudal acetabular and ischial area and the retracted muscles protect the sciatic nerve.

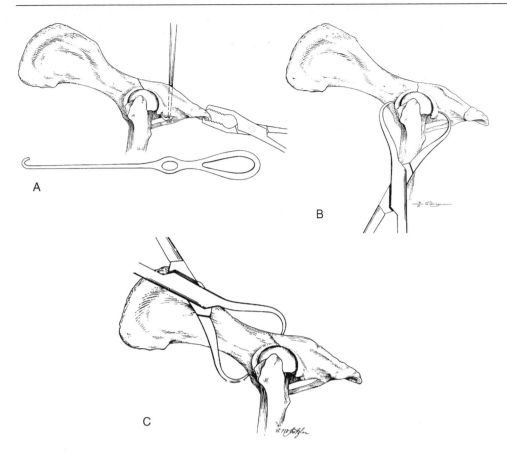

FIGURE 14–14. Aids to reduction of acetabular fractures. (*A*) Because the caudal fragment is always rotated and displaced ventrally, a small hook placed in the obturator foramen is helpful to elevate the ischium. Distraction and rotational control is gained by placing a bone-holding forceps on the ischial tuberosity after a short cutdown approach directly over the bone. (*B*) Compression of a transverse fracture can be achieved by application of a pointed reduction forceps across the acetabulum. The pointed jaws of the forceps can be introduced through soft tissues, taking care to avoid the sciatic nerve. (*C*) In a similar manner, the pointed reduction forceps is here seen compressing an oblique fracture. Avoidance of the sciatic nerve is again a consideration.

tures. Final reduction is checked by observing the fracture line, the acetabular rim, and the articular cartilage inside the acetabulum via a small capsule incision. Particular attention must be paid to rotational reduction to ensure that the central portion of the acetabular fossa is realigned.

Internal Fixation

BONE PLATES ■ The method of fixation varies with the type of fracture, but bone plates and screws have yielded the best percentage of success.[2,3,12] The various types of bone plates that may be contoured and used on acetabular fractures include standard straight, acetabular (Synthes Ltd. [USA], Paoli, PA) (Fig. 14–15), reconstruction (Synthes) (Fig. 14–16), cuttable (Synthes), and various small fragment plates. See Figure 2–74 for correct plate size relative to body weight. Reconstruction and acetabular plates lend themselves to easy contouring, which is helpful, since it is absolutely essential that the plate conform

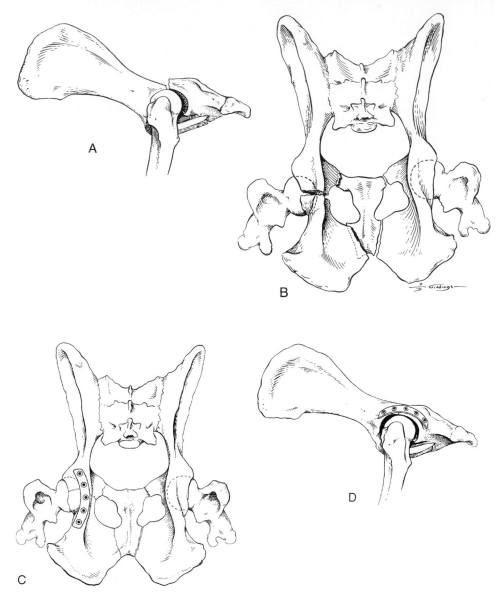

FIGURE 14–15. (*A, B*) Serrated transverse fracture of the acetabulum and fracture of the ischium and pubis. (*C, D*) With bone plate fixation, at least two screws should be inserted on each side of the fracture line. The plate should be contoured so that it fits the surface to which it is applied. In cases such as this, any one of the various types of plates could have been used: reconstruction, acetabular, regular, or small fragment.

perfectly to the bone surface. Failure to do so results in displacement of the fracture surfaces as the screws are placed and tightened. In multiple fragment fractures, the individual fragments are reduced and stabilized by K-wires preparatory to plate application (Fig. 14–16).

Lag Screws ■ Oblique two-piece fractures often present the opportunity to use lag screws as the primary fixation. When properly placed and inserted they provide very stable fixation. In order to attain the correct angle for screw insertion it may be necessary to work a tap sleeve through muscle to protect the

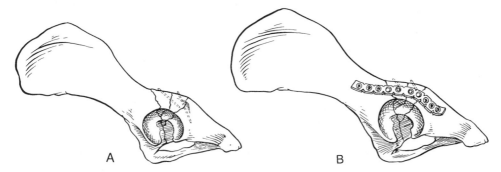

FIGURE 14–16. (A) Multiple fractures of the acetabulum; as pieces were reduced, they were skewered into place with Kirschner wires, one at a time. (B) Bone plate contoured and applied; the center two fragments are too small for screw fixation. A reconstruction plate contours very easily and is very adaptable to fractures of this type.

drill bit and tap. The two most common fracture types treated in this manner are seen in Figures 14–17 and 14–18.

Tension Band Wire ■ Tension band wire fixation (Fig. 14–19) can be used only on interlocking, stable two-piece fractures. The dorsal side of the acetabulum is used for tension band fixation, and it is essential that a small IM pin/K-wire cross the fracture line to prevent shearing motion at the fracture surfaces. Simply compressing the fracture will not prevent this type of motion. This type of fixation is not as stable as plate or lag screw, and is best reserved for small breeds, where plates and screws can be more difficult to insert.

Multiple Fractures

Fractures of the ilial body are the most common significant fracture to accompany acetabular fractures (Figs. 14–20B and 14–21A, B). Both fractures can be simultaneously reduced through the approach to the os coxae (Fig. 14–20A).[5] The ilial fracture is reduced and fixed first, as this will then give one stable fragment for reduction of the acetabular fracture. Fixation for each fracture is as detailed above (Figs. 14–20C and 14–21C). If the ilial body fracture is close to the acetabulum, a long reconstruction plate (see Fig. 14–16) can be used for both fractures. Because of the intricate contouring involved in fitting such a plate, considerable intraoperative time can be saved by contouring the plate to a similar size pelvic specimen preoperatively. Only minor corrections will then have to be made intraoperatively.

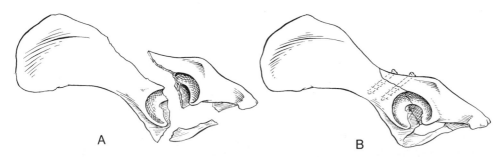

FIGURE 14–17. (A) Oblique fracture through the cranial part of the body of the ilium and acetabulum. (B) Two lag screws are preferable if there is room for insertion.

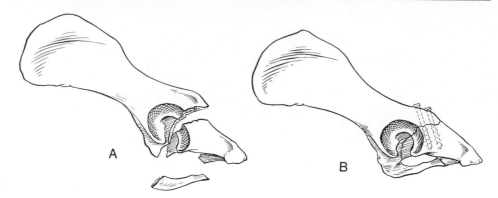

FIGURE 14–18. (*A*) Oblique fracture through the caudal part of the body of the ischium and acetabulum. (*B*) Two lag screws are inserted for fixation.

Closure of Soft Tissues

Secure soft tissue closure is important in restoring good stability to the hip joint. This consists of suturing the joint capsule, the deep gluteal muscle, and when cut, the combined tendons of the internal obturator and gemellus muscles. The osteotomized tip of the trochanter major is fixed with the tension band wire technique. The remaining muscles—the superficial gluteal, the biceps femoris, and tensor fasciae latae—are sutured in place, followed by the gluteal fascia, subcutaneous tissue, and skin.

Aftercare

Ideally the animal would be allowed early active use of the hip joint. This requires totally stable internal fixation, good owner compliance with confinement and exercise restrictions, and a patient that will not overstress the repair due to hyperactivity. If any of these elements are less than optimal, an off–weight-bearing sling (see Fig. 2–32) is advisable for 2 to 3 weeks. Exercise should be severely restricted for 6 weeks, with a gradual return to unrestricted activity at 10 to 12 weeks.

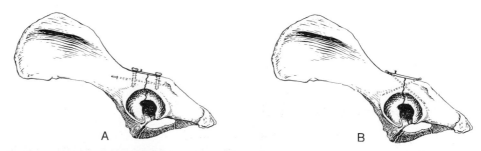

FIGURE 14–19. Additional fixation methods applicable to nonfragmented transverse fractures. (*A*) A tension band wire is place between bone screws inserted on each side of the fracture. It is *imperative* that a small pin or Kirschner wire be placed across the fracture surface to neutralize shear loads. (*B*) Similar fixation with only pins and tension band wire. At least one pin must cross the fracture line.

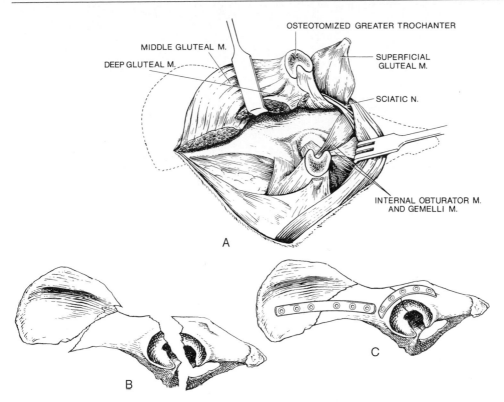

MIDDLE GLUTEAL M.

OSTEOTOMIZED GREATER TROCHANTER

DEEP GLUTEAL M.

SUPERFICIAL GLUTEAL M.

SCIATIC N.

INTERNAL OBTURATOR M. AND GEMELLI M.

A

B

C

FIGURE 14–20. Exposure and fixation of a common multiple fracture combination. (*A*) Oblique fracture of the ilia shaft and acetabular fracture. (*B*) This combination of fractures may be exposed by a combined lateral exposure to the ilium and dorsal approach to hip joint (approach to the os coxae[5]). (*C*) The ilial fracture is reduced first and fixed with a bone plate; the acetabulum is then reduced and stabilized with an acetabular plate.

FRACTURES OF THE ISCHIUM

Most fractures of the ischium accompany other fractures (e.g., the ilial body, acetabulum, or sacroiliac fracture-luxation).[2,3] If these fractures are properly reduced and immobilized, the ischium often needs no further treatment. When an ischial fracture is of primary concern (e.g., fracture of the ischial body and pubis with marked dislocation), reduction and fixation may be indicated when speed of recovery is important, when cosmetic concerns are present, when the animal is very painful, and if optimal athletic function is desirable. Ischial fractures are displaced ventrally by the powerful hamstring muscles and eventually heal in a markedly abnormal position.

Open Approach and Reduction

The cranial part of the ischial body can be exposed from the dorsolateral side by the approach to the caudal aspect of the hip joint and body of the ischium (Fig. 14–22).[5] A recently described approach involving osteotomy of the ischial tuberosity provides more exposure to the body.[13] The caudal body, ramus, and tuberosity are exposed from the caudomedial side by the approach to the ischium.[5]

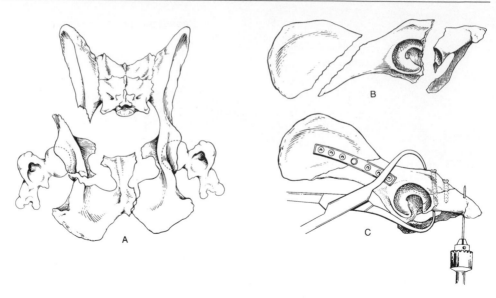

FIGURE 14–21. (*A, B*) Oblique fractures of the ilium, ischium, and acetabulum. (*B, C*) Reduction and fixation of the ilium rigidly stabilized one segment of the acetabulum, thereby facilitating reduction of the acetabular fracture. A pin through the tuber ischii and compression forceps assisted and maintained reduction while lag screws were inserted.

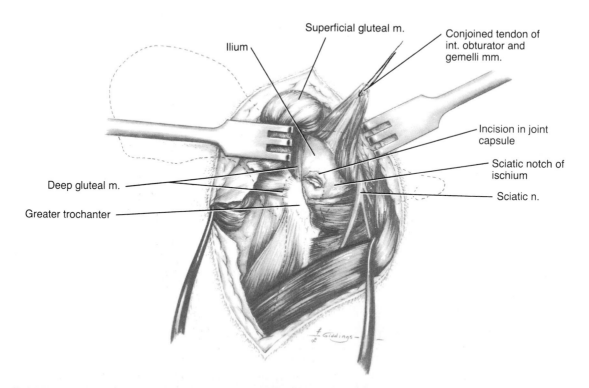

FIGURE 14–22. The caudal aspect of the acetabulum and body of the ischium can often be exposed without trochanteric osteotomy of the greater trochanter or tenotomy of gluteal muscles. (From Piermattei DL: Atlas of Surgical Approaches to the Bones and Joints of the Dog and Cat, 3rd ed. Philadelphia, WB Saunders Co, 1993, p 251, with permission.)

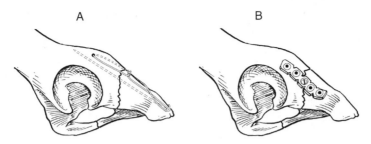

FIGURE 14–23. Fixation of ischial shaft fractures. (*A*) A pin from the ischial tuberosity and a tension band wire are biomechanically very effective. This is much easier to insert in the cat than in the dog. (*B*) The reconstruction plate (Synthes Ltd [USA], Paoli, PA) lends itself to the intricate contouring required in the ischiatic notch area.

Internal Fixation

ISCHIAL BODY ■ Fixation is usually accomplished by the use of an IM pin or Kirschner wire with a tension band wire, or small bone plate. Following open reduction, the pin is usually inserted in the region of the tuber ischium, and insertion is continued cranially beyond the fracture site until good anchorage is obtained (Fig. 14–23*A*). The addition of a tension band wire is important for stability due to the muscular bending forces; thus, the pin is less apt to loosen and work itself out prior to clinical union. The wire is usually inserted first, the pin next, and the wire then tightened. Space in this area is usually very limited because of the location of the sciatic nerve.

In larger dogs a small bone plate can be placed laterally in the ischiatic notch. The ischial tuberosity approach mentioned above would be advantageous here. Contouring of the plate is difficult; the reconstruction plate shown in Figure 14–23*B* is useful.

ISCHIATIC RAMUS AND TUBEROSITY ■ Most fractures of the ischiatic ramus and tuberosity respond satisfactorily to conservative treatment. In some patients, a sizable bone segment is fractured and pulled distally, causing considerable discomfort. The ventral surface of the ischiatic tuberosity gives rise to the powerful hamstring muscles—the biceps femoris, the semitendinosus, and the semimembranosus. Contraction of these muscles pulls the fracture segment distally (Fig. 14–24*A*). In these instances, surgical treatment may be indicated. The tuberosity fragment is fixed in place with pins, and a dorsal tension band wire is looped over a screw, or the fragment is fixed with screws alone in large breeds (Fig. 14–24*B*). Small Kirschner wires are used to hold the fragment in the reduced position while the fixation is inserted.

FRACTURES OF THE PELVIC FLOOR

As a result of traumatic injury, the os coxae may become separated at the pelvic symphysis. This may be accompanied by fracture-luxation of the sacroiliac articulation (Fig. 14–25*A*). With this injury, the animal loses the ability to adduct the legs; the rear legs abduct, and the patient is unable to stand. The condition is seen most frequently in an immature animal before the symphysis has ossified. If other fractures are present (e.g., in the ilium or acetabulum, or if there is fracture-separation of the sacroiliac articulation), proper treatment of these fractures usually gives sufficient stability so that surgery in the pelvic sym-

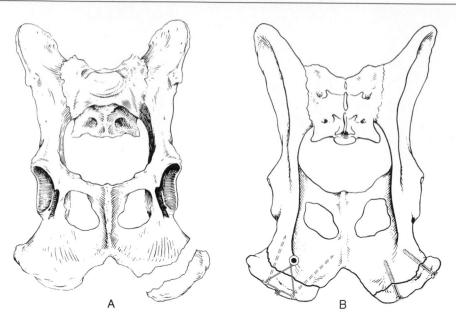

FIGURE 14–24. (*A*) The ventral surface of the ischial tuberosity gives rise to powerful hamstring muscles—the biceps femoris, the semitendinosus, and the semimembranosus. (*B*) This dorsal view shows the tuberosity fragment fixed in place with pins and a tension band wire looped over a screw on the left, or with screws only on the right. Temporary Kirschner wires were used to hold the fragment in reduced position while the screws were inserted.

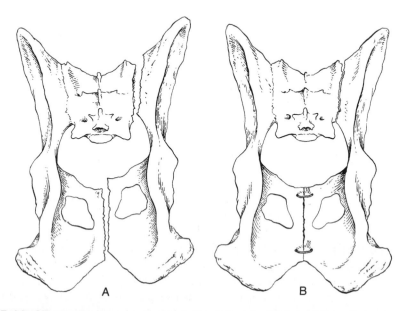

FIGURE 14–25. (*A*) Fracture-separation of pelvic symphysis and sacroiliac articulation; gross dislocation of the os coxae. (*B*) Reduction and fixation by use of two stainless steel wires. Two lag screws inserted to stabilize the sacroiliac articulation would achieve the same effect.

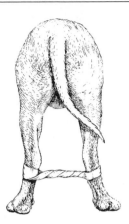

FIGURE 14–26. Rear legs hobbled together to restrict abduction until healing is under way and power of adduction is recovered.

physis area is not necessary. Primary treatment of these injuries is usually confined to adhesive tape hobbling of the hindlimbs to prevent abduction (Fig. 14–26). Usually about 1 week of hobbling will allow the animal to walk on a surface that is not slippery.

Infrequently, reduction and stabilization is accomplished by a ventral midline approach and insertion of interfragmentary wires (Fig. 14–25B).

MALUNION FRACTURES CAUSING COLLAPSE OF THE PELVIC CANAL

Healed fractures of the pelvis resulting in a marked decrease in size of the pelvic cavity are shown in Figure 14–27. This condition may be accompanied by constant or intermittent obstipation. Surgical treatment is indicated when medical treatment is ineffective in controlling bowel function.

One method of treatment involves a midline ventral approach to expose the pelvic symphysis area. The symphysis is split longitudinally with an osteotome, the two halves are carefully spread, and an allograft (body of ilium or rib) is inserted and fixed in place using two stainless steel wires. This markedly increases the diameter of the pelvic canal and returns defecation to normal, provided neurological control of defecation is normal.[2,3] Occasionally, it may be necessary to osteotomize the ilial shaft unilaterally to allow adequate spreading of the pelvis. Caution must be taken because the lumbosacral trunk may be incorporated in the bony callus on the medial side of the ilium. Plate fixation is used on the ilium.

Triple pelvic osteotomy (see Chapter 15) can also be used, although the ilial body malunion complicates fitting of the osteotomy plate.

POSTOPERATIVE MANAGEMENT OF PELVIC FRACTURES

Hemostasis prior to closure creates a smoother recovery period and minimizes complications in the operative area. A good anatomical closure by layers, particularly in the hip area, aids in rapid restoration of function and stability of the hip joint. A good skin closure is mandatory. Avascular necrosis of skin is a rare problem. If it occurs, however, it may be caused by the original trauma in the area, by unnecessary subcutaneous dissection in the operative process, or

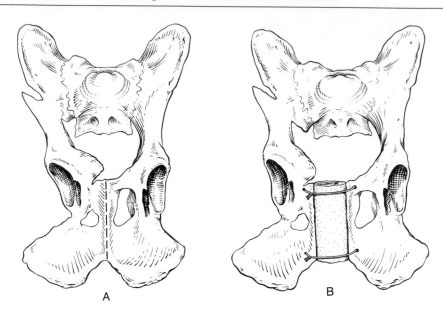

FIGURE 14–27. Healed, unreduced fractures collapsing the pelvic canal. (*A*) Healed fractures of the pelvis resulting in marked decrease in size of pelvic cavity, accompanied by constant or intermittent constipation or obstipation. (*B*). A midline ventral approach exposes pelvic symphysis area. The symphysis is split longitudinally with an osteotome. The two halves are spread, and an allograft (wing of ilium) is inserted and fixed in place using two wires. This increases the diameter of the pelvic canal and facilitates defecation.

by a combination of both. Conservative treatment is usually sufficient for a small area of necrosis, but debridement followed by secondary closure may be indicated if a large area is involved. Good nursing is an essential part of the aftercare. Particular attention must be paid to the patient's appetite, urination, defecation, and cleanliness. If the patient is temporarily nonambulatory, decubital ulcers may become a secondary complication. A dry, well-padded bed and frequent turning from side to side are good preventive measures.

Movement and restriction of activity will vary greatly with the individual case, the degree of trauma, and the stability of fixation. If good, rigid stability can be achieved, limited restricted movement should be encouraged. Local restriction of activity in the form of an Ehmer or non–weight-bearing sling (see Figs. 2–31 and 2–32) for 5 to 10 days is usually indicated in fractures involving the acetabulum and femoral head and neck or in a reduced coxofemoral dislocation. If adduction is a problem resulting from multiple fractures in the pelvic symphysis area or from muscle trauma, a restriction bandage or hobble is indicated for 5 to 7 days to limit abduction (Fig. 14–26). Marked restriction of activity is always indicated when many fractures are present. Fractures of the pelvis require the usual span of time for healing, which is normally 6 to 10 weeks. Some alteration in gait can be expected during this period. In general, bone plates and bone screws are not removed unless specifically indicated. Long-term follow-ups usually show no radiological indications of loosening or alteration in bone density.

References

1. Bookbinder PF, Flanders JA: Characteristics of pelvic fractures in the Cat. A 10 year retrospective review. Vet Comp Orthop Trauma 5:122–127, 1992.

2. Brinker WO: Fractures. In Canine Surgery, 2nd Archibald ed. Santa Barbara, American Veterinary Publications, Inc, 1974, pp 949–1048.
3. Brinker WO, Braden TD: Fractures of the pelvis. In Brinker WO, Hohn RB, Prieur WD (eds): Manual of Internal Fixation in Small Animals. New York, Springer-Verlag, 1984, pp 152–164.
4. Jacobson A, Schrader SC: Peripheral nerve injury associated with fracture or fracture-dislocation of the pelvis in dogs and cats: 34 cases (1978–1982). J Am Vet Med Assoc 190: 569–572, 1987.
5. Piermattei DL: An Atlas of Surgical Approaches to the Bones and Joints of the Dog and Cat, 3rd ed. Philadelphia, WB Saunders Co, 1993.
6. Radasch RM, Merkley DF, et al: Static strength evaluation of sacroiliac fracture-separation repairs. Vet Surg 19:155–161, 1990.
7. DeCamp C, Braden TD: The surgical anatomy of the canine sacrum for lag screw fixation of the sacroiliac joint. Vet Surg 14:131–134, 1985.
8. DeCamp C, Braden TD: Sacroiliac fracture-separation in the dog: A study of 92 cases. Vet Surg 14:127–130, 1985.
9. Montavon PM, Boudrieu RG, Hohn RB: Ventrolateral approach for repair of sacroiliac fracture-dislocation in the dog and cat. J Am Vet Med Assoc 186:1198–2001, 1985.
10. VanGundy TE, Hulse D, Nelson J: Mechanical evaluation of two canine iliac fracture fixation systems. Vet Surg 17:321–327, 1988.
11. Hulse D, VanGundy T, et al: Compression screw stabilization of oblique ilial fractures in the dog. Vet Comp Orthop Trauma 4:162–167, 1989.
12. Hulse DA, Root CR: Management of acetabular fractures: A long-term evaluation. J Comp Cont Ed 2:189, 1980.
13. Chalman JA, Layton CE: Osteotomy of the ischial tuberosity to provide surgical access to the ischium and caudal acetabulum in the dog. J Am Anim Hosp Assoc 26:505–514, 1990.

15

The Hip Joint

LUXATIONS OF THE HIP

Coxofemoral (CF) luxations in dogs and cats are generally the result of external trauma, with 59 to 83 percent due to vehicular trauma.[1,2] Most are unilateral injuries, and owing to the massive forces required to produce the luxation, about 50 percent have associated major injuries, often chest trauma.

Soft tissue damage varies considerably; however, in all luxations, a portion of the joint capsule and the round ligament is torn. In some of the more severe cases, one or more of the gluteal muscles may be partially or completely torn. Rarely, portions of the dorsal rim of the acetabulum are fractured, or a portion of the femoral head may be fractured. This is usually an avulsion fracture at the insertion of the round ligament.

The aims of treatment for this condition are to reduce the dislocation with as little damage to the articular surfaces as possible and to stabilize the joint sufficiently to allow soft tissue healing, with the expectation of normal clinical function. Most patients can be treated by closed reduction. More chronic cases and those with multiple injuries may require open reduction. Some of these may need supplementary fixation to maintain reduction. In certain cases hip luxation is irreparable because of pre-existing dysplasia, severe abrasion to the articular cartilage of the femoral head, and irreparable concomitant fractures of the acetabulum or femoral head. Such patients are generally treated with excision arthroplasty or total hip replacement, which will be covered later in this chapter.

Clinical Studies

Because of the usual history of trauma, clinical signs are associated with sudden onset, pain, deformity, crepitus, and limited or abnormal movement of the limb. The specific signs vary somewhat, depending on the location of the femoral head in relation to the acetabulum. (See Chapter 1 for a discussion of physical examination of the hip.)

Craniodorsal Luxation

This is the most common type of CF luxation, being seen in 78 percent of the time in dogs and 73 percent in cats.[1] The head of the femur rests dorsal and cranial to the acetabulum (Fig. 15–1A, B). The limb is shorter than the opposite limb when positioned ventrally and extended caudally. The thigh is adducted and the stifle is rotated outward and the hock inward (Fig. 15–1C).

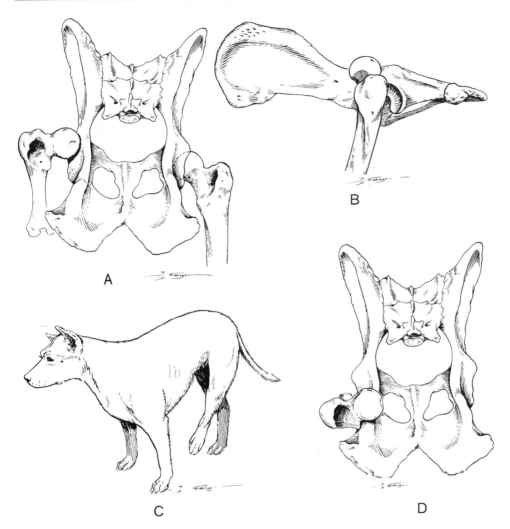

FIGURE 15–1. Luxation of the hip. (*A*) Craniodorsal luxation, dorsal view. (*B*) Craniodorsal luxation, lateral view. (*C*) Typical stance of a dog with a craniodorsal luxation. The leg is externally rotated and adducted. (*D*) Caudodorsal luxation, dorsal view. *Figure continued on following page*

On palpation, the trochanter major is elevated when compared with the normal side and the space between it and the tuber ischii is increased (see Figs. 1–3 and 1–4).

Caudodorsal Luxation

This is a rare condition and may simply be a craniodorsal luxation with a great deal of instability, allowing the femoral head to move caudally. In this case, the head of the femur rests caudal and dorsal to the acetabulum, and there is some risk of sciatic nerve injury (Fig. 15–1*D, E*). There is a slight increase in leg length when the limb is extended caudally but a decrease when the leg is positioned ventrally. The thigh is abducted, with inward rotation of the stifle and outward rotation of the hock. On palpation, there is a narrowing of the space between the trochanter major and the tuber ischii.

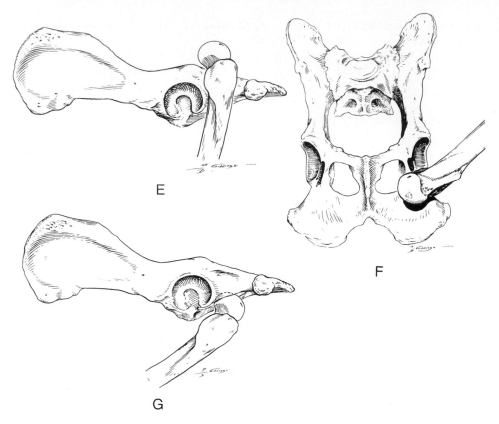

FIGURE 15–1. *Continued* (*E*) Caudodorsal luxation, lateral view. (*F*) Ventral luxation, ventral view. (*G*) Ventral luxation, lateral view.

Ventral Luxation

This relatively rare luxation (1.5 to 3.2 percent in reported case studies[3,4]) may occur as a separate entity or may be associated with an impaction fracture of the acetabulum. In nonfracture cases, the head of the femur rests ventral to the acetabulum, usually in the obturator foramen or cranial to it, hooked under the iliopectineal eminence. Cranioventral luxations are probably craniodorsal luxations that have been manipulated to the ventral position prior to diagnosis. Caudoventral luxations, however, occur spontaneously from trauma and not uncommonly are accompanied by fracture of the greater trochanter. The trochanter major is very difficult to palpate (Fig. 15–1F, G). There is a definite lengthening of the limb.

Diagnosis

Although the presence of a luxation can usually be determined on the basis of clinical signs, it is imperative that radiographs be made for each case in order to rule out several other injuries that present similar clinical signs and that will not respond to treatment for luxation. These injuries include fractures of the acetabulum, luxation of the hip and fracture of the acetabulum, and fracture of the capital femoral physis or fracture of the head or neck. Additionally, the presence of dysplasia or Legg-Calvé-Perthes disease will generally prevent stabilization of a dislocated hip after reduction. Avulsion fracture of the insertion of the round ligament (see Fig. 16–5) generally prevents successful closed reduction; furthermore, on the rare occasion when closed reduction is successful, the presence of the bone chip generally creates degenerative joint disease. All of the conditions mentioned require an open approach and specific treatment of the pathology present, as outlined in Chapters 14 and 16. If luxation follows trivial trauma (e.g., falling down two stairs), beware of underlying hip laxity associated with hip dysplasia.

Treatment

Closed Reduction

With craniodorsal luxation, the joint capsule can theoretically rupture in three places (Fig. 15–2): midway between the acetabulum and neck of the femur (type A), avulsion from the acetabulum (type B), or avulsion from the neck (type C). Type A is probably the most common type, and perhaps the kind that responds well to closed reduction. Type B results in a very unstable hip, since the fibrous lip or labrum of the acetabulum that normally aids femoral head coverage is missing. When type C is encountered, the joint capsule lies across the acetabulum like a "hammock" preventing deep-seated reduction. Upon closed reduction attempts, the femur moves to the right area but just doesn't "feel" right. It doesn't reduce with a "pop" or "snap."

When there are no complicating factors, most simple luxations can be reduced closed if they are treated within the first 4 to 5 days following the injury. As time passes, many factors will interfere with closed reduction. Reattachment of the round ligament to the gluteal muscles or to the shaft of the ilium will securely anchor the femoral head in some chronic cases. After several days, simple muscle contracture greatly limits the veterinarian's ability to reduce the luxation, particularly in large breeds. Soft tissue (such as joint capsule, hematoma, and hypertrophy of the round ligament and fat pad) within the acetabulum will block the acetabulum and prevent adequate reduction of the femoral head. For all these reasons, it is best to attempt closed reduction as soon as general anesthesia can be administered safely. Good relaxation of the animal is essential for the reduction process. For successful closed reduction to occur, the hole in the joint capsule and possibly torn muscle must be found and the femoral head returned through these holes to seat into the acetabulum.

The manipulative technique for the *craniodorsal* luxation begins by anesthetizing the animal and placing it in lateral recumbency with the affected hip

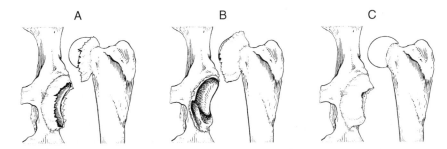

FIGURE 15–2. Types of capsular tears. (*A*) Type "A," capsule is torn midway. (*B*) Type "B," the capsule has avulsed from the dorsal rim of the acetabulum. (*C*) Type "C," the capsule has avulsed off the neck of the femur, resulting in a "hammock-like" obstruction to reduction.

uppermost. A soft cotton rope is placed in the groin area, where it can be grasped by an assistant or anchored to the rail of the surgical table and serve as countertraction. This gives the operator a fulcrum with which to exert traction on the affected leg. With one hand on the trochanter major and the other hand grasping the leg in the hock region, the stifle is rotated inward (Fig. 15–3A). An alternative method favored by many involves first externally rotating the femur, followed by traction and internal rotation (Fig. 15–3B) to clear the femoral head from rubbing on the pelvis. This is followed in both methods by abduction of the limb and firm pressure on the trochanter to guide the femoral head toward the acetabulum. With this firm downward pressure on the trochanter and sufficient abduction and internal rotation combined with traction on the limb, the femoral head can usually be felt to "pop" into the acetabulum. The movement can be felt by the hand on the trochanter. If reduction is not possible, traction is applied in different directions in order to find these "holes" in the soft tissues. Often if the head can be moved ventrally, lying cranial to the acetabulum, reduction may be accomplished by internally rotating the head while pushing up and caudally on the femoral head with the other hand. After reduction, the trochanter is pressed firmly toward the acetabulum with one hand while the hip is rotated, flexed, and extended with the other hand in order to force clots, folded joint capsule, or granulation tissue out of the acetabulum, all of which interfere with firm seating of the femoral head (Fig. 15–3B). Once this is accomplished, the hip joint is moved through a full range of motion with only light pressure on the trochanter major. In this way, the stability of the reduced joint can be determined.

A similar technique is used for *caudodorsal* luxations. If the femoral head stays in position through a full range of motion without pressure being exerted on the trochanter, the reduction is probably stable. If it luxates out of the acetabulum rather easily or seems to bind on flexion, indicating cranial reduction, additional measures need to be taken. These will be explained later in this chapter.

Closed reduction of *ventral* luxations varies with the type. Cranioventral luxations can be either manipulated directly back into the acetabulum, or else they can be converted to craniodorsal luxations and reduced as above. No attempt should be made to similarly manipulate caudoventral luxations, however, as damage may be done to bone and soft tissues. The limb is placed in traction with one hand (left hand for left limb, right hand for right limb), while the other hand applies countertraction against the ischium. The traction hand then applies a levering or lifting action on the proximal femur which is aided by the thumb of the opposite hand. The effect is to lift the femoral head laterally into the acetabulum.[4]

AFTERCARE ■ In most cases, it is appropriate to apply an Ehmer sling (see Fig. 2–31) for 5 to 7 days. If the femoral head snaps in somewhat loosely but seems to be reasonably stable, an Ehmer sling is always indicated and is generally left in place for 7 to 10 days.

To stabilize a ventral luxation, the leg is maintained in adduction by hobbling the rear legs together for 5 to 7 days (see Fig. 14–26). An Ehmer sling is contraindicated because the reduced head is forced ventrally where the joint capsule is ruptured.

PROGNOSIS ■ Failure rates of 47 to 65 percent have been reported for single attempts at closed reduction.[1,2] The presence of degenerative joint disease or hip dysplasia significantly lowers the chance of success in closed reduction,

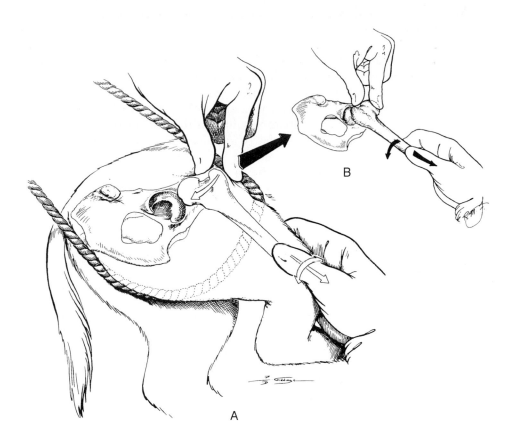

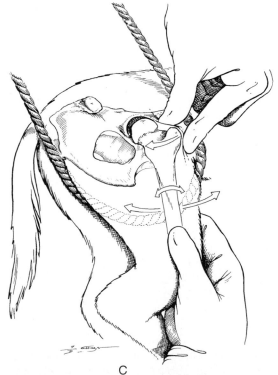

FIGURE 15–3. Closed reduction of a craniodorsal hip luxation. (A) The animal is secured to the table with a rope around the groin. The right hand pulls and internally rotates the femur to turn the femoral head toward the acetabulum while the fingers of the left hand are placed on the trochanter to help guide the femoral head. The right hand continues to pull and internally rotate the femur while abducting the limb. The left hand guides the trochanter and head over the acetabular rim. (B) Alternatively, the femoral head is first externally rotated as traction begins, followed by internal rotation. (C) Pressure is applied to the trochanter with the left hand while the femur is rotated, flexed, and extended to force soft tissue out of the acetabulum and to test stability of the luxation.

but attempts at closed reduction probably do not reduce the success of later open reduction procedures.

Open Reduction—Dorsal Luxations

Situations in which the hip remains very unstable following reduction or in which the femoral head cannot be reduced require an open approach. Open reduction is also necessary to deal with avulsion fractures of the femoral head and in situations in which immediate mobility of the patient is needed in order to better deal with concurrent injuries. If possible, the hip should be reduced prior to the approach, as it makes dissection much easier. The choice of approach varies with the situation. If the hip is reducible, the craniolateral approach is adequate. If the joint capsule cannot be adequately sutured, or if the hip cannot be reduced, the craniolateral approach is expanded by incising the gluteal tendon. If still insufficient the superficial gluteal tendon, and osteotomizing the trochanter major (dorsal approach) can be used. This approach is the method of choice for chronic luxations (over 5 to 6 days) or where extensive reconstruction is required.

After the joint has been exposed, the objectives are to remove or reduce any soft tissue that may be blocking the acetabulum, to reduce the femoral head into the acetabulum, and to stabilize the femoral head in the acetabulum. Exposure of the acetabulum is facilitated by placing a Hohmann retractor (or curved scissors) in or under the acetabulum and levering the proximal femur caudally. Soft tissue in the acetabulum should be carefully identified. Hematomas, hypertrophic round ligaments or fat pads, and muscle fragments are excised, but all joint capsule tissue is preserved. Avulsed bone fragments are removed, except in rare cases where they are large enough to be fixed in place (see Chapter 16). Following removal, a judgment must be made regarding the potential stability of the remaining femoral head. If it seems that the remaining head will not provide an adequate articular surface, a femoral head and neck excision arthroplasty or total hip replacement can be performed. Fortunately it is rare that the fracture fragment is too large to simply excise.

Following reduction, several choices are available to maintain reduction. If there is nonfrayed capsule on each side of the dislocation (type A; Fig. 15–2), simple closure with relatively heavy gauge synthetic absorbable, or nonabsorbable sutures (0 to 2-0) is used. If there is no capsule on which to anchor the sutures on the acetabular side (type B), bone screws and washers or holes drilled in the labrum can be used to attach the capsule to the pelvis. If the capsule avulses off the neck (type C), often the sutures may be attached to the muscles surrounding the trochanter major. If there is insufficient capsule on both sides, the anchorage techniques for types B and C may be used. Alternatively, suture can be anchored to the intertrochanteric fossa with a screw and washer, or holes made at the base of the trochanter major, or bony bridge of the neck (synthetic or prosthetic capsular repair). See the description in Figure 15–4 for details.

If the capsule can be closed securely, fixation will often be sufficient, although additional stability may be provided by reattaching the trochanter major distal and caudal to its original position (Fig. 15–4D). This causes a temporary retroversion and a relatively more varus position of the femoral head as a result of femoral abduction and thus seats it more deeply in the acetabulum.

When the capsule cannot be securely closed, additional measures must be taken to ensure stability of the joint until the capsule is repaired by fibroplasia. The method chosen should artificially provide stability for 3 to 4 weeks, by which time the joint should have been restored to its original stability. The

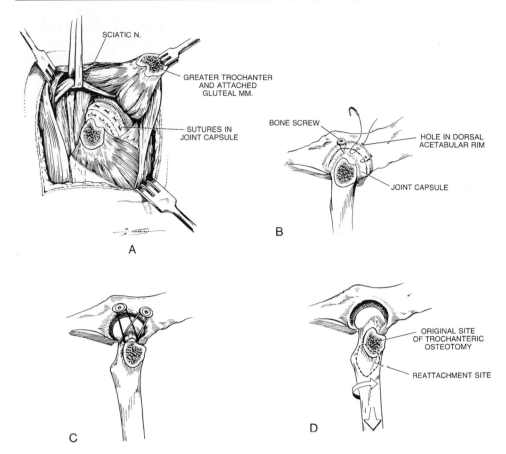

FIGURE 15–4. Open reduction of coxofemoral luxation. (*A*) The right hip has been exposed by osteotomy of the trochanter major.[6] The hip joint has been reduced and several mattress sutures are taken in the torn joint capsule. Size 3–0 to 0 synthetic absorbable or nonabsorbable suture material is used. (*B*) When the joint capsule cannot be reached to the acetabular side, a bone screw on the dorsal acetabular rim or holes drilled in the labrum can be used to anchor sutures. Nonabsorbable material is used with the bone screw, and synthetic absorbable material is used in the bone tunnels. Usually two screws are necessary to get good attachment of the entire capsule. (*C*) When no joint capsule is available on either side of the joint, two bone screws are placed on the dorsal acetabular rim, at the 11:00- and 2:00-o'clock (or 10:00 and 1:00 o'clock for the left hip) positions. A hole is then drilled transversely through the bony bridge of the femoral neck. Size 1–5 nonabsorbable sutures are tied with the limb abducted and internally rotated. Washers help prevent the sutures from slipping off the screw heads. (*D*) When the trochanter major is being reattached, additional stability may be gained by moving the trochanter slightly distal and caudal to its original site. Increased abduction and internal rotation of the femur results.

method chosen is not important to success, as all the methods suggested below have about the same rate of good to excellent results; the choice then is one that appeals to the surgeon and is compatible with the equipment at hand.

Synthetic Capsule Technique

This simple and effective technique is illustrated in Figure 15–4C. After reduction as explained above, two bone screws of suitable diameter (2.7 to 4.0

mm) are inserted in the dorsal rim of the acetabulum, at the 10:00- and 1:00-o'clock positions for the left hip and the 11:00- and 2:00-o'clock positions for the right hip. Care must be taken to ensure that the screws do not penetrate the articular surface. Metal or plastic washers are placed on the screws to prevent the suture from slipping off the head of the screws. Two lengths of size 1–5 braided polyester, monofilament nylon, or polypropylene suture are threaded through a hole drilled in the bony bridge between the trochanter and femoral head. The sutures are separated and then each is placed around a screw, under the washer. The femoral head is held firmly reduced with the hip at a normal angle of flexion and slightly abducted while the sutures are tied tightly. A few degrees of internal rotation of the limb is probably useful, as it creates femoral head retroversion, which adds stability, but external rotation must be avoided as the sutures are tied. A third screw and washer placed in the trochanteric fossa can be used to replace the drill hole.[7]

Toggle-Pin Fixation

If the capsule has been severely damaged or if the luxation is chronic, it may not be possible to stabilize the joint sufficiently by suturing the remnants. In this case, other techniques must be used in addition to reconstruction of the joint capsule.

A modified Knowles toggle-pin technique has worked well in a variety of situations, such as chronic luxations, multiple limb injuries, mild hip dysplasia, or where early use of the luxated limb is desirable.[8] The synthetic round ligament that is created is not expected to function indefinitely, but it will maintain stability until the soft tissue damage in the region of the hip joint has undergone healing with maturation of the scar tissue and reformation of the joint capsule. No evidence has ever been seen in which the suture material used to create the synthetic round ligament has created a problem in the joint. In those cases that have reluxated and been reoperated, the broken suture material has been encapsulated in the regenerating round ligament and thus was no longer intrasynovial.

Following a dorsal open approach with osteotomy of the trochanter major,[5] a hole is drilled through the femoral head and neck starting at the fovea capitis and continuing laterally to exit the femoral shaft in the region of the third trochanter (Fig. 15–5A). The size of the hole is either $7/64$ or $5/32$ inch (2.8 or 4.0 mm), depending on the size of the toggle pin used (Fig. 15–6). This relatively small hole minimizes additional devascularization of the femoral head. The drill is then used to create a hole in the upper end of the acetabular fossa (Fig. 15–5B).

The stainless steel toggle pin (Fig. 15–6) is attached to two lengths of size 0–5 braided polyester suture. The toggle pin is then placed in the acetabular hole and pushed through to the medial side (Fig. 15–5C). By means of alternate tugging on the suture ends, the toggle pin is made to turn 90 degrees to lock itself on the medial cortex of the acetabulum (Fig. 15–5D). These sutures are then pulled through the drill hole in the femoral neck (Fig. 15–5E) and held taut while the hip is returned to the reduced position (Fig. 15–5F). A hole is drilled from cranial to caudal through the lateral femoral cortex, slightly proximal to the exit hole of the sutures. One pair of sutures is pulled through the second drill hole and then tied to the opposite pair on the lateral side of the femoral cortex (Fig. 15–5G). The joint capsule is sutured to the extent possible (see Fig. 15–2A) and the trochanter major is reattached with two Kirschner wires or a tension band wire (see Fig. 16–6C, D).

Transarticular Pinning[9]

This technique pins the femoral head to the acetabulum. Complications such as pin breakage or colon/rectum penetration can occur, and this technique should be avoided if at all possible. This technique starts as described for the toggle pin, with a suitable size intramedullary pin or Kirschner wire (Table 15–1) being driven from the fovea capitis laterally through the neck and exiting the bone on the lateral femoral cortex distal to the third trochanter (Fig. 15–7A). Following reduction the femoral head is held firmly reduced with the hip at a normal angle of flexion and slightly abducted while the pin is driven through the acetabular wall into the pelvic canal. A few degrees of internal rotation of the limb is probably useful, as it creates femoral head retroversion, which adds stability, but external rotation must be avoided as the pin is driven. The entire point of the pin (5 to 6 mm) should be within the pelvic canal, and this is checked by rectal palpation by an assistant. The protruding (lateral) end of the pin is cut short but long enough to allow later removal (Fig. 15–7B). The joint capsule is closed to the extent possible.

An Ehmer sling is applied postoperatively for 10 to 14 days, at which time the sling and the pin are removed. If the hip is very unstable at the time of reduction, the pin and Ehmer sling are removed in 3 weeks.

AFTERCARE ■ Following all CF reduction techniques, the limb is usually supported in an Ehmer sling (see Fig. 2–31) for 7 to 10 days unless otherwise noted. Exercise is limited to the house or leash for 3 weeks, then gradually increased to normal over a 2- to 3-week period. Sometimes when limb fractures are on the opposite side, no sling bandage is used, and early, limited weight bearing is allowed. Bilateral luxations have also been repaired without the use of postoperative slings but require meticulous postoperative care, which includes towel support under the lower abdomen when outdoors, strict house inactivity, and avoidance of stairs.

PROGNOSIS ■ The prognosis for open reduction varies with the stability achieved following reduction and with the time interval between luxation and reduction. Cases that are reduced early with adequate stability carry a good prognosis, and essentially normal function may be anticipated in 70 to 75 percent of these cases. Those cases that have been luxated for a considerable length of time, most especially in skeletally immature animals, may result in increased degenerative joint disease and at times avascular necrosis of the femoral head. Occasionally, a hip may reluxate after reduction, although this is rare if reduction is maintained for 7 to 8 days unless there is pre-existing hip laxity (hip dysplasia). Varying degrees of osteoarthritis may develop if there has been sufficient damage to the acetabulum or femoral head. Hips that are even slightly dysplastic often will reluxate. Reluxation is an indication for femoral head and neck resection arthroplasty or for a prosthetic hip joint.

Open Reduction—Caudoventral Luxations

Although most caudoventral luxations can be handled by closed reduction,[4] nevertheless some cases require open reduction. Typically, a craniodorsal approach[5] is used if the greater trochanter is fractured, as it allows access to the acetabulum as well as to the trochanter. The joint is debrided as described above, the hip is reduced, and any available soft tissues are sutured. Once the greater trochanter is repaired (see Chapter 16), the joint is usually very stable.[3]

There are cases, however, that remain very unstable following reduction, and it has been suggested that a deficiency in the ventral transacetabular ligament is responsible.[10] A ventral approach will allow inspection of this area.[5] Two techniques have been reported for stabilizing these luxations. An autogenous corticocancellous bone graft from the iliac crest was implanted on the ventral acetabular region with success in four cases.[10] In another case, the pectineus muscle was used to stabilize the femoral head.[11] The muscle was detached dis-

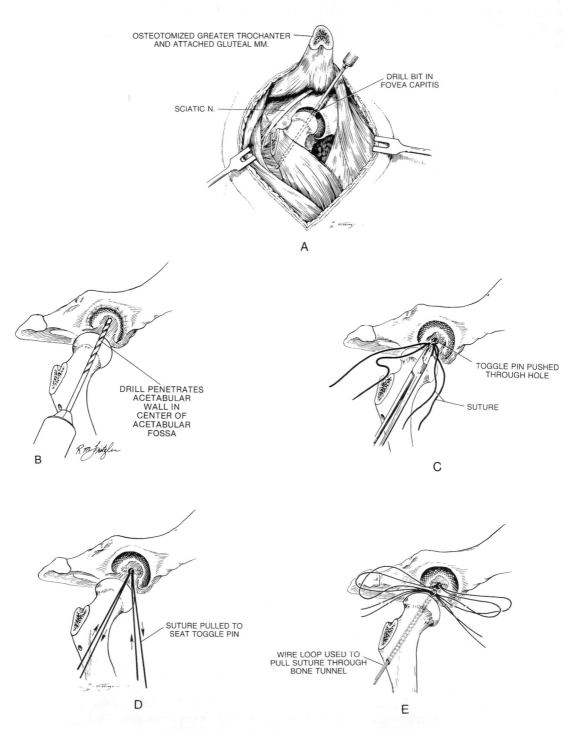

FIGURE 15–5. *See legend on opposite page*

tally and directed caudally ventral to the femoral neck, then dorsally and cranially over the femoral neck and deep to the gluteal muscles. The remaining free portion of the muscle was then sutured to any soft tissue available to hold the pectineus in position.

Remaining portions of the joint capsule are sutured and the hindlimbs are hobbled together (see Fig. 14–26) for 2 to 3 weeks postoperatively. Slow return to normal activity is allowed over the next 2 to 3 weeks. Owing to the small number of cases available for evaluation, the prognosis in this situation is uncertain.

HIP DYSPLASIA

Hip dysplasia is an abnormal development or growth of the hip joint, usually bilaterally. It is manifested by varying degrees of laxity of surrounding soft tissues, instability, malformation of the femoral head and acetabulum, and osteoarthrosis.

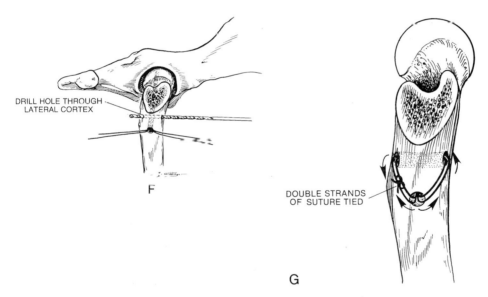

FIGURE 15–5. Toggle-pin fixation of a dislocated hip. (A) The right hip has been exposed by means of a dorsal approach with osteotomy of the trochanter major.[5] A hole is drilled from the fovea capitis, through the neck to emerge along the crest of the third trochanter. (For proper drill size, see Fig. 15–6.) (B) With the hip luxated the drill is passed through the acetabular fossa wall. Care must be taken not to penetrate too deeply. (C) The hip has been reluxated. Two strands of braided polyester suture, size 0–5, are threaded through the toggle pin (see Fig. 15–6). With the pin held in forceps, it is then pushed through the acetabular hole. (D) The ends of the suture are alternately pulled back and forth to cause the toggle pin to turn 90 degrees and seat against the medial cortex of the acetabulum. (E) All four ends of the sutures are pulled through the bone tunnel with a piece of bent wire. The sutures are pulled taut, and the hip is reduced. (F) A small hole is drilled in the lateral cortex in the craniocaudal direction between the osteotomy and the bone tunnel. (G) One set of sutures passed through the proximal bone tunnel and tied to the other suture set.

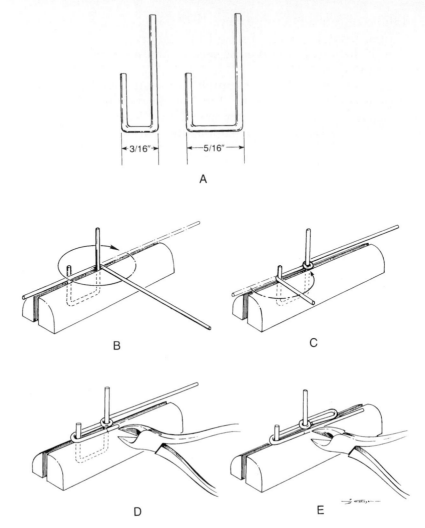

FIGURE 15–6. Fabrication of a toggle pin. Small pins are used in animals weighing up to 9 kg and large pins are used in animals weighing over 9 kg. (*A*) The pins are made from Kirschner wire bent around a jig that is clamped in a vise. The small jig is ³/₁₆ inch wide and is made of 0.035-inch Kirschner wire. The large jig is ⁵/₁₆ inch wide and is made of 0.045-inch Kirschner wire. (*B*) The pins are formed from the same-diameter wire as the jig. The long end of the wire is bent 360 degrees around the taller post of the jig. (*C*) The wire is repositioned on the jig. One end is bent 180 degrees around the short arm of the jig. (*D*) The wire is cut just short of the center hole. (*E*) The partially completed pin is rotated end-for-end and inverted to allow the second end to be formed, as in Figure 15–6D. The entire pin is then compressed with pliers to ensure that the small pin will pass through a ⅛-inch drill hole and that the large pin will pass through a ⁵/₃₂-inch drill hole.

Incidence

One of the most prevalent disorders of the canine hip, hip dysplasia is the most important cause of osteoarthritis of the hip in the dog. Incidence ranges from 0.9 percent in the borzoi to 47.4 percent in the St. Bernard in dogs radiographically evaluated by the Orthopedic Foundation for Animals.[12] This is not the true incidence for any breed or the general population, as most radiographs

TABLE 15–1. PIN SELECTION ACCORDING TO BODY WEIGHT*

Weight (kg)	Diameter (mm)	Diameter (inches)
4–7	1.6	1/16
8–11	2.0	5/64
12–19	2.3	3/32
20–29	2.7	7/64
≥30	3.1	1/8

*From Hunt CA, Henry WB: Transarticular pinning for repair of hip dislocation in the dog: A retrospective study of 40 cases. J Am Vet Med Assoc 187:828, 1985, with permission.

with recognizable dysplasia are not submitted, but it does indicate the relative incidence among the breeds, and most of the large working and sporting breeds are well represented.

The disease rarely occurs in dogs that have a mature body weight of less than 11 to 12 kg. Although hip dysplasia has been observed in toy breeds and cats, their unstable hips do not typically produce the bony changes common in heavier dogs. Coxofemoral luxation after trivial trauma is seen, however.

Pathogenesis

Recent comprehensive reviews of hip dysplasia have brought together most of the known facts regarding this disease and are the basis for most of the discussion that follows.[13–15] A book intended for the lay public is an excellent source for dog owners and breeders.[16]

Many observations have been made regarding the etiology of this complex disease. Among the more important are the following:

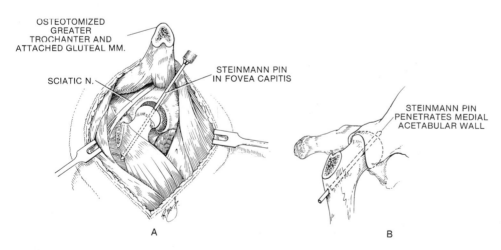

FIGURE 15–7. (*A*) Transarticular pinning of the hip joint. Following an open approach (here a dorsal approach with osteotomy of the trochanter major), cleaning of the acetabulum, and a trial reduction of the femur, a small Steinmann pin (see Table 15–1) is driven from the fovea capitis laterally through the head and neck. It should exit the lateral cortex distal to the trochanter major. (*B*) With the hip reduced and the limb fixed at a normal standing angle, the pin is carefully driven through the acetabular wall. It should protrude not more than ¼ inch (6 mm) into the pelvic canal. The joint capsule is then sutured to the extent possible before closing.

1. There is a polygenic predisposition to congenital dislocation of the hip with multiple factors that influence and modify the disease.

2. Environmental factors are superimposed on the genetic susceptibility of the individual.

3. The genes do not affect the skeleton primarily but rather the cartilage, supporting connective tissue, and muscles of the hip region.

4. The biochemical explanation of the disease is that it represents a disparity between primary muscle mass and disproportionately rapid skeletal growth.

5. The hip joints are normal at birth. Failure of muscles to develop and reach functional maturity concurrently with the skeleton results in joint instability. Abnormal development is induced when the acetabulum and femoral head pull apart and initiate a series of changes that end in the recognizable disease of hip dysplasia.

6. Bony changes of hip dysplasia are a result of failure of soft tissue to maintain congruity between the articular surfaces of the femoral head and acetabulum.

7. The disease is preventable if hip joint congruity is maintained until ossification makes the acetabulum less plastic and the surrounding soft tissues become sufficiently strong to prevent femoral head subluxation. Under usual circumstances, tissue strength and ossification progress sufficiently to prevent the disease by 6 months of age.

8. Dogs with greater pelvic muscle mass have more normal hip joints than those with a relatively smaller pelvic muscle mass.

9. The onset, severity, and incidence of hip dysplasia can be reduced by restricting the growth rate of puppies.

10. The occurrence of hip dysplasia can be reduced, but not eliminated, by breeding only dogs that have radiographically normal hips. Only 7 percent will be normal if both parents are dysplastic.[16]

History and Clinical Signs

Clinical findings in hip dysplasia vary with the age of the animal.[13] Very often, there are no signs appreciated by pet owners. There are two recognizable clinical groups of dogs:

1. Young dogs between 4 and 12 months of age.
2. Animals over 15 months of age with chronic disease.

Young dogs often show sudden onset of unilateral disease (occasionally bilateral), characterized by sudden reduction in activity associated with marked soreness of the hindlimbs. They will show sudden signs of difficulty in arising with decreased willingness to walk, run, jump upwards, and climb stairs, and the muscles of the pelvic and thigh areas are poorly developed. Often the client has noted a "bunny-hopping" gait in the rear quarters. Most will have a positive Ortolani sign (see Chapter 1). This is the click produced by the movement of the femoral head as it slips in and out of the acetabulum with adduction and proximal pressure applied to the femur followed by abduction (see Figs. 15–9C, D and 1–7). Radiographically, the conformation of the femoral heads usually appears normal; however, some degree of subluxation may be seen, and if the process has been present for a few months, the angle of inclination of the femoral neck may increase beyond 146 degrees (valgus), and occasionally some lipping of the ventral aspect of the femoral head will be seen radiographically.

The sudden onset of signs in young dogs is caused by occurrence of micro-fractures of the acetabular rims. When femoral heads are subluxated, the area of contact of the femoral head with the dorsal acetabulum is limited to the area between the 10- and 2-o'clock positions, with an extreme buildup of stress in that area. This eventually overloads the acetabular rim, producing tissue fatigue, loss of tissue elasticity and contour, and eventual microfracture. Pain results from tension and tearing of nerves of the periosteum. Sharpey's fibers rupture, bleed, and form osteophytes on the acetabulum and femoral neck. These usually do not become radiographically visible until 17 or 18 months of age, but may be seen as early as 12 months.[13] These fractures heal by the time of skeletal maturity, with the result that the hip joints become more stable and pain is markedly decreased. Most dysplastic dogs between 12 and 14 months of age walk and run freely and are free of significant pain, despite the radiographic appearance of the joint. Most exhibit a "bunny-hopping" gait when running.

Older dogs present a different clinical picture because they suffer from chronic degenerative joint disease and its associated pain (see Chapter 6). Lameness may be unilateral but is usually bilateral. The signs may have become apparent over a long period of time, or they suddenly occur after brisk activity that results in a tear or other injury of soft tissues of the abnormal joint. Most clinical signs result from prolonged degenerative changes within the joint. There is lameness after prolonged or heavy exercise, a waddling gait, and often crepitus and restricted range of motion of the joint. This crepitus is best detected by placing the examiner's ear or stethoscope bell directly on the proximal trochanter major region while applying proximal pressure during abduction/adduction maneuvers with different degrees of hip extension. The dog often prefers to sit rather than stand and arises slowly and with great difficulty. Thigh and pelvic muscles atrophy markedly with the result that the greater trochanters become quite prominent and even more so if the hip is subluxated. Concurrently, shoulder muscles hypertrophy because of the cranial weight shift and increased use of the forelimbs. The Ortolani sign is rarely present owing to the shallowness of the acetabulum and fibrosis of the joint capsule. There are two other common instances where the hip dysplasia seemingly "worsens:" (1) either full or partial cruciate ligament tears, or (2) spinal problems such as disks or degenerative myelopathy. Stifle palpation and radiographs help in detecting the additional knee problems, while a delayed or absent conscious proprioception test is helpful in distinguishing spinal problems.

Diagnosis

Radiographic Signs

Radiographic confirmation is essential in establishing a positive diagnosis. The Orthopedic Foundation for Animals has formed a hip dysplasia registry (University of Missouri, Columbia, MO) and, as a result of examining many radiographs, has established seven grades of variation in congruity of the femoral head and acetabulum. The dog must be over 2 years of age to apply these gradations. The first three are considered within the range of normal:

1. Excellent—Nearly perfect conformation.
2. Good—Normal conformation for age and breed.
3. Fair—Less than ideal but within normal radiographic limits.

4.   Borderline—A category in which minor hip abnormalities often cannot be clearly assessed because of poor positioning during radiographic procedures. It is recommended that another radiograph be repeated in 6 to 8 months.

Dysplastic animals fall into three categories:

1.   Mild—Minimal deviation from normal with only slight flattening of the femoral head and minor subluxation.
2.   Moderate—Obvious deviation from normal with evidence of a shallow acetabulum, flattened femoral head, poor joint congruency, and in some cases subluxation with marked changes of the femoral head and neck.
3.   Severe—Complete dislocation of the hip and severe flattening of the acetabulum and femoral head.

Dogs in moderate and severe grades are most likely to be clinically affected.

Radiographic evaluation of dysplasia requires adequate relaxation for proper positioning in dorsal recumbency with the femurs extended parallel to each other and to the cassette and the patellae centered on the femoral condyles. Evaluation of properly exposed radiographs is done by reference to several landmarks that are illustrated in Figure 15–8A. The more important points are:

- The femoral head should be congruent with the cranial acetabular margin, which should in turn be perpendicular to the midline.

- The intersection of the physeal scar with the dorsal acetabular rim defines the amount of the femoral head that is under the acetabular rim. At least 50 percent of the head should be covered by the acetabulum.

- Variable amounts of femoral head flattening and remodeling may obscure the fovea capitis. The head becomes more oval in outline as osteophytes build on the femoral neck at the insertion of the joint capsule. In later stages the acetabulum becomes filled with bone and the medial wall appears very thickened.

Reliability of radiographic evaluation for dysplasia is a function of age of the dog. In the German shepherd dog (Alsatian), it is 70 percent at 12 months, 83 percent at 18 months, and 95 percent at 24 months. In general, evaluation between 12 and 18 months has a reliability of 85 percent compared with evaluation at 24 months.[12]

Physical Examination

The ability to diagnose hip dysplasia early in life is economically useful to breeders and could eliminate considerable distress for owners who become very attached to a pet only to find later that the dog has hip dysplasia. Palpation of 6- to 8-week-old puppies for hip joint laxity by the method of Bardens[17] has been demonstrated to be statistically significant in predicting hip dysplasia in at-risk breeds.[18] Bardens reported an accuracy of 83 percent in predicting dysplasia in puppies. The technique is best done on 8- to 9-week-old puppies and requires deep sedation or light general anesthesia. With the pup on its side, the thumb of one hand is rested on the tuber ischii and the middle finger on the dorsal iliac spine. The index finger of the same hand is placed on the greater trochanter as the opposite hand lifts the femur laterally, raising the femoral head out of the acetabulum. The amount of lift can be estimated by observation of the index finger on the acetabulum. Although this is a very subjective measurement, a simple lever device has been described to allow an objective mea-

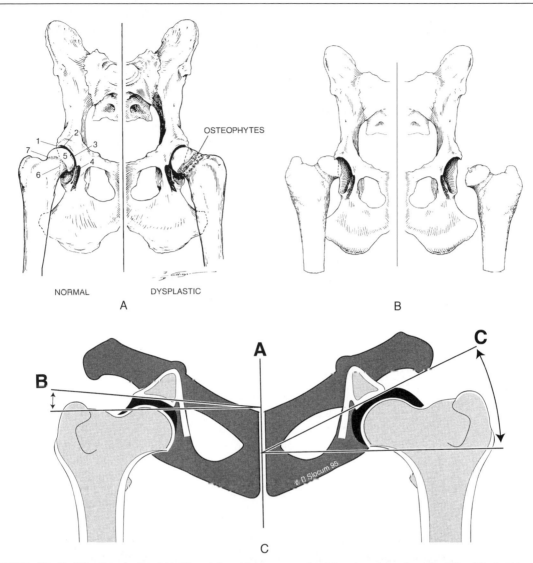

FIGURE 15–8. Hip dysplasia. (A) The right side is normal with several landmarks identified: (1) cranioiolateral rim; (2) cranial acetabular margin; (3) fovea capitis; (4) acetabular notch; (5) femoral head; (6) dorsal acetabular rim; and (7) physeal scar. (See text for details). The left side is dysplastic: The femoral head is flattened and not congruent with the cranial acetabular margin; the intersection of the physeal scar and the dorsal acetabular rim shows only about 40 percent of the femoral head under the acetabular rim; osteophytes have formed at the intersection of the joint capsule and the femoral neck, giving it a very thickened appearance. (B) The right side shows obvious subluxation. The craniodorsal rim is underdeveloped due to pressure upon subluxation. Dramatic incongruency is noted between the femoral head and the cranial acetabular margin, and the intersection of the physeal scar and dorsal acetabular rim shows less than one third of the femoral head under the acetabular rim. The femoral head has lost its spherical shape. The left side shows complete luxation with secondary changes of the femoral head and neck. (C) Dorsal acetabular rim (DAR) view of the pelvis, providing a tomogram-like cross-sectional view of the acetabuli. Line A is the sagittal plane of the pelvis. Lines B and C are tangent to the dorsal acetabular rims and form angles with a line perpendicular to the sagittal plane that define the angle of the dorsal acetabular rims. Normal dogs typically have an angle of not more than 15 degrees, as seen on the left, while dysplastic dogs show increased angulation. (Redrawn from Slocum B, Devine T: Pelvic osteotomy for axial rotation of the acetabular segment in dogs with hip dysplasia. Vet Clin North Am Sm Anim Prac 22:645–682, 1992; and Slocum B, Devine T: Dorsal acetabular rim radiographic view for evaluation of the canine hip. J Am Anim Hosp Assoc 26:289–296, 1990, with permission. Drawing courtesy of B Slocum.)

surement.[18] There is a correlation between the degree of laxity and the presence of hip dysplasia at 12 months of age.

The usefulness of the Ortolani sign (Figs. 15–9C, D and 1–7) as a predictor of dysplasia has not been documented in puppies of this age range, but a similar correlation would be expected, since both methods measure hip joint laxity. Palpation for joint laxity in mature animals is usually unrewarding owing to the fibrosis of the joint capsule and shallowness of the acetabulum. The general orthopedic and radiographic examination is more important in this situation.

The definitive diagnosis of hip dysplasia has to be based upon the radiograph. In young dogs, however, with beginning lameness, the radiographs may not show much change at all. Palpation for Ortolani is often helpful. In the older dog, listening for crepitus with the examiner's ear or stethoscope bell on the trochanter major is often helpful. Diagnosing the origin of lameness when there are concurrent problems such as cruciate ligament rupture or luxating patellas is problematic, especially when each of these conditions is known to occasionally be asymptomatic. If the dog has sustained a cruciate ligament injury, this problem is usually attended to first. After surgery recovery, if lameness is still present, the hips are then treated.

Treatment

Conservative Therapy

Many dogs with hip dysplasia show no signs of pain; others have only mild, intermittent signs. Indeed, in 68 dogs in which hip dysplasia was diagnosed at an early age, 76 percent had minimal gait abnormalities at a mean of 4.5 years later.[19] A large number of these animals can be treated by conservative methods that include minimizing exercise below the threshold level that the hips can tolerate without clinical signs of pain and fatigue. This might include retiring the dog from strenuous athletic competition, or moderating the amount of exercise demanded in some pet situations such as frisbee chasing or jogging with the owner. This will often cause relief of signs with no other treatment. Weight reduction is essential for obese animals. During acute flare-ups, exercise should always be curtailed.

The use of analgesics and other anti-inflammatory agents is indicated in many animals. Aspirin and sodium salicylate do much to improve the well-being of the dog and improve the quality of life. Buffered aspirin is generally the first choice in a twice-daily dose of 325 mg (5 grains) for a 25- to 30-pound animal (25 mg/kg). Phenylbutazone is useful and seems to be more effective than aspirin in some dogs. For chronic use, a therapeutic dosage is 1 mg/kg divided into two or three daily doses, but doses as high as 4 to 5 mg/kg can be used for short periods of time. Corticosteroids hasten degenerative changes in the joint and should be avoided for chronic use. Meclofenamic acid (Arquel, Fort Dodge) has worked well in dogs who tolerated it without gastric or intestinal irritation. It is available in tablet form and in an equine powder which works well mixed in dog food. Dosage is 1 mg/kg daily for 4 to 7 days, then ½ mg/kg. One teaspoon of the equine powder equals 160 mg.

Hannan and associates[20] have demonstrated a chondroprotective effect by polysulfated glycosaminoglycan (Arteparon, Luitpold Werk, Munich, FRG; Adequan, Luitpold Pharmaceutical Inc., Shirley, NY) following experimental meniscectomy. This is also supported by limited clinical experience in treating hip dysplasia. Dosage of 1 mg/kg intramuscularly every 4 days for six doses often

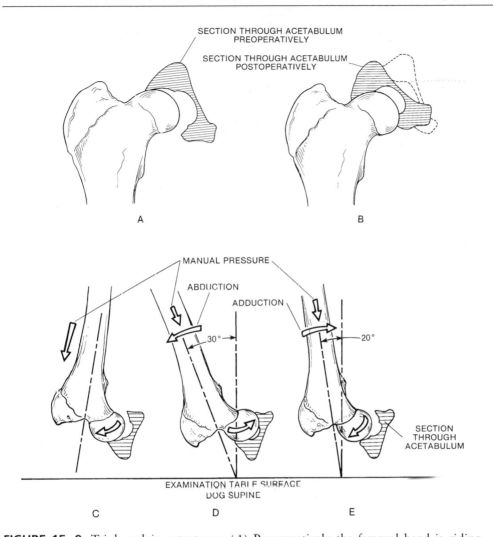

FIGURE 15–9. Triple pelvic osteotomy. (*A*) Preoperatively the femoral head is riding loosely in the acetabulum and contacting only a small area of the dorsal acetabular rim, setting the stage for the structural changes we identify as hip dysplasia. (*B*) Following osteotomy the acetabular portion of the pelvis has been rotated laterally over the femoral head, greatly increasing the contact area between head and acetabulum and thus decreasing local bone and cartilage loads. (*C, D, E*) Finding the acetabular rotation angle.[26,27] (*C*) With the dog supine, the Ortolani sign (subluxation of the femoral head) is elicited by *adduction* and pressure on the femur directed toward the table. This is most easily done bilaterally, which eliminates the problem of the dog rotating when pressure is applied. (*D*) While continuing to apply pressure to the femur, the femur is slowly *abducted*. At some point a distinct click or popping sensation will be felt and perhaps heard as the femur reduces into the acetabulum. In addition, a visible motion will be seen in the inguinal region as the femur returns medially. The angle of the femur relative to the sagittal plane (i.e., the plane 90 degrees to the table top) is identified as the reduction angle and represents the maximum angle the acetabulum would need to be rotated to stabilize the femur. In this example the angle measured 30 degrees. The optimal angle of rotation is about 5 to 10 degrees less than the angle of reduction. (*E*) With the femur in the reduced position, it is slowly *adducted* while maintaining pressure toward the table. Again a distinct point will be appreciated visually, audibly, and by palpation that represents the femur luxating from the acetabulum. This is measured as in *D* and is called the angle of luxation, 20 degrees here, and represents the minimum angle of rotation of the acetabulum. *Figure continued on following page*

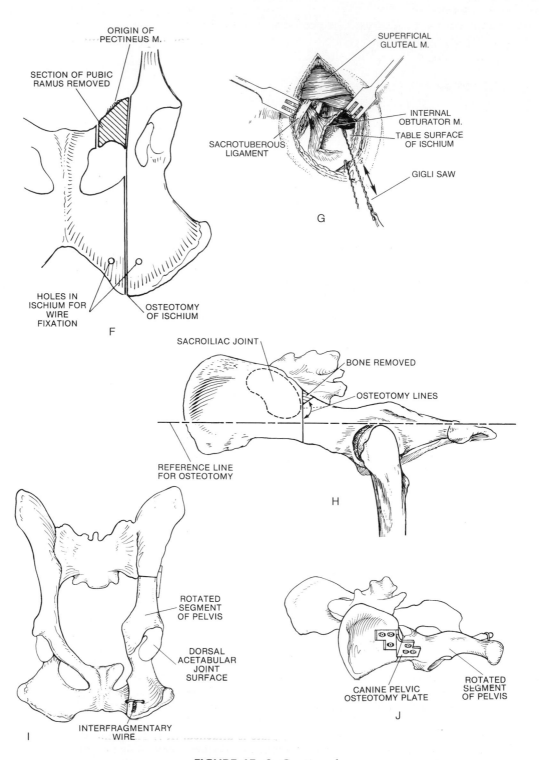

ORIGIN OF
PECTINEUS M.

SECTION OF PUBIC
RAMUS REMOVED

HOLES IN
ISCHIUM FOR
WIRE
FIXATION

OSTEOTOMY
OF ISCHIUM

F

SUPERFICIAL
GLUTEAL M.

SACROTUBEROUS
LIGAMENT

INTERNAL
OBTURATOR M.

TABLE SURFACE
OF ISCHIUM

GIGLI SAW

G

SACROILIAC JOINT

BONE REMOVED

OSTEOTOMY LINES

REFERENCE LINE
FOR OSTEOTOMY

H

ROTATED
SEGMENT
OF PELVIS

DORSAL
ACETABULAR
JOINT
SURFACE

INTERFRAGMENTARY
WIRE

I

CANINE PELVIC
OSTEOTOMY PLATE

ROTATED
SEGMENT
OF PELVIS

J

FIGURE 15–9. *Continued*

produces clinical improvement. This dose is then repeated to effect, usually every 4 to 6 weeks. The drug is not yet approved for use in dogs in the United States, so the equine variety must be used. In a double-blind study of dogs with advanced hip dysplasia arthritis, however, Adaquan did not improve clinical performance when compared to placebo.[21]

Surgical Therapy

The veterinary orthopedist is truly in a quandary when trying to decide on a course of treatment for an individual dog when the clinical signs of dysplasia develop at an early age. Although the results of triple pelvic osteotomy are very encouraging, they must be balanced against the observation of Barr, Denny, and Gibbs that 76 percent of dogs diagnosed with hip dysplasia at a young age never had serious clinical signs of dysplasia at follow-up 4½ years later.[19] One might ask if these dogs would not develop problems later in life. However, if these figures hold true, only between 10 and 17 percent of the affected puppies really will benefit from triple pelvic osteotomy or intertrochanteric femoral osteotomy (see below). Conversely, it is impossible to predict how any individual puppy will fare later in life, and so the decision to pursue early surgical treatment needs to be carefully considered, since the results are predictable. If the animal is destined to be primarily a house/yard pet, a conservative approach is probably rational. If pain becomes a problem, then femoral head and neck ostectomy, or total hip replacement are alternatives. If the dog is to be a sporting or working "canine athlete," a more aggressive approach should be pursued at an early age, when the chances for a reconstructive approach are best.

Surgical therapies can be broken down into two groups: those that provide relief from pain, and those that prevent or lessen the amount of future degenerative joint disease.

The preventative surgeries are performed on young, large, growing dysplastic dogs. The theory behind these surgeries is to realign the pelvis or femoral head so that the femoral head seats more deeply into the growing acetabulum. This results in better head coverage by the acetabulum, reducing the amount of subluxation present. Triple pelvic osteotomies or possibly intertrochanteric oste-

---

FIGURE 15–9. *Continued* (F, G) Pubic ostectomy and ischial osteotomy. (F) A section of the pubic ramus is removed via a ventral approach and detachment of the pectineus muscle at its origin (see text). (G) A caudal approach to the ischium allows elevation of the internal obturator muscle and osteotomy of the ischial table from the lateral border of the obturator foramen caudally on a line parallel to the midline. The results of this osteotomy are seen in F as are the 2-mm drill holes, through which 20- or 18-gauge (0.8- to 1-mm) wire is threaded but not tightened at this time. (H) Osteotomy of the iliac shaft. A horizontal reference line is created by passing a small blunted Steinmann pin from the dorsal surface of the tuber ischii cranially to a point one third the distance from the ventral to the cranial dorsal iliac spines. The transverse osteotomy is 90 degrees to the horizontal line and at the caudal aspect of the sacroiliac joint. The sciatic nerve must be protected when the osteotomy is made (see text). A triangular piece of bone will be removed dorsally after the plate is attached. (I, J) The completed triple pelvic osteotomy procedure. The iliac osteotomy is stabilized with a Canine Pelvic Osteotomy Plate (Slocum Enterprises) and the ischial osteotomy with a twisted interfragmentary wire. A standard 2.7- or 3.5-mm plate can be twisted to provide a similar effect. Note how the rotated acetabular segment would provide greater dorsal coverage for the femoral head.

otomies are examples of the latter. Pain relief may result from pectineal myectomy, femoral head and neck ostectomy, or total hip arthroplasty.

Pelvic Osteotomy

Pelvic osteotomy is indicated for young dogs with clinical signs of hip dysplasia, as discussed above, and who demonstrate signs of instability (laxity, subluxation) of the hip joint. The procedure provides axial rotation of the acetabulum to stabilize the femoral head within the acetabulum in a functional position (Fig. 15–9A, B), and has been shown to be a clinically effective method of treating dysplasia, especially in young animals.[22–24] Theoretical analysis has suggested that the procedure may reduce the magnitude of forces acting on the femoral head.[25] Force plate analysis has confirmed that weight-bearing forces improve in operated versus nonoperated hips.[26]

PATIENT SELECTION ■ The operation should be done early, most commonly between 4 and 8 months of age, in order to take advantage of the remodeling capacity of immature bone and before the articular cartilage is badly damaged. With instability and subluxation over a period of time, the acetabulum becomes filled with new bone that covers the original surface, thus preventing congruency and stability between the femoral head and acetabulum. These changes become increasingly severe by the age of 10 to 12 months. Age is, however, not the most important criterion determining success. The primary consideration is the condition of the joint surfaces (i.e., the degree of degenerative changes that have occurred). If the acetabulum is filled with bone, or the dorsal acetabular rim (labrum) is lost due to eburnation, or the cartilage of the femoral head is destroyed, pelvic osteotomy will not result in a successful outcome.[22,23]

Radiographic Examination[27,28] ■ In selecting patients for this procedure, standard ventrodorsal and lateral radiographs are taken and analyzed for the pathology described above (Fig. 15–8A, B). Of particular interest is the shape of the dorsal acetabular rim, which will become increasingly cupped or S-curved in its outline. This is probably a result of lack of development due to pressure from the subluxated femur and to abrasion from the femoral head. Osteophytes form first at the joint capsule insertion on the femoral neck and are responsible for the thickened appearance of the neck. Osteophytes on the acetabular rim are signs of advanced degenerative changes. Filling of the acetabulum with new bone is evidenced by a loss of definition of the original deep acetabular outline, replaced by a less well-defined surface that is farther from the medial acetabular cortex than normal. The lateral views are examined closely for signs of cartilage thickness loss. As the bright white lines of the subchondral bone approach each other without the intervening radiolucent cartilage they tell of cartilage thinning. Acetabular osteophytes are well defined in this view as a radiographic density dorsal to the acetabulum. The "frog-leg" view is used to determine the depth of the acetabulum. In dorsal recumbency, the femurs are abducted 45 degrees with the femurs perpendicular to the pelvis/spine. This stress forces the femoral head deeply into the acetabulum, and if the head is not deeply seated it indicates bony filling of the acetabulum or hypertrophy of the round ligament as a result of instability of the femoral head. Abduction of the femurs more than 45 degrees can cause the dorsal acetabular rim to contact the femoral neck, especially in the presence of acetabular osteophytes, and lever the femoral head ventrolaterally out of the acetabulum.

Additionally, the dorsal acetabular rim (DAR) view[27] is very helpful in ruling in or out a given animal for pelvic osteotomy. The animal is placed in sternal recumbency, the hips flexed, and the stifles fixed against the body wall with tape or a strap. When the tuber calci are elevated 2 to 4 inches (5 to 10 cm), depending on body size, above the table top the pelvis is vertical to the table and the x-ray beam can be directed through the long axis of the pelvis. The acetabuli can then be seen in cross section in the frontal plane (Fig. 15–8C). A line is drawn tangent to the curvature of the dorsal aspect of the acetabular surface where it contacts the femoral head. The angle formed by this line can be measured against a reference line drawn between the dorsal acetabular rims or against a vertical line drawn in the sagittal plane. Normal dogs will have a summed angle of 15 degrees from horizontal (165 degrees from vertical) or less; 15 to 20 degrees is suspicious of hip dysplasia, and animals with greater than 20 degrees will have the other signs of dysplasia mentioned above.[27,28] The normal acetabular rim is quite sharp, and wearing of the rim is evidenced by rounding and loss of definition and sclerosis. Most of the information gained from the DAR can be inferred from the other radiographs and the palpation discussed below, but the DAR is useful in documenting the acetabular changes.

Palpation ▪ Equally as important as the radiographs is palpation of the hips with the dog anesthetized or deeply sedated. The objective is to assess passive laxity (subluxation) of the hip both quantitatively and qualitatively. The *trochanteric compression test* is done with the dog on its side while moderate pressure is applied to the greater trochanter. If the hip is chronically subluxated it will be reduced by this pressure and the change in position of the trochanter will be sensed.

With practice one can recognize breakdown of the dorsal acetabular rim and the condition of the cartilage of the femoral head by the character of the "click" evidenced during testing for the *Ortolani sign*. The sign of Ortolani is elicited (Fig. 15–9C, D, E) with the dog on its back, with the femur held vertically, and the stifle flexed. The femurs are grasped distally, and gentle pressure is applied proximally (toward the pelvis) causing the femoral head to subluxate and rest on the dorsal acetabular rim due to capsular laxity. This movement may or may not be appreciated at this time; it will be more evident later in the test. As the femur is abducted with the pressure maintained, a distinct "click" or "clunk" is heard and felt when the femoral head reduces. The angle of the femur from vertical at this point is the *angle of reduction*. Reversing the procedure by adducting the femur results in another softer "click" when the head subluxates from the acetabulum, and the angle of the femur from vertical at this point is the *angle of subluxation*. If the articular cartilage is undamaged, these clicks will be appreciated as abrupt motions of the femoral head with a smooth and crisp feeling. The sensation of the reduction phase produces a very solid-feeling "clunk." The subluxation phase is less dramatic. Wearing of the cartilage of the femoral head and acetabular rim causes a muffling of the sounds and a less crisp, to a grating, fibrillated, or crepitant feeling as the femoral head glides over the acetabular rim. The reduction motion, particularly, is less abrupt and crisp when the dorsal rim is lost and the acetabulum becomes shallow due to filling with new bone.

The angle of reduction (AR) increases as capsular laxity increases, and the angle of subluxation (AS) increases as the acetabular rim is lost due to wear.[27] As the capsule becomes thickened due to fibrosis and the acetabulum fills with bone, the angles approach each other in value and the Ortolani sign cannot be elicited because the femoral head is permanently subluxated and supported mainly by the capsule. The femoral head cannot be reduced because there is no functional acetabulum. This is typical of the mature dog with hip dysplasia. Occasionally young dogs will show a positive AR (e.g., 15 degrees, with an AS of 0 degrees). This may represent a situation of passive laxity without functional laxity, and although in the absence of clinical signs it does not require pelvic osteotomy, it does merit monitoring for future degenerative changes. Although passive hip joint laxity is closely associated with development of degenerative joint disease,[29] there is apparently considerable difference between breeds regarding this correlation.[30]

The *ideal candidate for pelvic osteotomy* would be 5 to 7 months of age with clinical signs of hip dysplasia, and would show minimal or no signs of degenerative changes radiographically and on palpation. The trochanteric compression test would be negative and the summed DAR angles would be 20 degrees or less. The AR would be 30 degrees or less and the AS 10 degrees or less, indicating an acetabulum without filling and with an intact dorsal acetabular rim. As the AR goes above 30 degrees and the AS above 10 degrees the prognosis declines due to the pre-existing changes in the acetabulum. An AR/AS reading of 45/20 degrees is the highest to rate a good prognosis with pelvic osteotomy.[27]

CONTRAINDICATIONS ■ Pelvic osteotomy is contraindicated when there are radiographic or palpable signs of advanced degenerative joint disease, breakdown of the dorsal acetabular rim, shallow acetabulum, or neurological disease.

SURGICAL TECHNIQUE ■ The triple pelvic osteotomy (TPO) technique of Slocum and Devine has proven most dependable in our hands.[22,23,27] The AR represents the probable maximum angle the acetabulum needs to be rotated to achieve stability, while the AS represents the minimal angle of rotation of the acetabulum that will produce stability of the hip. These two angles are used to select the appropriate implant for axial rotation of the acetabular segment of the pelvis.[23] In order to prevent overrotation of the pelvis and subsequent impingement of the dorsal acetabular rim on the femoral neck and excessive narrowing of the pelvic canal, the angle selected should usually be *closer to the angle of luxation than to the angle of reduction, and should not exceed 45 degrees.*

Slocum has devised a bone plate for this procedure (Canine Pelvic Osteotomy Plate [CPOP], Slocum Enterprises, Eugene, OR), using 3.5-mm screws, which is made in three angles of rotation: a 20-degree plate with a fixed angle; a 30-degree plate that can be twisted to angles between 20 and 40 degrees; and a 45-degree plate that can be molded between 35 and 60 degrees. In practice it is rarely necessary to rotate the acetabulum more than 30 degrees, since further rotation usually causes difficulty in abduction as the femoral neck impinges on the dorsal acetabular rim. It is our practice to limit the rotation to 30 degrees, and supplement this with femoral neck lengthening (see below) when the Ortolani sign is not abolished by 30 degrees of rotation. The CPOP device has proved most satisfactory and easy to use and is our method of choice (Fig. 15–9I, J). It is superior to a twisted conventional bone plate because it provides eight potential points of fixation (six screws, two cerclage wires) and thus minimizes fixation failure. It also lateralizes the acetabular portion of the pelvis and so widens the pelvic canal. A standard five- to seven-hole, 2.7- or 3.5-mm straight plate can be used by twisting the plate in its midsection; however, recent studies have confirmed the advantages of the CPOP in providing superior dorsal acetabular coverage and minimal disruption of normal pelvic architecture compared to twisted plates.[31,32]

The procedure is performed in three stages. The limb is prepared and free draped so as to allow access to both the inguinal and lateral aspects of the pelvis. With the animal in dorsal recumbency and the limb held in a vertical position, the pubic ramus is exposed through a ventral approach[5] (Fig. 15–9F). The pectineus muscle is severed close to its origin on the iliopectineal eminence and the prepubic tendon. The muscle belly is allowed to retract and is not sutured. Elevation of the gracilis muscle caudally and the abdominal muscles and prepubic tendon cranially exposes the pubic ramus. Most of the ramus is removed after two cuts in the bone, one near the medial limit of the obturator foramen and the other at the junction of the pubis with the ilium, medial to the iliopubic eminence. It is important to make this cut as close as possible to the body of the ilium in order to minimize the length of the bone spike that will be turned into the pelvic canal.[33] The obturator nerve must be protected during this cut, as it lies very near the caudal limit of the cut. The abdominal muscles and prepubic tendon are sutured to the cranial border of the gracilis muscle and the rest of the tissues are sutured in layers.

The dog is returned to lateral recumbency and a second incision is made over the medial angle of the ischiatic tuberosity. After elevation of the internal obturator dorsally and the semimembranosus and quadratus muscles ventrally, the ischiatic table is osteotomized in a paramedian plane, beginning cranially at the lateral aspect of the obturator foramen (Fig. 15–9F, G). This can be done with a Gigli wire saw, a hand saw, or a power saw, but not with an osteotome, as there is a good chance of cutting into the ramus of the ischium. Drill holes are placed 5 mm from the cut edges, and a 1-mm (18-gauge) wire is threaded through the holes but not tightened.

A lateral approach is next made to the shaft of the ilium,[5] and the gluteal muscles are elevated from the body and ventral wing of the ilium. Taking care to protect the cranial gluteal, obturator, and sciatic nerves, all muscles are elevated from the iliac shaft ventrally, medially, and dorsally. An iliac osteotomy is performed just caudal to the sacrum (Fig. 15–9H). The cut is made perpendicular in both planes to a line between the dorsal side of the ischiatic tuberosity and the ventral third of the iliac crest. This line is established by inserting a small Steinmann pin from the dorsal surface of the tuber ischium cranially toward the cranial ventral iliac spine, where it is positioned by palpation one third of the distance between the ventral and dorsal iliac spines. The pin can then be used to establish the proper angle for the iliac osteotomy. The object of this exercise is to make the osteotomy perpendicular to the axis of rotation of the acetabular portion rather than perpendicular to the long axis of the ilium. The resulting angle of the osteotomy is approximately 20 degrees to the long axis of the ilium and allows for optimal contact of the bone surfaces, while minimizing decrease of pelvic inlet area and increasing in the interischiatic tuberosity distance and acetabular version.[31]

Following this osteotomy, the acetabular segment is moved cranially and laterally with bone-holding forceps and the sharp spike of ilium dorsal to the plate is removed to prevent irritation of the gluteal muscles. The plate is now attached to the caudal segment with 3.5-mm screws. If the CPOP is used, at least one of these screws is placed in the load position to compress the angular step against the bone. The acetabular segment is rotated laterally and the plate temporarily clamped cranially to the cranial iliac segment. The hip should now be stable with no Ortolani sign; if not, the plate is removed and twisted more or replaced with another plate of increased angle. If the Ortolani sign is eliminated but there is still lateral translational movement of the femoral head of more than a few millimeters, transposition of the greater trochanter (see Fig. 15–4D) can be used to augment the stability of the femoral head.[24] Another alternative in this situation is femoral neck lengthening as described below. Neck lengthening is the equivalent of adding 10 degrees of acetabular rotation.[27] Even without either of these ancillary procedures, most hips will stabilize within a few weeks due to the basic stability afforded by the pelvic osteotomy, and definitive guidelines for these procedures await longer term experience. After the proper angle is found for the acetabular segment, the ischial wire is tightened, and the plate is then fixed to the cranial iliac segment (Fig. 15–9I, J). In very young dogs, the screw fixation can be supplemented with a hemicerclage wire through holes in each end of the CPOP. The triangular bone fragment from the ilium or the pubic ramus fragment can be cut into small fragments and used as bone graft in the osteotomy site to hasten healing. Both surgery sites are closed routinely by layers.

AFTERCARE ■ Postoperatively, the dog is confined to the house or leash exercise for 4 to 6 weeks, at which time the opposite side is operated if indicated. In severely dysplastic 4- to 7-month-old puppies, the opposite side should be operated in 2 to 3 weeks, as the bony structures and joint cartilage are remodeling rapidly.

PROGNOSIS ■ Slocum has reported on follow-up evaluation of 138 dogs that underwent triple pelvic osteotomy. Of these dogs, 122 had hip dysplasia: 30 percent had grade 4 dysplasia; 33 percent grade 3; and 34 percent grade 2. In age at surgery, 13 percent were less than 6 months of age; 47 percent were 6 to 12 months; 22.5 percent were 1 to 2 years; and 17 percent were more than 2 years. At the time of postoperative evaluation, 86.2 percent were fully active with normal weight bearing and activity.[23] In another study, 92 percent of operated limbs showed remission of lameness at 28 weeks postoperatively, and progression of detectable degenerative joint disease was minimal, despite the fact that gross and microscopic degenerative changes were similar in treated and untreated hips.[26]

Femoral Neck Lengthening

In addition to the mechanical stability afforded the femoral head by a deep acetabulum with a normal dorsal acetabular slope, there is a dynamic component of hip stability that is due to muscular forces, primarily the internal and external rotator muscles. These muscles all insert on the greater trochanter, so increasing the length of the femoral neck increases the lever arm over which these muscles operate, and thus increases the medially directed force they apply to the femur.

INDICATIONS ■ Femoral neck lengthening has been proposed as primary treatment for dysplastic dogs that have adequate dorsal acetabular coverage, but whose hips are unstable due to insufficient muscular force to prevent the hip from subluxating.[34] These dogs typically have a short femoral neck, and some breeds such as the chow chow and the Akita are prone to this problem. Suitable candidates for primary neck lengthening should have an angle of subluxation of 0 degrees or less, and a normal dorsal acetabular rim angle.[35] The second indication for neck lengthening has been mentioned above in conjunction with triple pelvic osteotomy. If the acetabular rotation angle needed to obliterate the Ortolani sign (approximately equal to the angle of reduction) exceeds 30 degrees, it is probably better to add neck lengthening rather than exceed 30 degrees of rotation, since doing so creates problems with abduction of the hip. Neck lengthening has the same stabilizing effect as 10 degrees of acetabular rotation.[27]

SURGICAL TECHNIQUE ■ The proximal femur is approached by detaching the vastus lateralis muscle from its origin on the proximocranial aspect of the femoral neck and shaft.[5] A parasagittal osteotomy is made in the proximal femur, starting at the junction of the greater trochanter and the femoral neck, and ending distally at the lateral cortex 1 to 2 cm distal to the lesser trochanter (Fig 15–10A, B). Before the osteotomy is made, a 2-mm hole is drilled at the distal end of the intended osteotomy, and the osteotomy ends at this hole. The purpose of the hole is to prevent cracks from propagating beyond this point when the trochanter is forced laterally. A 3.5-mm cortical thread lag screw is placed transversely just distal to this hole as additional insurance against cracking the lateral cortex.

A second 3.5-mm cortical screw (typically about 35 mm long) is placed in the greater trochanter, threaded only in the first cortex. The tap hole is drilled only to the depth of the osteotomy. As the screw is tightened the tip of the screw contacts the trabecular bone of the femoral neck, and as tightening of the screw continues, the trochanter is distracted laterally. This distraction is slowly continued until the lateral translational laxity of the femoral head is abolished (Fig. 15–10C). At this point a third 3.5-mm cortical screw is placed 1 cm distal to the distracting screw (Fig. 15–10D), and is threaded in both cortices (positional screw). If the distracting screw protrudes lateral to the trochanter it is replaced with a shorter screw. The origin of the vastus lateralis muscle is sutured to the cranial border of the deep gluteal muscle.

AFTERCARE ■ Postoperatively, the dog is confined to the house or leash exercise for 4 to 6 weeks. The opposite side is operated after 3 or 4 weeks if indicated.

Intertrochanteric Varus Osteotomy of the Femur

The true angle of inclination of the canine femoral neck in relation to the diaphysis is about 146 degrees.[36] In animals with hip dysplasia, this angle increases as much as 30 to 35 degrees, leading to the condition known as coxa valga (Fig. 15–11C). This is due to subluxation of the hip joint and subsequent lack of normal stress on the femoral neck, which is necessary for development of the normal angle. This valgus angle of the head and neck contributes to further subluxation and instability, perpetuating a vicious circle. Additionally, the femoral neck inclines farther cranially (anteversion) from the normal angle of about 27 degrees and again contributes to subluxation and instability.[36]

The principle of varus derotational osteotomy for treatment of congenital hip luxation and instability is well established in humans and in the dog.[37,38] By making the femoral neck more perpendicular to the femoral shaft (varisation) and reducing anteversion, the femoral head can be placed more deeply within the acetabulum, and forces acting on any given area of the bone and cartilage of the acetabulum and femoral head can be reduced by distributing weight-bearing loads through greater congruency over a greater percentage of the articular cartilage. When the osteotomy is done in an immature animal with a high potential for bony remodeling, there can be permanent improvement in joint congruity. In the mature animal with degenerative joint disease and instability, pain may be relieved by reduced forces on the acetabulum and femoral

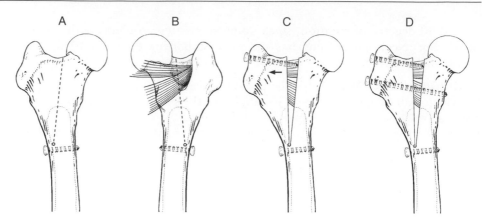

FIGURE 15–10. Femoral neck lengthening. (A) Cranial view of the femoral head and neck region showing the line of osteotomy. A 2-mm drill hole at the end of the osteotomy and a positional screw are placed to prevent distal fissuring of the bone. (B) Caudal view to show the osteotomy deep and medial to the insertions of the obturator-gemellus muscles on the greater trochanter. (C) A 3.5-mm screw is inserted to the osteotomy line after drilling and tapping only the lateral cortex. As the screw is tightened the tip of the screw bears against the bone of the femoral neck and the trochanter is distracted laterally along the screw threads. Distraction is continued until lateral translational motion of the femoral head is abolished. (D) A positional screw, threaded in both cortices, is placed distal to the distraction screw to maintain the lateralized position of the trochanter.

head and redistributing weight-bearing forces more uniformly over the diseased cartilage.

The purpose of intertrochanteric osteotomy is to improve the biomechanics of the hip and to reduce hip pain.[30] It is more effective when done before degenerative joint disease is present, between the ages of 4 and 10 months in most patients. Patient selection is identical to triple pelvic osteotomy, with careful radiographic evaluation and palpation of the joints to aid in evaluating the condition of the joint surfaces. Contraindications include degenerative joint disease that is radiographically obvious, shallow acetabulum, and loss of the dorsal acetabular rim. Since the amount of increased dorsal acetabular coverage does not seem to be as great as with TPO, we reserve intertrochanteric osteotomy for less severe cases.

FIGURE 15–11. (A) Finding angle of inclination of the femoral neck by the symmetric axis-based method.[39] Tracings are made from the ventrodorsal pelvic radiograph, with the hips extended, femurs parallel to the cassette, and the patellae centered (see Fig. 15–8A). Best fit circles are superimposed on the femoral head, the femoral neck-trochanter region, and the femoral condyles. Connecting the center points of the circles provides the angle of inclination. (B, C, D) Intertrochanteric varus osteotomy using AO/ASIF 3.5-mm double hook plates (Synthes Ltd. [USA], Paoli, PA). (See text for details.) (B) The hooks on the proximal end of the plate are placed in holes in the trochanter major. (C) Instability of the hip joint is created by the valgus angle of inclination of the femoral neck. Removal of the wedge of bone will create a slightly varus 135-degree angle and restore stability. (D) The bone wedge has been removed and the intertrochanteric osteotomy fixed with the double hook plate. Note the improved congruity of the joint surfaces and compare with Figure 15–9B. (E) In dogs too small for the double hook plate, a multiple pin and tension band wire fixation technique can be used.

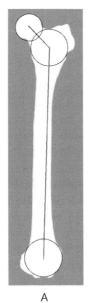

A

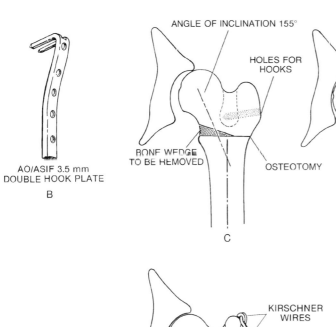

AO/ASIF 3.5 mm
DOUBLE HOOK PLATE

B

ANGLE OF INCLINATION 155°

HOLES FOR
HOOKS

BONE WEDGE
TO BE REMOVED

OSTEOTOMY

C

ANGLE OF
INCLINATION 135°

D

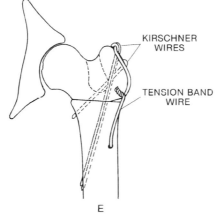

KIRSCHNER
WIRES

TENSION BAND
WIRE

E

FIGURE 15–11. *See legend on opposite page*

space for more bone cement and creates an irregular surface for the attachment of cement to the bone. Drilling into the iliac and ischiatic shafts and dorsal acetabular rim is another method of achieving this (Fig. 15–13C, D); long drill bits and drill sleeves to protect soft tissues are necessary. Once the acetabulum is prepared, a trial insertion of the prosthesis is done to ensure proper fit. The acetabular component is then cemented (Surgical Simplex P bone cement, Howmedica International, Ltd., London, England; Howmedica, Inc., Rutherford, NJ) in place, using a positioner to ensure proper orientation (Fig. 15–13E). The positioner must be oriented so the handle is aligned with a line from the ischiatic tuberosity to the dorsal iliac spine. Additionally, the shaft of the positioner must be vertical to the sagittal plane of the pelvis, and inclined caudally about 10 degrees.

Returning to the femur, the femoral canal is enlarged to the appropriate size with a powered drill and tapered reamer (Fig. 15–13F, G). Reaming is often facilitated by removing the thin bone of the caudal femoral neck that remains after excision of the head, thus opening the trochanteric fossa and allowing better centering of the reamer in the femoral shaft. This is followed by hand filing and rasping with a broach to fit the femoral component completely within the femoral medullary canal and firmly in contact with the femoral neck ostectomy (Fig. 15–13H, I, J). A trial prosthesis with a femoral head attached is inserted and the hip reduced and checked for stability (Fig. 15–13K). If the chosen femoral head is of the correct neck length the hip will be moderately difficult to reduce and there will be virtually no lateral translational movement of the head with vigorous pulls laterally on the femur. The femoral head prosthesis is replaced as necessary to achieve this goal. Once satisfied with the combination of trial femoral head and stem, the permanent implants are joined together; tapping the head with a mallet produces an interference fit that maintains the head on the stem. The head can be attached either before or after the femoral component is cemented. Bone cement is introduced into the femoral canal, preferably by injection of liquid phase cement, and the prosthesis is placed into the canal, with care to prevent anteversion. Following hardening of the cement, the hip is reduced, the joint capsule is closed with several interrupted sutures, and the remaining tissues are closed by layers.

AFTERCARE ■ No external support is used on the limb. Oral cephalexin is started as soon as possible and continued for 3 days. Close confinement and limited leash exercise are stressed for the first month postoperatively. Most dogs are walking comfortably by 2 weeks, and trotting easily at 4 weeks. At this time a physical evaluation for range of motion, evidence of pain, and degree of function is done, and if all is well the exercise is slowly increased over the second month. If functionally sound, the animal is released to return to normal activity, although it may take as much as 6 months for muscle atrophy to resolve and for maximal function to return. At this point it is not necessary to impose any limitations on the dog's activity. Decisions about the advisability of a second procedure on the opposite hip should be delayed until at least 6 months, as it is difficult to evaluate the unoperated leg until the operated leg achieves normal function. Should the nonoperated leg remain or become lame, the options are either another hip replacement or excision arthroplasty.

PROGNOSIS ■ Most dogs return to full function by 8 weeks postoperatively. Satisfactory function occurred in 95 percent of 362 cases followed 3 months or more.[44] This was defined as full weight bearing, normal range of motion, normal gait, and normal level of activity with no signs of pain in the hip. Another study reported good to excellent function in 96 percent of cases.[46] Similar results have been experienced at Colorado State University. Late aseptic loosening of the acetabular prosthesis currently accounts for most of the failures, with a 3 percent incidence reported.[44] Salvage of the limb is usually achieved by removal of the prosthesis and bone cement, and treating it as an excision arthroplasty, although revision by implanting a new prosthesis is possible. There seems to be no tendency for the prostheses to break down or loosen with time as in human patients, except as noted above. Thus, at this point, the procedure does not appear to be time limited, and this indicates that the technique has established itself as a reliable clinical procedure for the treatment of a variety of abnormal conditions of the hip.

Femoral Head and Neck Excision

Femoral head and neck excision to allow formation of a fibrous false joint is also termed *excision arthroplasty* or *femoral head and neck ostectomy* (FHO). Pain is relieved by elimination of bony contact between the femur and the pelvis as scar tissue interposes. Because of slight limb shortening and some loss of range of motion, some gait abnormality persists. The procedure may be performed bilaterally, preferably with procedures separated by an interval of 8 to 10 weeks.

PATIENT SELECTION ■ Excision arthroplasty is a nonreversible procedure and must be considered a salvage operation. Nevertheless, it is a valuable method for improving the quality of life for many pets by elimination of pain. Indications will vary with the skill of the surgeon, internal fixation devices available, and financial considerations. There is some tendency to overuse the procedure for conditions that are reparable.

Degenerative joint disease resulting from dysplasia is the most common indication for excision arthroplasty. The procedure is often the first choice of treatment for a mature animal that is basically a house or yard pet only; it is also the treatment of choice for Legg-Calvé-Perthes disease. More pragmatically, it may be used when financial constraints preclude expensive orthopedic reconstruction. Other common indications include chronic osteoarthrosis from any cause, comminuted fractures of the acetabulum or femoral neck, fractures of the femoral head, and chronic luxation of the hip with erosion of the femoral head. In summary, the procedure is suitable for any condition in which the integrity of the hip joint has been compromised and primary repair is not feasible or in which osteoarthrosis is well established.

SURGICAL TECHNIQUE ■ A craniolateral approach to the hip (Fig. 15–14A, B) is preferred because it does not involve transection of the gluteal muscles, as do the dorsal approaches.[5] Some surgeons favor a ventral approach (Fig. 15–14C, D) because it is more cosmetic. In the craniolateral approach, it is important to incise and reflect the joint capsule and origin of the vastus lateralis muscle to expose the cranial aspect of the femoral neck adequately. The gluteal muscles are retracted dorsally by inserting a Hohmann retractor inside the joint capsule. Bone-holding forceps attached to the region of the trochanter may be used to subluxate the femur. This facilitates cutting of the round ligament with curved scissors and elevation of the rest of the joint capsule from the femoral head.

The neck is best cut with an osteotome, with the leg externally rotated 90 degrees. In a large dog, this osteotome should be at least 1 inch wide (2.5 cm).

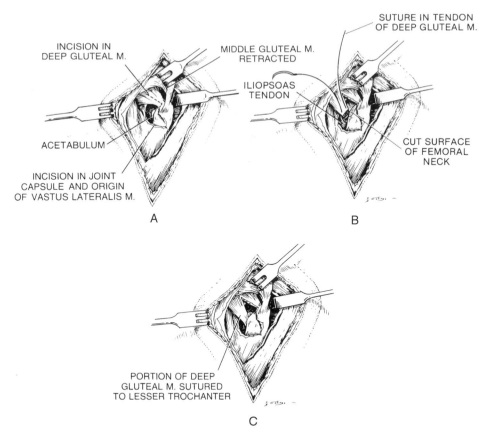

FIGURE 15–16. Provision for a soft tissue pad between the femoral neck and the pelvis. (*A*) Following a craniolateral approach[5] a pedicle of the deep gluteal muscle can be detached from the trochanter major, cutting close to the bone to leave as much tendon as possible on the muscle. (*B*) With strong external rotation of the femur, the pedicle is sutured through its tendinous end to the tendon of the iliopsoas muscle near its insertion on the lesser trochanter. (*C*) With the femur returned to a neutral position, the deep gluteal pedicle covers the cut surface of the femoral neck.

the animal to move about a confined area are encouraged until suture removal. After 2 weeks postoperatively, active exercise such as running and swimming is encouraged. Animals will ordinarily be toe-touching in 10 to 14 days, partially weight bearing in 3 weeks, and actively using the leg by 4 weeks. When bilateral operations are indicated, they should be done 8 to 10 weeks apart. In some cases, it will be necessary to delay the second surgery even further until active use of the first limb has been achieved. In cases of severe pain from bilateral hip problems, bilateral excisions can be done simultaneously. Aftercare is dif-

FIGURE 15–17. (*A*) Another method of soft tissue interposition involves freeing a pedicle of biceps muscle (*dashed line*). (*B*) A suture is attached to the muscle pedicle and is pulled under the gluteal muscles from a caudal to cranial direction. (*C*) The muscle pedicle is sutured to the elevated vastus lateralis in a position that holds it across the femoral neck ostectomy.

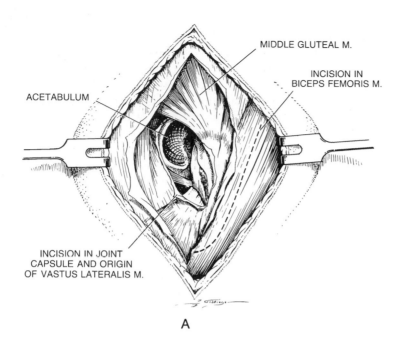

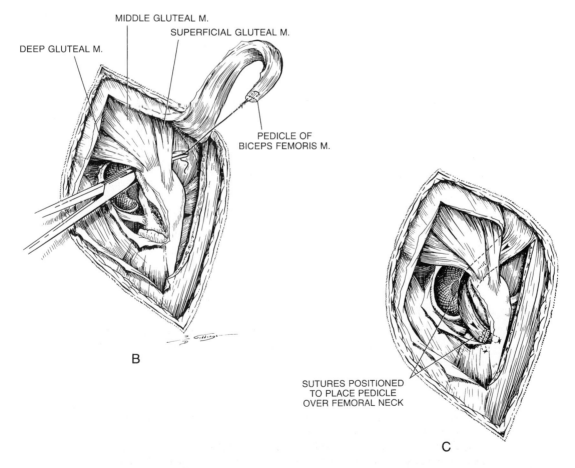

FIGURE 15–17. *See legend on opposite page*

ficult, as it takes several days for such animals to become ambulatory. This care is much easier in smaller breeds (e.g., <25 kg [55 pounds] in body weight).

PROGNOSIS ■   Return to active and pain-free use of the limb depends on surgical skill, length of time the hip pathology has been present, and severity of the pathology. Animals receiving operations for acute trauma, such as head and neck fractures, may be functional within 30 days. Those having chronic dysplasia with long-standing pain and muscle atrophy may require 6 months or more. These animals benefit particularly from swimming as an exercise. Patients with markedly displaced acetabular fractures and some with chronic dysplasia may never again regain good function.

Reported results vary considerably. Gendreau and Cawley's[50] analysis of 32 cases indicated only 37 percent excellent results and 26 percent good results, with only three of seven dogs weighing over 25 kg experiencing excellent results. Yet the Berzon series showed 90 to 100 percent use of the limb in 83 percent of all cases with no significant difference in results between large and small breeds.[47] It is pointless to assess results in this surgery by evaluating the postoperative gait. There is no doubt that smaller breeds experience less change in gait but the operation is usually successful in large breeds for relieving pain and restoring the animal's quality of life.

Pectineal Myectomy

A variety of operations on the pectineus muscle have been proposed to treat hip dysplasia and to prevent it. These surgeries include myectomy, myotomy, tenectomy, and tenotomy. All are designed to relieve tension produced by the muscle and transmitted to the hip joint. It has been speculated that this dorsal force on the femoral head pushes it against the dorsal acetabular rim and thus contributes to development of hip dysplasia.[51] Subsequent studies have indicated no effect in preventing dysplasia as a result of pectineal tenotomy[52] or myotomy.[53] Nevertheless, symptomatic improvement does result in many mature dogs for a variable length of time following pectineal resection.

Pectineal resection does not affect the radiographic changes associated with hip dysplasia; the degenerative changes progress at least as fast after surgery as would be expected without surgery. It is possible that increased abduction of the femur results, with a more varus position of the femoral head relative to the pelvis, which places the head more deeply in the acetabulum (see the discussion of the intertrochanteric varus osteotomy, above). Relief of pain possibly results from increasing the load-bearing areas of the femoral head and neck, thus decreasing the load per unit area of articular cartilage. Stress on the joint capsule may also be lessened. Because the joint is still unstable, however, degenerative changes continue and pain usually returns after a variable period of time ranging from a few months to years.

There is no way of predicting how long the effects of surgery will be beneficial; therefore, pectineal surgery has only limited value in treating hip dysplasia. It is useful under conditions in which short-term effects are acceptable, such as completing a field trial campaign.

SURGICAL TECHNIQUE ■   The pectineal muscles are exposed by means of the ventral approach to the hip joint. After the pectineus tendon is undermined and its origin cut, the abducted leg is adducted, thereby extruding the muscle through a proximal incision. The distal tendon is incised and the entire muscle is removed. Subcutaneous tissues and skin are closed only after attaining perfect hemostasis in the field.

AFTERCARE ■   Moderate exercise should be started 2 to 3 days after surgery to minimize the possibility of fibrous bands forming in the excision site which could restrict the femur. Such bands are minimized by total myectomy; however, they are not totally eliminated.

LEGG-CALVÉ-PERTHES DISEASE

Known by several other names such as Legg-Perthes or Calvé-Perthes disease, osteochondritis juvenilis, avascular necrosis, and coxa plana, Legg-Calvé-Perthes disease is noninflammatory aseptic necrosis of the femoral head and neck in small-breed dogs (Fig. 15–18). The cause of such necrosis is not known with certainty, but ischemia resulting from vascular compression[54] and precocious sex hormone activity[55] have been proposed. A genetic cause, homozygosity for an autosomal recessive gene, has been reported.[56]

In all cases, the bone of the femoral head and neck undergoes necrosis and deformation, during which time pain is manifested by the animal. The articular cartilage cracks as a result of the collapse of subchondral bone. Bone eventually returns to the necrotic area, but the femoral head and neck are deformed, with resulting joint incongruity and instability. This condition leads to severe degenerative changes within the entire hip joint and to development of marked osteoarthrosis.

Male and female animals are equally affected. Bilateral involvement has been reported as 16.5 percent[57] and 12 percent.[58] The toy breeds and terriers are most susceptible. The peak incidence of onset is 5 to 8 months of age, with a range of 3 to 13 months.[56]

Clinical Signs

Often the first abnormality noted is irritability. The animal may chew at the flank and hip area. Pain can be elicited in the hip, especially on abduction.

A   B

FIGURE 15–18. Legg-Calvé-Perthes disease. (*A*) Bony destruction early in the disease causes both radiographic lucency and actual loss of substance in the femoral head (gray circular spots) and neck. The epiphysis seems unaffected in this early stage. (*B*) At the end point of the process the femoral head has collapsed and deformed. Occasionally loss of bone will result in pathological avulsion fracture.

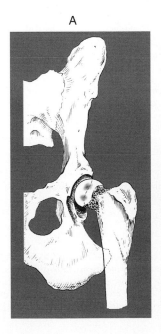
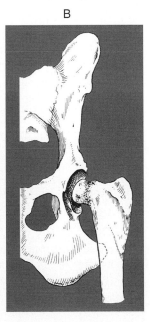

Later, crepitus may be present, with restricted range of motion and shortening of the limb. Atrophy of the gluteal and quadriceps muscles becomes apparent. Onset of lameness is usually gradual, and 6 to 8 weeks are required to progress to complete carriage of the limb,[57] although pain can be acute when there is fracture of the femoral head at lytic areas.

Radiographic signs (Fig. 15–18A, B) include increased joint space and foci of decreased bone density in the head and neck. The femoral head flattens where it contacts the dorsal acetabular rim, then distorts further to a variable degree. Osteophytes, as well as subluxation and fracture of the femoral head and neck, may be seen occasionally.

Treatment

Excision of the femoral head and neck produces more favorable results than does conservative treatment consisting of rest and analgesics.[57,58] Results are better, and recovery time is much shorter. With the proper surgical technique, virtually 100 per cent of these animals will become ambulatory and free of pain. A slight limp may remain because the leg is shortened by removal of the femoral head and neck, and the thigh and hip muscles remain somewhat atrophied. In rare instances where lucencies are seen without collapse of the femoral head an Ehmer sling may be tried for 3 to 4 weeks.

References

1. Basher AWP, Walter MC, Newton CD: Coxofemoral luxation in the dog and cat. Vet Surg 15:356, 1986.
2. Bone DL, Walker M, Cantwell HD: Traumatic coxofemoral luxation in dogs: Results of repair. Vet Surg 13:263, 1984.
3. Harari J, Smith CW, Rauch LS: Caudoventral hip luxation in two dogs. J Am Vet Med Assoc 185:312, 1984.
4. Thacher C, Schrader SC: Caudal ventral hip luxation in the dog: A review of 14 cases. J Am Anim Hosp Assoc 21:167, 1985.
5. Piermattei DL: An Atlas of Surgical Approaches to the Bones and Joints of the Dog and Cat, 3rd ed. Philadelphia, WB Saunders Co, 1993.
6. Allen SW, Chambers JN: Extracapsular suture stabilization of canine coxofemoral luxation. Cont Ed 8:457, 1986.
7. Braden TD, Johnson ME: Technique and indications of a prosthetic capsule for repair of recurrent and chronic coxofemoral luxations. Vet Comp Orthop Trauma 1:26, 1988.
8. Piermattei DL: A technique for surgical management of coxofemoral luxations. Small Anim Clin 3:373, 1963.
9. Hunt CA, Henry WB: Transarticular pinning for repair of hip dislocation in the dog: A retrospective study of 40 cases. J Am Vet Med Assoc 187:828, 1985.
10. Herron MR: Atraumatic ventral coxofemoral luxation in dogs (abstr.). Vet Surg 15:123, 1986.
11. Wadsworth PL, Lesser AS: Use of muscle transfer to prevent reluxation of the hip: Two case reports. Proc Vet Orthop Soc 14th Annual Meeting, 1986.
12. Corley EA: Hip dysplasia: A report from the Orthopedic Foundation for Animals. Semin Vet Med Surg 2:141, 1987.
13. Riser WH, Newton CD: Canine hip dysplasia as a disease. In Bojrab MJ (ed): Pathophysiology in Small Animal Surgery. Philadelphia, Lea & Febiger, 1981, pp 618–623.
14. Lust G, Rendano VT, Summers BA: Canine hip dysplasia: Concepts and diagnosis. J Am Vet Med Assoc 187:638, 1985.
15. McLaughlin R, Tomlinson J: Part 1—Symposium on CHD: Diagnosis and medical management. Vet Med Jan:25–53, 1996.
16. Lanting F: Canine Hip Dysplasia and Other Orthopedic Diseases. Loveland, CO, Alpine Publications, Inc, 1981.
17. Bardens JW: Palpation for the detection of joint laxity. Proc Canine Hip Dysplasia Symposium and Workshop, Orthopedic Foundation for Animals, St. Louis, 1972, pp 105–109.
18. Wright PJ, Mason TA: The usefulness of palpation of joint laxity in puppies as a predictor of hip dysplasia in a guide dog breeding programme. J Small Anim Pract 18:513, 1977.
19. Barr ARS, Denny HR, Gibbs C: Clinical hip dysplasia in growing dogs: The long-term results of conservative management. J Small Anim Pract 28:243, 1987.

20. Hannan N, Ghosh P, Bellenger C, Taylor T: Systemic administration of glycosaminoglycan polysulfate (Arteparon) provides partial protection of articular cartilage from damage produced by menisectomy in the canine. J Orthop Res 5:47, 1987.
21. deHaan JJ, Goring RL, Beale BS: Evaluation of polysulfated glycosaminoglycan for the treatment of hip dysplasia in dogs. Vet Surg 23:177–181, 1994.
22. Slocum B, Devine T: Pelvic osteotomy technique for axial rotation of the acetabular segment in dogs. J Am Anim Hosp Assoc 22:331–338, 1986.
23. Slocum B, Devine T: Pelvic osteotomy in the dog as treatment for hip dysplasia. Semin Vet Med Surg 2:107–116, 1987.
24. Schrader SC: Triple osteotomy of the pelvis and trochanteric osteotomy as a treatment for hip dysplasia in the immature dog: The surgical technique and results of 77 consecutive operations. J Am Vet Med Assoc 189:659–665, 1986.
25. Dejardin LM, Arnoczky SP, et al: The effect of triple pelvic osteotomy on the hip force in dysplastic dogs—a theoretical analysis (abstract). Proceedings, 4th ACVS Vet Symposium, 1994.
26. McLaughlin RM, Miller SW, et al: Force plate analysis of triple pelvic osteotomy for the treatment of canine hip dysplasia. Vet Surg 20:291–297, 1991.
27. Slocum B, Devine T: Pelvic osteotomy for axial rotation of the acetabular segment in dogs with hip dysplasia. Vet Clin North Am Sm Anim Pract 22:645–682, 1992.
28. Slocum B, Devine T: Dorsal acetabular rim radiographic view for evaluation of the canine hip. J Am Anim Hosp Assoc 26:289–296, 1990.
29. Smith GK, Popovich CA, et al: Evaluation of risk factors for degenerative joint disease associated with hip dysplasia in dogs. J Am Vet Med Assoc 206:642–647, 1995.
30. Popovich CA, Smith GK, et al: Comparison of susceptibility for hip dysplasia between Rottweilers and German shepherd dogs. J Am Vet Med Assoc 206:648–650, 1995.
31. Graehler RA, Weigle JP, Pardo AD: The effect of plate type, angle of ilial osteotomy, and degree of axial rotation on the structural anatomy of the pelvis. Vet Surg 23:13–20, 1994.
32. Koch DA, Hazewinkel HAW, et al: Radiographic evaluation and comparison of plate fixation after triple pelvic osteotomy in 32 dogs with hip dysplasia. Vet Comp Orthop Trauma 6: 9–15, 1993.
33. Sukhiani HR, Holmberg DL, Hurtig MB: Pelvic canal narrowing caused by triple pelvic osteotomy in the dog. Vet Comp Orthop Trauma 7:110–113, 1994.
34. Slocum B, Devine T: Femoral neck lengthening for hip dysplasia in the dog (abstract). Vet Surg 18:81, 1989.
35. Slocum B: Femoral neck lengthening (bulletin). Slocum Enterprises, Inc, Eugene, OR, Feb 1993.
36. Hauptman J, Prieur WD, Butler HC, Guffy MM: The angle of inclination of the canine femoral head and neck. Vet Surg 8:74, 1979.
37. Walker TL, Prieur WD: Intertrochanteric femoral osteotomy. Semin Vet Med Surg 2:117–130, 1987.
38. Braden TD, Prieur WD, Kaneene JB: Clinical evaluation of intertrochanteric osteotomy for treatment of dogs with early-stage hip dysplasia: 37 cases (1980–1987). J Am Vet Med Assoc 196:337–341, 1990.
39. Rumph PF, Hathcock JT: A symmetric axis-based method for measuring the projected femoral angle of inclination in dogs. Vet Surg 19:328–333, 1990.
40. Prieur WD: Double hook plate for intertrochanteric osteotomy in the dog. Synthes Veterinary Bulletin 1:1–4, 1984.
41. Brinker WO, Hohn RB, Prieur WD: Manual of Internal Fixation in Small Animals. Berlin, New York, Springer-Verlag, 1984.
42. Leger L, Sumner-Smith G, Gofton N, et al: A.O. hook plate fixation for metaphyseal fractures and corrective wedge osteotomies. J Small Anim Pract 23:209–216, 1982.
43. Olmstead ML, Hohn RB, Turner TT: Technique for total hip replacement. Vet Surg 10:44, 1981.
44. Olmstead M: Total hip replacement. Vet Clin North Am 17:943, 1987.
45. Olmstead M: The canine cemented modular hip prosthesis. J Am Anim Hosp Assoc 31: 109–124, 1995.
46. Massat BJ, Vasseur PB: Clinical and radiographic results of total hip arthroplasty in dogs: 96 cases (1986–1992). J Am Vet Med Assoc 205:448–454, 1994.
47. Berzon JL, Howard PE, Covell SJ, et al: A retrospective study of the efficacy of femoral head and neck excisions in 94 dogs and cats. Vet Surg 9:88, 1980.
48. Lippincott CL: Excision arthroplasty of the femoral head and neck utilizing a biceps femoris muscle sling. Part two: The caudal pass. J Am Anim Hosp Assoc 20:377, 1984.
49. Mann FA, Tanger CH, Wagner-Mann C, et al: A comparison of standard femoral head and neck excision and femoral head and neck excision using a biceps femoris muscle flap in the dog. Vet Surg 16:223, 1987.
50. Gendreau C, Cawley AJ: Excision of the femoral head and neck: The long term results of 35 operations. J Am Anim Hosp Assoc 13:605, 1977.
51. Bardens JW, Hardwick H: New observations in the diagnosis and cause of hip dysplasia. Vet Med Small Anim Clin 63:238, 1968.

52. Cardinet GH, Guffy MM, Wallace LJ: Canine hip dysplasia: Effects of pectineal tenotomy on the coxofemoral joints of German shepherd dogs. J Am Vet Med Assoc 164:591, 1974.

53. Bowen JM, Lewis RE, Kneller SK, et al: Progression of hip dysplasia in German shepherd dogs after unilateral pectineal myotomy. J Am Vet Med Assoc 161:899, 1972.

54. Gambardella PC: Legg-Calvé-Perthes disease in dogs. In Bojrab MJ (ed): Pathophysiology in Surgery. Philadelphia, Lea & Febiger, 1981, pp 625–630.

55. Ljunggren GL: Legg-Perthes disease in the dog. Acta Orthop Scand Suppl 95:7, 1967.

56. Pidduck H, Webbon PM: The genetic control of Perthes disease in toy poodles—a working hypothesis. J Small Anim Pract 19:729, 1978.

57. Lee R, Fry PD: Some observations of the occurrence of Legg-Calvé-Perthes disease (coxaplana) in the dog, and an evaluation of excision arthroplasty as a method of treatment. J Small Anim Pract 10:309, 1969.

58. Ljunggren GL: Conservative vs surgical treatment of Legg-Perthes disease. Anim Hosp 2:6, 1966.

16

Fractures of the Femur and Patella

The incidence for fractures of the femur is about 20 to 25 percent of all fractures in most veterinary practices; this rate is higher than for any of the long bones in the body. Additionally, femur fractures represent 45 percent of all long-bone fractures, a rate more than double that of other bones.[1] The femur also has the highest incidence of nonunion and osteomyelitis of all fractures. Open reduction and internal fixation is indicated in practically all femoral fractures.[2,3] Due to the eccentric loading of the femur during weight bearing (see Fig. 2–69), it is in this bone that the surgeon must be most cognizant of the tension/compression cortices and their effect on implants. Defects in the medial (compression/buttress) cortex place enormous bending loads on the implant, thus femoral fractures are the most severe test for an internal fixation device. In this chapter we suggest methods of treating various types of fractures as classified in the AO Vet Fracture Classification Scheme.[1] Patellar fractures are included with distal femoral fractures. Treatment recommendations are keyed to the Fracture Patient Scoring System detailed in Table 2–6 when applicable.[4,5]

FIXATION TECHNIQUES

Coaptation

This form of fixation has almost no application in femoral fractures because of the difficulty of immobilizing the hip joint in the dog and cat. A spica-type cast is required, but problems preventing the routine practical application of such a cast in small animals have not been solved.

For a period of about 20 years, starting in the early 1930s, the modified Thomas splint (see Fig. 2–25) was the most commonly used method of immobilizing femoral fractures.[6,7] With the advent of internal fixation this splint has rapidly faded from common usage as the sole method of immobilizing femoral fractures. When used as the sole method of fixation, the modified Thomas splint must be confined to greenstick fractures, fissure fractures, and fractures with minimal displacement in the very young patient. One must keep in mind that the ring, when properly applied, lies at the proximal third of the femur and may act as a fulcrum at the fracture site resulting in displacement of the proximal fragment. The splint also adds significant mass and elongates the distal lever arm, which can add to displacement of the distal fragment. The leg may be attached to the modified Thomas splint with the joints in various angles to exert the best mechanical advantage on the fracture. In most cases, however, the leg is splinted in the angulation of the normal standing position. Placing the leg in full extension over a period of time may lead to a decrease in range of joint movement in the stifle and to some loss of function or total dysfunction if fibrous ankylosis occurs in the hyperextended position. The splint must be frequently checked for pressure points, readjusted, and repaired during the healing period. It must be protected against moisture, both inside and out. Exercise must be restricted to help protect the splint from becoming loose or damaged. The presumed economic advantages of coaptation over internal fixation are seldom realized in the treatment of femoral fractures.

A long lateral molded splint (see Fig. 2–24) can also be applied to greenstick fractures, fissure fractures, and fractures with minimal displacement in the very young patient. The advantage over the Thomas splint is the absence of the ring proximally.

Intramedullary Pins and Wires

There are numerous types of intramedullary (IM) pins available with various types of points (see Fig. 2–54).[1,8] The round pins (Steinmann, Kirschner wire) are by far the most commonly used.

Steinmann Pin

When the Steinmann pin is used as the sole method of fixation of diaphyseal fractures, it should be reserved primarily for fractures that are inherently stable, such as type A1 and some type A3 (see Fig. 16–20). More instability can be tolerated in skeletally immature animals because of the rapidity of callus formation. Steinmann pins may be used for unstable fractures only with supplemental fixation such as an external fixator, multiple pins, cerclage wire, or lag screws.

PIN INSERTION ■ The pin may be inserted from the proximal end (normograde) by entering at the trochanteric fossa (Fig. 16–1) or by passing it retrograde from the fracture site proximally through the medullary canal (Fig. 16–2).

Normograde pin insertion is applicable to both closed and open reductions, and is preferred because it has the advantage over retrograde placement of positioning the pin more laterally in the trochanteric fossa and thus farther from the femoral head and sciatic nerve.[9] Additionally, less soft tissue is penetrated, facilitating cutting the pin shorter, which minimizes seroma formation and decreases patient discomfort. For midshaft and proximal femoral fractures it is best to simply extend the approach incision proximally for insertion of the pin. Transection of the tendon of insertion of the superficial gluteal muscle and elevation of the muscle before inserting the pin will allow for cutting the pin quite short at the conclusion of surgery. In other cases a short skin incision is made just dorsomedial to the greater trochanter. The pin is inserted through the subcutaneous fat and the gluteal muscles until the trochanter is felt on the tip of the pin. During the insertion process, the proximal femur is held in the angulation and rotation of the normal standing position. Keeping the pin chuck and pin axially oriented to the femur, the pin is "walked" medially off the trochanter into the trochanteric fossa, where it will center itself with some pressure through the pin chuck. When doing an open reduction the proximal femoral bone segment exposed in the open approach can be grasped with a bone-

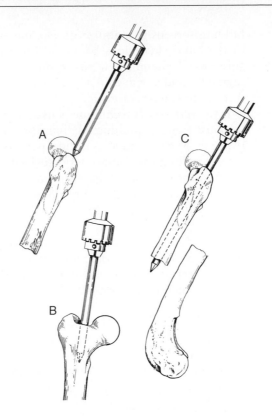

FIGURE 16–1. Normograde intramedullary pinning technique using Steinmann pin, with the proximal femur in the angulation and rotation of the normal standing posture. (*A*) The pin is inserted through the skin and underlying soft tissue at the eminence of the trochanter major. (*B*) The pin slides along the medial surface of the trochanter major into the trochanteric fossa, through the cortical bone, and down the medullary cavity. (*C*) The pin is held in axial alignment, and the bone fragment is held with bone-holding forceps to prevent rotation during pin insertion.

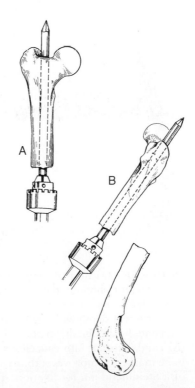

FIGURE 16–2. Retrograde technique intramedullary pinning technique using Steinmann pin, with the proximal femur in the angulation and rotation of the normal standing posture. Correct position of the proximal femur, particularly avoiding abduction, external rotation and excessive flexion of the hip, is essential to avoid potential sciatic neuropraxia. (*A*) The distal end of the proximal bone fragment is grasped with bone-holding forceps, and the pin is inserted proximally in the medullary canal. (*B*) As the pin is driven proximally an effort is made to direct it along the craniolateral surface of the medullary cavity. The proximal bone fragment is adducted until it is parallel to the surface of the table and held in the rotation and angulation of the normal standing position as the pin penetrates the proximal bone and soft tissues.

holding forceps to stabilize it. The pin is driven into the bone by quarter turns of the hand chuck in a back-and-forth motion, constantly applying firm pressure. Axial alignment is easily maintained by watching the proximal femoral segment, and the medullary cavity is quickly entered and the pin continued distally to the fracture site.

If the *retrograde* technique is used, care should be taken to have the proximal fracture fragment adducted (parallel to the table) and in the angulation and rotation of the normal standing position. On passing the pin proximally, it is directed along the craniolateral surface of the medullary cavity (Fig. 16–2). All of these precautions help keep emergence of the pin away from the femoral head and sciatic nerve. See the discussion below relative to sciatic nerve injury associated with IM pinning.

The method of seating the pin distally varies with the patient's bone type. Most dogs have pronounced cranial bowing of the femoral shaft (Fig. 16–3A). If the pin is allowed to follow its own course into the distal segment it will often penetrate the cranial cortex just proximal to the femoral trochlea (Fig. 16–3B). In this case simple pin retraction is not appropriate because postoperatively the pin often migrates distally through the pin track and re-enters the joint. The pin should be retracted to the fracture site, the fracture reangulated as described below, and the pin driven distally into unpenetrated trabecular bone. Even if the pin does not penetrate the cortex it is not stable fixation for fractures of the mid or distal segments. In these fractures it is important that the pin be seated in the dense trabecular bone of the distal metaphysis and condyles.

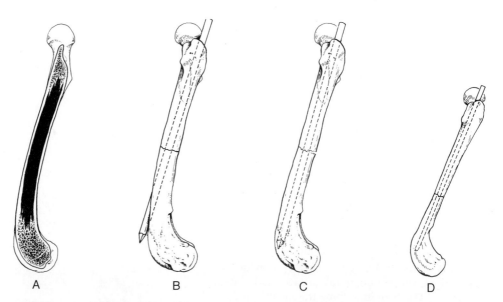

FIGURE 16–3. Effect of femoral shape on pin insertion. (*A*) Sagittal section through a canine femur showing the cortical bone, cancellous bone, and marrow cavity. (*B*) The canine femur has some cranial curvature, and the intramedullary pin cannot be inserted to a sufficient depth with the fracture reduced in perfect apposition. (*C*) With the fracture segments bent caudally at the fracture site, the intramedullary pin can be passed along the caudal cortex into cancellous bone at the distal end. This anchorage in cancellous bone markedly improves stability. (*D*) Anatomical reduction of a cat femur and insertion of a Steinmann pin for fixation. The diaphysis of a cat femur is straight.

After the fracture is reduced and as the pin is directed into the distal segment, it is best to angle both segments slightly caudally. This allows for deeper insertion of the pin in the cancellous bone of the distal metaphysis and for more stable fixation (Fig. 16–3C). When the bone is relatively straight, as in the toy dog breeds and in the cat, the pin naturally follows the medullary canal distally into the condyles (Fig. 16–3D). In any situation *the pin should penetrate distally at least to the proximal border of the patella* when the stifle is placed at the normal standing angle. With the pin chuck removed from the pin, another pin of the same length can be positioned external to the leg to verify the depth of insertion. Rotation of the distal femoral segment while seating the pin is neutralized by flexing the stifle and using the proximal tibia as a lever to control the femur. This also allows some compressive force to prevent distracting the fragments while driving the pin.

After the pin is inserted to the full depth with the point of the pin near, but not penetrating, the subchondral bone, it is cut as short as possible or it may be retracted 1 cm, cut off, then driven back into position by means of a countersink and mallet. Do not allow the fracture to distract during this type pin seating. A long pin in the gluteal area can lead to discomfort and seroma formation as well as to increasing the possibility of sciatic nerve entrapment by the tissue reaction incited by the pin (see discussion below). Some prefer that the depth of insertion be checked by taking a radiograph prior to cutting the pin. The incision may be closed, and taking precautions to maintain sterility of the protruding pin, a lateral radiograph is taken, and depth adjustments made prior to cutting the pin.

PIN DIAMETER ■ Ideally, pin diameter should approximate 75 to 80 percent of the marrow cavity. This is possible throughout the medullary canal in the cat and toy dog breeds because the femur is straight (Fig.16–3D); however, it is not possible in most dogs due to the cranial bowing of the femur (Fig. 16–3A), and to the narrowing of the canal at the midshaft. In these dogs, the pin should occupy about 75 to 80 percent of the marrow cavity diameter at the midshaft, which will give the pin 50 to 75 percent diameter relative to other areas of the medullary canal.

COMPLICATIONS ■ Horizontal shearing and rotary instability are the most common complications when a round pin is used. Any instability at the fracture site will invariably cause the pin to loosen due to bone resorption and to migrate proximally, sometimes completely out of the bone. Additional supplemental fixation should be added to guard against instability and movement at the fracture site. Supplemental fixation is described later in this chapter.

The *sciatic nerve* can become irritated or trapped over the top of the cut-off intramedullary pin either at the time of insertion, or more commonly, during the convalescent period if the precautions stated above are not observed. The incidence of such sciatic injury was 14.5 percent in one retrospective study.[10] Most cases are the result of excessive fibroplasia due to leg motion and an overly long and medially placed pin, rather than outright damage to the nerve during pin insertion. Clinical signs were delayed for 2 or 3 weeks postoperatively in 79 percent of cases, probably due to contracture of maturing fibrous tissue. Usual clinical signs included pain in the hip region on palpation, carrying of the leg with the hip flexed, and the proprioceptive reflex of the foot was diminished or lost. Immediate surgical intervention is in order in such a situation. After careful dissection down to the area, the pin is either cut shorter or removed if the fracture is healed. Enveloping fibrous tissue is dissected away from the nerve. Injury to the sciatic nerve is usually temporary, with no cases of permanent neurological deficit in a series of 14 cases.[10]

POSTOPERATIVE MANAGEMENT ■ Activity must be restricted until the stage of clinical union is reached. Union should be checked radiographically before removal of the pin. After clinical union is achieved, the pin may be removed by incising over its top and retracting it by pulling with quarter turns back and forth. This is usually done under a short-acting anesthetic, but in some cases, it may be removed under sedation and local anesthesia. Aseptic procedures are used for removal of the pin. If the pin has been cut sufficiently short to preclude soft tissue irritation, it is sometimes left in place with no ill effects. Occasionally, such a pin will loosen and migrate proximally, necessitating immediate removal.

Küntscher Nail

This nail has the advantage of affording rigid stability to both bending and torsion or rotation; however, insertion requires attention to the details in its use. Frequent complications include (1) the nail may jam in the medullary canal or split the bone, (2) longitudinal fracture lines already present may be opened up, or (3) if too small in diameter, it may not give sufficient stability. The Küntscher nail is rarely used in North America for small animals because of the aforementioned complications and the availability of other fixation methods.

Interlocking Nail

At the time of this writing, the interlocking nail (IN) is still in very limited use, but it appears to offer the promise of being a very effective fixation method for femoral fractures in large dogs (see Fig. 2–54).[11] Whereas standard Steinmann IM pinning is of no value in unstable fractures, the IN has the ability to provide both rotational and compression (buttress) stability heretofore available only by bone plate fixation.

Kirschner Wires

In reality only a small-diameter Steinmann pin, these "K-wires" are used as transfixation pins in a variety of femoral fractures, both as primary and supplemental fixation (see Figs. 16–7, 16–10, 16–12, 16–13, 16–14, 16–15, and 16–32).

Pins and Tension Band Wire

This method is widely applied for fractures/avulsions of the trochanter major (see Fig. 16–7C). The tendon of the superficial gluteal muscle is cut and the muscle elevated off the trochanter before placing the pins. The pins can either be anchored distally in the medial cortex distal to the lesser trochanter, or driven straight down the medullary canal, in which case they should be slightly longer for greater stability. Proximally, the wire is passed around the pins through the middle gluteal muscle close to the bone in order to prevent cutting of the muscle as the wire is tightened. The transverse hole for distal anchorage of the wire can be drilled through the distal end of the third trochanter without elevating the vastus lateralis muscle if the drilling proceeds from caudal to cranial, with internal rotation of the femur and strong retraction of the biceps femoris muscle. Careful bending of the protruding pins and seating them close to the bone is necessary to avoid soft tissue irritation, which can be a problem in thin dogs.

Cerclage Wires

These wires can provide very effective interfragmentary compression of larger fragments when a reconstructive approach is taken to the fracture repair (see Figs. 16–21, 16–24, 16–25, and 16–27). They are always used as a supplemental fixation and never as primary stabilization in shaft fractures.

Because of the insertion of the adductor magnus muscle on the diaphysis, most fragments from the caudal half of the femur have a viable periosteal blood supply. Great care should be taken in reducing such fragments to preserve the muscle attachment and its blood supply. Proof of the usefulness of this blood supply is provided by the observation that the first callus observed in femoral fractures is always along the caudal side of the shaft. Considerable effort must also be expended to pass the wire around the femur in the most atraumatic fashion in order to elevate a minimal amount of muscle from the bone. The use of a wire passer (Fig. 2–61) greatly assists in this maneuver. The passer is used as if it were a large needle and is inserted into adductor muscle as close as possible to the bone surface, then rotated around the bone to emerge cranially. The wire is inserted into the lumen in the tip of the passer and inserted until the tip of the wire is visible in the hole of the passer. The wire is grasped and the passer backed out through the same track.

Because the shaft of the femur is reasonably tubular there is no problem of wire slippage in the central portion of the bone. As the subtrochanteric and supracondylar areas are approached it may be necessary to notch the bone or otherwise prevent migration of the wires in these tapering areas (see discussion of cerclage wires in Chapter 2).

External Fixators

One is restricted to use of the unilateral type IA one-plane configuration on the femur. Double connecting bars are often indicated because of the bending load imposed in most unstable fractures. In general, the splint is well tolerated by the patient, although dogs are sometimes reluctant to bear weight on the limb, apparently due to the penetration of both the quadriceps (stifle extensor) and the biceps femoris (stifle flexor) muscles. This temporarily limits the range of stifle joint movement, which with the formation of adhesions may become a permanent limitation. Passive range-of-motion exercises may help minimize this problem. This temporary loss of function can be tolerated as long as there are no other limb fractures. In such a situation it is usually necessary to achieve early equalized load sharing between the limbs in order to minimize stress on the implants. This problem with function is not often encountered in the cat.

The splint may be applied with the fracture site closed or open. The latter is usually preferable because the reduction can be visualized during the insertion procedure. The muscle mass of the thigh makes closed reduction difficult in most animals. Because the splint is inserted on the lateral surface of the femur and penetrates large muscles, it is vulnerable to trauma, pin track drainage, and premature fixation pin loosening. This loosening can be partially overcome by inserting six or eight pins; however, the more fixation pins used, the greater the muscular impingement problem. Postoperative use of bulky dressings to stabilize the soft tissues has been advocated to reduce pin loosening due to muscular motion around the pins.[12]

When the external fixator is applied on femoral fractures as the sole method of fixation, it is used primarily on small breeds of young dogs and cats. These in general heal quite rapidly. When used on other femoral fractures, and especially in dogs, it is best to combine the fixator with the intramedullary pin.

External Fixator and Intramedullary Pin

The external fixator is added to the intramedullary pin fixation to help increase stability by reducing movement and rotation at the fracture site and helping to maintain length.[2,13,14] The unilateral type IA two-pin fixator (Fig. 16–4), is used primarily for transverse and short oblique fractures, and a four- or six-pin fixator is used on comminuted fractures. As a general rule it is advisable to use a minimum of four fixation pins; only with a Fracture Patient score of 9 to 10, and a body weight of less than 15 pounds (6.8 kg) should two pins be considered.[14]

The reasoning behind this combination of methods is that the presence of the IM pin will allow the fixator to be removed as soon as stabilizing callus is radiographically visible, typically at 4 to 6 weeks. Early removal allows greater weight bearing on the limb, which favors fracture healing and minimizes chances of permanent loss of motion in the stifle joint.

TECHNIQUE ■ The procedure for inserting the intramedullary pin (Fig. 16–4A, B) is the same as described earlier. When using this combined fixation, the IM pin can be reduced somewhat in diameter from the normal, to provide better clearance for the fixation pins that are inserted in the proximal and distal fragments. Following are the steps to use:

1.   Start the fixation pin insertion with the soft tissue in its normal position. The pin should pierce intact skin and preferably not enter on the incision line.

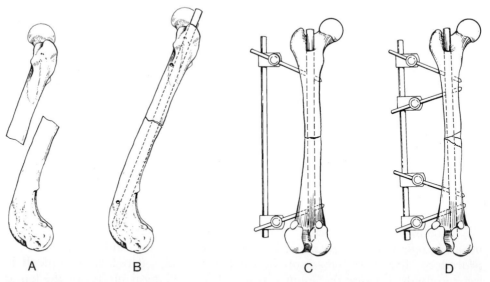

A   B   C   D

FIGURE 16–4. Insertion of an intramedullary pin and type 1A external fixator, 1/1 pins for fixation. (*A*) Transverse fracture of the femur. Fractures of this type have a tendency to rotate. (*B*) Self-locking bone-holding forceps holds fracture reduced during insertion of the Steinmann pin into the distal segment. Holding both fracture segments so that they do not rotate during the insertion process makes for a tighter fitting pin. The two circles show approximate location of fixation pins. Fixation pins can also be placed caudal to the IM pin. (*C*) Caudocranial view of reduced and fixed fracture. (*D*) Wedge fracture (caudocranial view) immobilized by use of an intramedullary pin and external fixator, 2/2 pins. Four pins are inserted for added stability.

2.   Insert the pins near the proximal and distal ends to obtain the best mechanical advantage. Placement of these pins to avoid the IM pin is facilitated by utilizing the greater trochanter proximally and the condylar region of the femur distally (Fig. 16–4B).

3.   Insert pins slightly off center to miss the intramedullary pin.

4.   Place the fixation pins at approximately a 70-degree angle to the long axis of the bone, penetrate both cortices, and connect the pins with single clamps and a connecting bar (Fig. 16–4C, D).

5.   When four or six fixation pins are used, the end pins are inserted first with two or four empty single clamps assembled on the connecting bar. The remaining pins are then inserted through the clamps into the bone.

The wound may be closed before or after application of the external fixator. Closure after application has the advantage of enabling visualization of the fracture site until all fixation is in place.

POSTOPERATIVE MANAGEMENT ■ Activity should be restricted during the healing period. The external fixator usually can be removed after a good primary callus is visible radiographically; this takes about 4 to 6 weeks. The intramedullary pin is removed when the fracture has reached the stage of clinical union.

Bone Plates

Bone plates are adaptable to practically all types of shaft fractures and have the distinct advantage of providing uninterrupted rigid internal fixation. In most cases, it is the fixation of choice in large dogs.[3] Depending on the fracture type the plate may be used as a tension band compression plate in short oblique, transverse, and some segmental fractures; as a neutralization plate in long oblique and reducible wedge fractures; and as a buttress or bridging plate in nonreducible wedge fractures. These functions are sometimes combined according to the fracture type (see Fig. 6–23). Figure 2–74 lists applicable plate sizes according to body weight.

The plate is usually applied on the lateral surface and contoured to fit that surface. Usually, the curvature pattern for contouring is taken from a craniocaudal radiograph of the opposite femur for buttress (bridging) application, or the plate may be contoured at the time of application for reducible fractures. A considerable lateral twist is necessary in the caudodistal end of the plate if it is necessary to extend the plate onto the condyle. Failure to do so will result in the craniodistal corner of the plate being elevated from the bone. A liberal exposure is necessary for application of the bone plate. In order to extend the plate distally to the condyle it is necessary to open the stifle joint as an extension of the approach to the shaft.

At least three or preferably four or more bone screws (penetrating six to eight or more cortices) should be placed in each of the proximal and distal bone segments. A simple transverse type A3 fracture can typically be stabilized with six cortices on each side of the fracture while eight cortices are minimum in buttress (bridging) applications. Whenever possible, the plate and screws should be inserted to develop compression at the fracture site. This has the distinct advantage of providing a more rigid fixation and making conditions more nearly optimal for healing.

Lag Screws

The primary site of application of lag screws as primary fixation is in proximal and distal zone fractures, where they are invaluable in providing rigid fixation (see Figs. 16–7, 16–10, 16–13, 16–17, 16–18, 16–34, and 16–35). Figure 2–74 lists applicable screw sizes according to body weight. Lag screws are never used as the sole method of fixation in immobilizing shaft fractures of the long bones. They can be used advantageously for interfragmentary compression in oblique, spiral, and butterfly segments and in certain types of multiple fractures when combined with a primary fixation method (see Figs. 16–22, 16–23, 16–26, and 16–27). If diaphyseal bone segments are large enough for bone screws to be used, they are to be preferred over cerclage wire. When properly inserted, bone screws are superior for compression and rigid fixation and are less apt to disrupt periosteal blood supply during their insertion.

PROXIMAL FRACTURES

Fractures of the proximal zone (Fig. 16–5) account for approximately 25 percent of femoral fractures[1] and offer significant challenges to provide adequate internal fixation. Very few of these fractures will respond to nonoperative treatment.

Fracture Type 31-A; Proximal, Trochanteric Region (Fig. 16–5A)

OPEN APPROACHES ■ Type A fractures of the trochanteric region are exposed by the approach to the greater trochanter and subtrochanteric region of the femur (Fig. 16–6A). Type B cervical and type C capital fractures are usually adequately exposed by the craniolateral approach to the hip (Fig.16–6B), sometimes combined with the trochanteric approach.[15]

Type A1, Avulsion

In most cases, this is a physeal separation at the trochanter accompanied by dislocation of the femoral head (Fig. 16–7A).[2] With the animal under anesthesia, a closed reduction of the femoral head is usually attempted first. If this can be accomplished and the reduction feels stable, fixation of the fracture is next

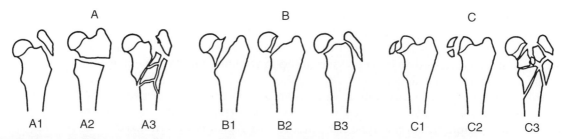

FIGURE 16–5. Proximal fractures of the femur. (*A1*) Avulsion, (*A2*) intertrochanteric simple, and (*A3*) multifragmentary. (*B1*) Basicervical, (*B2*) transcervical, and (*B3*) with trochanteric avulsion. (*C1*) Articular simple, (*C2*) articular multifragmentary, and (*C3*) multifragmentary cervical and trochanteric. (From Unger M, Montavon PM, Heim UFA: Classification of fractures of the long bones in the dog and cat: Introduction and clinical application. Vet Comp Orthop Trauma 3:41–50, 1990, with permission).

in order. If the dislocation cannot be reduced or is unstable on reduction, the open approach should include the coxofemoral joint.

Reduction and Internal Fixation

The following steps are observed:

1. If closed reduction of the hip was successful, or if there is no luxation, make the approach to the trochanteric region and proceed with fixation of the trochanter major. The trochanter major may be fixed by using two small pins or K-wires, and is sufficient for most animals under 4 months of age (Fig. 16–7B). These pins must be anchored in the medial cortex of the cervical region to provide good stability. Fixation by use of a tension band wire is usually the procedure of choice, particularly in larger dogs (Fig. 16–7C). Fixation with a cancellous bone screw is used only for animals approximately 4½ months of age or older (Fig. 16–7D). In our experience, this procedure has not significantly altered anatomical growth of the femur (length or shape) in dogs over 4½ months of age.

2. When open reduction and repair of the coxofemoral joint capsule are indicated, proceed directly with the approach to the hip joint.

3. Some of the origin of the vastus lateralis muscle is usually still attached to the lateral surface of the fractured trochanter major. Sever this origin with a tag end remaining attached to the trochanter major, to be sutured on closure.

4. After replacing the femoral head, obtain stability by closing the joint capsule. Abduction of the leg allows for easier and tighter closure of the joint capsule. Other measures for stabilizing the hip joint are discussed in Chapter 15.

5. Apply fixation of the trochanter major.

Aftercare ■ If the coxofemoral joint was luxated, place the leg in an Ehmer sling or off-weight-bearing sling (see Figs. 2–31 and 2–32) for 5 to 7 days, and limit exercise during the healing period of 4 to 6 weeks. No external support is needed for simple trochanter fracture.

Type A2 Intertrochanteric Simple

Reduction and Internal Fixation

Following exposure by the approach to the trochanter and subtrochanteric region of the femur, the pin and tension band wire method can be used for fixation in animals with a relatively high Fracture Patient score (e.g., 8 to 10). Although similar in principle to the method described above for the trochanter (Fig. 16–7C), some modification of pin size is needed. Rather than small flexible K-wire, larger Steinmann pins are used, and they are driven distally as is usual for Steinmann pins (Fig. 16–8). Because of their diameter it may not be possible to bend the proximal end of these pins; in this situation they are driven as closely as possible to the bone surface without the wires slipping over the end. Carefully passing the wire through the middle gluteal muscle close to the bone will help prevent slipping over the pins. Rush pins can also be used in place of Steinmann pins, and their hooked end eliminates the problems described above. Drilling of the distal hole for the tension wire will require elevation of the vastus lateralis muscle. The position of the hole is adjusted to cause the wire to cross close to the fracture line.

Other possible fixation methods for lower Fracture Patient scores (<8) involve external fixators or bone plates, as described below for type A3 fractures.

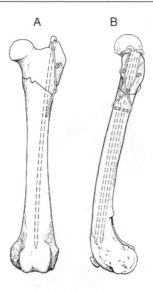

FIGURE 16–8. Fixation of a type A2 intertrochanteric simple fracture of the proximal femur. (*A, B*) The fracture is pinned with two small Rush or Steinmann pins from the eminence of the greater trochanter. A tension band wire is then applied, anchored around the protruding ends of the pins and through a drill hole distally. The drill hole is positioned to cause the figure-of-8 wire to cross close to the fracture line.

Both external fixators and bone plates offer suitable fixation. The *external fixator* is a type IA, single plane, with at least two, but preferably three pins in each major bone segment (Fig. 16–9). One pin can be inserted deeply into the femoral head, but with care to not penetrate the articular surface. The remaining proximal pins penetrate the calcar region medially. *Bone plate* fixation is similar to that shown for type C3 fractures (see Fig. 16–18), with some of the plate screws probably acting as lag screws to stabilize fragments. Double hook plates, as used for intertrochanteric osteotomy (see Chapter 15) have also been applied to these subtrochanteric fractures.[16] Autogenous cancellous bone graft should be used in any unreduced fracture gaps.

Aftercare ■   No external support is required, only restriction of exercise for the healing period. The external fixator is removed when clinical union is verified. Removal of the bone plate after clinical union may be necessary if soft tissue irritation or loosening of the implant is noted. An additional reason to

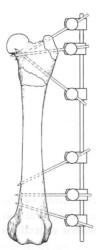

FIGURE 16–9. Fixation of a type A3 multifragmentary fracture of the proximal femur by means of a type IA external fixator. A double connecting bar is used for very large breeds or when significant fracture gaps remain.

remove the plate is that because the plate ends in the diaphysis and creates a stress raiser, there is an increased risk of accidental fracture at the end of the plate.

Fracture Type 31-B Proximal, Simple Cervical (Fig. 16–5B)

In these fractures, the fracture line varies and is usually simple; however, it may be multiple in nature. Various degrees of embarrassment to the blood supply of the head and neck may occur in connection with the original injury.[3,17,18] Considerable mechanical damage from abrasion can be done to the fracture surfaces if the animal starts actively walking on the limb before fixation is accomplished. This abrasion can destroy the irregular surfaces of the fracture and make accurate reduction very difficult. The incidence of unfavorable complications can be markedly reduced by (1) early surgery, (2) accurate reduction, (3) rigid uninterrupted fixation with compression at the fracture site, and (4) careful supervision of the postoperative care. In general, if these points can be complied with, the prognosis is favorable. Because of this, excision of the femoral head and neck or total hip replacement is usually considered a second choice in most fresh fractures of the femoral neck in larger breeds. Technical difficulties arise in repairing neck and head fractures in small breeds, and because of their excellent function with femoral head and neck excision, many consider this the best treatment in cats, toy, and miniature breeds.

Note: Repair of a fractured femoral neck or of a fracture of the proximal femoral epiphysis in a young growing animal may result in shortening of the femoral neck and instability of the hip joint, which may give rise to alterations of the hip joint characteristic of hip dysplasia.

OPEN APPROACHES ■ The craniolateral approach to the hip joint (Fig 16–6B) is preferred for open reduction, as it is generally more sparing of blood supply to the bone than the dorsal approaches.[18]

Type B1, Basicervical; Type B2, Transcervical

Both of these fracture types are handled in a similar manner. An impacted fracture with no displacement may heal with external immobilization and restricted exercise. The safer and preferred procedure is to apply fixation using a bone screw or multiple pins without further disturbing the position. Fractures showing various degrees of displacement respond best to an open approach with reduction and fixation. Mechanical studies indicate that a lag screw or three parallel 2.0-mm ($^5/_{64}$-inch) K-wires were able to resist a force of three times body weight, equivalent to the forces placed on a normal hip during walking exercise. Two K-wires, either parallel or divergent, were not as strong.[19] See Figure 2–74 for appropriate screw sizes.

Reduction and Fixation

After making the approach, temporary reduction is usually carried out to see if reduction and fixation are feasible. This usually can be accomplished by grasping the trochanter major with vulsellum or pointed reduction forceps and manually maneuvering the fracture segments back into position (see Fig. 2–15A, B). Abduction of the femoral shaft is usually necessary to accomplish reduction.

LAG SCREW FIXATION ■ A cortical lag screw is preferred over partially threaded screws for fixation, as it eliminates the necessity for ensuring that all the threads are in the neck/head fragment.

1.   The gliding hole is first drilled through the femoral neck (Fig. 16–10A, B). Note carefully the angle of the drill relative to the femoral shaft. The hole is started at the distal end of the third trochanter in order to keep the screw entirely within the femoral neck. The screw is commonly started too high on the trochanter, with the result that the screw is too acutely angled to the shaft.

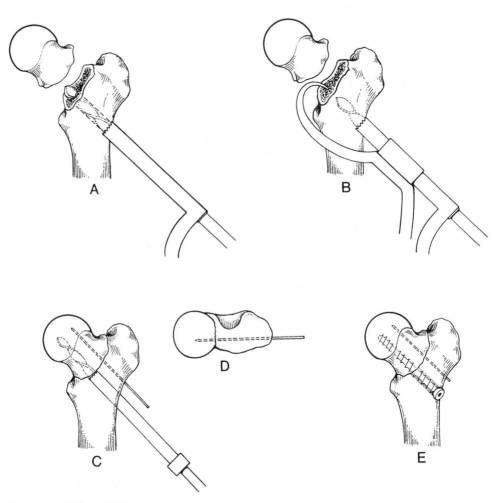

FIGURE 16–10. When a cortex screw is used for cervical fracture fixation, the gliding hole is drilled up through the femoral neck before reduction so that the hole is properly placed. (A) Drilling the hole using regular drill guide. (B) Drilling the hole using a pointed drill guide. This is advantageous in placing the hole properly. (C, D) The fracture is next reduced, and small Kirschner wire is inserted to aid in stabilizing the fragments. The appropriate drill sleeve is inserted into the femoral gliding hole. This functions as a guide for drilling the appropriate size hole in the femoral head. (E) After the hole is measured and tapped (unless a self-tapping screw is used), the appropriate size and length of screw is inserted. This serves as a lag screw in compressing the fragments. A cancellous screw could be used to accomplish the same objective if all of the threads are on the far side of the fracture line.

This results in high bending loads on the screw, with subsequent failure or loosening.

2.   With the fracture segments reduced and compressed either by a pointed reduction forceps or by medial pressure on the trochanter, one or more Kirschner wires (0.045 to 0.062 inch; 1.2 to 1.6 mm) are inserted through the trochanter, femoral neck, and head. Unlike the screw, the Kirschner wire should traverse the dorsal bridge of bone between the trochanter major and femoral head, not the trochanteric fossa, for maximum holding power (Fig. 16–10C, D). The pin is positioned proximally so that it does not interfere with insertion of the bone screw. It will assist in maintaining reduction and will help keep the femoral head from turning during the drilling, tapping, and insertion of the bone screw. Maintenance of reduction is assisted by applying pressure at the fracture site using bone forceps attached to the trochanter major.

3.   An appropriate size drill sleeve is next inserted through the glide hole; this serves as a guide for centering and drilling the appropriate size tap hole in the femoral head. Ideally, the depth of the hole should be to the subchondral bone; this depth can be estimated by visualizing and measuring the head and neck segment before reduction and by measurement from the radiograph. Before the drill bit is removed, a check for penetration of articular cartilage should be made by rotation and flexion-extension of the hip joint to check for crepitus. A curved hemostat can also be passed along the surface of the femoral head through a small joint capsule incision. The depth of the hole is measured, tapped, and the appropriate size cortical screw is inserted (Fig. 16–10D). Compression of the fracture line should be confirmed visually during tightening of the screw. The Kirschner wire is usually left in place. When the basicervical fracture line is quite oblique, as in Figure 16–11, special attention must be paid to reduction because there may not be good contact at the distal part. Elevation of a portion of the vastus lateralis off the fractured neck allows visualization of the reduction. Application of reduction forceps during fixation in the distal calcar area is essential in most cases of this type. It may be possible to insert a second lag screw from the midpoint of the third trochanter into the calcar.

KIRSCHNER WIRE FIXATION ■   After reduction as described above, the K-wires are best placed with a low-speed power drill; they are difficult to accurately drill with a hand chuck. The angle of insertion is as described above for the screw (Fig. 16–12). The outer wires are placed as proximally and distally in the neck as possible, and the central pin is then placed between.

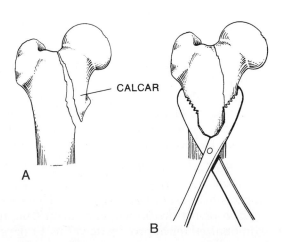

FIGURE 16–11. (*A*) Oblique type B1 fractures of the femoral neck require care (*B*) to reduce and compress the calcar region prior to bone screw fixation.

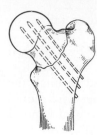

FIGURE 16–12. Fixation of a type B1 femoral neck fracture using Kirschner wires. This method is used primarily for small dogs and cats.

Aftercare ■ At the completion of surgery, radiographs should be taken from two ventrodorsal views; one view should show the legs flexed at the hips (frog-leg position), and another should show the rear legs extended. The frog-leg position is particularly useful to visualize the depth of the screw in the head and neck. The leg is usually placed in an off-weight-bearing or Ehmer sling (see Figs. 2–31 and 2–32) for 7 to 10 days. Exercise is restricted for the next month or until the stage of clinical union is reached as evaluated radiographically, then activity is slowly returned to normal over the next month. The bone screw and pin are not usually removed.

Type B3, Cervical with Trochanteric Avulsion

A combination of the methods described above for A1 and B1 and B2 fractures is applied to these fractures.

Fracture Type 31-C Proximal, Capital or Multifragmentary Cervical (Fig. 16–5C)

Type C1, Articular Simple

This group of fractures includes both fractures through the articular surface (Fig. 16–13), and those involving the physis only (Fig. 16–14).

Avulsion Fracture of the Femoral Head

With this fracture, a small portion of the femoral head remains attached to the round ligament, and the femoral head is dislocated in the craniodorsal position (Fig. 16–13A). The fracture segment remaining attached to the round ligament varies in size and is usually visible on a radiograph. Treatment varies with the individual case, depending primarily on the size of the fragment and the exact location of the fracture line. Presented here are several suggestions of courses that may be followed.

CLOSED REDUCTION ■ An Ehmer sling (see Fig. 2–31) is applied for approximately 2 weeks, and activity is restricted for an additional 2 to 4 weeks. Success of this procedure depends on perfect reduction at the fracture site and maintenance of the reduction until the fracture segments have healed. Both of these conditions must be met if this procedure is to be successful, but this is difficult to accomplish unless the fragment is very small.

SURGICAL EXCISION OF THE BONE FRAGMENT AND REDUCTION OF THE FEMORAL HEAD ■ The avulsed segment is removed through a craniolateral approach to expose the hip joint. The femoral head is replaced and stabilized by one of the methods discussed in Chapter 15; following closure, the leg is immobilized for approximately 7 to 14 days (e.g., by means of an Ehmer sling).

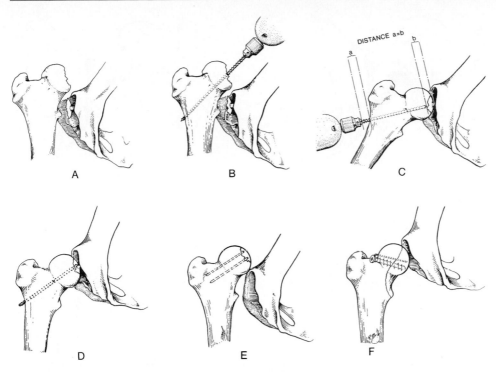

FIGURE 16–13. Fixation of a type C1 avulsion fracture of the femoral head. (*A*) Avulsion fracture with dislocation of the femoral head. (*B*) A small double-pointed thread pin is inserted in the center of the fracture surface and passed retrograde through the head and neck, emerging at the base of the trochanter major. (*C*) A pin chuck is attached at a distance from the bone (*a*) corresponding to thickness of avulsed segment (*b*); fracture segments are reduced and compression is applied during insertion of the pin. (*D*) About ⅛ inch of the pin is left protruding so that removal is possible. (*E*) Alternate method is to cut the round ligament, reduce the fracture, and stabilize by inserting two or more countersunk Kirschner wires. (*F*) Occasionally, a portion of the femoral head and neck is fractured off in an oblique fashion. If the fragment is large enough, it may be fixed using a small screw and Kirschner wire.

If the removed avulsed segment is too large, the remaining portion of the femoral head may not remain stable in the acetabulum, and dislocation will occur. Development of significant degenerative joint disease is to be anticipated if the fragment is large.

OPEN REDUCTION AND FIXATION[2,3] ■　A dorsal open approach with osteotomy of the trochanter major is necessary to expose the hip joint (see Fig. 14–13).[15] A small threaded K-wire is started in the center of the fracture surface of the femoral head and passed retrograde through the head and neck, emerging at the base of the trochanter major (Fig. 16–13B). The pin is inserted until it is flush with the fracture surface, and the chuck is attached on the opposite end at a distance from the bone corresponding to the thickness of the avulsed fragment (Fig. 16–13C). The fracture is held in reduction and compressed during insertion of the threaded pin. The pin is then cut off about ⅛ inch beyond the bone (Fig. 16–13D). If the fracture segment is large enough, two pins are inserted. Following closure, the leg is immobilized in a non–weight-bearing or Ehmer sling (see Figs. 2–31 and 2–32) for about 10 to 14 days. Exercise is restricted until healing is complete.

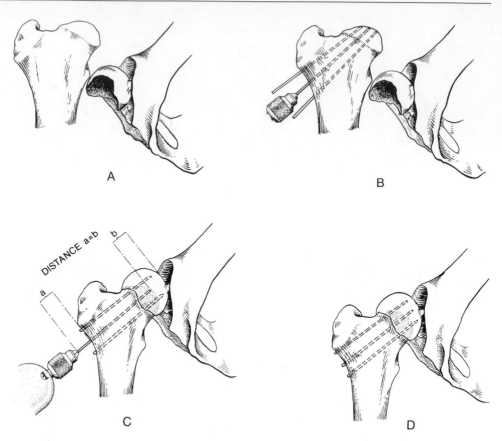

FIGURE 16–14. Normograde fixation of a proximal femoral type C1 physeal fracture with multiple Kirschner wires. (*A*) Physeal fracture. (*B*) Two to four Kirschner wires are driven from the base of the trochanter major up through the femoral neck to the fracture surface. (*C*) After reduction, a pin chuck is set at a distance from the bone corresponding to the thickness of the epiphysis; pins are driven into the epiphysis. (*D*) All pins are deeply seated into the epiphysis but do not penetrate the articular cartilage.

Another method of fixation worth consideration is to cut the round ligament, reduce the fracture fragments, and stabilize by use of two or more small countersunk Kirschner wires (Fig. 16–13*D*). Miniscrews (1.5 to 2.0 mm) can also be used from the articular surface as illustrated in Figure 16–16. In some cases, the ventral portion of the head and neck is fractured obliquely and may be reduced and fixed in place using a miniscrew and Kirschner wire placed from the edge of the articular surface (Fig. 16–13*F*).

TOTAL HIP REPLACEMENT ■ When the femoral head cannot be reconstructed and saved, total hip replacement (see Chapter 15) should be considered as an option.

EXCISION OF THE FEMORAL HEAD AND NECK ■ Excision arthroplasty is usually considered a last resort because the intact joint should be maintained if possible (see Chapter 15).

Fracture of the Femoral Capital Physis

This condition is limited to young animals in which the capital physis is still present (Fig. 16–14*A*). It usually occurs between the ages of 4 and 11 months.

In most cases, it is primarily a separation at the epiphyseal line (usually Salter-Harris I, occasionally II); the joint capsule can be attached to the epiphysis, partially detached, or completely stripped off, which undoubtedly affects healing. Fortunately, in most cases there is some attachment. If open reduction and internal fixation are to be done, they should be performed as soon as possible, preferably within the first 24 hours, to avoid the danger of thrombosis occurring in the kinked capsular vessels at the junction of the femoral head and neck, and to avoid further injury to the surface of the neck due to abrasion from the epiphysis. The femoral neck also undergoes demineralization quite rapidly, and this change is usually evident on the radiograph within 7 to 10 days. Internal fixation is primarily indicated in large-breed dogs, as small dogs and cats have excellent and predictable function with excision arthroplasty (femoral head and neck excision).

The *prognosis* of internal fixation depends on the age of the patient, concurrent injuries of the hip joint, early accomplishment of surgery, preservation of blood supply in the operative procedure, accurate reduction at the fracture site, rigid uninterrupted fixation, and restriction of early weight bearing. The percentage of success decreases with each day's delay in surgery. A good healing response is possible for patients treated within 4 days. Success has been achieved in patients treated within 10 days; however, after this period of time, rigid fixation is difficult to obtain because of demineralization and abrasion of the femoral neck. All dogs will show evidence of degenerative joint disease at some point postoperatively.[20] Arthritic changes are more pronounced in animals that are 4 months of age or less at time of injury, and in animals that have concurrent ipsilateral injury to the coxofemoral joint.[21] Although radiographic narrowing of the femoral neck occurs in about 70 percent of cases following internal fixation, this seldom results in collapse of the neck.[21]

KIRSCHNER WIRE OR PIN FIXATION ■ The pin techniques described below are preferable to use of a lag screw in most cases and particularly in younger animals (<7 months of age) because they are less apt to bring about premature closure of the physeal plate and resultant femoral neck shortening. Figure 16–14 shows the surgical procedure for fixation of a proximal femoral physeal fracture.[2,3] The exposure of the area should be conservative to minimize destruction of blood supply. Reduction of the fracture is best accomplished by grasping the trochanter major with vulsellum or pointed reduction forceps and moving the femur distally and medially into position (see Fig. 2–15A, B). The capitus is usually rotated in relation to the neck due to the round ligament and may cause some difficulty in reduction. Medial pressure on the trochanter while flexing and extending the hip joint with the femur abducted will usually cause the epiphysis to derotate and lock into the femoral neck in the reduced position. Small pointed reduction forceps applied with finger pressure only can be attached to the periphery of the capitus to assist in the derotation. Maintaining medial pressure will maintain reduction while fixation is applied.

Note: A review of the contour of the epiphysis and epiphyseal line is most helpful prior to undertaking anatomical reduction.

Two to four small smooth pins are inserted for immobilization. Pin size corresponds with the size of bone and may range from a 0.035-inch Kirschner wire to a ⁵/₆₄-inch Steinmann pin (1 to 2 mm). The pins may be inserted in antegrade (Fig. 16–14) or retrograde (Fig. 16–15) fashion. The former is preferred in most cases. The pins may be inserted parallel or in a converging-diverging fashion; mechanical studies indicate superior strength of parallel placement over

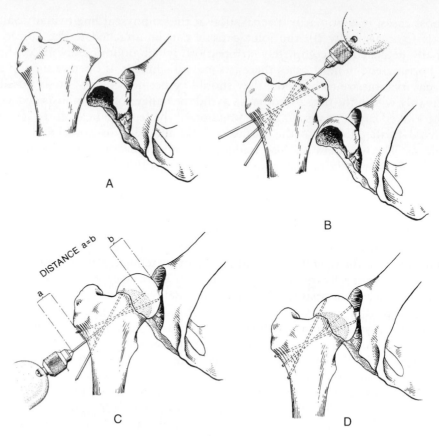

FIGURE 16–15. Retrograde fixation of a type C1 proximal femoral physeal fracture with multiple Kirschner wires. (*A*) Physeal fracture of the proximal femur. (*B*) Two to four double-pointed Kirschner wires are driven retrograde from the fracture to exit distal to the trochanter major on the lateral femoral surface. (*C*) After reduction, a pin chuck is set at a distance from the bone corresponding to the thickness of the epiphysis; pins are driven into the epiphysis. (*D*) All pins are deeply seated in the epiphysis but do not penetrate the articular cartilage. The converging/diverging pins may not be as strong as parallel pins.[19]

diverging pins.[19] The main objective is to have the pins well distributed at the fracture surface. The pin chuck is set on the pin so that the distance from the chuck to the lateral femoral cortex corresponds with the thickness of the epiphysis (Figs. 16–14C and 16–15C). With the fracture compressed in the reduced position, the pins are inserted into the epiphysis one at a time (Figs. 16–14C, D and 16–15C, D). The pins should not penetrate the articular cartilage. Pin penetration can be checked by careful movement of the femoral head in the acetabulum after each pin is inserted and by palpation of the femoral head using a small curved hemostat.

Aftercare ■   At the completion of surgery, radiographs should be taken from two ventrodorsal views; one view should show the legs flexed at the hip (frog-leg), and the second should show the rear legs extended. The frog-leg view is superior for judging depth of penetration of the pins. Follow-up radiographs should be taken at about 6 weeks. At this time, they should reveal healing or any complications.

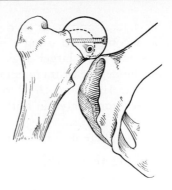

FIGURE 16–16. Fixation of a type C1 physeal fracture with lag screws from the articular surface. Two 1.5 to 2.0-mm screws are used, with the screw heads countersunk below the cartilage surface. One screw is in the fovea capitus and the second is near the cranial border of the epiphysis.

An Ehmer or non–weight-bearing sling (see Figs. 2–31 and 2–32) is applied to the leg for about 7 to 10 days. Exercise should be limited for the next 5 weeks. The pins are usually left in place unless indicated otherwise.

LAG SCREW FIXATION ■ Fixation can also be achieved by lag screw application through the articular surface (Fig. 16–16).[22] The epiphysis must be freed of soft tissue attachments and removed from the acetabulum. After reduction onto the metaphysis, a K-wire is inserted through the fovea capitus for temporary stabilization while a 1.5- to 2.0-mm screw is inserted in lag fashion cranial to the fovea. The head of the screw must be countersunk below the articular surface. The K-wire is removed and replaced with a second screw.

In those animals approximately 7 months of age or older, the epiphysis may be reattached by use of lag screw fixation through the femoral neck (Fig. 16–17), although there is no significant mechanical advantage over pin fixation,[19] and the technique is technically more difficult due to the thin cross section of the epiphysis.

Type C2, Articular Multifragmentary

Successful internal fixation of these fractures is very unlikely, and degenerative joint disease is the almost inevitable consequence of such attempts. Most of these animals are candidates for either total hip replacement or excision arthroplasty, which are covered in Chapter 15.

Type C3, Multifragmentary Cervical and Trochanteric

For these fractures there is no option of closed reduction; reduction is accomplished by performing an open approach. The exposure of choice is usually a combination of the craniolateral approach to the hip joint (Fig. 16–6B) and

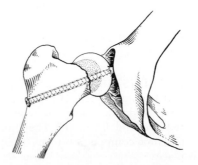

FIGURE 16–17. Lag screw fixation of a type C1 physeal fracture of the femoral head. Care must be taken in tightening the screw because the threads in the epiphyseal end are in cancellous bone.

the lateral approach to the femur (see Fig. 16–19). Fixation can usually best be accomplished using a bone plate and bone screws.[2,3] Fractures of this type in some of the larger dogs are amenable to the use of a hook plate.[16] Depending on the degree of fragmentation, the pin or external fixator techniques shown in Figures 16–8 and 16–9 may be applicable, as a screw for the femoral neck can be accommodated in both instances.

Bone Plate and Lag Screws

In Figure 16–18, a craniolateral approach to the hip joint and a lateral approach to the femur are performed to expose the fracture site. The approach procedure is modified to fit the individual fracture. Reduction is usually accomplished by starting at the proximal end and working toward the distal end. Bone-holding forceps, Kirschner wires, lag screws, and cerclage wire help hold the fragments in the reduced position. The bone plate is contoured. An easy and helpful procedure is to pre-bend the plate to the curvature of the lateral surface of the opposite femur, as shown from a craniocaudal view on the radiograph. The use of a compression plate (DCP) has the added advantage of allowing oblique insertion of the bone screw proximally into the femoral neck and head along with affording compression of the various fracture segments. Usually, the first bone screw is inserted through the base of the trochanter major and neck, and into the femoral head. The trochanter major is then reduced and fixed in position (Fig. 16–18A, B). The remaining bone screws are inserted as indicated (Fig. 16–18C, D). In some cases, additional bone screws that produce a lag effect may be used advantageously to assist in compressing at the fracture site.

Aftercare ■   Following closure, an off-weight-bearing sling (see Fig. 2–32) may be indicated for 3 to 7 days. Exercise is severely restricted for 6 to 8 weeks. Radiographs taken at 6 to 8 weeks are used to evaluate the healing, and if satisfactory, a gradual resumption of normal activity is started.

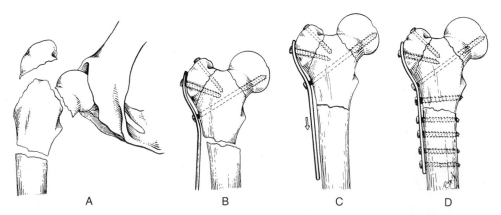

         A   B   C   D

FIGURE 16–18. Fixation of type C3 fractures of the femoral neck, trochanter major, and femoral shaft. (*A*) Fracture as seen in a craniocaudal radiograph. (*B*) The plate is contoured, and a long lag screw is placed in the femoral neck. The trochanter major is reduced and fixed. (*C*) The subtrochanteric fracture is reduced. A tension device or dynamic compression plate (DCP) is used to obtain compression. (*D*) Fixation plate in place.

Complications in Proximal Femoral Fractures

Most complications in femoral head and neck fractures are caused by:

1. Embarrassment of the blood supply to the femoral head and neck that occurs at the time of the initial injury or during the surgical procedure.
2. Poor bone reduction.
3. Inadequate fixation.
4. Premature weight bearing.

The most frequently occurring complications are:

1. Delayed union or nonunion.
2. Avascular necrosis.
3. Secondary osteoarthritis.
4. Cessation of neck growth in young animals as a result of premature closure of the physis, leading to subluxation of the hip.

Radiographic Signs

Radiographic evidence of a complication may show up as a loss of density in the femoral neck or along the fracture line in contrast to the surrounding bony tissue. Such a sign points toward disturbance in blood supply, demineralization, and possible movement at the fracture site. In long-standing cases, a mottled appearance of the femoral head indicates replacement of some areas of necrotic bone by new bone. In some instances, the femoral neck may disappear partially or completely in 3 to 6 weeks, leading to varying degrees of segmental collapse of the neck. In most cases, clinical and radiographic evidence of complications is evident within 6 weeks. However, about 6 months should elapse before the clinician attempts to determine the ultimate fate of the femoral head and neck, even in those patients that appear to be healing initially. Most cases of coxofemoral dislocation, physeal separation, or femoral neck fracture that made a good recovery show some temporary demineralization and slight narrowing of the femoral neck.

Treatment

If reduction and fixation are satisfactory, restricted activity and more healing time are indicated. In some cases, a more rigid internal fixation with restriction of activity is indicated. Those beyond salvaging with a functional hip joint are subjects for excision arthroplasty of the femoral head and neck or for total hip replacement, as discussed in Chapter 15.

DIAPHYSEAL FRACTURES

These fractures are usually the result of direct trauma and are accompanied by various degrees of soft tissue damage and hematoma.[2,3] The fracture pattern may be quite variable: transverse, oblique, spiral, multiple, fragmented, or, occasionally, greenstick in the young animal. As discussed above, external fixation is rarely adequate. Treatment recommendations are keyed to the Fracture Patient Scoring System detailed in Table 2–6 when applicable.[4,5] The internal methods of fixation include use of:

1. Intramedullary Steinmann pin alone.
2. Intramedullary Steinmann pin plus auxiliary fixation.

3. Interlocking intramedullary nail. Although still in the early stages of clinical use, the IN holds promise of being as useful in femoral fractures as bone plates have been in the past.

4. Unilateral external fixator with an intramedullary pin and other auxiliary fixation as indicated. The caveats applicable to external fixators used on canine femoral fractures are discussed above in the section Fixation Techniques.

5. Plate with or without lag screws or cerclage wires. The multiple and very unstable fractures, in general, respond best to bone plate and screw fixation. In large dogs, almost all femoral shaft fractures make a better functional response and are accompanied by fewer complications with bone plate and screw fixation.

OPEN APPROACH AND REDUCTION ■   With few exceptions, a lateral approach is used to expose the femoral shaft for reduction and internal fixation (Fig. 16–19).[15] In mid to proximal femoral fractures, the proximal fragment rotates caudally, allowing excessive anteversion of the femoral head. This must be remembered when applying fixation, especially in comminuted fractures (see Fig. 16–25). Oblique or multiple wedge fractures develop considerable overriding, and can be very difficult to reduce, especially in large breeds or when several days have elapsed since the injury. The use of fracture distractors or reduction by means of an intramedullary pin is helpful (see Figs. 2–18 and 2–19).

Fracture Type 32-A; Diaphyseal Simple or Incomplete
(Fig. 16–20A)

Type A1, Incomplete

The temptation to treat these fractures by external splintage should be resisted, for the reasons mentioned above in the discussion of fixation techniques. Additionally, these fractures occur primarily in growing animals, and immobilization of the limb in these animals often leads to development of coxa valga and resulting instability of the coxofemoral joint. Fracture Patient scores typically are in the 9 to 10 range. It is very simple to insert a Steinmann pin in a normograde manner, often without open approach (Figs. 16–1 and 16–3). The pin adequately stabilizes the fracture against the bending forces of the hamstring muscles, and allows early weight bearing. The pin can be smaller diameter than

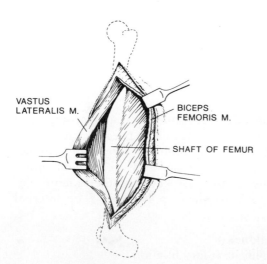

VASTUS
LATERALIS M.

BICEPS
FEMORIS M.

SHAFT OF FEMUR

FIGURE 16–19. Open approach to expose the femoral shaft.[15] The belly of the biceps femoris muscle is reflected caudally and the vastus lateralis muscle and fascia lata are reflected cranially, exposing most of the femoral shaft.

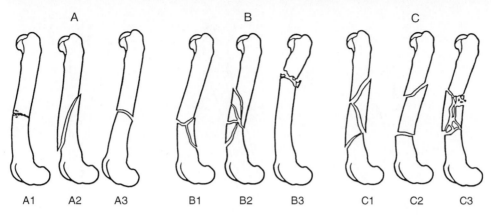

FIGURE 16–20. Diaphyseal fractures of the femur. (*A1*) Incomplete, (*A2*) oblique, (*A3*) transverse. (*B1*) One reducible wedge, (*B2*) reducible wedges, (*B3*) nonreducible wedges. (*C1*) Reducible wedges, (*C2*) segmental, and (*C3*) nonreducible wedges. (From Unger M, Montavon PM, Heim UFA: Classification of fractures of the long bones in the dog and cat: Introduction and clinical application. Vet Comp Orthop Trauma 3:41–50, 1990, with permission.)

usual, and should be seated close to the bone in the trochanteric fossa to minimize compromise of hip joint function. Because of bone growth it may not be possible to remove the pin after healing.

Type A2, Oblique

Reduction and Fixation

A long oblique fracture of the femur is shown in Figure 16–21. A Fracture Patient score of 8 to 9 would be expected. Following a lateral open approach, the Steinmann pin is inserted in the proximal segment, the fracture is reduced and maintained by using self-retaining bone forceps, and the pin is then inserted into the distal segment. In long oblique fractures with a fracture line length equal to twice the bone diameter, cerclage wires are inserted at about 1-cm

FIGURE 16–21. (*A*) Type A2 long oblique fracture of the femur. (*B*) Following a lateral open approach, an intramedullary pin is inserted into the proximal segment. The fracture is reduced and maintained by self-retaining bone forceps; the pin is inserted into the distal segment. (*C*) In long oblique fractures, cerclage wires are inserted at 1- to 2-cm intervals; after clinical union, the intramedullary pin is removed and cerclage wires are left in place. If there is any doubt in regard to stability after applying the above, an external fixator may be added at the time of surgery.

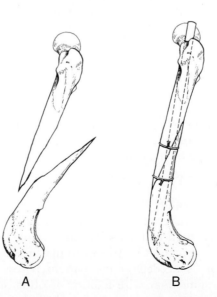
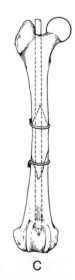

A   B   C

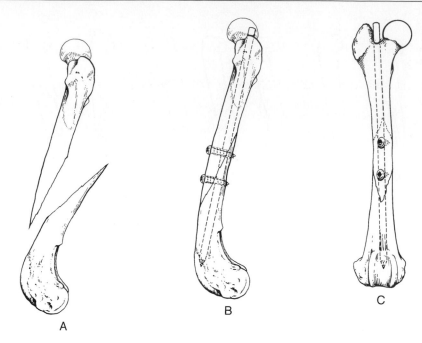

FIGURE 16–22. (*A*) Type A2 long oblique fracture of the femur. (*B*) After reduction and insertion of an intramedullary pin, lag screws may be inserted to bring about interfragmentary compression. (*C*) Lag screws may be inserted off center to avoid the intramedullary pin. After clinical union, intramedullary pin is removed and lag screws are left in place.

intervals (Fig. 16–21*B*, *C*). After clinical union, the intramedullary pin is removed, and the cerclage wires are left in place.

Figure 16–22 presents another instance of a long oblique femoral fracture with a Fracture Patient score of 8 to 9 in a large- or giant-breed dog. After reduction and insertion of the Steinmann pin, one or more lag screws may be inserted to bring about interfragmentary compression (Fig. 16–22). In this case, an intramedullary pin slightly smaller in diameter is used. The lag screws are inserted off center to avoid the intramedullary pin. After clinical union, the intramedullary pin is removed, and the lag screws are left in place.

Type A3, Transverse

Providing rotational stability is the primary concern in these fractures, and in large breeds this could easily drive the Fracture Patient score down to 7 to 8. Although considered a "simple" fracture, this type is one of the most common types to result in nonunion, no doubt due to underestimating the biomechanical forces involved. Age and size of the patient are important determinants as to type of fixation.

Internal Fixation

STEINMANN PIN ■ If the patient is less than approximately 6 months of age, the exuberant callus expected will compensate to a considerable degree for lack of rotational stability, and simple Steinmann pin fixation would be adequate (Figs. 16–1 to 16–3). In mature dogs, however, some additional auxiliary fixation is needed. If the patient is less than 15 to 20 pounds (7 to 9 kg), interfragmentary wire fixation is often adequate. These patterns are described in Chapter 2 (see Fig. 2–62). Such wire fixation must be very carefully applied in order to ensure that the wire is truly tight, and this author is very conservative in recommending them.

STEINMANN PIN AND EXTERNAL FIXATOR ■ In larger breeds, a type 1A fixator combined with the pin is much more secure than pin and wire fixation (Fig. 16–4). The technique is descibed above in the section Fixation Techniques.

INTERLOCKING NAIL ■ The interlocking medullary nail (see Fig. 2–54E) shows promise of being a very useful fixation in large breeds.[11]

BONE PLATE ■ Compression bone plate fixation is a very simple and highly effective method of treatment in all size animals, and especially in large and giant breeds. Six to eight cortices should be captured by the plate screws (see Fig. 2–74 for choice of plate size).

Aftercare ■ See aftercare suggestions at the end of this section (Diaphyseal Fractures).

Fracture Type 32-B; Diaphyseal Wedge (Fig. 16–20B)

Increasing degrees of instability characterize these fractures, hence simple intramedullary Steinmann pinning is less applicable. Fracture Patient scores range from 3 to 7.

Type B1, One Reducible Wedge

Reduction and stabilization of the wedge by means of cerclage wires or lag screws converts these fractures to type A3 transverse fractures, so primary fixation is as described for those fractures. Fracture Patient scores typically are 6 to 7.

Internal Fixation

BONE PLATE AND LAG SCREWS ■ Figure 16–23 illustrates the combination of lag screw and compression plate fixation.

STEINMANN PIN, CERCLAGE WIRES, AND EXTERNAL FIXATOR ■ After reduction and cerclage wire stabilization of the wedge, this fixation can be completed as shown in Figure 16–4.

INTERLOCKING NAIL AND CERCLAGE WIRES ■ After reduction and cerclage wire stabilization of the wedge, the interlocking nail would be appropriate fixation in large breeds.

Type B2, Several Reducible Wedges

Increasing instability and complexity cause Fracture Patient scores to drop to 4 to 6.

Internal Fixation

The methods of fixation are an extension of those for type B1 fractures. Figure 16–24 illustrates stabilization by multiple *cerclage wires, Steinmann pin,* and *type 1A external fixator.* Bone plates are typically applied to function as *neutralization plates* rather than compression plates. A minimum of six cortices must be captured by plate screws in each of the proximal and distal segments. Either cerclage wires under the plate or lag screws are used to secure the wedges.

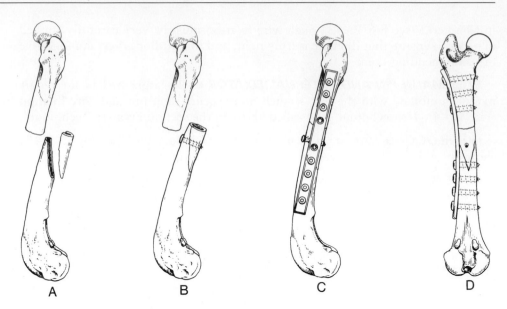

FIGURE 16–23. (*A*) Type B1 femoral shaft fracture with butterfly fragment. (*B*) Reduction of fracture and fixation in place using a lag screw for interfragmentary compression. (*C*, *D*) Contoured bone plate applied on lateral surface of the femur.

Type B3, Nonreducible Wedge

Although not all the fragments can be reduced and stabilized, nevertheless, the bone is able to assume some buttress function, and shortening of the bone is not the major problem as long as the major diaphyseal sections are held in alignment. It is best to take a biological fixation approach to these fractures, since total reduction is not possible; on the other hand, a bridging or buttress fixation isn't needed.

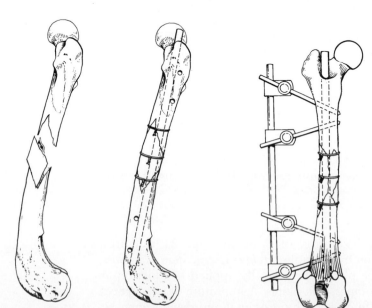

FIGURE 16–24. (*A*) Type B2 fracture of the femur. (*B*, *C*) Rigid fixation by use of an intramedullary pin, three cerclage wires, and an external fixator.

Reduction and Internal Fixation

BONE PLATE ■   The principles of biological fixation can be respected during plate fixation only if the temptation to attempt reduction of the fragments is resisted. The fracture hematoma and fragments should be disturbed as little as possible consistent with reduction of the major diaphyseal fragments. It is usually possible to place the fracture under compression with the plate, and this will add stability. Six to eight cortices must be captured by plate screws in each major segment.

The *major problem with plate fixation* occurs when the nonreducible fragments are on the medial cortex, which is the natural buttress cortex of the femur. Failure to bone graft this area (see Chapter 3) can lead to plate failure due to repetitive bending stresses applied to the plate over a very short segment of the plate. If the fragmented area of the medial cortex is relatively small, autogenous cancellous bone graft will stimulate early callus formation and relieve the bone plate of bending stress. Larger nonreduced areas on the medial cortex can be physically reinforced by onlay or inlay grafts supplemented with autogenous cancellous graft (see Fig. 3–3E). Fragmentation of the caudal cortex usually does not need grafting, since the fragments have intact periosteal blood supply from the adductor magnus muscle if they are not stripped away from the muscle.

INTERLOCKING NAIL ■   Because bending stresses are more evenly distributed over the length of the IN than in the bone plate, loss of the medial cortex is not as critical. Autogenous cancellous bone grafting is still a useful procedure to ensure early callus formation. Minimal exposure of the fracture site may be necessary to ensure passage of the pin into the distal segment. This method is restricted to large and giant breeds.

STEINMANN PIN AND TYPE 1A EXTERNAL FIXATOR ■   As in the case of the IN, bending stresses due to loss of the medial cortex are less critical with this fixation than with plates. This is a very useful alternative to plate fixation in the cat, and slightly less satisfactory in the dog due to the problems with function mentioned above in the section Fixation Techniques. Minimal exposure of the fracture site may be necessary to ensure passage of the pin into the distal segment. A minimum of six fixation pins are advisable, and a double-bar configuration (see Fig. 2–43E) is used in animals larger than approximately 45 pounds (20 kg).

Aftercare ■   See aftercare suggestions at the end of this section (Diaphyseal Fractures).

Fracture Type 32-C; Diaphyseal Complex (Fig. 16–20C)

These segmental fractures represent the most challenging fixation problems of all long-bone fractures due to the magnitude of the mechanical forces acting at the fracture site. Fracture Patient scores are very low, in the 1 to 3 range.

Type C1, Reducible Wedges

Reduction and Internal Fixation

As may be anticipated, fixation is a combination of methods described above. The fracture is intermediate in Fracture Patient score relative to the other two

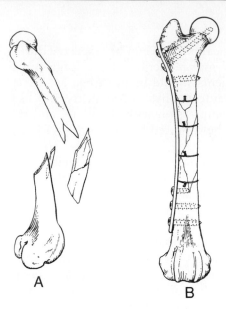

FIGURE 16–25. (*A*) Type C1 fracture of the femoral shaft with numerous fissure fractures present. (*B*) Reduction of fracture segments, one by one. Cerclage wires immobilize fragments and reconstruct femur. Neutralization plate applied; screw holes in plate directly overlying fracture lines are left vacant.

fractures in this group. Either cerclage wires (Fig. 16–25) or lag screws (Fig. 16–26) are used to join the wedges, followed by a primary fixation.

BONE PLATE ■   This is probably the most widely used form of fixation in this situation. The function of the plate will vary, depending on the obliquity of the proximal and distal fracture lines. If all the fracture lines can be compressed by cerclage wires or lag screws, the plate functions as a pure neutralization plate (Figs. 16–25 and 16–26). If the proximal and/or distal fracture line is greater than 45 degrees relative to the long axis, the plate can be placed in some degree of compression, typically with one screw placed in the load position in the plate hole.

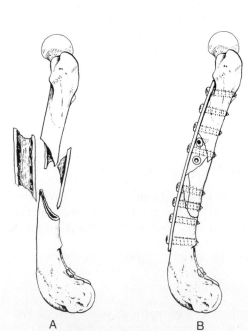

FIGURE 16–26. (*A*) Type C1 fracture of the femur. (*B*) Fracture reduced; interfragmentary compression achieved by use of lag screws through the bone alone and through the plate. A neutralization plate is applied to overcome rotary, bending, and compressive forces. In this case, it was more advantageous to apply the plate on the cranial surface.

STEINMANN PIN AND TYPE 1A EXTERNAL FIXATOR ■ If the wedges can be stabilized with cerclage wires, a type 1A external fixator and Steinmann pin can be used as primary fixation. Due to the instability inherent to these fractures, a minimum of six fixation pins are advisable, and a double-bar configuration (see Fig. 2–43E) is used in animals larger than approximately 45 pounds (20 kg).

INTERLOCKING NAIL ■ If the wedges can be stabilized with cerclage wires, the IN can be used as primary fixation.

Type C2, Segmental

This is the most stable fracture within this group, consisting of only two fracture lines (Fig. 16–27).

Reduction and Internal Fixation

BONE PLATE ■ Depending on the obliquity of the fracture line, the plate can function in compression or neutralization mode. If both fracture lines are transverse, the plate is applied with compression at both ends (see Fig. 2–71D, E, F). If the fractures are oblique, they can be compressed with either cerclage wires or lag screws, and the plate applied in the neutralization mode. In some

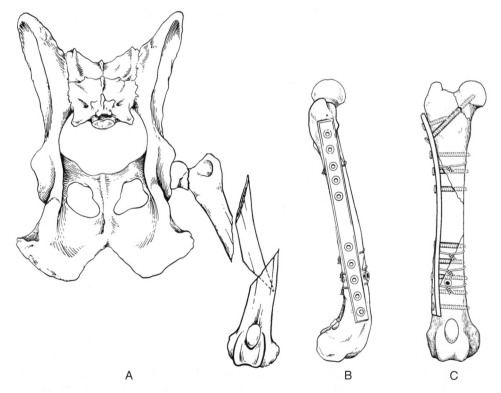

A   B   C

FIGURE 16–27. Type C2 multiple fracture of the femoral shaft and neck in 1-year-old Border collie. (A) Upon open approach, numerous fissures were noted in the various fracture segments. (B, C) The femoral shaft was first reconstructed and fixed together with one lag screw and four cerclage wires. A neutralization plate was applied with a 4.5-mm lag screw to immobilize the femoral neck fracture. Note the twist in the distal plate necessary in the supracondylar region. The plate was removed at 7 months; shaft lag screw and cerclage wires were left in place.

cases the plate is applied in compression at one end of the intermediate segment and in neutralization at the other end. At least six cortices must be captured by plate screws in each of the proximal and distal segments.

STEINMANN PIN AND TYPE 1A EXTERNAL FIXATOR ■ Due to the instability inherent to these fractures, a minimum of six fixation pins are advisable, and a double-bar configuration (see Fig. 2–43E) is used in animals larger than approximately 45 pounds (20 kg). If the fracture lines are oblique enough, cerclage wires or lag screws can be used to compress these fractures before the fixator is applied.

INTERLOCKING NAIL ■ If the fracture lines are oblique enough, cerclage wires can be used to compress these fractures before the IN is applied in large dogs.

Type C3, Nonreducible Wedges

Bridging osteosynthesis is applicable to these fractures, whose Fracture Patient scores range from 1 to 3.

Reduction and Internal Fixation

Maximal advantage of bridging osteosynthesis is taken when the fracture is reduced either in a closed manner, or with minimal open approach and no manipulation of fragments. Minimal disruption of blood supply to the bone fragments and fracture hematoma is caused by such a method; therefore, early callus formation is encouraged. Care must be taken to ensure rotational alignment when closed or minimal open reduction is done.

BONE PLATE ■ Although a much larger exposure is needed to apply the plate in buttress or bridging function, nevertheless bone plates work well in this application if proper care is taken. Application of a bridging plate is illustrated in Figure 16–28. The temptation to disrupt and manipulate the wedges must be overcome. "Neat freaks" have a distinct disadvantage here! The plate is

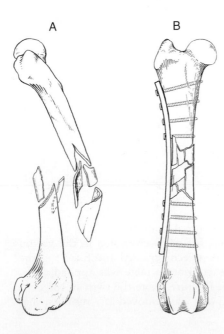

A   B

FIGURE 16–28. Biological osteosynthesis with a bone plate. (*A*) A complex type C diaphyseal fracture of the femur. (*B*) The plate is contoured from the radiograph of the opposite femur and attached proximally and distally without any handling or reduction of the fragments, which will tend to be pulled into the fracture gap by muscular forces. It is important to restore bone length as accurately as possible to allow the fragments to drift into position. Eight cortices proximally and distally should be engaged by plate screws for this type fixation of the femur.

contoured from a craniocaudal radiograph of the normal femur and applied to the proximal segment, ideally ensuring at least eight cortices are captured by plate screws. Proximal screws placed deeply in the femoral neck are counted as two cortices; six cortices can be accepted in the proximal segment if necessary. The distal segment is attached to the plate with bone-holding clamps and best possible length is attained by traction, the fracture distractor (see Fig. 2–18), or IM pin distraction (see Fig. 2–19). The proximal segment must be rotated cranially to eliminate excessive anteversion before the plate is clamped to the distal segment. The distal screws are then applied through the plate, with at least eight cortices captured. Autogenous cancellous bone graft (see Chapter 3) is applied to the fracture area, taking care to not disturb the wedges.

STEINMANN PIN AND TYPE 1A EXTERNAL FIXATOR ■ The aims of bridging osteosynthesis are respected by the use of the pin and type 1A fixator, applied as described above. This is a very useful alternative to plate fixation in the cat, and slightly less satisfactory in the dog due to the problems with function mentioned above in the section Fixation Techniques. Because there will be no load sharing of the bone with the fixator, a minimum of six fixation pins are advisable, and a double-connecting-bar configuration (see Fig. 2–43E) is used in animals larger than approximately 45 pounds (20 kg).

INTERLOCKING NAIL ■ Because of its ability to act as a buttress, the IN is a good choice here if the patient is large enough. Minimal exposure of the fracture site may be necessary to ensure passage of the pin into the distal segment.

Aftercare of Diaphyseal Fractures

Ideally the animal would be allowed early limited active use of the limb. This requires totally stable internal fixation, good owner compliance with confinement and exercise restrictions, and a patient that will not overstress the repair due to hyperactivity. If any of these elements are less than optimal, an off-weight-bearing sling (see Fig. 2–32) is advisable for 2 to 3 weeks. Exercise should be severely restricted for 4 to 6 weeks, with a gradual return to unrestricted activity at 8 to 12 weeks. Radiographs should be taken at 4 to 8 weeks for intramedullary pins and external fixators and 8 to 10 weeks for plates to confirm clinical union before any significant increase in exercise is allowed.

DISTAL FRACTURES

Fractures of the distal segment (see Fig. 16–29) represent about 25 percent of all femoral fractures, and 11 percent of all diaphyseal fractures.[1] Fractures involving the distal femoral physis are relatively common in young animals between the ages of 4 and 11 months. Salter type I and II fractures are seen most frequently.[2,3,23] Supracondylar fractures are seen most frequently in the mature animal: both fracture types present similar biomechanical problems relative to reduction and fixation and will be discussed together. See Chapter 21 for further discussion of physeal injuries. Articular fractures are relatively rare, accounting for about 17 percent of all distal segment fractures.[1]

OPEN APPROACHES ■ Arthrotomy of the stifle joint is necessary to expose all these fractures. The exact approach varies with the extent of the pathology,

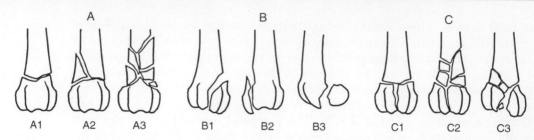

FIGURE 16–29. Distal fractures of the femur. (*A1*) Simple, (*A2*) wedge, and (*A3*) complex. (*B1*) Lateral condyle sagittal, (*B2*) medial condyle sagittal, and (*B3*) frontal unicondylar. (*C1*) Simple, metaphyseal simple or wedge, (*C2*) simple, metaphyseal complex; and (*C3*) multifragmentary. (From Unger M, Montavon PM, Heim UFA: Classification of fractures of the long bones in the dog and cat: Introduction and clinical application. Vet Comp Orthop Trauma 3:41–50, 1990, with permission.)

but the lateral approach is most common, as it is suitable for all the nonarticular fractures (see Fig. 16–30).[15] Medial and bilateral approaches are used for articular fractures, and osteotomy of the tibial tuberosity is sometimes useful for type C fractures.

Fracture Type 33-A; Distal, Extra-articular (see Fig. 16–29*A*)

The distal segment is usually displaced caudally and accompanied by a sizeable hematoma (see Fig. 16–31*A*). The objectives of treatment should include (1) anatomical reduction and (2) rigid uninterrupted fixation so that the animal is free to move the stifle joint during the healing period. Suggested methods of treatment include Rush pins, or small transfixation pins/K-wires inserted across

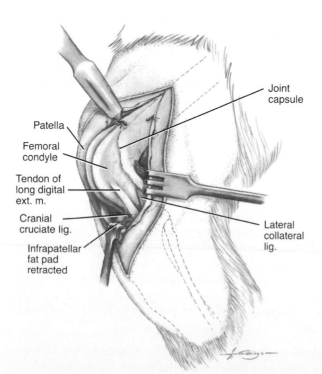

Patella

Femoral condyle

Tendon of long digital ext. m.

Cranial cruciate lig.

Infrapatellar fat pad retracted

Joint capsule

Lateral collateral lig.

FIGURE 16–30. Approach to the distal femur and stifle joint through a lateral incision. (From Piermattei DL: An Atlas of Surgical Approaches to the Bones and Joints of the Dog and Cat, 3rd ed. Philadelphia, WB Saunders Co, 1993, p 275, with permission.)

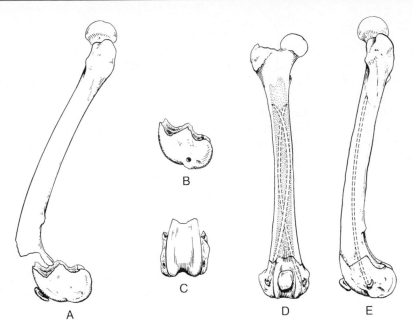

FIGURE 16–31. Rush pin fixation of type A1 distal femoral physeal fractures. (*A*) Salter-Harris type 1 fracture of the distal femoral physis. (*B, C*) Position on femoral condyles of entry holes for Rush pins. These holes should be the same diameter as Rush pins and placed in the caudal half of the physis (condylar area). (*D, E*) After reduction of the fracture, double Rush pins are driven into the femoral medullary canal. Pins should be two thirds to three fourths of the length of the femur. The pins bend in two planes as they are driven, thus storing energy that is transferred to the bone as compression.

the fracture line in a crossing or parallel pattern. In type A2 (Salter II) fractures in which a portion of the metaphysis is attached to the distal epiphysis, it may be advantageous to insert a lag screw transversely to attach the metaphyseal wedge.

Type A1, Simple and A2, Wedge

Closed Reduction and Fixation

In early cases with minimal displacement, and especially in cats and small dogs, closed reduction is sometimes possible if the case is seen within the first 24 hours. The fracture is reduced by flexing the stifle joint with the tarsus extended and applying distal traction on the caudal surface of the proximal part of the tibia. With the femur stabilized, flexion of the stifle with proximal pressure on the tibia usually maintains the reduction. Immobilization is applied, holding the stifle in flexion by means of a modified Thomas splint (see Fig. 2–25) or Ehmer sling (see Fig. 2–31). With splint fixation, padding, gauze, and adhesive tape are applied to maintain caudal traction on the femur and cranial traction on the tibia. Reduction should be confirmed radiographically. This treatment may result in some stiffness of the stifle because the joint is not free to move during the healing period and intra- and extra-articular adhesions are more likely to form during immobilization of the joint. Removing the fixation at 2 weeks will minimize this problem.

Open Reduction

The patient is placed in the dorsal recumbent position. A lateral approach to the stifle joint is made and the fascia lata incision is extended proximally to allow separation of the biceps femoris muscle from the quadriceps muscles, exposing the fracture site.

The same basic maneuvers described above for closed reduction are used, but reduction can be aided by levering the epiphysis back into position. A flat bone skid or scalpel handle can be used to assist in this. The most proximal edge of the epiphysis containing the trochlear groove is quite fragile and must be protected from secondary fracture. Grasping the epiphyseal segment with a bone-holding forceps should be avoided if possible. If necessary, a pointed reduction forceps or vulsellum forceps can be applied to the medial and lateral surfaces of the condyles, off the gliding surfaces. If a week or more has elapsed since fracture, it may be necessary to remove a small amount of bone from the distal end of the proximal segment. Perfect reduction is ideal; however, if this is not possible, the distal segment should be overreduced cranially to avoid patellar impingement during extension of the stifle. Failure to adequately reduce the epiphysis was the main cause of poor results in a study of 47 distal femoral fractures.[24]

Internal Fixation

Although retrograde insertion of small Steinmann pins has been an accepted fixation in the past, this method was more likely to be associated with sciatic nerve impingement, as discussed above in the section Fixation Techniques.[10] Other methods are suggested here for this reason.

RUSH PINS ■ Two Rush pins are inserted by first drilling diagonal holes (20 degrees to the sagittal plane of the femur) into the medial and lateral surfaces of the condyles just proximal to the gliding surfaces (Fig. 16–31B, C). The two pins are then inserted and driven into the femoral shaft simultaneously (Fig. 16–31D, E). Note that the pins are also aimed cranially, so that they curve in both the frontal and sagittal planes. This requires that the holes be drilled as far caudally on the condyles as possible, near the collateral ligaments. Care must be taken so that the holes in the distal segment are not split out in the drilling and insertion process. In most cases, no additional fixation is necessary. Healing is rapid, and the pins are removed in 3 to 5 weeks if they are used in a young, growing animal. Alternatively, in young animals, the hook end is cut off after pin placement, which lessens the chance of causing premature closure of the growth plate. If the animal is near to skeletal maturity, the pins are routinely left in situ because they have very little tendency to loosen and migrate. Using true Rush pins, this method is most applicable to large breeds of dogs, where 3/32- or 1/8-inch (2.4- to 3.2-mm) pins are most common. In cats and toy breeds of dogs, 0.045- to 0.062-inch (1.2- to 1.5-mm) Kirschner wires can be used in a manner similar to that for Rush pins. The hook end can be bent before setting the pin against the condyle.

TRANSFIXATION PINS OR KIRSCHNER WIRES ■ For this simple nailing fixation, the pins can be applied in a crossed or parallel position (Fig 16–32). Pin size varies from 0.045-inch (1.2-mm) K-wires to 3/32-inch (2.4-mm) Steinmann pins. This method is particularly advantageous in brachycephalic breeds, where the extreme curvature of the distal femur and condyles makes other methods difficult. When using cross pins, they are usually started in the metaphyseal

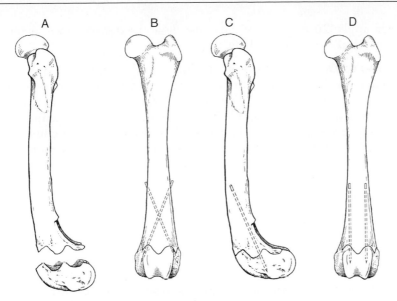

FIGURE 16–32. (*A*) Distal femoral type A1 physeal fracture. (*B*, *C*) After reduction, fixation may be accomplished by the use of two transfixation cross pins. These may be inserted from proximal to distal without penetration of the articular cartilage, or from the condyle into the opposite cortex with the pin cut and seated flush with the cartilage. Note the caudal angulation of the pins to ensure their being seated well into the condyle. (*D*) An alternative method of pinning is placing the pins parallel to each other.

area and extend distally into the opposite condyles (Fig. 16–32*B*, *C*). Parallel pins are similar, except that they are driven into the ipsilateral condyle (Fig. 16–32*D*). Note that the pins must be started far enough medially and laterally in the femur to avoid the quadriceps muscle, which must be free to glide. A common error is failure to angle the pins caudally sufficiently to enter the large part of the condyles. Both methods avoid penetration of the articular cartilage, thus no pin ends are in the joint. Crossing pin fixations cause more complications than did single Steinmann pin or modified Rush pin fixation in one study due primarily to the fact that the fracture could be more easily fixed while still underreduced than with the other fixations.[24]

Crossing pins are driven from the articular surface by some surgeons, and this method has the disadvantages both of having the pins protrude into the joint and often less stable fixation. The latter is due to the flare of the condyles relative to the shaft; starting the pin into the condyle at an angle sufficient to cause the pin to "bite" in the bone creates a more acute pin angle relative to the shaft than is desirable. The result is that the pin exits the metaphyseal cortex too close to the fracture line to provide optimal stability.

LAG SCREWS ■ Bone screws can be substituted for the transfixation pins described above, and provide additional stability, especially in large breeds. Care must be taken to ensure a lag effect for maximum stability. Insertion from proximal to distal is advisable.

Aftercare ■ Activity should be restricted, and no additional fixation is usually indicated. Healing is rapid in physeal fractures, usually being clinically united in 2 to 3 weeks. Nonphyseal fractures take 3 or 4 more weeks to clinical union. If there is considerable trauma in the area, it may be advisable to have the owner apply 20 to 30 gentle passive flexion-extension movements of the stifle joint two to three times daily.

Prognosis of Distal Fractures ■   Relative to physeal fractures, some degree of disturbance of femoral growth is common, and most likely in animals that are younger, with more potential bone growth, than those that are closer to skeletal maturity. Functional problems relative to femoral shortening were seen in 18 percent of the animals in that study.[25] Good to excellent clinical function was reported in 88 percent of 48 fractures, with adequacy of reduction being the main determinant of outcome in another study.[24]

Type A3, Complex

There is no possibility for closed reduction of these fractures; they must be handled by open approach and internal fixation.

Reduction and Fixation

BONE PLATE ■   Neutralization plate fixation can be considered if the fragments are large enough to reduce and fix by any method. The reconstruction plate (Synthes Ltd. [USA], Paoli, PA) is adaptable to this location because it can be contoured to curve from the shaft onto the condyle (Fig. 16–33A).[26] It is important that the fragments be reduced and that the plate is truly a neutralization plate because this plate is not stiff enough to function as a buttress plate. Conventional straight plates are rarely useful, as it is difficult to get sufficient screws into the distal segment due to the curvature of the bone. The hook plate used for intertrochanteric osteotomy (see Chapter 15) can be made to function as a buttress plate in large dogs by placing the two hooks and one screw in the distal segment.

A problem with plate fixation of any type is that the plate is intra-articular at its distal end. This can lead to irritation of the joint and varying degrees of lameness; therefore, these plates are usually removed after several months. Additionally, a very secure closure of the lateral parapatellar retinaculum is needed to prevent dehiscence and medial patellar luxation.

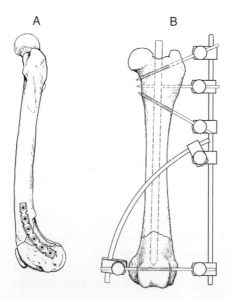

A   B

FIGURE 16–33. Fixation of type A3 complex distal femoral fractures. (*A*) Reconstruction plate (Synthes Ltd. [USA], Paoli, PA) contoured on edge to closely fit the femoral condyle. (*B*) A hybrid type I-II external fixator with a curved connecting bar controls rotation and length while the IM pin provides axial stability. The double clamp on the connecting bar can be avoided by attaching it to the third fixation pin with a single clamp.

EXTERNAL FIXATOR ■ A hybrid fixator (Fig. 16–33B) can be used when the fragments are irreducible and buttress or bridging fixation is needed. The Steinmann pin is placed in conventional manner with care to seat it as deeply as possible in the condyle, and a center-threaded, positive-thread-profile fixation pin is placed transversely through the condyle. This pin is attached to the straight lateral connecting bar, and a curved connecting bar is used to attach the medial end of the pin to the lateral bar. The Steinmann pin and fixation pin provide stability in both axes of the condyle.

Fracture Type 33-B; Distal, Partial Articular (Fig. 16–29B)

Type B1, Lateral Condyle, Sagittal and Type B2, Medial Condyle, Sagittal

Condylar fractures (Fig. 16–34) are quite rare; when they occur, the medial condyle is the one most frequently involved. In most instances, the caudal cruciate ligament and the medial collateral ligament are attached to the fractured segment. In some cases, the fractured condyle is a single segment; in others, it is multiple in nature. The latter may be difficult to treat and restore to good function. A good functional recovery depends on anatomical reduction, rigid fixation, and movement of the joint during the healing period.

Reduction and Fixation

An open approach is performed as already described. If the fracture is primarily in one piece, and particularly if it includes attachments of the cruciate and collateral ligaments, reduction and fixation should be attempted. Reduction is usually accomplished by use of a hook to pull the segment cranially, and levering is used for final reduction. If reduction is impossible, especially if the

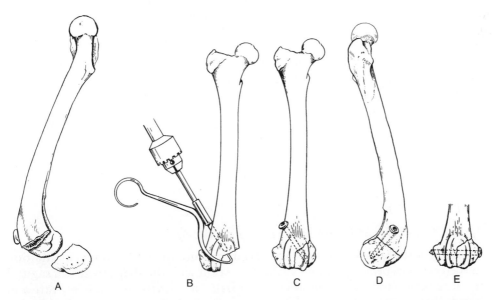

FIGURE 16–34. (A) Type B1 condylar fracture of the femur. (B) Fixation by drilling and inserting a cancellous bone screw diagonally from proximally into the fractured segment. (C, D) Craniocaudal and lateral views of the fracture reduced and cancellous bone screw in place. (E) If the fractured condylar segment is large enough, it may be immobilized by a transcondylar bone screw (cancellous or cortical screw with lag effect).

injury is several days old, a partial horizontal capsulotomy in addition to the standard vertical parapatellar incision allows room for maneuvering the caudally displaced condyle (approach to the caudomedial or caudolateral parts of the stifle joint[15]). Exposure can also be improved in some cases by osteotomy of the origin of the collateral ligament.

Lag screw fixation may be accomplished by two general methods, depending on the exact location and direction of the fracture line. In many cases it is necessary to drill and insert a bone screw diagonally from proximally in the opposite metaphyseal cortex into the fractured condyle (Fig. 16–34B, C, D). In larger dogs, it is advantageous to insert two bone screws. If the intercondylar fracture surface is large enough, the screw may be inserted in a transcondylar fashion (Fig. 16–34E). Before closure, the joint should be inspected for small fragments of loose bone and cartilage that should be removed.

Aftercare ■ Every effort should be made to keep the joint moving. Passive range-of-motion exercises, 20 to 30 cycles, two to three times a day, should be started as soon as the animal will tolerate them. If external support is needed, an off-weight-bearing sling (see Fig. 2–32) is preferred to any immobilization, as some limited motion will be possible.

Type B3; Frontal Unicondylar

As in the sagittal fracture, the medial condyle is most often involved. Open approaches are similar to those described above for type B1 and B2 fractures.

Reduction and Fixation

Lag screw fixation is indicated, but it is difficult to place the screws so that the head of the screw does not interfere with joint function. It is preferable to direct the screw from cranial to caudal by starting the screw just outside the trochlear ridge, then across the fracture line. The other possibility is lag screw or K-wire fixation directed from the condyle surface cranially into the metaphysis. Obviously the head of the screw or end of the K-wire must be countersunk below the articular cartilage unless it is possible to place the screw/pin outside the gliding surface. The miniscrews in 1.5- or 2.0-mm sizes are easiest to countersink.

Aftercare ■ The postoperative consideration are similar to those detailed above for type B1 and B2 fractures.

Fracture Type 33-C; Distal, Complex Articular
(Fig. 16–29C)

Type C1, Simple, Metaphyseal Simple or Wedge

This is a supracondylar and bicondylar fracture in combination. In addition to the condyles being fractured at their junction with the shaft, there is a sagittal fracture between the condyles (Fig. 16–35A). This fracture is relatively rare and is usually accompanied by displacement, extensive soft tissue damage, and hemarthrosis. The joint should be checked for ligament and meniscal damage. Anatomical reduction, rigid fixation of the fracture segments, and early postoperative movement of the stifle joint are essential to ensure good return of function.

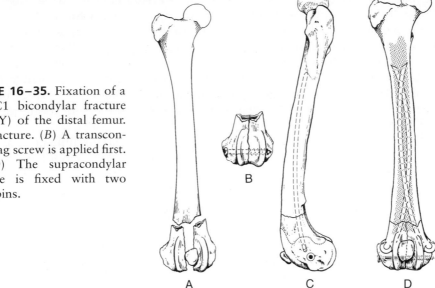

FIGURE 16–35. Fixation of a type C1 bicondylar fracture (T or Y) of the distal femur. (*A*) Fracture. (*B*) A transcondylar lag screw is applied first. (*C, D*) The supracondylar fracture is fixed with two Rush pins.

Reduction and Fixation

An open approach is performed as described above. The fractured condyles are reduced and held together by vulsellum or pointed reduction forceps. Because the fracture involves an articular surface, anatomical reduction is essential. A hole is drilled transversely through the condyles, and a cancellous or cortical screw inserted with a lag effect will compress the fracture site (Fig. 16–35B). Essentially, the fracture has now been converted into a supracondylar type A1 or A2 fracture. The condyles are attached to the femoral shaft using two Rush pins (Fig. 16–35C, D), two crossing or parallel transfixation pins (Fig. 16–32B, C, D), or a curved reconstruction plate (Fig. 16–33A).

Aftercare ■ Every effort should be made to keep the joint moving. Passive range-of-motion exercises, 20 to 30 cycles, two to three times a day, should be started as soon as the animal will tolerate them. If external support is needed, an off-weight-bearing sling (see Fig. 2–32) is preferred to total immobilization, as some limited motion will be possible.

Type C2, Simple, Metaphyseal Complex and Type C3, Multifragmentary

Surgical exposure, reduction, and fixation of this group is a combination of methods described above. A transcondylar lag screw (Fig. 16–35B) is always the first step, converting the remaining fracture to a type A3 fracture, which is treated as in Figure 16–33. Multiple lag screw and K-wire fixation of small articular fragments is accomplished as the situation demands. Aftercare is as described above.

PATELLAR FRACTURES

Fractures of the patella are rarely encountered in small animals. Being a sesamoid bone located between the tendon of the quadriceps femoris muscle and the patellar ligament, the bone fragments are subjected to strong distracting forces. Internal fixation is indicated in simple two-piece fractures when the fragments are of approximately equal size. Due to the strong tension forces over the cranial cortex, tension band wire fixation is indicated. Use monofilament stainless steel wire of sufficient strength for immobilization. Wire of 22 gauge (0.025 inch; 0.635 mm) is suitable for toy breeds and cats, 20 gauge (0.032 inch; 0.812 mm) for average dogs, and 18 gauge (0.040 inch; 1.02 mm) diameter for large breeds. It is always safest to err on the side of too large wires, rather than too small.

Apical fragments of less than one third of the patella are difficult to stabilize and are best treated by excision and reattachment of the tendon/ligament to the remaining fragment. Some multifragmentary fractures may need total patellectomy (see Chapter 17), but an attempt should be made to salvage at least one large fragment as this will often provide better function than a total patellectomy.

Undisplaced Fissure Fracture

Figure 16–36 shows a fissure fracture of the patella immobilized by use of two tension band wires. The first wire is inserted through the quadriceps tendon and patellar ligament close to the patella. Passage of the wire through the tissue can be facilitated by first passing a bent hypodermic needle and then inserting a wire through it. The second wire is inserted in a similar or figure-of-8 fashion but in a more cranial position. The wires are then tightened.

Transverse Fracture

Figure 16–37 illustrates a transverse fracture fixed with one Kirschner wire and a tension band wire in a small- or medium-size dog—in large breeds a second wire is used (Fig. 16–38). A medial or lateral parapatellar incision is made for examination of the fracture line and articular surface. A retrograde hole is drilled with a 1.5-mm drill bit in the proximal patellar segment (Fig. 16–37B). The fracture is reduced and held in position by use of pointed re-

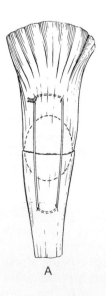

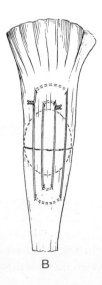

A   B

FIGURE 16–36. Fissure fracture of the patella immobilized by two tension wires. (A) One wire is inserted through the quadriceps tendon and patellar ligament close to the patella. Passage of the wire through the tissue can be facilitated by first passing a bent hypodermic needle and then inserting a wire through it. (B) The second wire is inserted in a similar or figure-of-8 fashion, but in a more cranial position. The wires are then tightened.

FIGURE 16–37. Transverse fracture fixed with one Kirschner wire and a tension band wire. (*A*) A medial or lateral parapatellar incision is made to enable examination of the fracture line and articular surface. (*B*) With a 1.5-mm drill bit, a retrograde hole in the proximal patellar segment is drilled. (*C*) The fracture is reduced and held in position by compression forceps. The hole is extended into the distal segment by drilling, and a Kirschner wire is inserted. (*D, E*) The tension wire is inserted and tightened, and the pin is cut distally. The joint capsule, retinaculum of the quadriceps, and skin are sutured.

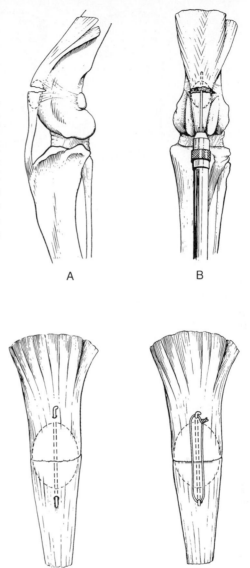

duction forceps. The hole is extended into the distal segment by reversing the drill, and a Kirschner wire is inserted (Fig. 16–37C, D). The tension band wire is inserted and tightened, and the pin is cut distally (Fig. 16–37E). The joint capsule, retinaculum of the quadriceps, and skin are sutured.

Multifragmentary Fracture

Figure 16–38 shows a multifragmentary fracture of the patella fixed with one Kirschner wire and two tension band wires. If too small to be reduced and fixed, the small chips are removed. A Kirschner wire is inserted after drilling a 1.5-mm hole. A tension band wire is applied and tightened (Fig. 16–38B). In larger dogs, an additional tension band wire is inserted through the tendon of the quadriceps and patellar ligament for increased stability (Fig. 16–38C).

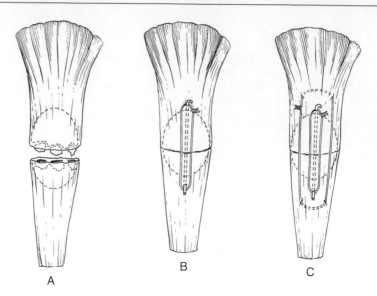

FIGURE 16–38. Multifragmentary fracture of the patella fixed with one Kirschner wire and two tension wires. (*A, B*) If indicated, the small chips are removed. A Kirschner wire is inserted after drilling a 1.5-mm hole. A tension wire is applied and tightened. (*C*) In many cases, an additional tension wire is inserted through the tendon of the quadriceps and patellar ligament for more stability.

Postoperative Care

Additional auxiliary fixation, such as a modified Thomas splint (see Fig. 2–25) or off-weight-bearing sling (see Fig. 2–32), may be indicated in some cases to relieve the operative area of excessive tension during the early healing period (1 to 2 weeks). Activity should be restricted until clinical union at 4 to 6 weeks. The Kirschner wires and tension wires may need to be removed at this time if there is any migration of implants or soft tissue irritation.

References

1. Unger M, Montavon PM, Heim UFA: Classification of fractures of the long bones in the dog and cat: Introduction and clinical application. Vet Comp Orthop Trauma 3:41–50, 1990.
2. Brinker WO: Fractures in Canine Surgery, 2nd Archibald ed. Santa Barbara, American Veterinary Publications, Inc, 1974, pp 949–1048.
3. Olmstead ML: Fractures of the femur. In Brinker WO, Hohn RB, Prieur WD (eds): Manual of Internal Fixation in Small Animals. Springer-Verlag, New York, 1984, pp 165–175.
4. Palmer RH, Hulse DA, Aron DN: A proposed fracture patient score system used to develop fracture treatment plans (abstract). Proc 20th Ann Conf Vet Orthop Soc, 1993.
5. Palmer RH: Decision making in fracture treatment: The fracture patient scoring system. Proc (Sm Anim) ACVS Vet Symposium, 1994, pp 388–390.
6. Schroeder EF: Fractures of the femoral shaft of dogs. North Am Vet 14:38, 1933.
7. Leonard EP: Feline therapeutics and hospitalization. North Am Vet 19:58, 1938.
8. Rudy RL: Principles of intramedullary pinning. Vet Clin North Am 5:209–228, 1975.
9. Palmer RH, Aron DN, Purington PT: Relationship of femoral intramedullary pins to the sciatic nerve and gluteal muscles after retrograde and normograde insertion. Vet Surg 17:65–70, 1988.
10. Fanton JW, Blass CE, Withrow SJ: Sciatic nerve injury as a complication of intramedullary pin fixation of femoral fractures. J Am Anim Hosp Assoc 19:687–694, 1983.
11. Dueland RT, Johnson KA et al: Forty two interlocking nail fracture cases in the dog. Proc Vet Orthop Soc 21:51–52, 1994.
12. Aron DN, Dewey CW: Application and postoperative management of external skeletal fixators. Vet Clin North Am Sm Anim Pract 22:69–98, 1992.

13. Brinker WO, Flo GL: Principles and application of external skeletal fixation. Vet Clin North Am 5:197–208, 1975.
14. Foland MA, Schwarz PD, Salman MD: The adjunctive use of half-pin (type I) external skeletal fixators in combination with intramedullary pins for femoral fracture fixation. Vet Comp Orthop Trauma 4:77–85, 1991.
15. Piermattei DL: An Atlas of Surgical Approaches to the Bones and Joints of the Dog and Cat, 3rd ed. Philadelphia, WB Saunders Co, 1993.
16. Lewis DD, Bellah JR: Use of a double-hook plate to repair a subtrochanteric femoral fracture in an immature dog. J Am Vet Med Assoc 191:440–442, 1987.
17. Daly WR: Femoral head and neck fractures in the dog and cat: A review of 115 cases. Vet Surg 7:29, 1978.
18. Kaderly RE, Anderson WD, Anderson BG: Extraosseous vascular supply to the mature dog's coxofemoral joint. Am J Vet Res 43:1208, 1982.
19. Lambrechts NE, Verstrate FJM, et al: Internal fixation of femoral neck fractures in the dog—an in vitro study. Vet Comp Orthop Trauma 6:188–193, 1993.
20. Gibson Kl, vanEe Rt, Pechman RD: Femoral capital physeal fractures in dogs: 34 cases (1979–1989). J Am Vet Med Assoc 198:886–890, 1991.
21. DeCamp CE, Probst CW, Thomas MW: Internal fixation of femoral capital physeal injuries in dogs: 40 cases (1979–1987). J Am Vet Med Assoc 194:1750–1754, 1989.
22. Tillson DM, McLoughlin RM, Roush JK: Evaluation of experimental proximal femoral physeal; fractures repaired with two cortical screws placed from the articular surface. Vet Comp Orthop Trauma 7:140–147, 1994.
23. Grauer GF, Banks WJ, Ellison GW, et al: Incidence and mechanism of distal femoral physeal fractures in the dog and cat. J Am Anim Hosp Assoc 17:579–586, 1981.
24. Hardie EM, Chambers JN: Factors influencing the outcome of distal femoral physeal fracture fixation: A retrospective study. J Am Anim Hosp Assoc 20:927–931, 1984.
25. Berg RJ, Egger E, Blass CE, et al: Evaluation of prognostic factors for growth following distal femoral physeal injuries in 17 dogs. Vet Surg 13:1172–1180, 1984.
26. Lewis DD, vanEe RT, et al: Use of reconstruction plates for stabilization of fractures and osteotomies involving the supracondylar region of the femur. J Am Anim Hosp Assoc 29: 171–178, 1993.

17

The Stifle Joint

PATELLAR LUXATION

Patellar luxations occur frequently in dogs and occasionally in cats and are commonly seen in most small animal practices. These luxations fall into several classes:

1. Medial luxation—toy, miniature, and large breeds.
2. Lateral luxation—toy and miniature breeds.
3. Medial luxation resulting from trauma—various breeds (rare).
4. Lateral luxation—large and giant breeds (genu valgum).

Categories 3 and 4 will be discussed separately below.

Medial Luxation in Toy, Miniature, and Large Breeds

Most luxations are termed "congenital" because they occur early in life and are not associated with trauma. Although the luxation may not be present at birth, the anatomical deformities that cause these luxations are present at that time and are responsible for subsequent recurrent patellar luxation. The only well-researched investigation into the cause of these luxations concluded that the occurrence of medial patellar luxation is characterized by coxa vara (a decreased angle of inclination of the femoral neck) and a decrease in femoral neck anteversion (relative retroversion).[1] These basic skeletal changes were considered to be the cause of the complex series of derangements of the pelvic limb that characterize medial patellar luxations in the small breeds. The changes are depicted in Figure 17–1A and B. Patellar luxation in these breeds should be considered an inherited disease. Breeding of affected animals is not advisable.[2]

Medial luxation is far more common than lateral luxation in all breeds, representing 75 to 80 percent of cases, with bilateral involvement seen 20 to 25 percent of the time. We have noted a dramatic increase in medial luxation in large and giant breeds in recent years, especially in the Akita, Labrador, husky, and malamute. Concurrent rupture of the cranial cruciate ligament is present in 15 to 20 percent of the stifles of middle-aged and older dogs with chronic patellar luxation. In this situation, the cruciate ligament is placed under increased stress because the quadriceps mechanism is ineffective in stabilizing the joint. The leg is also internally rotated, which stretches the cruciate ligament. In the cat, medial luxation is also more common than lateral luxation. One series of 21 cases included 52.4 percent bilateral medial, 33.3 percent unilateral medial, and 14.3 percent unilateral lateral luxations.[3]

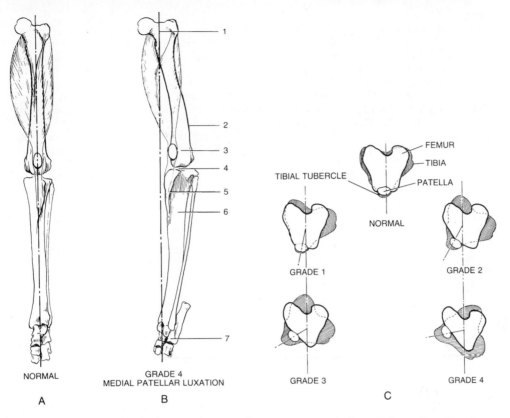

FIGURE 17–1. Skeletal abnormalities with severe congenital medial patellar luxation. (*A*) Normal left hindlimb, cranial view. Note that the quadriceps mechanism is centered over the femur and that the dashed line through the proximal femur and distal tibia also runs through the patella. (*B*) Deformities typical of medial patellar luxation. Note the position of the quadriceps mechanism and patella; the dashed line from proximal femur to distal tibia lies well medial to the stifle joint. (*1*) Coxa vara. (*2*) Distal third of femur bowed medially (genu varum). (*3*) Shallow trochlear sulcus with poorly developed or absent medial ridge. (*4*) Medial condyle hypoplastic; joint tilted. (*5*) Medial torsion of the tibial tubercle, associated with medial rotation of the entire tibia. (6) Medial bowing of the proximal tibia. (*7*) Internal rotation of foot despite lateral torsion of distal tibia. (*C*) Position of the tibia relative to the femur and shape of femoral trochlea in grades 1 through 4 of medial patellar luxation. The femoral cross section in the region of trochlear sulcus is shown in dark outline, and the proximal tibial cross section is shaded. Progressive medial rotation of the tibia and deformity of the medial trochlear ridge are noted. (See the text for a complete explanation of grades 1 through 4, according to Singleton.[4])

A method of classifying the degree of luxation and body deformity is useful for diagnosis and for deciding on the method of surgical repair. Such a classification was devised by Putnam[1] and adapted by Singleton.[4] The following is adapted from Singleton (see Fig. 17–1C).

Grade 1

Intermittent patellar luxation causing the limb to be carried occasionally. The patella easily luxates manually at full extension of the stifle joint, but returns to the trochlea when released. No crepitation is apparent.

When the patella is reduced, deviation of the tibial tubercle from the midline is minimal. After the patella is reduced, flexion and extension of the stifle is in a straight line with no abduction of the hock.

Grade 2

Luxation occurs more frequently than in grade 1. Lameness signs are usually intermittent and of a mild nature. The patella luxates easily, especially when the foot is rotated (internally for medial luxation, externally for lateral luxation, while the patella is pushed. Reduction occurs with opposite maneuvers.

The proximal tibial tuberosity may be rotated up to 30 degrees with medial luxations, and less so with lateral luxations. With the patella luxated medially, the hock is slightly abducted with the toes pointing medially ("pigeon-toed"). With lateral luxation, the hock may be adducted with the toes pointing laterally ("seal-like").

Many cases in this grade "live" with the condition reasonably well for many years, but the constant luxation of the patella over the medial lip of the trochlea can cause erosion of the articulating surface of the patella and also the proximal area of the medial lip. This results in crepitation becoming apparent when the patella is luxated manually. Increased discomfort may result in the dog's throwing its weight to the forelimbs upon ambulation.

Grade 3

The *patella is permanently luxated* (ectopic) with torsion of the tibia and deviation of the tibial crest of between 30 degrees and 60 degrees from the cranial/caudal plane. Although the luxation is not intermittent, many animals use the limb with the stifle held in a semiflexed position.

Flexion and extension of the joint causes abduction and adduction of the hock.

The trochlea is very shallow or even flattened.

Grade 4

The tibia is medially twisted and the tibial crest may show further deviation with the result that it lies 60 degrees to 90 degrees from the cranial/caudal plane.

The *patella is permanently luxated* (ectopic).

The patella lies just above the medial condyle (if medial luxation) and a "space" can be palpated between the patellar ligament and the distal end of the femur.

The limb may be carried if unilateral, or the animal moves in a crouched position, with the limbs partly flexed.

The trochlea is shallow, absent, or even convex.

Clinical Signs

Four classes of patients with patellar luxation are identifiable:

1. Neonates and older puppies often show clinical signs of abnormal hindleg carriage and function from the time they start walking; these represent grades 3 and 4 generally.

2. Young to mature animals with grade 2 to 3 luxations usually have exhibited abnormal or intermittently abnormal gaits all their lives but are presented when the symptoms worsen.

3. Older animals with grade 1 and 2 luxations may exhibit sudden signs of lameness because of further breakdown of soft tissues (such as cruciate rupture) as a result of minor trauma or because of worsening of degenerative joint disease pain.

4. Dogs that are asymptomatic.

Signs of lameness vary from animal to animal. Lameness may be intermittent or continuous. Usually it is a mild to moderate weight-bearing lameness with occasional carrying of the limb. A few dogs will carry their leg most of the time. Dogs with lateral luxations have in general more ambulation problems than with medial luxations. The owner may see the dog stretch its leg backwards in its effort to reduce the patella. Reluctance to jump may be noted.

Signs may worsen as the animal gains weight, articular cartilage erosion occurs, the luxation becomes permanent, the cruciate ligament ruptures, or the hip becomes luxated.

When examining the limb for patellar luxation, it is best performed in lateral recumbency. Gentle palpation usually does not cause pain. In small animals or severely deformed legs, the patella is best located by starting at the tibial tuberosity and working proximally along the patellar ligament. The foot should be internally/externally rotated while trying to push the patella medially/laterally.

Observations should include:

1. Instability in both directions.
2. Presence of crepitus.
3. Degree of tibial tuberosity rotation.
4. Limb torsion or angulation.
5. Inability to reduce the patella.
6. Location of the reduced patella within the trochlea. In straight-legged dogs such as the Akita or Shar pei, the patella occasionally rides proximal in the trochlea ("patella alta"), while chondrodystrophied dogs' patellas ride distal in the trochlea ("patella baja").
7. Inability to extend the limb to a normal standing angle (in puppies with severe contracture accompanying patellar ectopia).
8. Presence/absence of drawer movement.

Each of these features affects the types of steps needed for surgical repair.

Surgical Repair of Patellar Luxation

Often asymptomatic patellar luxation is found during routine physical examinations. We don't recommend immediate surgery, but instead counsel owners on subtle signs indicative of problems such as kicking the leg out behind, reluctance to jump, and reluctance to exercise vigorously. These dogs still respond well to late surgical repair, even if cruciate ligament rupture subsequently occurs. However, there are two exceptions where we recommend surgery on the "asymptomatic" animal. In young puppies with patellar ectopia, it is well to consider repair early (3 to 4 months) prior to irreparable contracture. In medium to large breeds, surgery is recommended early prior to erosion and deformity to the trochlea. Surgical choices are then more restricted and the prognosis more guarded.

Arthroplastic techniques applicable to stabilization of patellar luxations can be divided into two classes: soft tissue reconstruction and bone reconstruction. Considerable judgment and experience are necessary to decide the best procedure or combination of procedures for a given case. After the descriptions of various surgical techniques, we have attempted an algorithmic approach of progressive surgical procedures to use to achieve patellar stability (treatment plan).

A cardinal principle is that skeletal deformity, such as deviation of the tibial tuberosity and shallow trochlear sulcus, must be corrected by bone reconstruction techniques. Attempting to overcome such skeletal malformation by soft tissue reconstruction alone is the most frequent cause of failure. Soft tissue procedures, by themselves, *must be* limited to obvious grade 1 cases. Failure to transpose the tibial tubercle is perhaps the most common cause of failure. The surgeon must be aggressive in deciding to move the tubercle without moving it too great a distance. Sometimes 2 to 3 mm is a sufficient amount to realign the quadriceps mechanism with the femoral trochlea and thus stabilize the patella. Both stifles are routinely operated on at the same time in small dogs and cats, regardless of the types of procedures done. With practice, the surgeon will not find these to be lengthy procedures, and the extra costs and dangers of a second operation outweigh the slightly more difficult postoperative course with bilateral surgery.

Soft Tissue Reconstructive Procedures

OVERLAP OF THE LATERAL OR MEDIAL RETINACULUM (Fig. 17–2) ■

This method can be used on either the lateral side for a medial luxation or on the medial side for a lateral luxation. The retinacular fascia and joint capsule are incised 3 to 5 mm from and parallel to the patella. This incision extends from the tibia proximally to a point 1 to 2 cm above the patella. An incision of the fascia lata continues to the midfemur level (Fig. 17–2A). With size 2–0 or 3–0 nonabsorbable suture, the cut edge of the fascia attached to the patella is sutured beneath the more lateral fascia with several mattress sutures placed through the fornix of the capsule (Fig. 17–2A, B). The superficial layers of fascia and capsule are next sutured to the fascia that remains attached to the patella. In some cases, this fascia will extend beyond the cranial midline of the joint and will be sutured to fascia on the opposite side of the patella (Fig. 17–2B). Suturing continues the length of the fascial incision (Fig. 17–2C).

This technique can be combined with patellar and tibial antirotational suture ligaments (see Fig. 17–4). For lateral luxation, a similar procedure is performed on the medial side. The fascial incision is made through fascia between the

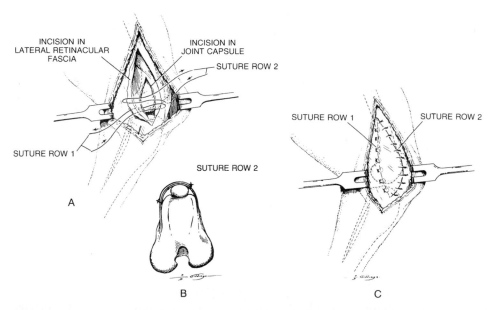

FIGURE 17–2. Lateral retinacular overlap. (A) A lateral parapatellar incision has been made through lateral fascia and joint capsule. The superficial fascia (fascia lata) has been incised from the tibia to the midfemoral level. Suture row 1 is started well back from the edge of the fascia caudally; it passes through the fornix of the joint capsule, through the cranial fascia close to the incision, and back through the caudal fascia like a mattress suture. All these sutures are placed before row 2 is placed. Size 2–0 or 3–0 nonabsorbable suture is preferred. (B) A cross-sectional view shows the two suture rows. Note that row 2 may actually be medial to the midline, depending on the looseness of the caudal fascia. (C) Row 1 and 2 sutures are complete. The biceps creates increased tension on the patellar ligament, the patella, and the distal half of the quadriceps.

caudal belly of the sartorius and the vastus medialis and cranial belly of the sartorius.

FASCIA LATA OVERLAP (Fig. 17–3) ■ This technique[5] is applicable only to medial luxations; when the procedure is used alone, it is indicated only in the limb that has normal conformation (grade 1 luxation). This overlap is opposite that of the retinacular overlap. It can be combined with patellar and tibial antirotational sutures (See Fig. 17–4).

Subcutaneous tissues are reflected to expose the lateral retinaculum and fascia lata to the midpoint of the femur. The fascia lata is incised at its junction with the biceps femoris muscle from the level of the patella proximally as far as possible. Distal to the patella, the incision runs parallel to the patellar ligament over the tendon of the long digital extensor (Fig. 17–3A). The fascia lata proximal to the patella is reflected cranially and bluntly elevated off the underlying vastus lateralis until the white aponeurosis between the vastus lateralis muscle and the rectus femoris muscle is visualized. Nonabsorbable size 2–0 and 3–0 sutures are placed between the cranial edge of the biceps muscle and the exposed aponeurosis. The first suture is in the patellar tendon at the proximal end of the patella, with three to four more sutures placed proximally (Fig. 17–3A, B). If the patella can still be luxated, one or two more sutures are placed just proximal to the patella to further tighten the biceps muscle. Distal sutures are placed in the patellar ligament. The cranial fascia lata is pulled caudally over

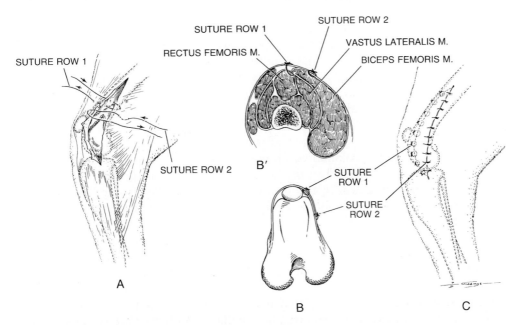

FIGURE 17–3. Fascia lata overlap. (*A*) A lateral parapatellar incision has been made through the fascia lata and joint capsule. This incision follows the cranial edge of the biceps muscle proximally, and distally it ends over the long digital extensor tendon. The cranial fascia is reflected and elevated in order to identify the white aponeurosis between the rectus femoris and vastus lateralis muscles. Row 1 sutures are placed to pull the biceps to this aponeurosis proximal to the patella and to the lateral border of the patella and patellar ligament distally. Row 2 sutures complete the overlap. (*B, B′*) Two cross-sectional views show the relationship of the biceps muscle and fascia lata to the rectus femoris muscle and patella. The biceps has been pulled cranially to exert lateral tension on the quadriceps and patella. (*C*) Suture rows 1 and 2 are completed.

the surface of the biceps muscle and sutured in place with a combined simple pattern and a Lembert pattern (Fig. 17–3B, C).

PATELLAR AND TIBIAL ANTIROTATIONAL SUTURE LIGAMENTS ■ An adaptation of Rudy's technique creates a synthetic lateral patellar ligament by anchoring the lateral fabella to the patella with nonabsorbable suture (Fig. 17–4A, B). Medial tibial rotation can be prevented by another suture passing from the lateral fabella to the tibial tubercle or distal patellar ligament (Fig. 17–4B). The two sutures can also be combined, as in Figure 17–4C. Similar placement of sutures around the medial fabella is used for lateral patellar luxations. Such sutures are most commonly used in conjunction with trochleoplasty in grade 2 older dogs and also work well as primary treatment in neonates as young as five days.[6]

The fabella is the center of the arc of rotation of the patella; hence, the suture remains relatively taut during both flexion and extension of the stifle. By adjusting the point of insertion on the distal patellar ligament or tibial tubercle (Fig. 17–4B), the surgeon can make the suture taut at whatever degree of flexion produces the most medial tibial rotation. In many cases, particularly in dogs that are several years old before patellar luxation occurs, the tibial tubercle is not truly displaced or rotated relative to the rest of the tibia and foot (grades 1 and 2). In this situation it will be noted that when the patella luxates medially, the whole tibia rotates medially. This phenomenon is particularly noticeable in lateral luxation, a condition in which the tibia rotates laterally. Prevention of tibial rotation will markedly reduce the tendency of the patella to luxate. These sutures will probably break or loosen eventually in most cases; however, the fibrous tissue formed around the suture, plus realignment of soft tissues, will maintain the new position of the tibia or patella.

This fascia lata is incised along the cranial edge of the biceps muscle to allow retraction of the biceps caudally (Fig. 17–4A). Braided polyester (suture size 2–0 to 0 for small breeds, 0 to 2 for large breeds) is placed around the fabella (see Fig. 17–12 for details on technique for needle placement) on a half-circle Mayo catgut or Martin's uterine suture needle. The needle passes around the fabella in a distal-to-proximal or cranial-to-caudal direction most easily. The joint capsule can be opened on the lateral side to allow inspection of the joint and to perform trochlear arthroplasty if indicated. The suture is attached around the patella in semi–purse-string fashion by a bite taken into the quadriceps tendon from lateral to medial at the proximal end of the patella. The suture is then passed distally along the medial border of the patella and laterally along the distal end of the patella (Fig. 17–4A).

All bites are placed deeply and as close to the patella as possible. With the suture passing medial to the patella, it cannot pull out. The lateral joint capsule is closed and sometimes imbricated if there is redundant tissue. The patellar suture must not lie on exposed articular cartilage. With the patella in place, the suture is tied with enough tension to prevent patellar dislocation.

The same method can be used on the medial side for lateral luxation. An incision is made along the cranial border to the caudal belly of the sartorius muscle, which is retracted caudally to expose the medial fabella. Suture placement is similar to that described for medial luxation.

The tibial antirotational suture is placed around either the medial or the lateral fabella. The suture can be attached either to the distal patellar ligament or through a hole in the tibial tuberosity (Fig. 17–4B). The leg is positioned in various degrees of flexion to find the angle of maximal tibial rotation. The

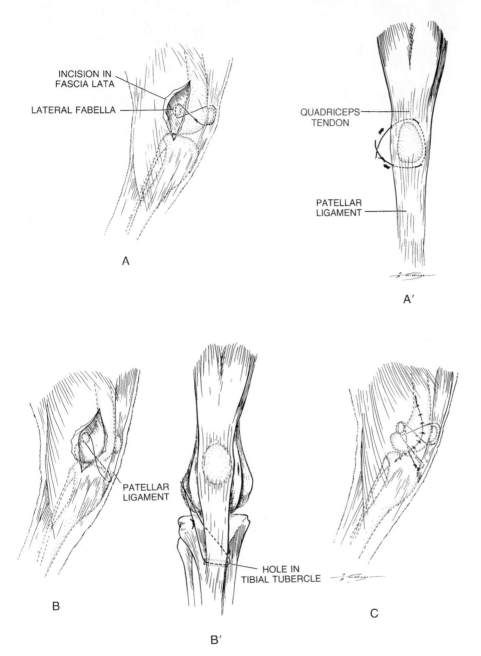

FIGURE 17–4. Patellar and tibial antirotational suture "ligaments."[6] (A) The fascia lata is opened along the cranial border of the biceps muscle to expose the lateral fabella by caudal retraction and elevation of the biceps. Braided polyester suture material (size 2–0 in toy breeds to size 2 in large breeds) is passed behind the lateral fabella and around the patella, as shown in A'. The suture is tied just tight enough to stabilize the patella. (B) To prevent medial tibial rotation, a suture can be passed around the fabella as in A, then placed either in the distal patellar ligament or in the tibial tuberosity (B'). Various locations are tried in order to find one that results in the suture's being tightest when the stifle is flexed to the degree that causes greatest internal tibial rotation. The suture is tied tight enough to prevent rotation. (C) The two sutures can be combined. The caudal fascia lata has been overlapped in closing.

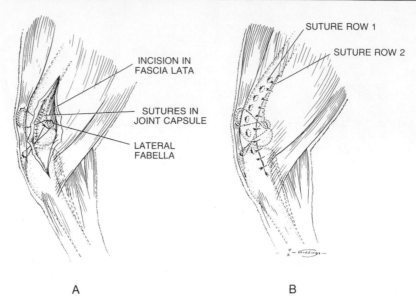

INCISION IN
FASCIA LATA

SUTURES IN
JOINT CAPSULE

LATERAL
FABELLA

SUTURE ROW 1

SUTURE ROW 2

A

B

FIGURE 17–5. Combining patellar and tibial suture "ligaments" with fascia lata over-lap. (*A*) The lateral fascia has been incised (see Fig. 17–3). The joint capsule has been sutured before the suture "ligaments" are placed to prevent suture material from rubbing on articular cartilage. (*B*) After the fascia lata overlap, the suture "ligaments" are almost completely covered by fascia, emerging only for a short distance before being inserted around the patella or in the patellar ligament.

suture material is then tied tightly enough to prevent tibial rotation. In addition, lateral or medial retinacular overlap can be performed to imbricate the joint (Figs. 17–2 and 17–4C), or the fascia lata overlap method can be used (Fig. 17–5).

DESMOTOMY-CAPSULECTOMY ■ Rarely used alone, these are steps frequently used in combination with other steps. Desmotomy means a simple release of the contracted medial or lateral retinaculum on the side toward which the patella is luxated (see Fig. 17–7E). The incision commences at the tibial plateau and continues proximally through both layers of the joint capsule and retinacular tissues proximal enough to relieve all tension on the patella. The incision is usually left open to prevent tension from redeveloping. Synovium will quickly seal the joint to prevent synovial fluid leakage. Sutures connecting the edge of the patella with the deep fascia helps prevent rocking of the patella. Capsulectomy means removing an elliptical piece of stretched joint capsule and retinaculum on the side opposite the direction of the patellar luxation. Suturing the edges together brings about imbrication or tightening of the joint capsule.

QUADRICEPS RELEASE ■ In some grade 3 and most grade 4 luxations, the quadriceps is so misaligned that it causes displacing tension on the patella after reduction of the luxation. In this situation, the entire quadriceps mechanism must be dissected free to the midfemoral level.

Bilateral parapatellar incisions are made through the joint capsule and retinaculum, as in the bilateral approach to the stifle joint.[8] These indications are continued proximally along the borders of the quadriceps muscle groups. Laterally, the separation is made between the vastus lateralis and biceps muscles; medially, it is made between the vastus medialis and caudal belly of the sartorius. The entire quadriceps is then elevated from the femur, freeing the insertion of the joint capsule proximal to the trochlea. The superficial fascial incisions are sutured after the rest of the reconstructive procedures are completed.

Bone Reconstructive Procedures

TROCHLEOPLASTY ■ Trochleoplasties are techniques that deepen a shallow, absent, or convex trochlea. There are three different ways to achieve this, each involving injury to the articular cartilage and should be avoided if possible, especially in the larger dog. Small dogs and cats tolerate these procedures well, although lameness recovery may be somewhat delayed.

To assess sufficiency of trochlear depth, the patella is reduced. Upon reluxating the patella, there should be an obvious "catch" or impedance to luxation, especially at the level of the trochlea where luxation occurs. If this is not the case, more aggressive deepening is performed.

1.   *Trochlear chondroplasty*[9,10] ("cartilage flap" technique) is useful only in puppies up to 10 months of age. As an animal matures, the cartilage becomes thinner and more adherent to the subchondral bone, making flap dissection difficult. A cartilage flap is elevated from the sulcus (see Fig. 17–6A), the sub-

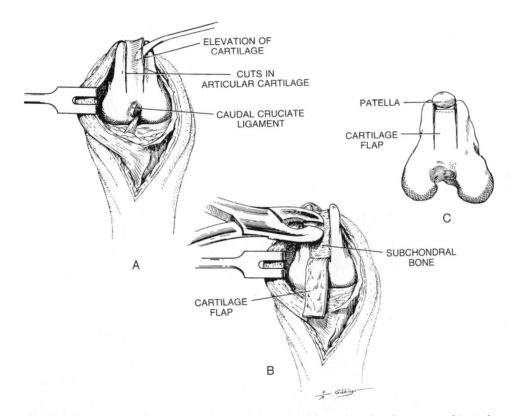

FIGURE 17–6. Trochleoplasty techniques. (*A*) Trochlear chondroplasty. For this technique, the animal must be less than 10 months old. The new sulcus is outlined by cuts through the thick adolescent cartilage. The proximal transverse cut is at the level of the proximal trochlear ridges. A sharp periosteal elevator is used to raise cartilage from subchondral bone. (*B*) The cartilage flap is hinged distally to allow removal of subchondral bone with rongeurs. (*C*) When the cartilage flap is replaced, the sulcus is deep enough to retain the patella. Fixation of the cartilage is not required. *Figure continued on following page*

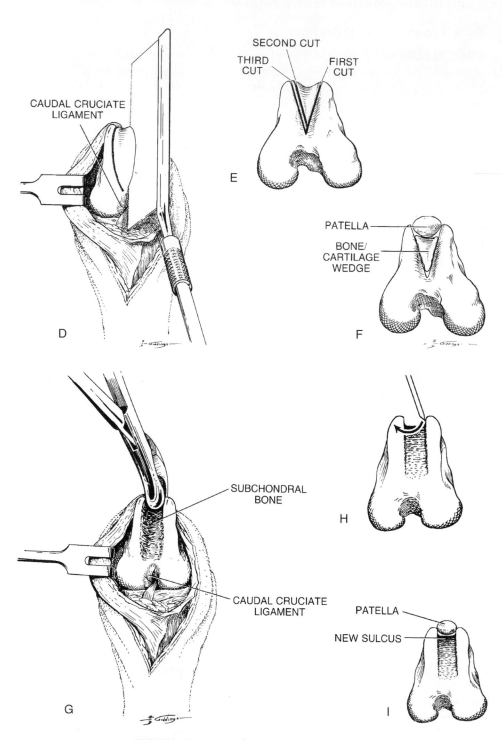

CAUDAL CRUCIATE LIGAMENT

D

SECOND CUT
THIRD CUT
FIRST CUT

E

PATELLA
BONE/CARTILAGE WEDGE

F

SUBCHONDRAL BONE

CAUDAL CRUCIATE LIGAMENT

G

H

PATELLA
NEW SULCUS

I

FIGURE 17–6. *See legend on opposite page*

chondral bone removed from beneath it (Fig. 17–6B), and the flap pressed back into the deepened sulcus (Fig. 17–6C). If not deep enough, the process is repeated. This results in a deepened trochlea with maintenance of articular cartilage in the sulcus, and fibrocartilage or fibrous tissue at the incisional gaps. The cartilage flap survives and experimental dogs have shown no ill effects from the procedure.[9]

2. *Recession sulcoplasty*[11] ("taco shell"). A V-shaped wedge, including the sulcus, is removed from the trochlea with a saw (Fig. 17–6D). The resulting defect in the trochlea is widened by another saw cut on one edge to remove a second piece of bone (Fig. 17–6E). When the original bone wedge is replaced, it is recessed into the defect, creating a new sulcus composed of hyaline cartilage[12] (Fig. 17–6F). The sides of the defect become lined with fibrocartilage. This method is preferred in mature animals.

3. *Trochlear sulcoplasty*[7] (curretage technique). Articular cartilage is removed to the level of subchondral bone to create a sulcus deep enough to prevent patellar luxation (Fig. 17–6G, H, I). By cutting completely through articular cartilage to subchondral bone, fibroplasia will result in a sulcus lined with fibrocartilage, which is an acceptable substitute for hyaline cartilage in non–weight-bearing areas. The width of this new groove must accommodate the width of the patella, and must be smooth. This can be accomplished by scraping the convex surface perpendicularly with an osteotome (Fig. 17–6H) or by using a rasp. Others prefer to use high-speed dental drills. While destructive to the entire cartilaginous trochlear sulcus, it nonetheless results in good function in small dogs and cats.

Owing to the relatively wide patella in the cat, it does not fit into the trochlea well. The patella can be narrowed by removing bone from the medial and lateral sides.

TRANSPOSITION OF THE TIBIAL TUBEROSITY[13,14] ■ When the tuberosity is deviated, relocation to a more cranial position on the leg helps patellar stability. Degree of deviation can best be assessed by placing the animal in dorsal recumbency with the surgeon standing at the end of the table near the animal's feet (Fig. 17–7A).

FIGURE 17–6. *Continued* (D) Modified recession sulcoplasty.[11] A thin-blade hobby saw (X-Acto, Long Island City, NY), ethylene oxide or chemically sterilized, is used to cut a V-shaped wedge from the trochlea, extending from the caudal cruciate origin to the proximal trochlear ridges. (E) Cuts made in the indicated order create a V-shaped defect and slightly smaller wedge. (F) When the original bone and cartilage wedge is replaced in the defect, it is recessed and hence creates a deeper sulcus. No fixation of the wedge is required. (G, H) Trochlear sulcoplasty ("curettage"). An outline of the proposed sulcus is made in the cartilage with a scalpel along the condylar ridges. Then articular cartilage and bone is removed (G, I) within the outlined area to create a straight-sided, flat-bottomed trough as shown in H. (H) After removal of cancellous bone, the bed is made smooth by scraping across the groove with an osteotome. Others prefer a rasp. The distal end of the trough is near the origin of the caudal cruciate ligament, and it extends to the proximal trochlear ridges. The trough should be deep enough so that the patella does not touch bone in the bottom of the trough and wide enough so that the patella rides deeply in the new sulcus. Done in this manner, articular cartilage of the patella is not damaged by abrasion on subchondral bone, and fibrocartilage can fill in the gap and conform to the excursions of the patella.

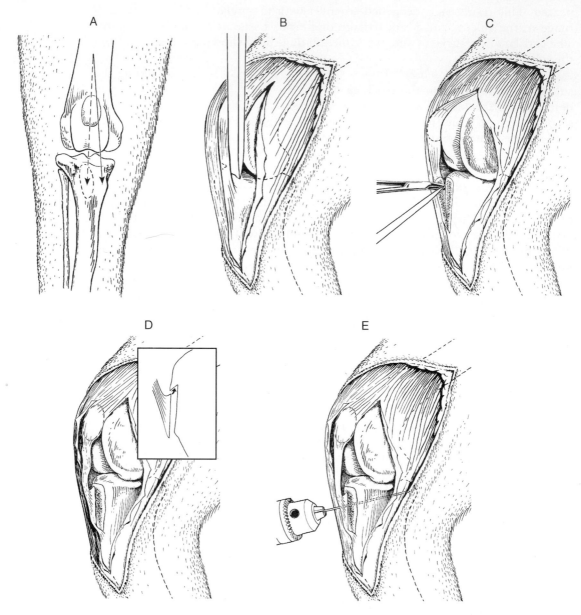

FIGURE 17–7. Tibial tuberosity transposition.[13] (A) Evaluating the amount of transposition needed. The dotted line demonstrates the correct relocation of the deviated tuberosity (*solid line*). (B) The tuberosity crest osteotomy is started 3 to 4 mm from the insertion of the patellar ligament. (C) With the tuberosity and crest retracted with a hemostat, a triangular piece of tibia is removed from the lateral aspect of the tibial crest (assuming medial luxation). (D) The notch made on the side of the tibia is similar in shape to the flange of bone left proximal to the patellar ligament insertion (see *inset*). With the knee hyperextended, the tuberosity is placed into the notch. (E) With the tuberosity held in place with thumb forceps (omitted for clarity), a pin is driven toward the caudal medial tibial condyle, with great care taken not to drive it proximally into the joint. *Figure continued on following page*

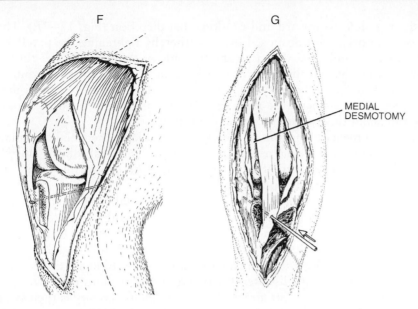

F   G

MEDIAL
DESMOTOMY

FIGURE 17–7. *Continued* (F) The pin is cut so that there is 1/8 inch pin protrusion to prevent the bone from slipping off the pin. Alternatively, the pin may be bent prior to being cut if the tuberosity is thick enough. (G) An alternative method for transposing the tuberosity involves incising lateral and medial attachments to the tuberosity but leaving the distal bone and periosteum intact. The tuberosity is swiveled and pinned.[14] (Note: this is the opposite leg.)

A medial skin incision is made for lateral or medial luxations.[8] For medial luxations a lateral arthrotomy with or without a capsulectomy is used. For lateral luxations, a medial arthrotomy is performed. An incision is made in the periosteum medially along the tibial tuberosity and crest including the distal attachment. The exact insertion of the patellar ligament is found by knicking the joint capsule along the medial aspect of the patellar ligament (the beginning of the desmotomy). To osteotomize the tuberosity, an osteotome as wide as the tuberosity should be used to avoid splitting it. The bone is cut starting 3 to 4 mm proximal to the insertion of the patellar ligament, which leaves a flange of bone that will be shaped similar to the notch of bone that will be cut on the tibia (Fig. 17–7B, D). The osteotome should not be twisted (keep flat side parallel with the patellar tendon) in order to avoid an asymmetric osteotomy.

After the tuberosity crest is loosened medially and distally, it is pushed laterally while the tibialis cranialis muscle is dissected away from the lateral aspect of the tibia. The soft tissues are *not* removed from the lateral aspect of the osteotomized tuberosity crest. To expose the area for the notch to be made along the lateral side of the tibia, a curved hemostat is levered between the tuberosity and caudal tibia (Fig. 17–7C). A triangular notch is usually made 5 to 8 mm distal from the proximal end of the osteotomy. If the tuberosity is markedly deviated, this notch is placed farther caudal and lateral on the tibia. For lateral luxations, the tubercle is osteotomized the same way, but the bed for the tubercle to relocate medially is made larger than the lateral notch.

To relocate the tuberosity, the knee is hyperextended to relax the extensor mechanism, and the top of the tuberosity is placed in the notch and held tightly (Fig. 17–7D, *inset*) while drilling 0.035- to 0.062-inch Kirschner wires (depending on animal size). The pin is driven through the thickest part of the tubercle in a slightly upward and caudomedial direction (Fig. 17–7E). The tuberosity has now been transposed distally (thereby tightening the patellar ligament), laterally, and twisted so that the flat side of the tuberosity is flush with the side of the tibia. Realignment is checked, and if satisfactory the pin is cut 2 to 3 mm from the tuberosity (Fig. 17–7F). In large dogs, two pins may be used. Some surgeons bend the pins, prior to cutting them, but this should be avoided in small tuberosities to prevent splitting.

Closure commences by suturing the external fascia of the tibialis cranialis to the periosteum on the medial aspect of the tibia. The lateral joint is closed and the patella checked for stability. If still unstable the groove may have to be deepened, or the tuberosity rotated farther.

In dogs with severe deformity, the lateral and medial attachments to the tuberosity may have to be incised in order to move the tuberosity to the area of the fibula. In cases of "patella alta," the tuberosity may have to be moved more distally after freeing more of the soft tissues proximal to the patella.

Another technique for osteotomizing the tuberosity is to incise the periosteum medially and tibialis cranialis laterally, freeing up both sides of the tuberosity. However, the tuberosity is left attached distally. The tuberosity is then swiveled laterally and pinned to a newly made notch[14] (Fig. 17–7G).

PATELLECTOMY ■ Patellectomy should be used only in very rare occasions where erosion is severe, and the dog has not improved clinically with successful realignment procedures. It is accomplished by incising vertically over the midline of the patella. With a sharp scalpel blade, the quadriceps tendon, retinaculum, and joint capsule and patellar ligament are peeled off the patella in quadrants, leaving as much soft tissue as possible. After the patella is removed there is a large defect over the femoral trochlea (Fig. 17–8A) that is closed by simple interrupted or purse-string sutures using nonabsorbable sutures. If there is a large void of soft tissue and fear of tissue breakdown, a vertically placed locking loop suture pattern may be used (Fig. 17–8B).

OSTEOTOMY ■ In rare cases with severe deformity, after the extensor mechanism has been relocated to a more normal cranial position, the osteotomized tibial tuberosity lies above the proximal end of the tibia due to muscle contracture and cannot be pinned. In a few instances the femur has been os-

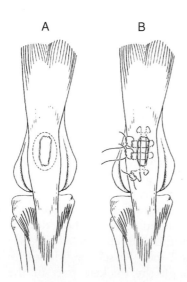

FIGURE 17–8. Patellectomy. (A) After exposure with a medial parapatellar skin incision, a vertical incision has been made on the midline of the patella. The patella is "shelled" out in quadrants with a sharp scalpel, leaving an oval hole (the dotted line represents the previous location of the patella). (B) Closure of the hole in the soft tissue can be accomplished by two horizontal mattress or interrupted sutures with nonabsorbable suture. If there is fear of dehiscence, a vertical locking loop suture pattern may be added.

teotomized, 1 or more cm of bone removed, and then repaired with intramedullary pins (or plated if trochleoplasty interferes with proper seating of the pins). This relaxes the extensor mechanism and allows the tibial tuberosity to be moved distally for pinning to the tibia. In cases of severe torsion of the tibia and femur, realignment osteotomies have been reported, but are complex, and we have not used them. In such cases, arthrodesis is probably a more feasible procedure.

FEMORAL OSTEOTOMY FOR LATERAL LUXATION ■ In the large and giant breeds, lateral luxation (see further discussion below) may be associated with valgus deformity and rotation of the femur (Fig. 17–9A, B), and if these deformities are severe enough the bone corrective procedures described above may not be sufficient to stabilize the patella. In such a situation a midshaft opening wedge osteotomy is done, the femur is derotated and placed in sufficient varus position to allow the patella to center in the trochlear sulcus, and a bone plate is used for fixation (Fig. 17–9C). The defect created in the lateral cortex is filled with autogenous cancellous bone graft (see Chapter 3). Lateral desmotomy, various soft tissue reconstructions, and recession trochleoplasty as detailed above, may be necessary in addition to the osteotomy.

Aftercare for All Surgical Techniques

External splinting is usually not needed in any of the procedures mentioned. Early, active use of the limb is beneficial if trochlear sulcoplasty has been performed, but exercise should be limited for 3 to 4 weeks, and jumping should in particular be prevented. Since many of these breeds are "jumpers," padded bandage support for 10 to 14 days may be useful in the active patient. If bilateral surgery has been performed, postoperative pain may seriously inhibit attempts to use the limbs. Appropriate aspirin or phenylbutazone dosage for 5 to 7 days is useful.

Because toy and miniature breeds are not especially tolerant of pain, some difficulties are occasionally encountered. If the dog is not starting to bear weight by 4 weeks, active physiotherapy must be started. Swimming is best but often

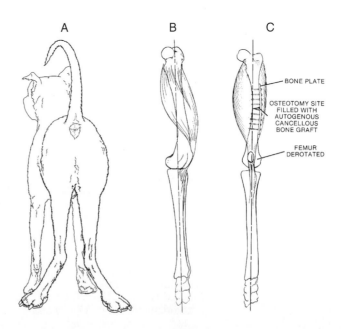

FIGURE 17–9. (A) Large Great Dane puppy with genu valgum. Note the wide hips, narrow stifles and hocks, with the toes pointing outward. (B) Femur and tibia from a large Great Dane with genu valgum showing valgus angulation and torsion of the femoral condyles. (C) Surgical correction involves a midshaft transverse osteotomy, internal rotation of the distal femur, creating a varus bowing of the femur sufficient to realign the quadriceps mechanism, and stabilization with a bone plate. The osteotomy gap is filled with autogenous cancellous bone graft.

BONE PLATE

OSTEOTOMY SITE FILLED WITH AUTOGENOUS CANCELLOUS BONE GRAFT

FEMUR DEROTATED

is not possible. Passive flexion-extension, 20 to 30 times, four times a day may be helpful. Leash walking, ball throwing, and other activities to tempt the animal into a running gait are also useful. Taping a small plastic syringe cap or glass marble between the toes and metatarsal pad of the opposite limb for a few hours at a time also works very well on some dogs. Placing the opposite leg in an Ehmer sling for several days may be done as a last resort.

Prognosis

Willauer and Vasseur have reported on the follow-up evaluation of medial patellar luxation repair in 52 stifles.[15] No lameness was observed in 92 percent of the stifles, although 48 percent had persistent, palpable patellar luxation. The recurrent luxations were always of a lesser grade than the preoperative grade, 17 of the 25 being grade 1. Regardless of the degree of lameness or stability of the patella, most dogs had radiographic signs of degenerative joint disease. It must be inferred from these findings that stability of the femoropatellar joint is not essential to good function in the small breeds, and this conforms to the common clinical observation in small-breed dogs with medial patellar luxations who never show clinical signs. Early correction of severe deformities will undoubtedly go a long way toward ensuring good function.

Medial Luxation Treatment Plan

Although not all cases can be fitted into rigid categories, we have attempted to outline procedures that may be useful for each grade of luxation. Treatment is aimed at reducing the anatomical defects. The procedures are done in the following order until patellar stability is achieved.

Grade 1
1. If the extensor mechanism is straight:
   a. Lateral fascia lata overlap (see Fig. 17–3).
   b. Tibial antirotational suture (see Figs. 17–4B and 17–5).
2. If the tubercle is deviated:
   Tibial tubercle transposition (see Fig. 17–7), with or without capsulectomy, retinacular or fascia lata overlap (see Figs. 17–2 and 17–3).

Grade 2
1. Medial desmotomy if the medial retinaculum prevents easy patellar reduction (see Fig. 17–7F).
2. Tibial tubercle transposition (see Fig. 17–7) and lateral capsulectomy retinacular or fascia lata overlap (see Figs. 17–2 and 17–3).
3. If the patella is still unstable, add:
   Trochleoplasty (see Fig. 17–6).

Grade 3
1. Medial desmotomy (see Fig. 17–7F).
2. Tibial tubercle transposition (see Fig. 17–7).
3. Trochleoplasty (see Fig. 17–6).
4. Capsulectomy, lateral retinacular or fascia overlap (see Figs. 17–2 and 17–3).
5. Lateral patellar and tibial antirotational sutures (see Figs. 17–4 and 17–5) if the patella is still unstable.

Grade 4
1. Procedures for grade 3.
2. Release of quadriceps.
3. If still unstable, consider:
   a. Femoral (see Fig. 17–9B, C) and tibial osteotomy, or
   b. Arthrodesis (see Figs. 17–30 and 17–31).

The limiting factor in grade 4 luxation repair is flexure contraction at the stifle. If the joint cannot be extended to a near normal angle, arthrodesis may be the only viable option.

Lateral Luxation Treatment Plan

Surgical treatment is as follows:

Grade 1
1. Medial retinacular overlap or capsulectomy (see Fig. 17–2) in all cases.
2. Medial tibial antirotational suture (see Fig. 17–4B) if the patella is still unstable after 1.

Grades 2 and 3
1. Lateral desmotomy if the lateral retinaculum prevents easy patellar reduction (see Fig. 17–7F).
2. Medial tibial tubercle transposition (see Fig. 17–7).
3. Medial retinacular overlap (see Fig. 17–2).
4. If the patella is still unstable, add:
   a. Trochleoplasty (see Fig. 17–6).
   b. Medial patellar and tibial antirotational sutures (see Figs. 17–4B and 17–5).

Combined Medial and Lateral Luxation Treatment Plan

Surgical procedures are as follows:

The tubercle is usually in straight alignment
1. Trochleoplasty (see Fig. 17–6).
2. Combined medial and lateral retinacular overlap (see Fig. 17–2), or capsulectomies.

Medial Luxation Resulting from Trauma

All breeds are subject to this relatively rare injury, although minor skeletal changes and mild patellar instability predispose to the problem. Traumatic luxation of the hip can be accompanied by medial patellar luxation. In our experience, we have not seen traumatic lateral luxation.

Clinical Signs

Mechanically, the situation is similar to that of a grade 1 luxation, with signs of acute inflammation superimposed. Pain is severe, and anesthesia or deep sedation is usually required for palpation. The limb is carried in flexion and internal rotation. Joint effusion and swelling of soft tissue are evident.

Radiographic examination to rule out hip luxation, patellar fracture, and avulsion or tearing of the patellar ligament is indicated. (See Chapter 16 for a discussion of these injuries.)

Treatment

Closed reduction and immobilization in a sling or Schroeder-Thomas splint may be indicated if the patella is reasonably stable following reduction. If the patella is markedly unstable or if luxation recurs after immobilization, surgical treatment should be undertaken.

1. Fascia lata overlap.
2. Lateral patellar suture (see Figs. 17–4 and 17–5) if stability is not achieved by 1.

Lateral Luxation (Genu Valgum) in Young Large and Giant Breeds

Also called genu valgum, this condition is seen in the same breeds that are affected by hip dysplasia. We have noted an unusual incidence in certain strains of flat-coated retrievers. Rudy[6] postulated a genetic pattern of occurrence and noted Great Danes, St. Bernards, and Irish wolfhounds as being the most commonly affected. Sten-Erik Olsson proposes that genu valgum of large and giant breeds of dogs is due to osteochondrosis of the distal femur.[16]

Components of hip dysplasia, such as coxa valga (increased angle of inclination of the femoral neck) and increased anteversion of the femoral neck,[17] are related to lateral patellar luxation. These deformities cause internal rotation of the femur with lateral torsion and valgus deformity of the distal femur, which displaces the quadriceps mechanism and patella laterally (see Fig. 17–9A, B). Early treatment consists of slowing the puppies' growth rate by feeding adult dog food. If patellar luxation occurs, then surgical correction is necessary.

Clinical Signs

Bilateral involvement is most common. Animals appear to be affected by the time they are 5 to 6 months of age. The most notable finding is a knock-knee (genu valgum) stance. The patella is usually reducible, and laxity of the medial collateral ligament may be evident. The medial retinacular tissues of the stifle joint are often thickened, and the foot can often be seen to twist laterally as weight is placed on the limb.

Treatment

The following procedures are used:

1. Mildly affected—lateral luxation without marked rotational deformity of the femur.
   a. Trochleoplasty (see Fig. 17–6).
   b. Tibial tubercle transposition (see Fig. 17–7).
   c. Retinacular overlap (see Fig. 17–2).
2. Markedly affected—lateral luxation with marked valgus deformity of femur.
   a. Corrective osteotomy of the femur (see Fig. 17–9C).

RUPTURE OF THE CRANIAL CRUCIATE LIGAMENT

Cranial cruciate ligament ruptures are one of the most common injuries in the dog and the major cause of degenerative joint disease in the stifle joint. The ligamentous injury may be a complete rupture with gross instability or a partial rupture with minor instability. In either case, untreated animals show degenerative joint changes within a few weeks and severe changes within a few months. The severity of degeneration seems to be directly proportional to body size, with those animals over 15 kg showing the most changes. Indeed, Vasseur has consistently demonstrated degenerative changes and decline in material properties (strength) of the ligament in dogs over 5 years of age.[18] The intensity of the changes became worse with age, but animals of less than 15 kg body weight had significantly less change in material properties than did larger dogs. This confirms the earlier observations of Paatsama[19] and Rudy.[6] Systemic inflammatory joint diseases, such as rheumatoid arthritis, have been known for years in humans and dogs to be associated with rupture of the cranial cruciate ligament.[20]

Recently,[21,22] synovial fluid analysis of partial cruciate tears demonstrated increased nucleated white cells, suggesting a moderate inflammation compared to the typical noninflammatory changes seen with complete tears and degenerative joint disease. There was no historical evidence of systemic (i.e., multiple joints/limbs) joint disease.

The function of the cranial cruciate ligament is to constrain the stifle joint so as to limit internal rotation and cranial displacement of the tibia relative to the femur and to prevent hyperextension.[23] The ligament is composed of two functional parts: the small craniomedial band (CMB) and the larger caudolateral band (CLB). Mechanisms of injury can be related to these normal functions: most commonly the ligament is injured when the stifle is rotated rapidly with the joint in 20 to 50 degrees of flexion or when the joint is forcefully hyperextended.[24] The former happens when the animal suddenly turns toward the limb with the foot firmly planted. This causes extreme internal rotation of the tibia with stress on the cranial cruciate ligament. Hyperextension probably occurs most commonly by stepping into a hole or depression at a fast gait.

The medial meniscus may be torn acutely at the time of injury but is more often damaged as a result of chronic instability of the joint, producing folding and eventual shredding of the caudal horn of the medial meniscus. Some type of meniscal injury is present in about 50 percent of the animals we have seen. These injuries are discussed later in this chapter. Concurrent patellar luxation is fairly often seen in toy breeds of dogs. It seems most likely in these cases that the patellar luxation is probably the initial condition and that the cruciate ligament ruptures are due to the tibial instability produced by the luxated patella and subsequent stretching of the crucial ligament. Partial cruciate ligament disease is becoming more frequently diagnosed, and is seen especially in straight-legged dogs, and will be discussed separately.

Clinical Signs and Diagnosis

Although pain is noted early with non–weight-bearing, most animals will start to use the limb within 2 to 3 weeks and apparently improve for several months until a gradual or sudden decline in the use of the limb is noted, often as a result of secondary meniscal damage. At this time, the degenerative changes of osteoarthrosis are present and functional decline is continuous. Diagnosis is based upon demonstration of cranial drawer motion (see Chapter 1). Drawer motion should be tested in both flexion, normal standing angle, and extension. With acute injuries and gross instability, drawer motion may be evident. Joint effusion may be noted for several days after injury. With chronic injuries and with partial tears, drawer motion is much less evident and requires very careful examination. With chronic cruciate ligament instability, periarticular tissues become thickened and fibrotic with only limited stretching possible. Drawer motion in these cases may be almost imperceptible, but any motion that ends gradually as a result of tissue stretching is abnormal. In skeletally immature dogs especially, slight drawer motion may be possible, but such motion stops abruptly as the ligament is stretched taut. This abrupt stoppage of cranial drawer motion is also noted in cases of isolated caudal cruciate rupture.

With partial cruciate ruptures, a small amount of drawer motion will be appreciated only in flexion, emphasizing the need to check drawer in extension, neutral, and flexion. This injury and its diagnosis are discussed in more detail later in this chapter. Testing the joint for increased internal rotation of the tibia is also helpful in chronic cases and in partial rupture cases. The amount of torsion of the tibia can be compared with the opposite limb.

Fibrosis of the joint capsule and associated structures partially stabilizes the joint but not sufficiently to prevent its continual deterioration. In animals of all ages there is often firm swelling of tissues on the medial surface of the joint between the medial collateral ligament and the tibial tubercle. The significance of this swelling is uncertain, but we believe it to be associated with chronic meniscal injury.

Radiographs are of little value in the typical cruciate ligament rupture other than to document the amount of osteoarthrosis present. These are better appreciated upon arthrotomy. If radiographs are taken, observations should include:

1. Osteophytes—this is seen especially around the distal patella, the supratrochlear region, and the tibial and femoral margins.

2. Fat pad sign—on the lateral projection, there is a normal triangle of radiolucent fat that is present from the distal patella to the femur and tibia (Fig. 17–10). The cruciates and menisci account for the normal radiodensity just

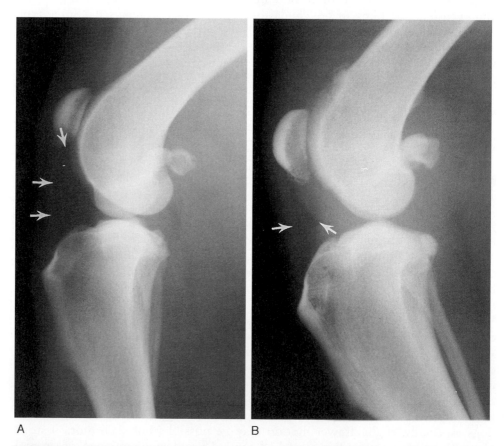

A   B

FIGURE 17–10. (A) On a lateral projection of a normal stifle, the fat pad is represented by a triangle of dark lucency (*arrows*) that reaches the femoral condyle. (B) On a lateral projection of a swollen stifle, the "fat pad sign" is represented by a smaller triangle (*arrows*) of dark lucency that does not reach the femoral condyle. The increased soft tissue density caudal to the lucency is due to fluid, or fibrosis of the fat pad.

FIGURE 17–11. Tibial position in neutral and cranial drawer positions. (*A*) In a neutral position, a straight line made from the fabella, end of the femoral condyle, and tibia/fibula will touch the head of the fibula/tibia. (*B*) With significant cranial drawer, this line will not touch the fibula. *Note:* unless there is a meniscus wedging the tibia forward, it is rare to find cranial drawer upon radiography of the unstressed stifle.

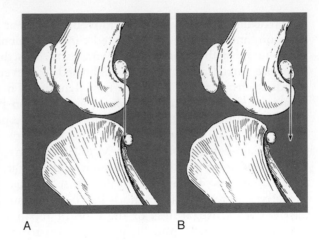

A   B

caudal to this triangle. With synovial effusion or fibrosis of the fat pad region, the area cranial to the femur becomes whiter (Fig. 17–10*B*). Good-quality soft tissue technique films are necessary to define this change.

3.   Cranial drawer—normally with cruciate rupture the unstressed leg lies in a neutral drawer position (Fig. 17–11*A*). If cranial drawer is detected on the radiograph (Fig. 17–11*B*), it may mean the presence of a torn meniscus wedging the tibia forward.

4.   Avulsions—seen rarely and usually occur in the young animal.

Modes of Therapy

It is well agreed that once instability resulting from cranial cruciate insufficiency occurs, progressive degenerative changes such as periarticular osteophytes, articular erosions, and meniscal damage begin within a few weeks. Controversy exists regarding the best treatment for ruptured cranial cruciate ligament.

Conservative treatment by splintage has been advocated. Close confinement for 4 to 8 weeks was reported to yield satisfactory function in the majority of small dogs (body weight <20 kg).[26] Vasseur reported similar results.[27] He found that dogs of 15 kg or less had satisfactory function several months after injury, while larger breeds uniformly functioned poorly. All animals had evidence of degenerative joint disease, and one has to speculate how well they would function several years later. Despite this evidence to the contrary, if the owner wants the best treatment for his or her pet, our clinical experience leads us to recommend surgical treatment of all dogs and cats with this injury.

There is no surgical technique that consistently stops the development or the progression of degenerative joint disease (DJD). It is hoped that less DJD develops due to the surgical stabilization than when no surgery is performed. Clinically, most authors cite an 85 to 90 percent clinical "success" rate after surgery, even after dogs have been lame for months.

Most stifle joints should be opened, explored, and "cleaned up" regardless of the stabilization technique. A medial arthrotomy is most helpful for examining and removing the commonly ruptured medial meniscus. It may be accomplished through a lateral arthrotomy if the stabilization technique dictates a lateral approach. The synovium ought to be inspected, rough or voluminous periarticular osteophytes are removed to prevent physical irritation to the synovium, and menisci are inspected carefully (meniscectomy is discussed later). The stump of the cruciate ligament, as well as the remainder of a 20 percent or more partial cruciate tear, is debrided to prevent degenerative inflammatory products from irritating the synovial lining. The joint is then closed (unless contraindicated due to the type of stabilization procedure used) with nonabsorbable sutures and the stabilization procedure performed.

Extracapsular methods embrace a wide variety of stabilization techniques for the cruciate-deficient stifle joint. Most of these involve use of heavy-gauge suture to decrease joint instability, although some rely instead on transposition of soft or bony tissues. The indication for these approaches as opposed to the reconstructive intra-articular methods has been the subject of endless debates in the last 30 years. Regardless of the type of repair done, most published reports indicate between 85 and 90 percent good to excellent function at follow-up. Intracapsular methods usually involve anatomic (or nearly) replacement of the cruciate ligament with autogenous or autologous grafts or synthetic materials. An in vitro examination of various methods of repair indicated that intra-articular methods of repair result in more normal joint motion than extra-articular methods.[25] This seems to be particularly important in dogs weighing over 17 to 20 kg and most especially in the acute injury to the athletic animal. Extra-articular methods work well in smaller breeds but have often been considered not as satisfactory in the larger, athletic animal with an acute cruciate rupture. In a recent study[28] in dogs undergoing experimental cranial cruciate ligament repair, there was essentially no functional difference in peak vertical forces measured by force plate analysis (see Chapter 1) between the dogs' preoperative and 20-week postoperative evaluations following an extracapsular technique (modified retinacular imbrication technique). Dogs undergoing an under-and-over intracapsular technique still had significant decreased vertical peak forces 20 weeks postoperatively. Stability with extracapsular suture techniques is attributed to thickening of the joint capsule and retinaculum owing to inflammation from the surgical procedure and implanted sutures. Recent experience of one of us (DLP), however, suggests that the fibular transposition method discussed later in this chapter is highly satisfactory for large dogs. On the other hand, one of us (GLF) uses the suture technique exclusively, including performance dogs. A high percentage of patients with ACL surgery, however, are household pets. Recent experience also indicates that extra-articular techniques are the method of choice when the cruciate injury is chronic. In this situation the inflammatory response and chronic changes within the joint create an adverse environment for transposed autologous tissue. Synthetic replacements for the cranial cruciate ligament have had some success in humans, but none of the available protheses are economically feasible for widespread veterinary use.

A question arises as to the advisability of operating a symptomatic animal with very chronic instability and severe degenerative joint disease. Simply providing stability will not cause the degenerative joint disease to disappear, but the animal usually improves dramatically in function. Because most chronic cases suffer from torn menisci, they will be greatly improved, and inflammatory reaction in the joint will decrease in intensity, if the torn meniscus is removed (see discussion later in this chapter). Attention must be given to medical management of the joint disease as discussed in Chapter 6.

The following surgical section will review extracapsular techniques (imbrication, retinacular, modified retinacular imbrication, three-in-one, and fibular head transposition), intracapsular techniques (Paatsama, over-the-top, under-and-over), and a combination (four-in-one over-the-top).

Postoperative care may or may not (surgeon preference) include a soft bandage for 2 weeks followed by 6 weeks of strict leash walks of only 5 to 10 minutes' duration. After that the animal's activity is slowly increased over the next 4 to 8 weeks pending physical demands. Weight reduction (usually indicated) is attempted by lowering caloric intake, and clients are warned that there is a 30 percent chance that the opposite cranial cruciate ligament will rupture in the next 2 years.

Extracapsular Techniques

Imbrication Technique

An older technique for stabilizing drawer movement involves the placement of Lembert sutures on the medial and lateral aspects of the joint capsule.[29] In our experience, this, by itself, stretches out. However, it is the basis for combination techniques that we perform.

Retinacular Technique

The retinacular technique as first described by DeAngelis and Lau[30] involves placing one or two large nonabsorbable sutures around the lateral fabella and anchoring to the distal patellar ligament (see Fig. 17–13B). This becomes a restraint to drawer movement.

Modified Retinacular Imbrication Technique (MRIT)

This technique[31] borrows from the previously described techniques. Instead of one or two sutures around the lateral fabella that are anchored to the patellar ligament, mattress sutures are passed around both the lateral and medial fabellae and anchored to a hole in the tibial tuberosity. Another suture is passed from the lateral fabella to the retinaculum along the side of the lateral aspect of the patella and acts as an imbrication suture (Fig. 17–12A). A landmark for finding the fabella is the distal third of the patella. The suture material we presently use for both the MRIT and the "three-in-one" is monofilament nylon fishing leader material (20- to 80-pound test available [material size approximates the weight of the animal]; Hard Nylon leader, Mason Tackle Co, Otisville, MI). Very few reactions have been encountered compared to other suture materials used. Breakage occasionally occurs. This material is carefully rinsed, and sterilized with ethylene oxide or a "cold cycle" of steam. Large braided polyester suture (size 0 for small breeds and 2 to 4 for larger breeds) can be substituted and is recommended if sutures are placed in the patellar ligament rather than the tibial tuberosity (see Fig. 17–13B), which may be more suitable for toy and miniature breeds of dogs and cats. Soaking braided imbrication sutures in chlorhexidine solution a few minutes before implantation reduces the number of infections and draining tracts associated with burying large-gauge braided nonabsorbable sutures, which has been reported as high as 21 percent.[32]

SURGICAL TECHNIQUE ■ A medial arthrotomy is performed to remove remnants of the cruciate ligament and inspect the menisci. Inspection and removal of damaged medial menisci are more difficult through a lateral arthrotomy (see below). The arthrotomy is closed with interrupted nonabsorbable or synthetic absorbable simple interrupted or continuous sutures prior to the sta-

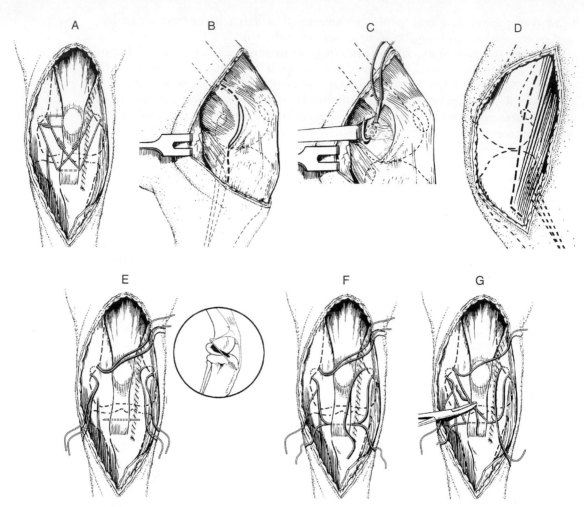

FIGURE 17-12. Modified retinacular imbrication technique (MRIT).[31] A medial approach[8] to the stifle joint has been performed, remnants of the cruciate ligament and torn menisci removed, and joint closed. Stabilization is accomplished with variations of the placement, size, and numbers of heavy-gauge mono-filament nylon sutures (see text). (*A*) Final placement of three sutures—one lateral fabellar/tuberosity, one medial fabellar/tuberosity, and one imbrication suture adjacent to the patella (sometimes omitted or rerouted to the tuberosity in large dogs). (*B*) A slightly curved incision at the biceps insertion is made to identify the fabella and to allow tightening of the suture without trapping muscle. The dotted line indicates extension of the fascial incisions if biceps muscle advancement is desired at closure. (*C*) Half the length of suture material is threaded through a heavy half-curved needle and passed around the proximal third of the lateral fabella. It is then cut close to the needle, which then forms two strands. (*D*) The medial fabella is exposed by incising along the cranial edge of the caudal belly of the sartorius muscle and partially detached at its insertion if later muscle advancement is desired. The medial suture is placed similar to C. (*E*) A horizontal hole is made with a 3/32- or 5/64-inch pin in the tuberosity, 1 cm caudal and distal to the patellar ligament insertion (see *A*). *Inset* shows the relationship of the mattress sutures with the plane of the cranial cruciate ligament when the hole in the tubercle is properly placed. (*F*) The caudal strand of the medial suture is passed from medial to lateral. The caudal strand of the lateral suture is passed through the same hole. (*G*) With all drawer movement removed by an assistant (see text), the first throw of the lateral suture is tightly tied and grasped with a smooth tipped forceps (ground down old needle holder works well). If drawer is eliminated, the knot is completed. If not, the forceps is released, and the suture is retightened and tied. The medial suture is similarly tied. An additional support suture is placed adjacent to the patella, being careful not to create a lateral luxating patella (see *A*). Closure of the deep fascia, subcuticular, and skin layers is routine.

bilization technique. To gain easier access to the fabella, a cutdown is made. The distal biceps femoris insertion on the fascia lata is incised just enough so that a large needle may be retrieved around the back of the fabella (Fig. 17–12B). In those techniques using advancement of muscle for active counter-traction to drawer movement (see three-in-one) the biceps femoris distal insertion is incised more proximally and distally (Fig. 17–12B). The fabella is identified by passing a curved mosquito forceps around and under the fabella. The forceps is quickly elevated several times so that the junction of the femur-fabella is delineated. A stout half-curved needle (Martin's uterine needle) is passed from cranial to caudal at the level of the proximal fabella (Fig. 17–12C). To achieve needle passage, the needle tip must be inserted perpendicular to the fabellar-femoral junction, and once it is inserted 5 to 6 mm, the needle arcs around and hugs the fabella to avoid injury to the fibular nerve, which lies about 2 to 3 cm caudally. Just after the needle emerges, the suture is cut behind the eye of the needle. Now there are two sutures around the fabella with one pass. The medial fabellar area is approached by longitudinally incising the cranial fascial insertion of the caudal belly of the sartorius (Fig. 17–12D). With the muscle reflected caudally, the needle and suture is similarly passed around the medial fabella. The hole on the tibial tuberosity is made with a $5/64$- or $3/32$-inch Steinmann pin 1 cm distal and 1 cm caudal to the proximal and cranial surface of the tibial tubercle in a 40-pound dog (Fig. 17–12E, E1). This ensures that the mattress suture is in the same plane as the cruciate ligament. The sutures are threaded through these holes by first bringing the medial suture from a medial to lateral direction (Fig. 17–12F). It is then taken back toward the medial fabella either under or over the patellar tendon. Likewise, the lateral suture is passed from the lateral to the medial side and then passed under or over the patellar tendon. Placing the sutures under the tendon avoids pressure on it. The knots may be placed near the hole on the tibial tuberosity or near the patellar ligament depending on how the sutures are brought through the tuberosity (i.e., the top part of the medial suture is brought through from lateral to medial, or the bottom part of the suture is brought through from medial to lateral). The surgeon should be consistent in order to facilitate their removal, if necessary.

To make the sutures effective, all slack and drawer movement must be removed from the joint as the sutures are tied tightly. To do this, an assistant finds the stifle angle of most drawer movement, and while keeping this angle, externally rotates the tibia, and pushes it in "caudal" drawer. The first throw of the lateral suture is held gently with a smooth forceps (a filed down old needle holder works well) (Fig. 17–12G) and drawer motion checked. If drawer remains, the suture is released, retightened, and regrasped with the forceps and checked again for drawer, and then tied completely. The medial fabellar suture is similarly tied, with the assistant holding the leg in the same overreduced position. The fabellar sutures lie on top of the patellar ligament and should not be tied so tightly that the ligament is appreciably indented. The lateral imbrication suture, which passes from the lateral fabella to the retinacular fascia adjacent to the lateral aspect of the patella, is lastly tied (Fig. 17–12A) with care not to overtighten and cause patellar luxation.

The number, placement, and size of these sutures are modified depending on the degree of drawer movement, size and function of animal, and the existence of concurrent patellar luxation. For instance, a 120-pound dog may have two lateral and two medial fabellar sutures placed without the imbrication suture. Dogs with minimal drawer may only get one lateral fabellar-to-tibial tubercle suture and one imbrication suture.

Three–in–One Technique

The technique shown here is a slight modification of the MRIT procedure described above. The major differences are the addition of advancement of the caudal sartorius muscle medially and the biceps femoris laterally to add some immediate postoperative support to the repair, and the position of the knots on the fabellar sutures. In small breeds (<30 pounds; 15 kg) the medial fabellar suture is eliminated. See the comments above in the MRIT section relative to suture material considerations.

SURGICAL TECHNIQUE ■   A medial arthrotomy is performed.[8] Fragments of the cruciate ligament are removed and menisci are inspected and removed only if severely torn or fragmented (see discussion of meniscus below). The medial joint capsule is closed with synthetic absorbable suture material (Fig. 17–13A). To expose the medial fabella, an incision is made through the fascia on the cranial edge of the caudal belly of the sartorious muscle and extended

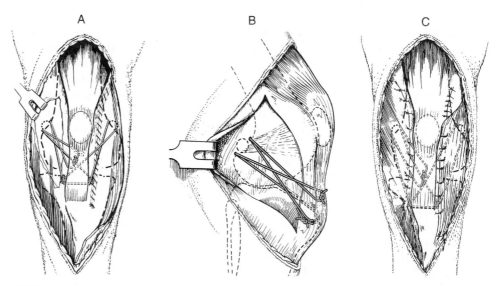

FIGURE 17–13. The three-in-one technique, a modification of the MRIT method of Figure 17–12. The changes include advancement of the biceps femoris and caudal sartorius muscles for additional muscle traction to combat drawer motion, and method of suture placement and position of the knots. (*A, B*) After closure of the medial arthrotomy, part of the distal insertion of the caudal belly of the sartorius muscle is detached from the tibia for later advancement (see also Fig. 17–12D). A medial fabellar suture is placed as in Figure 17–12C. Laterally an incision is made in the fascia lata starting proximal to the fabella and ending distally at the tibia, paralleling the patellar ligament. A transverse hole has been placed in the tibial tuberosity (see Fig. 17–12E) and a lateral fabellar suture placed as in Figure 17–12C. The proximal end of the suture is placed from lateral to medial through the drill hole, and the distal end of the suture is brought under the patellar ligament. A similar but opposite maneuver is used on the medial suture. The knots are tied distally, with the lateral suture tied first. The second lateral suture, placed in the distal patellar ligament and tied under tension to produce slight caudal displacement of the ligament, is optional. (*C*) The detached portion of the caudal sartorius is sutured to the patellar ligament proximally to the level of the patella. The fascia of insertion of the biceps femoris muscle is overlapped over the patellar ligament distally to place the muscle under increased tension.

distally into the proximal portion of this muscle's insertion on the tibial crest (Fig. 17–12D). A monofilament nylon suture is passed around the medial fabella with a half-circle Mayo catgut or Martin's uterine suture needle as shown in Figure 17–12C.

The skin is next undermined and reflected laterally to expose the lateral side of the joint (Fig. 17–13B). The fascia lata is incised on a line from the cranial edge of the biceps femoris muscle toward the patella, where the incision is angled toward the proximal tibia, paralleling the patellar ligament. The fascia lata is reflected caudally to expose the lateral fabella and collateral ligaments without incising the synovial capsule. Two sutures are placed around the lateral fabella as in Figure 17–12E if the patellar ligament imbricating suture is to be used (see below); if not, only one suture is placed. A small hole is drilled transversely through the tibial tuberosity near the insertion of the patellar ligament (Fig. 17–12E). The more proximal end of the medial suture is brought through the bone tunnel from a medial to lateral direction, and the distal part is passed under the patellar ligament to emerge laterally near the hole in the tuberosity, resulting in a figure-of-8 pattern (Fig. 17–13A). A similar but opposite maneuver is performed with one of the two lateral sutures. With the stifle held at a standing angle and all drawer motion removed (i.e., the tibia externally rotated and forced caudally), these sutures are then tied snugly, thus eliminating drawer movement. Having the sutures placed so that the knots are tied as if a horizontal mattress suture helps maintain tension within the knot while placing the second throw, thus more easily done by surgeon without an assistant. The lateral suture is tied first. The second lateral suture may be used, if desired, to further imbricate the joint by placing it in the lateral third of the distal end of the patellar ligament (Fig. 17–13B). The fascia lata is closed by overlapping it onto the patellar ligament and quadriceps fascia to increase tension on the muscle. The previously detached portion of the caudal belly of the sartorius and medial fascia are sutured to the patellar ligament medially. The proximal portion of the medial fascial incision is closed conventionally. The final closure (Fig. 17–13C) has the fabellar sutures completely covered, except for the knots, by muscle and fascia. This may help prevent seroma formation and contamination of these large sutures from partial disruption of the skin incision during the first few days postoperatively.

POSTOPERATIVE CARE ■ The limb is not splinted postoperatively. Very restricted exercise is allowed for the first 4 weeks with a slight increase in activity between 4 and 8 weeks and then unrestricted activity after 8 weeks.

Clinical experience tells us that if the lameness doesn't improve over the next 8 to 12 weeks, or if it improves but then worsens, these suggest that there is either a torn meniscus and/or a suture breakage or reaction. It is therefore important for the surgeon to know exactly where the knots were placed in order to expedite suture removal. Such removal of the imbricating sutures after 3 months postoperatively does not increase drawer motion, as the fibrosis created by surgery provides long-term stability.

Fibular Head Transposition

An alternative extra-articular technique that has gained increasing acceptance is the fibular head transposition (FHT) of Smith and Torg.[33] By freeing the fibular head and attached lateral collateral ligament (LCL), the fibula can be moved cranially and attached to the tibia. The LCL is placed under tension and functions similarly to the sutures in the MRIT or three-in-one method. Drawer motion and internal tibial rotation are resisted by the transposed ligament. Biomechanical studies have confirmed that the stiffness of the LCL is sufficient to stabilize the stifle joint.[34] Further mechanical studies following transposition of the LCL indicated a gradual increase in structural qualities, reaching approximately 135 percent of their original values 10 months postoperatively.[35]

Smith and Torg found the method produced good to excellent clinical grades in 90 percent of the cases, and the experience of one of us (DLP) with the FHT over a 7-year period is similar. The clinical results are very similar to intra-articular methods, but there is the major advantage of significantly decreased recovery time (see below). The effectiveness of the technique has been questioned in one experimental study that concluded that this method did not control drawer motion or rotational stability, did not prevent progression of degenerative joint disease, and was associated with meniscal damage in 25 to 50 percent of the dogs in the study.[36] Objectively, these are not impressive results, but they are more an indication of the state of the art in stabilizing the cruciate-deficient stifle than a condemnation of the technique. If all the currently used methods were subject to such a rigorous evaluation it seems certain that they would all show similar results. In point of fact, relative to the incidence of postsurgical meniscal injuries requiring second surgeries in 665 stifles stabilized with three methods (lateral retinacular imbrication, intra-articular over-the top, and FHT), significantly fewer dogs with FHT returned with meniscal injuries (8.6 percent) than with the other two methods (16.5 and 19 percent).[37]

SURGICAL TECHNIQUE ■   This surgery is more demanding than will be appreciated from the following description, and should be thoroughly practiced on cadavers before attempting it in a patient. Once familiarity is gained, the level of difficulty, operating time required, and incidence of postsurgical complications are very similar to the over-the-top procedures. Potential intraoperative problems include fracture of the fibular head or neck, accidental transection or avulsion of the collateral ligament, and injury of the peroneal (fibular) nerve. Wire breakage and pin migration are the most common late complications, but are minimal with good technique.

The technique described is slightly modified from the original description.[33] The anatomical relationships of the lateral collateral ligament and the fibular head are illustrated in Figure 17–14A. A lateral skin incision and medial parapatellar approach (to allow better exposure if meniscectomy is required) to the joint is made. Following inspection of the joint, with removal of the remnants of the cranial cruciate ligament and inspection of the meniscus (see discussion below), the medial capsule and retinaculum are closed, including the caudal belly of the sartorius muscle in the closure, as in Figure 17–13C. The fascia lata is next incised so that the incision continues distally along the lateral edge of the tibial tuberosity for 2 to 3 cm, avoiding the underlying fascia of the tibialis cranialis muscle. Caudal retraction of the fascia lata and biceps femoris muscle, after sharp elevation of the fascia from the tibia, exposes the fibular head, collateral ligament, and the underlying muscles (Fig. 17–14B). The peroneal (fibular) nerve *must* be identified and protected. The nerve is most readily seen if all fat and areolar tissue is elevated from the fascia of the peroneus longus muscle; the nerve and an accompanying vessel enter the muscle caudally 1 to 2 cm distal to the fibular head.

The first incision is into the fibularis longus muscle along the caudal side of the fibula, starting just proximal to the peroneal nerve, and continuing proximally along the caudal border of the collateral ligament. The muscle is elevated from the fibular head. Sharp dissection is used to free the cranial border of the collateral ligament from underlying joint capsule. Undermining and freeing of the ligament from the joint capsule is done from the caudal side of the ligament by blunt dissection using a curved forceps or scissors and a spreading action. The incision made to free the cranial border of the ligament is continued distally into the intermuscular fascia between the peroneus longus and tibialis cranialis muscles, and then cranially through the origin of the tibialis cranialis until the tendon of the long digital extensor muscle is exposed. The tibialis cranialis muscle and the tibial origin of the peroneus longus muscle are elevated from the tibia.

The ligaments of the fibular head are incised to free it from the tibia by working from the cranial aspect of the fibular head while retracting the peroneus longus muscle. The dissection plane between the tibia and fibular head is approximately 45 degrees caudal from the sagittal plane of the tibia (Fig. 17–14C). Incision of the ligaments can be done with a variety of instruments such as a scalpel, a sharp periosteal elevator, or osteotome, but the most useful instrument has been a canine meniscus knife (Veterinary Instrumentation, Sheffield, England; Jorgensen Laboratories Inc., Loveland, CO; see Fig. 17–21E). This instrument follows the plane between the bones without cutting bone and greatly reduces the chance of accidental fracture of the fibular head. It is only in more chronic cases that this dissection is difficult, as osteophytes may protrude into the interosseous plane.

After the proximal fibula is freely movable, a 0.62-inch (1.5-mm) Kirschner wire is driven into the center of the head of the fibula and is then used to help move the fibula laterally and then cranially under the caudal edge of the tibialis cranialis muscle. A 5/64-inch (2-mm) pin is used in very large breeds (>80 pounds; 35 kg). Use of larger pins will not allow them to bend easily, which is essential to the technique as described here. The tibia is externally rotated, and the stifle is held at a standing angle with drawer movement removed during the transposition maneuver. A Schroeder vulsellum forceps or an AO/ASIF pointed reduction forceps (Synthes Ltd. [USA], Paoli, PA) is useful to maneuver and hold the fibula in the desired position. One jaw of the forceps is placed caudal to the fibular head, and the other jaw is engaged on the tibial tuberosity. Be certain that the jaw of the forceps does not trap the peroneal nerve or penetrate the insertion of the collateral ligament, as this will cause tearing of the ligament. The forceps fixes the fibular head and collateral ligament and allows testing of drawer motion before drilling the Kirschner wire into the tibia. Most, but not all, of the motion will be neutralized at this time.

The Kirschner wire is then driven into the tibia to penetrate the transcortex (Fig. 17–14D, E). The K-wire should not be cut short yet. A 3/32-inch (2.5-mm) hole is drilled in the tibial tuberosity by laying the pin on the surface of the fibula and penetrating the tibialis cranialis muscle. A 16-gauge hypodermic needle is passed caudally through the bone hole and the tibialis cranialis muscle toward the surface of the fibula where the Kirschner wire penetrates it. A 16- to 18-gauge (1.2- to 1.0-mm) eyelet wire is inserted into the needle, which is then withdrawn, leaving the wire in place. The larger wire, 16-gauge or 1.2-mm, is used for dogs over 80 pounds (35 kg). The cranial end of the wire is looped laterally around the tuberosity and then passed back through the tibialis cranialis muscle toward the K-wire.

The free end of the wire is passed through the eyelet, which is positioned to face cranially by bending the wire around the pin. As the wire is tightened, the pin will bend cranially and produce more tension on the collateral ligament, thus the need for a small-diameter bendable pin. When cranial drawer motion is abolished, the wire is bent over and cut, the cut end being buried in the tibialis cranialis muscle. Substituting a twisted wire for the eyelet wire is possible, but is slightly more difficult to tighten without breaking the wire, due to the large number of turns required to move the fibula. A second wire is placed in a similar manner through a second hole in the tibial tuberosity, except that

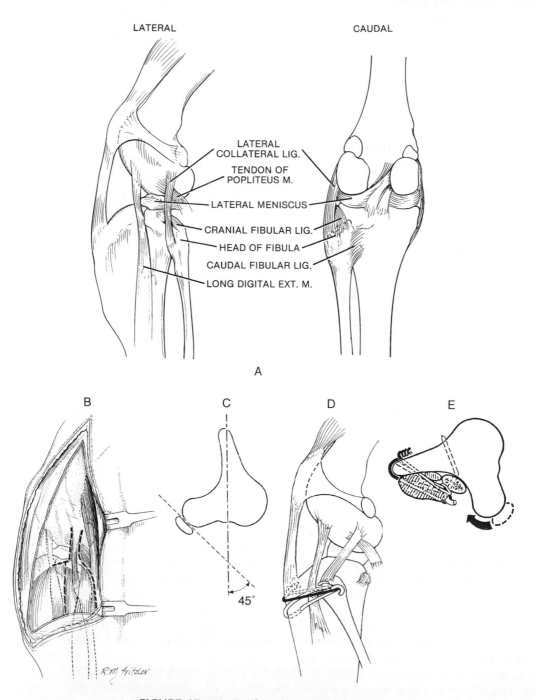

LATERAL   CAUDAL

LATERAL
COLLATERAL LIG.

TENDON OF
POPLITEUS M.

LATERAL MENISCUS

CRANIAL FIBULAR LIG.

HEAD OF FIBULA

CAUDAL FIBULAR LIG.

LONG DIGITAL EXT. M.

A

B   C   D   E

45°

R.M. Fritzler

FIGURE 17–14. *See legend on opposite page*

this wire is secured by twisting on the craniomedial aspect of the tuberosity and bent flat against the bone. Overtightening of this wire should be avoided, as it will loosen the first wire. This could also be an eyelet-type wire if desired. We have seen some wire breakage when a single wire is used, hence the addition of the second wire. A hook is now bent in the Kirschner wire, which is then driven flush with the fibula, taking care not to entrap the fibular nerve. The end of the K-wire protruding from the medial side of the tuberosity is cut flush with the bone. For very large dogs, over 100 pounds (45 kg), a second pin is used, placed caudal to the fibular head and driven into the tibia. The second wire is placed around this pin as described above.

Addition of a large monofilament nylon lateral fabella–to–tibial tuberosity suture, as described above in the MRIT and three-in-one sections, has clinically proven to be a useful addition to this procedure. Based on the work of Dupuis et al.,[35] the transposed collateral ligament undergoes elongation after transposition, but this all occurs in the first 3 weeks postoperatively. If the lateral suture can serve as a protector of the ligament during this period, there should be better long-term stability of the joint, and this has been borne out in practice, with very minimal long-term drawer motion observed. Following placement of the imbrication suture the fascia lata is sutured by advancing it as far craniomedially as possible, thereby placing the biceps femoris muscle under tension (see Fig. 17–12C).

AFTERCARE ■ The limb is not splinted postoperatively. Only very restricted exercise is allowed for 4 weeks, followed by a gradual increase of activity and full resumption of activity at 8 weeks. Most animals will be partially weight bearing within the first week, and walking comfortably with only a slight limp at 3 to 4 weeks.

FIGURE 17–14. Fibular transposition technique, modified from method of Smith and Torg.[33] (A) The lateral collateral ligament and tibial ligaments of the fibular head. The collateral ligament will be dissected free from the joint capsule and the ligaments of the fibula incised to free it from the tibia. (B) A lateral skin incision and medial parapatellar approach to the joint has been made. The medial capsule and retinaculum have been closed as in the three-in-one technique, but without a suture around the medial fabella (see Fig. 17–13C). The fascia lata is incised as in Figure 17–13B except that the incision continues distally along the lateral edge of the tibial tuberosity for 2 to 3 cm. After sharp elevation from the tibia, caudal retraction of the fascia lata exposes the fibular head, collateral ligament, and the underlying muscles. The peroneal (fibular) nerve must be identified and protected. See text for further description of the depicted incisions. (C) The dissection plane for incising the tibiofibular ligaments is 45 degrees to the sagittal plane of the tibia. (D, E) A 0.62-inch (1.5-mm) Kirschner wire is driven into the center of the head of the fibula and is then used to move the fibula cranially under the caudal edge of the tibialis cranialis muscle. When the collateral ligament is taut and most drawer motion abolished, the Kirschner wire is driven into the tibia to penetrate the transcortex. A hole is drilled in the tibial tuberosity for a 16- or 18-gauge (1.2- to 1.0-mm) eyelet cerclage wire, which is passed cranially through the tibialis cranialis muscle, around the tuberosity, and back through the muscle (see text for details). As the wire is tightened, the pin will bend and produce more tension on the collateral ligament; when cranial drawer motion is abolished, the wire is cut and the end is buried in the muscle. A twisted wire is then placed around the pin through a second bone tunnel and is tightened on the craniomedial aspect of the tibial tuberosity.

Intracapsular Techniques

Paatsama

One of the first intracapsular techniques was developed by Saki Paatsama[19] in the 1950s and is still a popular cruciate surgery performed by practitioners. The technique involves harvesting a 1- to 2-cm-wide strip of fascia lata from the thigh and leaving it attached distally. Holes are drilled in the femur and tibia at the anatomical origin and insertion of the ruptured anterior cruciate ligament. Care must be taken to avoid injury to the caudal cruciate ligament. The end of the fascia lata strip is threaded through each of these two holes using looped wire. The graft is then pulled tightly and anchored with sutures along the patellar ligament.

Over-the-Top

This procedure, developed by Arnoczky and co-workers,[38] involves harvesting a cruciate replacement composed of the medial third of the patellar ligament, part of the patella, and quadriceps tendon. It should only be considered in acute injuries of athletic dogs over 25 to 30 kg. Harvesting this graft is technically demanding, as significant injury to the patella can occur. The graft is brought through the joint and then over the top of the lateral condyle and sutured. This avoids improper hole placement and possible fraying of the graft from bony edges as with the Paatsama technique.

Following a medial arthrotomy the medial third of the patellar ligament is split away from the rest of the ligament but is left attached to the tibia and patella. Incisions in the patellar tendon and fascia lata continue proximally (Fig. 17–15A). A portion of the medial edge of the patella is split away from the patella with a small osteotome. Care should be taken not to penetrate the articular cartilage of the patella. The attachments of the patellar tendon proximally and patellar ligament distally must be preserved (Fig. 17–15B). When the bone fragment is free, dissection is continued proximally into the fascia lata, where the strip is prepared (Fig. 17–15C) as described below in the Four-in-One Over the Top. The fascia-bone-ligament strip needs to be only two times as long as the tibial tubercle–patella distance. The medial capsule incision is continued as far proximally as necessary to allow lateral luxation and retraction of the patella and exposure of the lateral condyle. The fascial strip is pulled through the joint similarly to Figure 17–16D, E except that the forceps is passed from inside the joint capsule. Following fixation of the fascial strip to periosteum, fascia, and the lateral collateral ligament (see Fig. 17–16H, I), the joint is closed as in Figure 17–16F.

AFTERCARE ■ No postoperative splinting is used with the over-the-top technique, but very restricted exercise (confining the animal to the house and walking the animal with a leash) is ordered for 12 weeks, followed by gradual return to activity and freedom for moderate exercise after 18 weeks. Intensive training of working dogs should not start until 6 months postoperatively.

The Under-and-Over Technique

This technique utilizes a fascia lata strip harvested like the Paatsama technique. However, the strip goes all the way to the tibia. A tunnel is made under the intermeniscal ligament and the graft passed under the intermeniscal ligament into the interior of the joint. It is then pulled through the joint and over the top of the lateral condyle/fabellar region. After it is pulled tight enough to

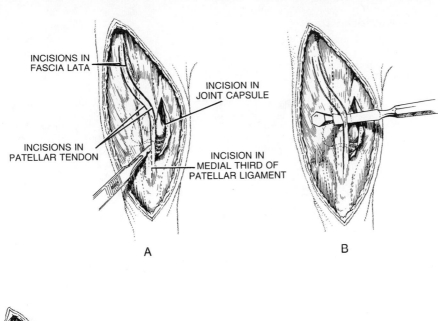

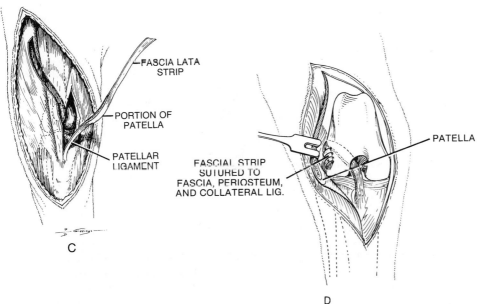

FIGURE 17–15. Intra-articular cranial cruciate stabilization: over-the-top technique.[38] (*A*) A medial approach[8] with a lateral skin incision has been made to the right stifle. The medial arthrotomy is made on the medial edge of the patellar ligament and patella and continues proximally into the cranial sartorius and vastus medialis. The medial third of the patellar ligaments is split away from the remainder of the ligament. Incisions in the patellar tendon and fascia lata define the fascial strip proximal to the patella. (*B*) A portion of the patella is removed with an osteotome, and care is taken not to cut into the articular surface. The patellar ligament attachment distally and the patellar tendon proximally must be preserved. (*C*) The patellar ligament–patella–fascia lata strip is freed. (*D*) The medial incision is continued as far proximally as necessary to allow lateral luxation and retraction of the patella and exposure of the lateral condyle. The fascial strip is pulled through the joint as in Figure 17–16*D, E*, except that the forceps are passed from inside the joint capsule. Following fixation of the fascial strip to the periosteum, fascia, and the lateral collateral ligament (see Fig. 17–16*H, I*), the joint is closed as in Figure 17–16*F*.

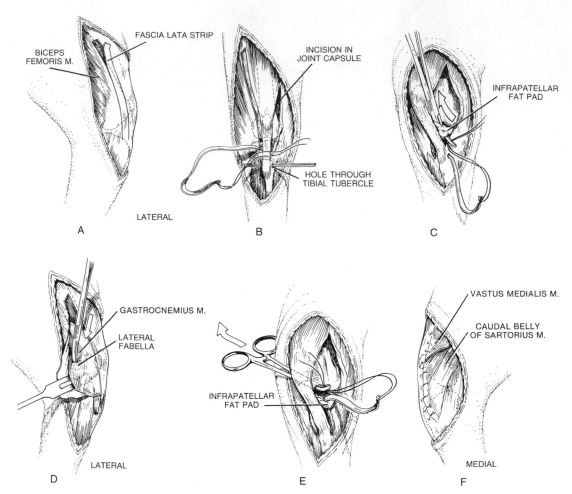

FIGURE 17–16. Intra- and extracapsular cranial cruciate stabilization: four-in-one over-the-top.[40] (*A*) Lateral view of right stifle. A medial arthrotomy has already been performed, the ligament remnants removed, and the joint explored. A fascia lata strip is developed, based on the tibial-patellar ligament junction. The strip is 1 to 1.5 cm wide at the base and slightly wider proximally. Its total length is 2.5 to 3 times the distance from the tibial tubercle to midpatella. (*B*) A 5/32- to 3/16-inch hole has been drilled transversely through the tibial tubercle, close to the tibial plateau. A heavy monofilament suture has been attached to the fascial strip, which is then reflected distally and pulled through the hole from lateral to medial. (*C*) The fascial strip is pulled into the joint by tunneling it through the fat pad. (*D*) The lateral edge of the fascia lata incision is dissected and retracted to expose the lateral fabella. The portion of the gastrocnemius muscle originating proximal to the fabella is elevated, and a curved forceps is passed medial to the fabella, through the caudal joint capsule, and into the intercondylar notch of the femur. (*E*) The curved forceps must emerge in the intercondylar space lateral to the caudal cruciate ligament. One end of the monofilament suture attached to the fascial strip is grasped so that the strip can be pulled proximally through the joint. (*F*) The medial arthrotomy is closed in one layer. The caudal sartorius muscle is partially detached from the tibia, then sutured with the joint capsule and medial fascia to the patellar ligament, creating increased tension in the muscle (see also Fig. 17–13C). *Figure continued on opposite page*

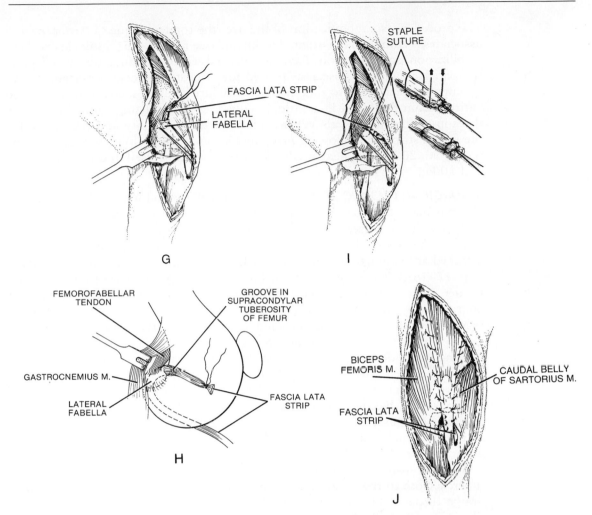

FIGURE 17–16. *Continued* (G) Two sutures of No. 2–4 nonabsorbable material are placed from the lateral fabella to the distal patellar ligament or tibial tuberosity and tied under tension with drawer motion reduced (see Fig. 17–13). (H) The femorofabellar ligament is elevated from the supracondylar tuberosity of the femur to allow a groove to be produced in the cortical bone of the tuberosity by rongeur, rasp, or osteotome. A wire loop can then be used to fish the suture attached to the fascia strip through this opening. (I) The fascial strip is pulled tight and attached to joint capsule or patellar ligament with the suture attached to its end. The strip is then sutured to the femorofabellar tendon, fascia, and joint capsule with 3–4 cruciate "staple" sutures (see *inset*). (J) This cranial view shows the bilateral closure that places caudal traction on the tibia as a result of increased tension from the biceps femoris and caudal sartorius muscles. Because of the removal of the fascial strip, the lateral closure places the biceps femoris muscle under tension.

eliminate drawer, the graft is attached to the lateral femoral condyle with a spiked washer and screw.[39]

Intra- and Extracapsular Technique

Four-in-One Over the Top

This technique involves using the three-in-one plus a fascia strip used in over-the-top fashion. This technique[40] is indicated for animals weighing over 15 kg and can be used for smaller breeds if they are athletic, such as hunting beagles.

The procedure is a modification of the over-the-top technique of Arnoczky and associates.[38] Although the original technique (see Fig. 17–15) results in excellent stabilization, some surgeons have experienced technical difficulties in collecting the patellar ligament–fascia strip used for cruciate ligament replacement. An attempt has been made to simplify the procedure by using a fascia strip collected entirely from the fascia lata. Additionally, lateral stabilizing sutures (as in the three-in-one technique, above) provide immediate stability and protection for the fascial strip. The following procedure is described as done in dogs weighing more than 20 kg. The next smaller suture sizes can be used in dogs between 15 and 20 kg.

SURGICAL TECHNIQUE ■   A medial arthrotomy following a lateral skin incision is made to allow inspection of the joint, removal of ligament fragments, and meniscectomy (see Fig. 17–21) when needed. A strip of fascia 1.5 to 2 cm wide at the base is isolated from the lateral aspect of the joint and remains attached at the junction of the patellar ligament with the tibial tubercle distally (Fig. 17–16A). The strip is fashioned by cutting its cranial edge from the lateral border of the patellar ligament and is continued proximally a few millimeters lateral to the patella. This incision, which is made with a scalpel, is ended just proximal to the patella, and the caudal edge of the strip is formed by incising 1.5 to 2 cm caudal and parallel to the first incision. Care is taken to avoid incising the underlying synovial membrane. Proximal to the patella, the fascia lata is easily elevated from the quadriceps and dissection is continued with scissors. The caudal cut is continued proximally first and follows the cranial border of the biceps femoris muscle. The cranial border from the proximal patella is cut next, taking care to maintain or slightly increase the strip's width at the proximal end. The length of this strip is equal to 2.5 to 3 times the distance from the tibial tubercle to the midpatella.

A $5/32$- to $3/16$-inch (4- to 4.8-mm) hole is drilled transversely through the tibial tubercle close to the tibial plateau, and the proximal end of the fascial strip is drawn through the hole, thus transferring the strip to the medial side of the tibia (Fig. 17–16B). Size 0 to 1 monofilament suture is attached to the fascia strip to aid in pulling it through the bone. The graft is pulled into the medial arthrotomy through the fat pad into the joint, medial to the patellar ligament (Fig. 17–16C).

On the lateral side of the joint, the lateral edge of the fascia lata incision is dissected and retracted to expose the lateral fabella. The portion of the gastrocnemius muscle originating proximal to the fabella is elevated from the femur and a 7-inch curved Crile or Kelly hemostatic forceps is passed through this opening medial to the fabella with the curve facing cranially, through the caudal joint capsule, and into the intercondylar notch of the femur (Fig. 17–16D). The tips of the forceps are positioned lateral to the caudal cruciate ligament, where one end of the suture attached to the fascial strip is grasped within the jaws of the forceps (Fig. 17–16E). The forceps is pulled proximally, and the suture is used to pull the graft "over-the-top" of the lateral fabella.

The medial arthrotomy is now closed in one layer. The insertion of the caudal belly of the sartorius is partially detached from the tibia and sutured to the patellar ligament along with the joint capsule and medial fascia as far proximally as the patella. From that point proximad, the sartorius is not included in the remainder of the medial closure (Fig. 17–16F).

Two sutures of size 2 to 4 braided polyester or monofilament suture material are placed from the lateral fabella to the distal portion of the patellar ligament and tied tightly to eliminate drawer movement and to act as internal splints (Fig. 17–16G). The femorofabellar ligament is elevated from the supracondylar tuberosity of the femur to allow a groove to be produced in the cortical bone of the tuberosity by rongeur, rasp, or osteotome (Fig. 17–16H). A wire loop can then be used to fish the suture attached to the fascia strip through this opening. The fascial strip is pulled taut and then sutured to the femorofabellar fascia and joint capsule with a "staple" suture (Fig. 17–16I). The lateral fascial incision is closed. Because of the strip of fascia removed, this closure results in tightening of the lateral retinaculum (Fig. 17–16J).

Four separate procedures have served to stabilize the joint: Advancement of the caudal sartorius and biceps muscles creates caudal traction on the tibia; fabellar-patellar ligament sutures prevent drawer motion immediately and serve as an internal splint for the fascial strip; and the fascial strip replaces the cruciate ligament.

Evaluation of Over-the-Top Procedures ■ These techniques generally provide a more anatomically placed pseudoligament than does Paatsama's original method involving the fascia lata.[16] Although in theory Paatsama's technique should result in anatomical placement of the fascial strip, in fact it has proved difficult for most surgeons to accurately drill from the lateral surface of the condyle to the point of the ligament's femoral origin. Additionally, the fascia usually made a sharp bend as it emerged from the bone tunnel and then turned distally, thus subjecting it to shearing forces. Arnoczky and colleagues demonstrated that the fascial strip placed "over-the-top" almost perfectly mimics the normal ligament, remaining taut during the complete range of motion of the stifle.[38] Because the pseudoligament is subjected only to tension and not shearing stress, it is not as apt to break. The fascial strip becomes vascularized, then undergoes fibroplasia and reorganization of collagen to resemble a normal ligament. This process appears to take 5 to 6 months; however, the animal is at risk until the tissue transfer regains strength and is the reason for using the lateral support sutures in the four-in-one procedure. Occasionally, an animal will stretch the "ligament" between 3 and 6 months postoperatively and will redevelop drawer motion. Such cases have undergone reoperation using extra-articular stabilization because the remaining fascia was unfit for use again. Previously these cases were reoperated by replacing the lateral sutures and adding a medial suture, as in the three-in-one technique described above. More recently, reoperation has been done with the fibular transposition method.

PARTIAL RUPTURE OF THE CRANIAL CRUCIATE LIGAMENT

A surprising number of stifle lamenesses are due to partial rupture of the cranial cruciate ligament. The veterinarian has only to explore joints in the face of minimal physical findings to verify this. There is an increasing number of dogs (especially Labrador retrievers and Rottweilers) that sustain partial tears at a young age (6 to 24 months of age). Often, it is bilateral and mimics hip dysplasia clinically, which may also be a concurrent problem. It is our experience that cruciate problems cause more clinical signs than the hip dysplasia and should be attended to first before it is deemed necessary to do anything surgically to the hips. Clinical signs and history mimic those of complete rupture but are not as dramatic, and secondary arthrosis is much slower in developing, probably because the meniscus is not damaged as often as in complete ligament rupture. Degenerative changes can be extensive given enough time.

The cranial cruciate functionally is composed of two parts: the small craniomedial band (CrMB) and the larger caudolateral band (CLB). The CrMB is taut in both flexion and extension, while the CLB is taut only in extension. The ability to diagnose these injuries by examination for drawer motion depends on which part of the ligament is damaged. If the injury is due to hyperextension, it is most likely to damage the CLB, and no drawer motion will be present, since the CrMB is intact. An injury caused by rotation or twisting with flexion is more likely to injure the CrMB. Under these circumstances there is a small amount of drawer motion in flexion (the CLB is relaxed) but no motion in extension (the CLB is taut). Partial rupture of the CrMB in a single case was first reported by Tarvin and Arnoczky,[41] and more recently a series of cases has been described by Scavelli and associates.[42] In this series partial ruptures accounted for 8 percent of 320 cases of isolated cranial cruciate rupture. Drawer motion was detected in 52 percent of the cases and, when present, was found in flexion only 69 percent of the time. At surgery 80 percent of the injuries were to the CrMB, 4 percent were CLB, and 16 percent were interstitial tears (grade 2 sprain), where the ligament was grossly intact but had suffered damage sufficient to render it functionally incompetent. Medial meniscus damage requiring surgical treatment was present in only 20 percent of these cases.

As can be seen from these figures, the incidence of partial tears of the cranial cruciate ligament is not insignificant and should be carefully considered as a cause of lameness in midsize to large breeds with pain in the stifle region and minimal or no drawer motion. Radiographs demonstrating the "fat pad sign" (Fig. 17–10) or osteophytes are truly significant. When operating these injuries they should be handled as if they were complete ruptures, since the ligament is no longer functional.[24]

AVULSION OF THE CRANIAL CRUCIATE LIGAMENT

As with most avulsions, this is a condition of skeletally immature dogs. Ligamentous attachments to bone by means of Sharpey's fibers are in some cases stronger than the bone; hence, an avulsion rather than a tear of the ligament results (Fig. 17–17). Usually seen as an avulsion of the insertion, this lesion is very rare in the dog.

Physical examination findings are similar to those described for rupture of the ligament, except that drawer motion is very obvious and joint effusion is marked. Radiographs demonstrate the avulsed bone fragment in the intercondylar space.

Surgical Technique

The joint is exposed by a medial approach.[8] Hematoma and granulation tissue are removed from the bone fragment so that it can be identified (Fig. 17–17A). Two small holes are drilled from the medial and lateral sides of the tibial defect toward the medial tibial cortex (Fig. 17–17B). Stainless steel wire (size 20 to 22 gauge; 0.8 to 0.6 mm) is placed through the ligament close to the bone. Each end is then passed through the bone tunnels and twisted tightly on the medial tibial cortex. Alternatively, three diverging Kirschner wires can be used (Fig. 17–17C). In rare instances, the bone fragment is large enough to

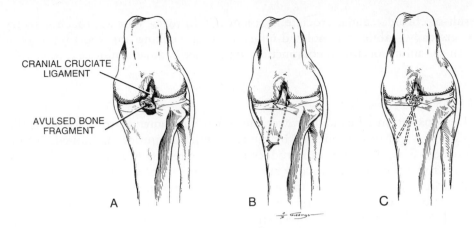

CRANIAL CRUCIATE
LIGAMENT

AVULSED BONE
FRAGMENT

A   B   C

FIGURE 17–17. Avulsion of the tibial insertion of the cranial cruciate ligament. (*A*) A bone fragment with the cranial cruciate attached has been elevated from the tibial plateau of the left tibia. A medial approach to the stifle is used for exposure.[8] Lag screw fixation is ideal if the bone fragment is large enough (see Fig. 17–19 *B*). For smaller fragments: (*B*) stainless steel wire, 20 to 22 gauge, is placed through the ligament insertion and through two drill holes that exit through the medial tibial cortex where the wire is twisted. (*C*) Three Kirschner wires, inserted at diverging angles, provide good fixation.

allow lag screw fixation (see Fig. 17–19*B*). If the fragment is comminuted, or if stretching of the ligament has also occurred, it may be well to pursue standard stabilization techniques, especially after 5 to 6 months of age.

AFTERCARE ■ The limb must be immobilized for 4 weeks to allow healing of the fracture. A Thomas splint (see Fig. 2–25) or a long lateral splint is suitable (see Fig. 2–24). The stifle must be fixed at the standing angle to minimize complications of immobilization such as periarticular fibrosis and quadriceps contracture. Full exercise should not be allowed until 4 weeks after splint removal.

RUPTURE OF THE CAUDAL CRUCIATE LIGAMENT

The caudal cruciate ligament is slightly larger than the cranial ligament and is an important stabilizer of the joint. It is the primary stabilizer against tibial caudal subluxation (drawer movement) and combines with the cranial ligament to limit internal tibial rotation and hyperextension.[23]

Little is known about the handling of ruptures of this ligament because it is a relatively uncommon injury. Most cases are due to severe trauma and are accompanied by rupture of the medial collateral and cranial cruciate ligaments. Medial meniscal injury is also common in this situation. Isolated caudal cruciate ruptures do occur, however. It has been suggested that the caudal cruciate is not functionally significant because the normal standing angle of the dog's stifle tends to work against caudal drawer motion,[43] and experimental severing of the ligament by Harari and co-workers did not create any functional or pathological changes in seven dogs observed postoperatively for 6 months.[44] In the absence of any clinical series reports it is difficult for the clinician to decide on the best method of handling a case. We have seen chronic lameness cases as a result of chronic caudal cruciate ligament (CCL) tears. Our approach is to try to surgically stabilize an isolated injury only in working and sporting dogs or when the injury occurs in conjunction with other ligament injuries of the stifle.

Clinical Signs

Demonstration of caudal drawer motion is fundamental to diagnosing this injury. This can be complicated by the concomitant injuries mentioned. Testing for caudal drawer motion can produce confusing results because the tibia seems always to be subluxated caudally at rest from the pull of the hamstring muscles. Therefore, what may appear to be cranial drawer motion is actually the reduction of tibial subluxation. From this reduced position, we can then demonstrate caudal motion. Therefore, unlike testing for cranial motion, it is more important to note the relative position of the thumbs as they grasp the femur and tibia *before* motion is applied to the tibia (see Chapter 1). With isolated CCL tears, drawer movement is less than that with full cranial cruciate rupture. Often a definitive end point ("thud") may be detected upon drawering cranially, as the cranial cruciate tightens, especially with the leg in flexion. Drawer may disappear when the leg is tested in a neutral position. With both cranial cruciate and CCL rupture, there is a severe amount of instability, unless the menisci are torn so badly that they impede adequate palpation.

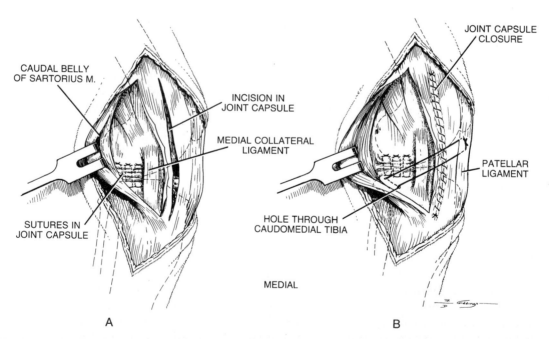

FIGURE 17–18. Rupture of the caudal cruciate ligament. (A) The left stifle has been exposed by a medial approach to the stifle joint combined with an approach to the medial collateral ligament and caudomedial compartment of the joint.[8] The caudomedial joint capsule has been imbricated with mattress sutures of nonabsorbable material (size 3/0–0) placed vertically to the joint caudal to the medial collateral ligament. (B) Following closure of the joint capsule, a heavy-gauge (size 0–4) braided polyester suture is placed between the proximal patellar ligament and a drill hole in the caudomedial corner of the proximal tibia. This suture is tightened with the stifle at a normal standing angle and with drawer motion reduced. *Figure continued on opposite page*

Diagnosis

Radiographs are important in caudal cruciate injuries because of these injuries' frequent association with other traumatic injuries and because of a higher percentage of avulsion injuries than with the cranial cruciate. This is probably due to the fact that the caudal ligament is larger and stronger than the cranial and therefore resists rupture but predisposes to avulsion. The definitive diagnosis is made upon arthrotomy. The CCL stump is evident in the intercondylar notch of the femur. Often it is covered by a proliferative mass that has to be debrided before the rest of the joint can be inspected.

Surgical Treatment

Little has been documented concerning clinical management of caudal cruciate injuries. No really satisfactory technique exists for large, active dogs. The technique shown here (Fig. 17–18) is satisfactory for small breeds and cats but is not always as useful in large breeds. Avulsion injuries are well stabilized by wire or screw fixation (Fig. 17–19). Repair of collateral meniscal injuries is described next.

Technique for a Ruptured Ligament

A medial or lateral arthrotomy is combined with approaches to the medial and lateral caudal compartments of the stifle joint.[8] Fragments of ligament are

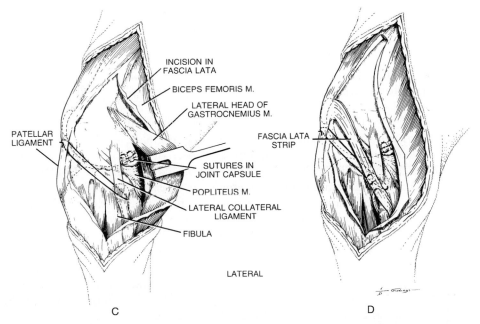

FIGURE 17–18. *Continued* (C) The skin is retracted laterally to allow incision of the fascia lata and retraction of the biceps femoris. This reveals the lateral collateral ligament and caudolateral joint capsule.[8] The joint capsule is imbricated caudal to the lateral collateral ligament and a heavy-gauge braided polyester suture is placed around the head of the fibula to the proximal patellar ligament. This suture is tied tightly with the stifle in a normal standing angle. (D) For further augmentation, a strip of fascia lata may be dissected free proximally and left attached to the lateral border of the patella distally. This strip is passed around the fibular head, pulled taut, and then sutured to itself and to the surrounding fascia.

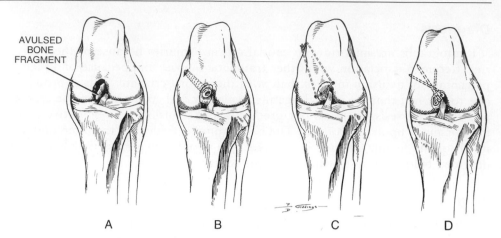

FIGURE 17–19. Avulsion of the femoral origin of the caudal cruciate ligament. (*A*) A fragment of bone with the attached ligament has been avulsed from the medial femoral condyle. (*B*) A lag screw has been used to fix the fragment. A lateral approach to the stifle gives best exposure.[8] (*C*) Stainless steel wire (20 to 22 gauge) is threaded through the ligament close to the bone fragment. Two parallel holes are drilled at opposite points on the edge of the femoral defect; the wire is passed through these holes, then twisted on the medial surface of the condyle. (*D*) Three Kirschner wires can be inserted at diverging angles to stabilize the fragment.

excised and meniscectomy is performed when indicated. The joint capsule is then sutured and collateral ligament repairs are made if needed. Stabilization is commenced on the medial side with placement of mattress sutures (size 2–0 to 0 nonabsorbable material), to imbricate the caudomedial joint capsule (Fig. 17–18*A*). A large imbricating suture of size 0 to 3 braided polyester material or heavy monofilament nylon (see MRIT, above) is then placed from the medial half of the proximal patellar ligament to a hole drilled through the caudomedial corner of the tibia (Fig. 17–18*B*). This suture is tied tightly, with drawer motion reduced and the stifle positioned at the standing angle.

Similar sutures are placed on the lateral aspect of the joint (Fig. 17–18*C*), but the large suture is anchored around the fibular head. The fibular nerve should be protected during suture placement. A fascia lata transfer is also used on the lateral side. The strip is based on the lateral side of the patella and is long enough to be pulled around the head of the fibula and sutured to itself (Fig. 17–18*D*).

The fascia strip and large imbricating sutures are similar to those used in the technique of DeAngelis and Betts.[45] However, they are positioned more distally at the patellar end to more closely approximate the angle of caudal ligament. Imbrication of the caudomedial and lateral joint capsule is based on the technique of Hohn and Newton for cranial cruciate rupture.[43]

AFTERCARE ■   No splint is used unless the medial collateral ligament was repaired. Exercise is severely restricted for 4 weeks, then gradually increased through the eighth week.

Technique for Avulsion

Most avulsions occur at the *femoral origin* of the ligament and are easily accessible for lag screw or wire fixation (Fig. 17–19*A*). If the fragment is large enough, fixation with a lag screw is preferred (Fig. 17–19*B*). Wire fixation can also be used if the bone fragment is small. The wire should pass through the ligament close to the fragment and then pass through bone tunnels to the medial condylar cortex, where it is twisted tightly (Fig. 17–19C). Another fixation method involves placing two or three Kirschner wires through the fragment at diverging angles. These pins should penetrate the opposite condylar cortex.

Avulsion of the *tibial insertion* is treated similarly, although the fragment is much more difficult to expose. Best exposure is probably afforded by the approach to the caudomedial compartment of the joint.[8] The medial head of the gastrocnemius muscle and popliteal vessels must be strongly retracted.

AFTERCARE ■ A Thomas splint (see Fig. 2–25) or long lateral splint (see Fig. 2–24) is maintained for 4 weeks, and exercise is severely restricted. After splint removal, activity is slowly increased through the eighth week.

MENISCAL INJURIES

In mammalian stifle joints there are two menisci, which are fibrocartilaginous structures interposed between the femur and tibia. The inner two thirds of the meniscus is avascular, and healing, when injured, is poor.

Unlike the situation in humans, damage to the meniscal cartilages of the dog and cat rarely occurs as a primary injury; in almost all cases, one or more stifle ligaments are torn or stretched. Most commonly, the caudal horn of the medial meniscus is damaged as a result of the cranial tibial drawer motion that results from rupture of the cranial cruciate ligaments. Because the medial meniscus is firmly attached to the tibia by the caudal tibial ligament and to the medial collateral ligament, it moves with the tibia. Cranial drawer motion displaces the caudal horn cranial to the femoral condyle and subjects the caudal horn to injury as a result of crushing and shear forces. Cranial drawer motion in extension is much more injurious to the meniscus and joint capsule than is drawer motion in flexion.[46] Isolated tears of the lateral meniscus have been seen by us, but rarely.

The two most common injuries to the canine and feline meniscus include the caudal longitudinal tear (so-called bucket-handle tear in man) (Fig. 17–20A, E) which separates the circumferential fibers completely from the tibial to the femoral surfaces and the "crush" of the caudal horn or limb of the meniscus, which is just an incomplete longitudinal tear (Fig. 17–20C, D). Other abnormalities include the double "bucket handle" tear (Fig. 17–20F), degenerative "fringe" tears (Fig. 17–20G) seen in the degenerate knee below an old femoral osteochondritic lesion, a rare transverse tear and congenital lateral discoid menisci (Fig. 17–20I). Occasionally, we as well as others have seen calcified menisci. Peripheral detachments (Fig. 17–20H) or avulsions are usually seen in the significantly traumatized (i.e., automobile) knee with multiple ligament derangement.[47,48] The incidence of meniscal injuries following rupture of the cranial cruciate ligament can run as high as 53 percent.[48,49] This incidence reflects a predominance of chronic cases as seen in a referral practice. Early surgical repair of the cruciate injury results in a much lower incidence of meniscal injury.

Clinical Signs and Diagnosis

Usually dogs and cats with meniscal injury along with cruciate tears have more pain and lameness in the subacute or chronic stages than just with cruciate

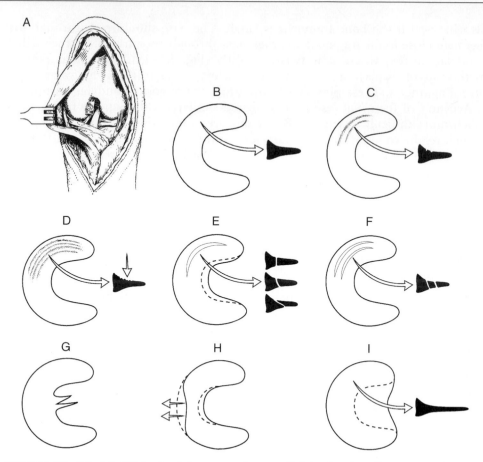

FIGURE 17–20. (*A*) With the joint opened, a medial bucket handle tear can be seen between the cranial horn of the meniscus and the femoral condyle. Vision and displacement of the torn part are assisted by levering a protected hemostat between the intermeniscal ligaments and femoral condyle (see Fig. 17—21*B*). (*B*) A dorsal and cross-sectional view of a normal meniscus. (*C*) Early fraying of the superficial layers of the meniscus. (*D*) A crushed caudal horn. (*E*) A longitudinal tear or so-called bucket handle tear. (*F*) A double "bucket handle" tear. (*G*) A degenerate fringe tear. (*H*) A peripherally detached meniscus seen with traumatic stifles. (*I*) A congenital lateral discoid meniscus. Dotted lines represent normal boundaries of the meniscus.

rupture alone. Often there is a history of improving lameness after the cruciate rupture followed by worsening as the meniscus subsequently is injured by the instability. An owner or observer may hear a "click" in 10 to 15 percent of dogs with meniscal injury. This click or grating sensation is often "felt" (and sometimes heard) when flexing, extending, performing the drawer test, or performing the cranial tibial thrust. Often there is a firm swelling at the medial joint line.

The definitive diagnosis is made upon observing the abnormally displaced meniscus or portion of it. If, upon arthrotomy, the caudal horn is reduced and injury unobservable, the tibia is levered forward by placing a curved mosquito hemostat forceps, guarded with a 1-inch piece of discarded sterilized suction tubing, under the cranial intermeniscal ligament. As the knee is brought into more extension (45 degrees of flexion), the curved hemostat is levered against the femoral condyle. If the caudal horn becomes visible and/or luxates forward of the femoral condyle (normally the caudal horn is not visible when drawer motion is produced this way), it is deemed abnormal and removed. Excessive force should not be used, as it will cause a normal meniscus to be displaced forward. Other surgeons use a Hohmann retractor placed through the interior of the joint to the back of the tibia and similarly levers the tibia forward. Often with this maneuver, a normal meniscus will be pushed forward towards the front of the femoral condyle. Only if the meniscus (or parts of it) luxates totally in front of the condyle should it be considered abnormal when using this technique.

If drawer motion is slight due to chronicity or partial tears, observation of the caudal horn may be difficult.

Radiography has not been a reliable diagnostic method for this condition. Arthroscopy may become important at some point, but at present, it is not useful for routine examination of the canine stifle joint. Surgical exploration remains the most common and useful method of definitive diagnosis.

Treatment

Meniscectomy

Indications

The outer 25 to 30 percent of the meniscus is avascular, and tears do not heal for all practical purposes.

Removal of a normal medial meniscus in otherwise intact stifles results in regenerative material but does create some degenerative joint disease.[50-52] Therefore, meniscectomy should not be performed unless pathological changes are seen. However, leaving a pathological meniscus in place often results in persistent lameness.

In man, total or partial meniscectomy was performed depending on surgeon preference. As long-term clinical follow-ups became available, it was apparent that some patients developed severe degenerative joint disease on the side of the joint where the meniscus was removed. With the development of arthroscopic surgery, the meniscal damage can be totally assessed. The top and bottom surfaces may be visualized and the meniscus probed for stability. Only the abnormal tissue can selectively be removed. In the last decade, with further refinement of arthroscopic techniques, tears in the outer vascular areas may be healed if sutured. This is usually only considered in the young (<40 years of age), athletic patient. It is a much more involved surgical procedure, and has a more extensive rehabilitation program than just plain meniscectomy.

In dogs and cats arthroscopy is not a readily available technique and thorough evaluation of the entire meniscus is impossible.

A partial meniscectomy means removing that strip of pathological meniscus that has flipped forward of the femoral condyle. A total or subtotal meniscectomy means removing the meniscus at its perimeter, more peripheral than the actual tear in the parenchyma.

Reasons some surgeons prefer total to partial meniscectomy include:

1. It is easier to perform without iatrogenic articular cartilage damage during the surgical procedure.
2. It does not leave an unseen double or multiple bucket-handle tear (seen in about 10 percent of meniscal tears).
3. More precise removal of the "crushed" meniscus.

4. Possibly better regeneration (debatable since the vascular portion is violated).

5. There doesn't seem to be a clinical problem in our hands with dogs returning years later with debilitating degenerative joint disease. The life span between dogs and humans may be the reason.

Technique

A medial arthrotomy[8] is preferred for medial meniscectomy because it provides better exposure and allows a transverse joint incision if exposure from the medial parapatellar incision proves inadequate. Visualization of the caudal meniscal horns is aided by joint instability.

Total medial meniscectomy begins by cutting of the intermeniscal and cranial tibial ligaments (Fig. 17–21, B).[49] All cutting is done with great care to avoid injury to articular cartilage of the tibia and femur. Number 11 and 15 blades or No. 64 Beaver miniblades (R. Beaver, Inc., Belmont, MA) are the most useful sizes for the procedure. A Kocher forceps or meniscus clamp (Ascott Enterprises, Missassauga, Ontario) is attached to the freed cranial horn. It is pulled laterally (axially) while the medial joint capsule is retracted medially (abaxially). The meniscus is dissected away from the joint capsule with the blade in a vertical position to avoid cutting the medial collateral ligament (Fig. 17–21C). When beginning the dissection, it is well to keep in mind the abaxial edge of the medial femoral condyle. Incising more medial (abaxial) may lacerate the medial collateral ligament and fibrous joint capsule. Dissection continues caudal to the medial collateral as strong traction is applied to the clamped meniscus in a craniolateral direction. Cutting the caudal synovial attachment is the most difficult part of the procedure and may require additional exposure, as discussed below. Fortunately, with traction most pathological menisci will tear in the right area at the caudal peripheral attachments. If the meniscus is "normal," it will not do this. A small curved meniscus knife (Veterinary Instrumentation, Sheffield, England; Jorgensen Laboratories Inc., Loveland, CO) greatly simplifies this part of the surgery. The knife is worked around the periphery of the meniscus, freeing it from the synovial membrane and collateral ligament. If these attachments can be freed at this point (Fig. 17–21D), the entire meniscus can be pulled cranially and the caudal tibial ligament can be cut (Fig. 17–21F) to free the meniscus.

If additional exposure is required, a medial transverse joint incision is made from the medial collateral ligament cranially to join the parapatellar incision (Fig. 17–21G). The medial collateral ligament is elevated to allow the incision to be extended caudally deep to it. The meniscus is dissected away from the caudal joint capsule and medial collateral ligament. Care is taken to avoid the popliteal vessels immediately caudal to the capsule. After the caudal capsular attachments are freed, the caudal tibial ligament is cut as described above to free the meniscus.

If by mistake, a cranial hemimeniscectomy has been created by inadvertently cutting too axially into the bucket handle, the abnormal caudal horn should be removed. Often this "lost" portion may be retrieved by levering the tibia forward and then sweeping a curved mosquito forceps caudally and along the inside of the medial collateral ligament. Another technique is to sweep the forceps from the caudal tibial attachment area outward towards the abaxial side or medial joint capsule. Once the horn is displaced forward the material is grasped and carefully incised.

AFTERCARE ■ No specific aftercare is required for meniscectomy. The care is usually dictated by repair of associated ligament damage. Heavy exercise should be withheld for 6 months, if possible, to allow for regeneration of the meniscus[48,52] before extreme stress is placed on the joint. Hannan and associates[52] have demonstrated a chondroprotective effect by polysulfated glycosaminoglycan (Arteparon, Luitpold Werk, Munich, FRG; Adequan, Luitpold Pharmaceutical Inc., Shirley, NY) following experimental meniscectomy. Dosage of 2 mg/kg body weight subcutaneously three times per week for 3 weeks, then twice weekly until the dogs were killed at 23 weeks, significantly improved the biochemical and morphological parameters studied in articular cartilage.

COLLATERAL LIGAMENT INJURIES

Ligament injuries that overstress the structure and damage ligament fibers are known as sprains (see Chapter 7). Such injuries may be minor (first degree) or more severe, with stretching and rupture of ligament fibers (second degree); or they may result in tearing or avulsion of the ligament (third degree).[54] Only third-degree and some second-degree injuries require surgical therapy.

Damage to collateral ligaments of the canine stifle occurs relatively infrequently. Severe injury is usually associated with traumatic incidents, such as being hit by an automobile or direct blows. Meniscal and cruciate damage should always be suspected with any collateral ligament injury severe enough to produce instability of the joint.

An understanding of the functional anatomy of these ligaments is necessary to diagnose the resulting instability.[55] Both ligaments are taut in extension and function with the cruciate ligaments to prevent internal tibial rotation. In extension, the collateral ligaments are the primary stabilizers of lateral (valgus) and medial (varus) angulation of the tibia. In flexion, the lateral ligament relaxes and allows internal tibial rotation to be limited only by the cruciates while the medial ligament remains taut and limits external tibial rotation. Since the cruciates do not limit external tibial rotation, the medial collateral is the primary stabilizer of this motion.

Clinical Signs

Injury to the medial ligament is more common than injury to the lateral side. Tearing of the cranial cruciate and medial meniscus commonly accompanies the collateral damage. Joint effusion and tenderness with no weight bearing are the obvious signs. Tibial angulation is checked with the joint in extension, and any drawer motion is reduced. Varus instability is present with lateral laxity, and valgus instability is present with medial laxity. When the medial collateral is completely torn, marked external tibial rotation is possible with the stifle flexed.

Physical examination will usually provide the diagnosis, but radiographs with the joint stressed to accentuate the instability are often useful.

Surgical Treatment

Injuries that produce observable instability in large, active dogs should be surgically repaired as early as possible. Even if the ligament is grossly intact and even if it heals by fibroplasia, it will always remain loose and will allow joint laxity.

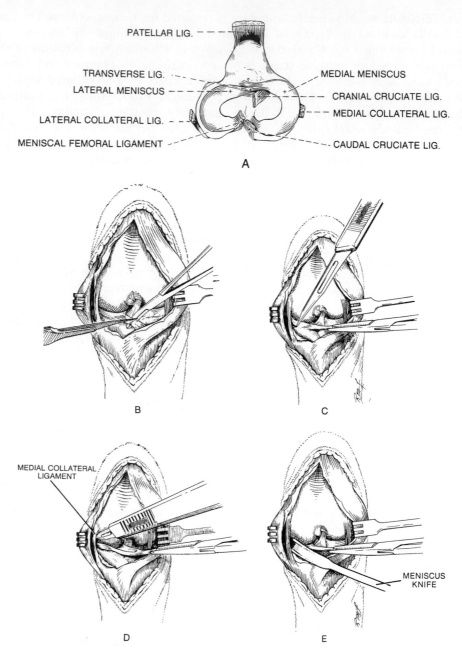

FIGURE 17–21. Medial meniscectomy.[49] (*A*) Menisci and meniscal ligaments of the left stifle joint, dorsal aspect. (*B*) The left stifle has been exposed by a medial parapatellar approach.[8] The cranial tibial and intermeniscal ligaments are severed with a hemostat inserted to protect the underlying cartilage. (*C*) Strong craniolateral traction is applied to the meniscus, and the medial joint capsule is retracted to allow dissection of the cranial horn free from the joint capsule. The scalpel blade is oriented vertically and aimed at the abaxial edge of the femoral condyle to avoid cutting the medial collateral ligament. The medial collateral ligament is normally not visualized but is inserted here for orientation. (*D*) Continued traction allows the caudal joint capsule attachments to be cut. (*E*) A small curved meniscus knife (Veterinary Instrumentation, Sheffield, England; Jorgensen Laboratories Inc., Loveland, CO) simplifies freeing the meniscus caudal to the collateral ligament. *Figure continued on opposite page*

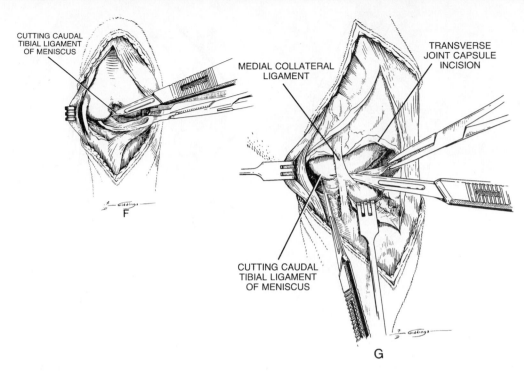

FIGURE 17–21. *Continued* (F) The caudal tibial ligament of the meniscus is cut with the blade held parallel to the tibial surface. (G) For additional exposure of the caudal peripheral attachments, a medial transverse joint incision is made from the parapatellar incision, extending caudally deep to the medial collateral ligament. Caudal capsular attachments can be easily cut, but care must be taken to avoid the popliteal vessels. The meniscus is dissected free of the deep portion of the medial collateral ligament. The caudal tibial meniscal ligament is cut, as in *F*. The transverse incision is closed with mattress sutures, followed by interrupted sutures in the parapatellar arthrotomy.

Stretched ligaments (second-degree injury) are tightened by suture imbrication, torn ligaments are sutured, and avulsed ligaments are reattached or synthetically replaced (Fig. 17–22; see also Figs. 7–6 and 7–7). Exposure of either ligament is readily done, either primarily or during an approach to the stifle joint.[8] Collateral ligaments of the stifle, especially the lateral ligament, must always be sutured or reattached with the stifle in extension to prevent shortening of the ligament, which either limits extension or overstresses the repair when the animal extends the joint.

AFTERCARE ■ All injuries are immobilized in a Thomas splint (see Fig. 2–25) or long lateral splint (see Fig. 2–24) for 4 weeks, followed by 2 more weeks of leash-only exercise. Activity can be slowly increased after 7 or 8 weeks.

LUXATION OF THE STIFLE JOINT

Total derangement of the knee, with rupture of all four major ligaments, is a disastrous injury seen on occasion. Cats appear to suffer a higher incidence than do dogs. Vascular integrity of the limb distal to the stifle must be carefully evaluated as the popliteal vessels may become entrapped by the tibial luxation.

More commonly seen is injury of the cranial and caudal cruciate and medial collateral ligaments. Also damaged to varying degrees are the secondary re-

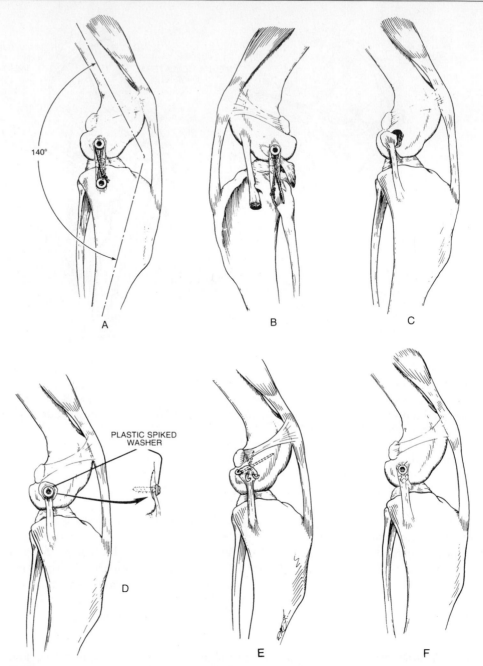

FIGURE 17–22. Surgical repair of collateral ligament injuries. (*A*) A midportion medial collateral tear has been sutured, using a locking loop pattern (see Fig. 7–6). The ligament repair is protected by heavy-gauge (0–3) braided polyester suture placed between two bone screws placed in the origin and insertion areas. This suture is tied with the joint extended or at a standing angle. (*B*) A midportion lateral collateral tear has been sutured as in *A*. Only one bone screw is needed, since a bone tunnel drilled in the fibula functions well for the distal insertion of the protective suture. (*C*) Avulsion of the origin of the medial collateral ligament. (*D*) The avulsion has been secured using a plastic spiked washer on a 3.5-mm screw. (*E*) Reattachment is also possible with three diverging Kirschner wires placed through the fragment. (*F*) This tear close to the origin of the medial collateral ligament was sutured with a locking loop pattern, and the suture was then secured around a bone screw. When possible, a bone tunnel can be used rather than a screw, as in *B*. *Figure continued on opposite page*

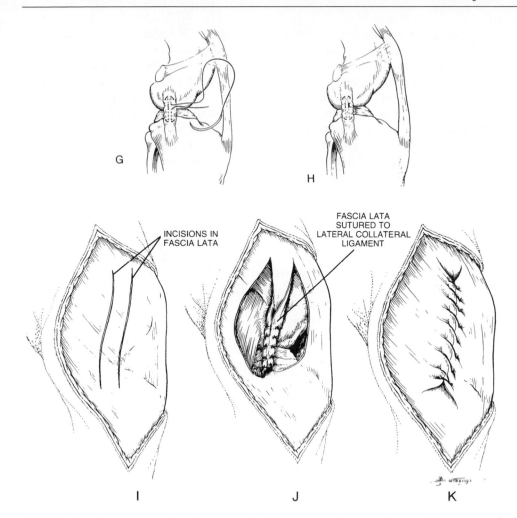

INCISIONS IN
FASCIA LATA

FASCIA LATA
SUTURED TO
LATERAL COLLATERAL
LIGAMENT

G

H

I

J

K

FIGURE 17–22. *Continued*   (*G*) A stretched ligament is being imbricated by means of a modified locking loop suture pattern. (*H*) Tying the suture results in shortening of the ligament between the suture loops. (*I*) Fascial lata reinforcement of a lateral collateral ligament injury[6] commences by elevating a strip of fascia that is left attached at each end. (*J*) The fascia is sutured to the repaired ligament. (*K*) The fascial defect is sutured.

straints of the joint such as joint capsule, menisci, and patellar ligament. Additionally, most have a variety of other traumatic injuries such as fractures or ruptured viscera. Despite the magnitude of this injury, good function can be obtained if a meticulous repair is made of each injury.[56] Paramount to attempting such repairs is a thorough preoperative assessment of the stifle joint. Such an examination can be done adequately and humanely only under general anesthesia in this circumstance. Owing to the multiple derangements of the joint, palpation can be confusing, and the diagnoses reached must always be regarded as presumptive.

Surgery should start with a thorough exploration of the joint, and this requires adequate surgical exposure. Meniscal injuries in this instance do not often require meniscectomy; most damage is usually done to meniscofemoral or meniscotibial ligaments or the joint capsule attachments. These can usually be sutured and should be done first, while the exposure is greatest. The collateral ligament injury should be stabilized next, as this will restore basic alignment to the joint and simplify the remaining surgery. Stabilization of the cruciate instability follows. The authors have usually used extracapsular methods. It is most helpful to temporarily place a small K-wire (0.062-inch) across the joint with the joint held in a neutral, reduced position prior to tightening the sutures or tissues so that the tibia is not stabilized in a deviated position. Hulse and Shires attribute much of their success in these problems to intra-articular stabilization.[56] Extra-articular repair of the cruciate ligament injuries and postoperative support with transarticular external skeletal fixators was successful in 13 cases reported by Aron.[58] The final step is careful imbrication of all available joint capsule and periarticular tissue to further stabilize the joint.

A newer stabilization procedure[57] for luxated stifles in cats and small dogs (after joint exploration) is to temporarily cross the femoral-tibial joint with a $\frac{1}{8}$- to $\frac{3}{16}$-inch pin with the leg held at a functional angle of 30 to 40 degrees of flexion. A reinforced bandage or cast is recommended until pin removal in 5 to 7 weeks. We have used this method successfully in selected small animals where cost constraints or open wounds were of concern.

Aftercare consists of exercise limitation as described above for each of the individual procedures. Surprisingly good function has been seen in these patients, both by us and others.[56,58] A consistent finding is reduction of 30 to 40 degrees in range of motion in the stifle joint. Arthrodesis is a possible option for a chronically unstable and painful joint (see Fig. 17–29A, B), but amputation results in better overall function of the animal.

OSTEOCHONDRITIS DISSECANS OF THE FEMORAL CONDYLE

The pathophysiology of osteochondrosis and osteochondritis dissecans (OCD) is discussed in Chapter 6.

The shoulder joint is most commonly involved, but the stifle is occasionally involved and is often overlooked. OCD is seen in all large breeds of dogs, especially the retrievers. Signs are usually first noted at 5 to 7 months of age. Early surgical treatment is indicated to remove loose cartilage and minimize osteoarthrosis. The prognosis is more guarded than for lesions of the shoulder, but about 75 percent will be normally functional if surgical treatment is done at an early age. Some degree of osteoarthrosis is to be expected.

Clinical Signs

Lameness varies from minimal to severe. Measurement of the diameter of the thigh muscles may demonstrate evidence of mild disuse atrophy. Palpation of the joint is not often rewarding, although very slight drawer motion movement may be noted if muscle atrophy is present. Joint effusion can often be noted. If a joint mouse has formed from detachment of the cartilage flap, popping or crepitus can be present.

Radiographic Findings

Radiographs are necessary for diagnosis, and technically high-quality films are necessary to detect a small lesion. Mediolateral and caudocranial views are needed, the latter in two different degrees of flexion-extension. Lesions are most commonly found on the medial aspect of the lateral femoral condyle (Fig. 17–23A, B), although the medial condyle can be affected. Slight flattening of the articular surface and subchondral sclerosis are the most common findings. Care must be taken not to mistake the radiolucent area of the extensor fossa (where the long digital extensor tendon inserts craniolateral on the distal end of the femur) for an OCD lesion (Fig. 17–23C). On the lateral radiograph, there may be a saucer-shaped lucency seen at the joint line (Fig. 17–23A).

Diagnosis

The diagnosis may be made based on the findings of lameness, stifle swelling, and the typical radiographic lesions in dogs over 4½ months of age. At an earlier age, the osteochondrotic lesion may not become a flap and could spontaneously heal. However, joint effusion and large radiographic OCD lesions merit a joint exploration.

Surgical Treatment

Either a lateral or medial parapatellar approach provides adequate exposure (Fig. 17–24A). The cartilage flap is excised, and the edges of the defect are trimmed to make a clean vertical border (Fig. 17–24B) and to make certain that the cartilage left is firmly adhered to the subchondral bone. Multiple drilling of the defect with a Kirschner wire may aid in early revascularization of a sclerotic lesion. If lesions are very deep, curettage with or without cancellous bone grafting may be indicated.

If a flap is not seen in surgery, it may mean that osteochondrosis, not osteochondritis dissecans, is present. Multiple drill holes (0.045-inch Kirschner wire) have been successful in "tacking" down the cartilage and preventing the flap from forming.

We have seen several cases of degenerate lateral meniscal lesions under presumed old OCD lesions in the lateral condyles of 4- to 6-year-old dogs. Meniscectomy in such cases has helped the lameness.

Aftercare/Prognosis

A light bandage is applied for 2 weeks to protect the arthrotomy followed by 2 more weeks of restricted activity. The prognosis for large weight-bearing lesions is guarded to fair, depending on size and lesion location.

RUPTURE OF THE PATELLAR LIGAMENT

Rupture of the patellar ligament is a rare injury. If both the ligament and the joint capsule are torn, the patella rides at the top of the trochlea or proximal to it ("patella alta"). Repair of the ligament utilizing 0–2 nonabsorbable suture material is accomplished with a tendon suture pattern (see Figs. 7–6 and 7–7) as well as simple interrupted sutures in the joint capsule. A supporting figure-of-8 wire is also inserted (Fig. 17–25) from the proximal quadriceps tendon region to the tibial tubercle.

Additional auxiliary fixation such as a modified Thomas splint for 1 to 2 weeks relieves tension at the anastomosis site. Wire removal should be contemplated after 5 to 7 weeks if seroma or lameness is present.

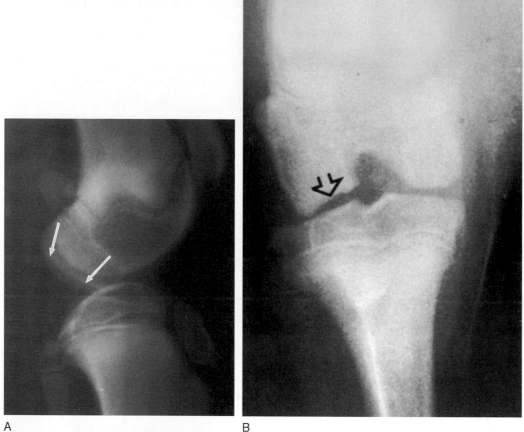

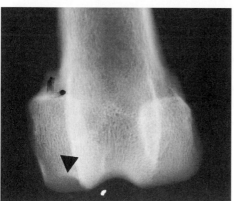

FIGURE 17–23. (*A*) Lateral radiograph of the distal femur. Note the saucer-shaped radiolucency (*white arrows*) indicative of osteochondrosis in this 4-month-old dog. This large radiographic lesion was explored and found to be mostly intact in spite of joint effusion. The cartilage and bone were drilled with several pin holes and the cartilage never became a flap. (*B*) Craniocaudal view of an osteochondritis dissecans (OCD) lesion of the lateral femoral condyle. (*C*) Craniocaudal view of a normal distal femur demonstrating the radiolucent area on the lateral femoral condyle (*black arrowhead*) that is at times mistaken for an osteochondritis dissecans lesion.

AVULSION OF THE PROXIMAL TENDON OF THE LONG DIGITAL EXTENSOR MUSCLE

Although it occurs infrequently, avulsion of the origin of the long digital extensor (LDE) muscle is a disabling injury resulting in degenerative joint disease.[59] Avulsion is a disease of skeletally immature, long-legged breeds such as sighthounds and Great Danes in the age range of 5 to 8 months, but rupture of the tendon can occur in mature animals, especially those with lateral patellar luxation.

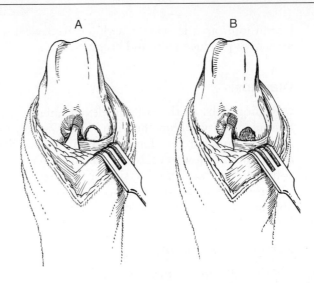

FIGURE 17–24. Osteochondritis dissecans of the femoral condyles. (*A*) A lesion of the lateral femoral condyle has been exposed by a medial parapatellar approach.[8] (*B*) The cartilage flap has been excised, and the edges of the lesion are debrided by curettage.

The LDE muscle originates in the extensor fossa of the lateral femoral condyle. The tendon crosses the joint and passes deep to the cranial tibial muscle through a sulcus in the proximolateral tibia. It is apparently not important to stability of the stifle joint. The detached bony fragment rapidly hypertrophies to several times its original size. The injury rarely is associated with known significant trauma. Surgical treatment produces gratifying results if performed before degenerative joint disease becomes evident.

Clinical Signs

Pain and joint effusion are seen immediately after the injury. Pain is the most pronounced in the craniolateral aspect of the joint. Lameness is variable and subsides quickly. If not operated, a chronic low-grade lameness may result. Loss of toe function does not seem to be a common problem. Firm thickening of the

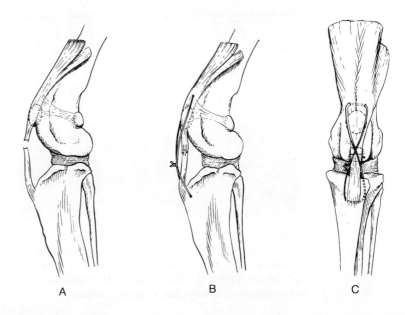

FIGURE 17–25. Rupture of the patellar ligament. (*A*) Lateral view of rupture. (*B*) Lateral view of ligament sutured, with a supporting figure-of-8 wire in place. (*C*) Cranial view with sutures in place.

lateral joint area is evident within 2 to 3 weeks, and pressure applied over this area may produce pain and crepitus.

Diagnosis

Radiographs of the stifle in flexed lateral and caudocranial views reveal an opaque density within the joint (Fig. 17–26). On the lateral view, the opacity is seen cranial to the femoral condyle and distal to the extensor fossa. The caudocranial view reveals the calcified mass to be just lateral to the femoral condyle. The radiographic size of the mass is much less than actual size, since a portion of it is cartilaginous and secondarily fibrotic. An early lesion may appear only as a sliver on bone owing to this cartilaginous nature.

Surgical Treatment

Reattachment of the avulsed fragment is the treatment of choice in recent injuries. If the fragment is so hypertrophic that the outline of the original fragment is no longer discernible, it is better to detach the bone fragment and reattach the tendon to adjacent soft tissue.

Exposure of the lesion is by way of a lateral approach to the stifle joint.[8] The avulsion is immediately visible when the joint capsule is incised (Fig. 17–27A). If the injury is recent and the avulsed fragment is not hypertrophied or covered with granulation tissue, it is reattached with a 3.5- or 4.0-mm lag screw and plastic spiked washer (Fig. 17–27B) (Synthes Ltd. [USA], Paoli, PA). Three diverging Kirschner wires can also serve as fixation.

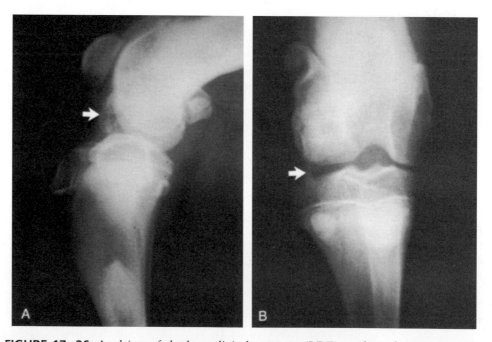

FIGURE 17–26. Avulsion of the long digital extensor (LDE) tendon of origin from the lateral femoral condyle. (*A*) The avulsed osteochondral fragment that was the origin of the tendon can be seen opposite the arrow in the cranial compartment of the stifle joint; mediolateral view. (*B*)The fragment can also be seen in the lateral aspect of the joint in the craniocaudal view, but it is less obvious.

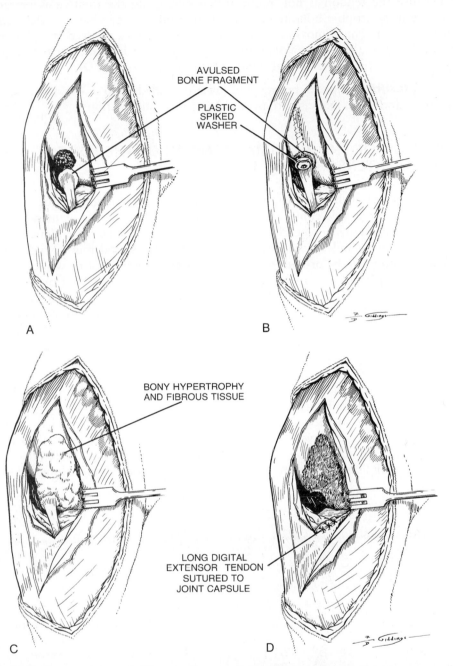

FIGURE 17–27. Avulsion of the tendinous origin of the long digital extensor muscle. (*A*) A fresh avulsion fracture has been exposed by a lateral approach to the femur. The bone fragment and attached tendon have pulled away from the femur. (*B*) A 4.0-mm lag screw and plastic spiked washer (Synthes Ltd. [USA], Paoli, PA) has been used to attach the avulsed fragment. (*C*) An example of a case of several weeks' duration, with bony hypertrophy and fibrous tissue covering the avulsed fragment. The bone fragment is not reattached in this situation. (*D*) The hypertrophic avulsed fragment has been resected and the tendon sutured to the joint capsule. The fascia of the cranial tibial muscle can also be used for attaching the tendon.

Because the tendon is not important in stabilizing the joint, it is better to exercise hypertrophic bone than to try reattachment and chance a delayed or fibrous union. This removes the mechanical irritation of the hypertrophic fragment. The bone can be cut free and the tendon can be attached to the joint capsule or fascia of the cranial tibial muscle (Fig. 17–27C, D).

AFTERCARE ■   Special precautions are not needed. Two weeks of house confinement and leash exercise are needed for soft tissue healing.

LUXATION OF THE PROXIMAL TENDON OF THE LONG DIGITAL EXTENSOR MUSCLE

This unusual problem, wherein the tendon displaces caudally out of the tibial sulcus, causes variable clinical signs. The dog may show marked lameness, with the leg occasionally not bearing weight,[60] or there may be no lameness at all but a clicking sound accompanying each step. This sound mimics a meniscal click and often can be produced on palpation by flexing the stifle while pushing proximally on the foot to simulate weight bearing and can be felt by placing a hand on the limb while the animal is walking. Surgical repair carries a good prognosis. We have also seen luxation of the long digital extensor tendon accompany patellar luxation.

Surgical Treatment

Although an acute injury may respond to external immobilization for 2 to 3 weeks, most cases are chronic when seen and require surgery.

A vertical skin incision is made between the tibial tubercle and the fibula. Dissection will easily reveal the tendon and the tibial sulcus. Nonabsorbable sutures are used to create a "roof" over the sulcus to trap the tendon (Fig. 17–28). If possible, the suture is placed through a bone tunnel along the edge

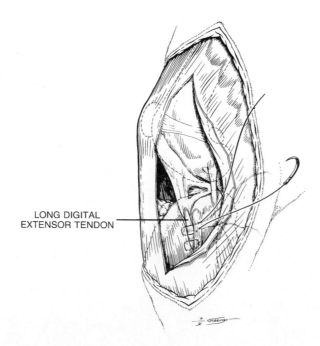

LONG DIGITAL
EXTENSOR TENDON

FIGURE 17–28. Luxation of the proximal tendon of the long digital extensor muscle. Two mattress sutures are placed across the tibial sulcus to prevent luxation of the tendon.

of the sulcus. Where there are no suitable points for bony anchorage, the suture is placed through periosteum and fascia. In some instances, it may be necessary to deepen the sulcus to obtain adequate reduction of the tendon.

AFTERCARE ▪ External immobilization is not required; exercise should be restricted for 2 to 3 weeks.

ARTHRODESIS OF THE STIFLE JOINT

A general discussion of indications for and principles of arthrodesis is found in Chapter 7. Strict attention to detail to establish proper joint angle and rigid internal fixation is necessary for success.

Arthrodesis of the stifle is an alternative to amputation for severely comminuted intra-articular fractures, acute total luxation (Fig. 17–29), chronic luxation or subluxation from a variety of causes, severe osteoarthritis, and severe patellar luxations that have not responded to conventional repair.

Function of the limb is markedly affected; however, when the fusion is at the proper angle (135 to 140 degrees in the dog and 120 to 125 degrees in the cat), function is satisfactory for pet animals. With fusion, the limb is sometimes circumducted, especially at faster gaits when the limb becomes relatively too long compared with the opposite limb. Knuckling of the toes may also occur at these times. Overall function of the fused limb is not as good in most dogs as with amputation. Bone plate fixation is the most suitable fixation for large breeds and is useful in all sizes of animals (see Fig. 17–30). Lag screws and tension band wire are suitable for small- to medium-sized animals (see Fig. 17–31A). Pins with tension band wire are satisfactory in cats and small breeds (see Fig. 17–31B).

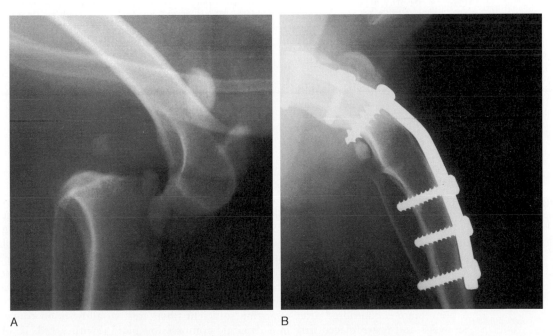

A   B

FIGURE 17–29. A 4-year-old 20-kg mixed-breed dog sustained a vehicular accident resulting in a dislocated stifle and multiple small fractures surrounding the joint. (A) Preoperative lateral radiograph. (B) 19 months after plate arthrodesis.

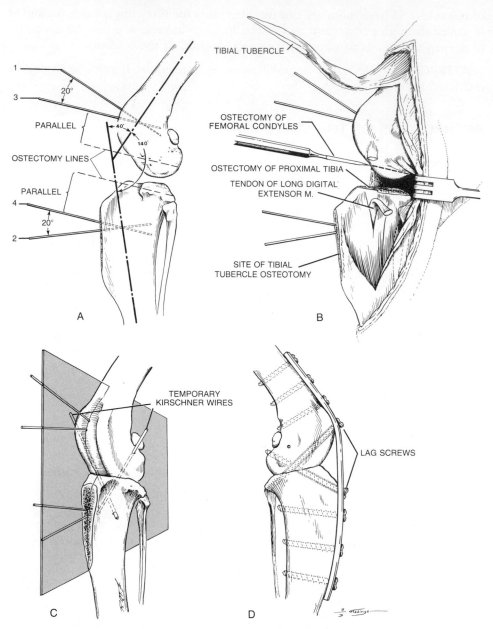

FIGURE 17-30. Arthrodesis of the stifle by bone plate fixation. (*A*) Planning of the ostectomies. Kirschner wires 1 and 2 are placed perpendicular to the femoral and tibial shafts. The joint angle chosen—140 degrees—has a complementary angle of 40 degrees. Dividing this by 2 gives a result of 20 degrees, so that pins 3 and 4, placed at an angle of 20 degrees to pins 1 and 2, are parallel to the ostectomy lines desired. (*B*) The tibial ostectomy is complete. The femoral cut is made with an osteotome held parallel to pin 3. An oscillating saw can also be used. (*C*) The joint is temporarily fixed by crossed pins. Kirschner wires 1 through 4 are kept in alignment with the sagittal plane to prevent rotation of the lower limb. The wires are removed after the crossed pins are placed. (*D*) A bone plate is contoured after removing sufficient tibial crest to allow good contact. Screws 3 and 6 are placed first in a dynamic compression plate (Synthes Ltd. [USA], Paoli, PA) to supply compression, or a separate compression device can be used in the tibia. At least one lag screw should cross the joint, and two are preferable, as shown here.

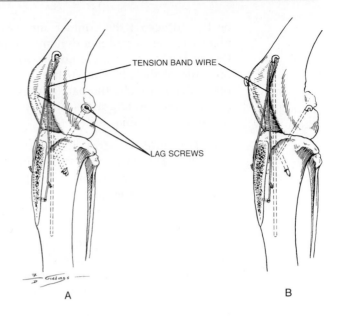

FIGURE 17–31. Arthrodesis of the stifle by lag screw or pin fixation. (*A*) After the contact surfaces are prepared, crossed lag screws are placed from the femoral condyles to the proximal tibia. A small pin is driven from the proximal trochlear sulcus into the proximal tibia, and a tension band wire is placed from the head of the pin to the tibial crest. (*B*) Pins can be substituted for lag screws in small dogs and cats.

Surgical Technique

Bone Plate

Because of the large size of the contact surfaces at the fusion site, it is difficult to change the angle of the joint after the initial cut to remove articular cartilage and subchondral bone without sacrificing large amounts of bone and thus shortening the limb. It is therefore worth the effort to do very precise planning of the initial ostectomy cuts.

A bilateral approach is made to the stifle, and the tibial tuberosity is osteotomized to allow proximal retraction of the entire quadriceps group.[8] The meniscal cartilages are completely excised. Although the collateral ligaments can be sacrificed at this time, maintaining them simplifies intraoperative manipulation of the limb. Kirschner wires are driven into the distal femur and proximal tibia, perpendicular to the long axis of each bone (wires 1 and 2, Fig. 17–30*A*). Both of these pins should lie in the sagittal midline plane of the limb. The selected joint angle is subtracted from 180 degrees to obtain the complementary angle. In the illustrated case, the chosen angle is 140 degrees and the complementary angle is 40 degrees. Since bone can easily be removed from both the femur and tibia, a 20-degree wedge of bone is removed from each. The plane of these ostectomies is parallel to Kirschner wires placed at angles of 20 degrees to the original wires (wires 3 and 4, Fig. 17–30*A*).

The initial ostectomies are performed with an osteotome (Fig. 17–30*B*) or an oscillating saw held parallel to pins 3 and 4. The popliteal vessels must not be severed. Rongeurs or a rasp is used to smooth the contact surfaces. Once the proper angle has been established, the bones are temporarily stabilized with two Kirschner wires placed in an "X" fashion (Fig. 17–30*C*). Pins 1, 2, 3, and 4 should be maintained in the sagittal midline plane during placement of the "X" pins to ensure that the lower limb is not rotated; pins 1 through 4 are then removed.

A bone plate that will allow at least four screws in each fragment is contoured to the cranial bone surfaces. Some of the tibial tuberosity and crest is removed to allow better contact of the plate (Fig. 17–30*D*). At least one screw should be lagged across the contact surfaces after compression is obtained with the plate screws inserted in a dynamic compression plate (Synthes Ltd. [USA], Paoli, PA) or with a separate compression device. The tibial tuberosity is pinned to one side of the plate in such a position that the patella does not contact the plate. Alternatively, the patella may be excised. The X-pins can be removed or left in place. Bone graft is not needed because of the large contact surfaces of the femur and tibia.

AFTERCARE ■   Most dogs and cats do not require external support of the limb. Because the plate is functioning as a tension band, it provides very rigid fixation. However, because the plate is angled and because there is a natural fulcrum at the stifle joint, the plate or screws may break if activity is excessive. External support of the limb should be used if there is any question about the owner's ability to restrict the animal's activity. About 8 weeks is required for radiographic signs of fusion, and activity should be restricted during this period. Fracture of the tibia at the distal end of the plate sometimes occurs and is probably a good reason to remove the plate 6 to 9 months postsurgically. Pins, wires, and screws are not removed unless they loosen.

Screw and Pin Fixation

These procedures begin as just described above. After the contact surfaces are prepared, lag screws or pins are placed in an X fashion across the joint (Fig. 17–31A, B). The pins or screws must penetrate the tibial cortices for best holding power. Pins 1, 2, 3, and 4 are removed. A pin is then driven from the proximal trochlear sulcus into the proximal tibia emerging on the cranial cortex distal to the tibial crest. A hole is drilled transversely through the proximal tibial crest and a tension band wire (size 18 to 22 gauge; 1.0 to 0.6 mm) is placed between the pin and the tibial crest.

AFTERCARE ■   External support using a Thomas splint (see Fig. 2–25) or a long lateral splint (see Fig. 2–24) is advisable for 4 weeks postoperatively. Exercise is severely restricted until radiographs show advanced fusion, usually about 8 to 10 weeks postoperatively.

References

1. Putnam RW: Patellar luxation in the dog. M.Sc. Thesis. Presented to the faculty of graduate studies, University of Guelph, Ontario, Canada, January 1968.
2. Priester WA: Sex, size, and breed as risk factors in canine patellar dislocation. J Am Vet Med Assoc 160:740, 1972.
3. Johnson ME: Feline patellar luxation: A retrospective case study. J Am Anim Hosp Assoc 22: 835, 1986.
4. Singleton WB: The surgical correction of stifle deformities in the dog. J Small Anim Pract 10: 59, 1969.
5. Flo GF, Brinker WO: Fascia overlap procedure for surgical correction of recurrent medial luxation of the patella in the dog. J Am Vet Med Assoc 156:595, 1970.
6. Rudy RW: Stifle joint: In Archibald J (ed): Canine Surgery, 2nd ed. Santa Barbara, American Veterinary Publications, 1974, pp 1104–1159.
7. Vierheller RC: Surgical correction of patellar ectopia in the dog. J Am Vet Med Assoc 134: 429, 1959.
8. Piermattei DL: An Atlas of Surgical Approaches to the Bones and Joints of the Dog and Cat, 3rd ed. Philadelphia, WB Saunders Co, 1993.
9. Flo GL: Surgical correction of a deficient trochlear groove in dogs with severe congenital patellar luxations utilizing a cartilage flap and subchondral grooving. M.S. Thesis, Michigan State University, East Lansing, MI, 1969.
10. Whittick WG: Canine Orthopedics. Philadelphia, Lea & Febiger, 1974, pp 319–321.
11. Slocum B, Slocum DB, Devine T, et al: Wedge recession for treatment of recurrent luxation of the patella. Clin Orthop Rel Res 164:48, 1982.

12. Boone EG, Hohn RB, Weisbrode SR: Trochlear recession wedge technique for patellar luxation: An experimental study. J Am Anim Hosp Assoc 19:735, 1983.
13. Brinker WO, Keller WE: Rotation of the tibial tubercle for correction of luxation of the patella. MSU Vet 22:92, 1962.
14. Singleton WB: The diagnosis and treatment of some abnormal stifle conditions in the dog. Vet Rec 69:1387, 1957.
15. Willauer CC, Vasseur PB: Clinical results of surgical correction of medial luxation of the patella in dogs. Vet Surg 16:31, 1987.
16. Olsson SE: Osteochondrosis in the dog. In Kirk RW (ed): Current Veterinary Therapy VI. Philadelphia, WB Saunders Co, 1977, pp 880–886.
17. Olmstead MR: Lateral luxation of the patella. In Bojrab MJ (ed): Pathophysiology in Surgery. Philadelphia, Lea & Febiger, 1981, pp 638–640.
18. Vasseur PB, Pool RR, Arnoczky SP, et al: Correlative biomechanical and histologic study of the cranial cruciate ligament in dogs. Am J Vet Res 46:1842, 1985.
19. Paatsama S: Ligament injuries in the canine stifle joint. A clinical and experimental study. Thesis. Royal Veterinary College, Stockholm, 1952.
20. Newton CD, Lipowitz AJ: Canine rheumatoid arthritis: A brief review. J Am Anim Hosp Assoc 11:595–599, 1975.
21. Griffen DW, Vasseur PB: Synovial fluid analysis in dogs with cranial cruciate ligament rupture. J Am Anim Hosp Assoc 28:277–281, 1992.
22. Pedersen NC, Pool RC, Castles JJ, et al: Noninfectious canine arthritis: Rheumatoid arthritis. J Am Vet Med Assoc 169:295–303, 1976.
23. Arnoczky SP, Marshall JL: The cruciate ligaments of the canine stifle: An anatomical and functional analysis. Am J Vet Res 38:1807, 1977.
24. Arnoczky SP: The cruciate ligaments: The enigma of the canine stifle. J Small Anim Pract 29: 71, 1988.
25. Arnoczky SP, Torzilli PA, Marshall JL: Biomechanical evaluation of anterior cruciate ligament repair in the dog, An analysis of the instant center of motion. J Am Anim Hosp Assoc 13: 553, 1977.
26. Pond MJ, Campbell JR: The canine stifle joint. I. Rupture of the anterior cruciate ligament. An assessment of conservative and surgical management. J Small Anim Pract 13:1, 1972.
27. Vasseur PB: Clinical results following conservative management for rupture of the cranial cruciate ligament in dogs. Vet Surg 13:243, 1984.
28. Jevens DJ, DeCamp CE, Hauptman J, et al: Use of force-plate analysis of gait to compare two surgical techniques for treatment of cranial cruciate ligament rupture in dogs. Am J Vet Res 57:389–393, 1996.
29. Childers HE: New method for cruciate repair. Mod Vet Pract 47:59–60, 1966.
30. DeAngelis M, Lau RE: A lateral retinacular imbrication technique for the surgical correction of anterior cruciate ligament rupture in the dog. J Am Vet Med Assoc 157:79–84, 1970.
31. Flo G: Modification of the lateral retinacular imbrication technique for stabilizing cruciate ligament injuries. J Am Anim Hosp Assoc 11:570, 1975.
32. Dulisch M: Suture reaction following extra-articular stifle stabilization in the dog; Part I: A retrospective study of 161 stifles. J Am Anim Hosp Assoc 17:569, 1981.
33. Smith GK, Torg JS: Fibular head transposition for repair of cruciate-deficient stifle in the dog. J Am Vet Med Assoc 187:375, 1985.
34. Dupuis J, Blackketter D, Harari J: Biomechanical properties of the stifle joint collateral ligament in dogs. Vet Comp Orthop Trauma 5:158–162, 1992.
35. Dupuis J, Harari J, et al: Evaluation of the lateral collateral ligament after fibular head transposition in dogs. Vet Surg 23:456–465, 1994.
36. Dupuis J, Harari J, et al: Evaluation of fibular transposition for repair of experimental cranial cruciate ligament injury in dogs. Vet Surg 23:1–12, 1994.
37. Metalman LA, Schwartz PD, et al: An evaluation of three different cranial cruciate ligament surgical stabilization procedures as they relate to postoperative meniscal injuries. Vet Comp Orthop Trauma 8:118–123, 1995.
38. Arnoczky SP, Tarvin GB, Marshall JL, Saltzman B: The over-the-top procedure, a technique for anterior cruciate ligament substitution in the dog. J Am Anim Hosp Assoc 15:283, 1979.
39. Shires PK, Hulse DA, Liu W: The under-and-over fascial replacement technique for anterior cruciate ligament rupture in dogs: A retrospective study. J Am Anim Hosp Assoc 20:69–77, 1984.
40. Piermattei DL, Moore RW: A preliminary evaluation of a modified over-the-top procedure for ruptured cranial cruciate ligament in the dog. 8th Annual Conference, Veterinary Orthopedic Society, Snowbird, Utah, 1981.
41. Tarvin GB, Arnoczky SP: Incomplete rupture of the cranial cruciate ligament in a dog. Vet Surg 10:94, 1981.
42. Scavelli TD, Schrader SC, Matthiesen DT: Incomplete rupture of the cranial cruciate ligament of the stifle joint in 25 dogs (abstr). Vet Surg 18:80, 1989.
43. Hohn RB, Newton CD: Surgical repair of ligamentous structures of the stifle joint. In Bojrab MJ (ed): Current Techniques in Small Animal Surgery, Philadelphia, Lea & Febiger, 1975, pp 470–479.

44. Harari J, Johnson AL, Stein FL, et al: Evaluation of experimental transection and partial excision of the caudal cruciate ligament in dogs. Vet Surg 16:151, 1987.
45. DeAngelis MP, Betts CW: Posterior cruciate ligament rupture. J Am Anim Hosp Assoc 9:447, 1973.
46. Stone EA, Betts CW, Rudy RL: Folding of the caudal horn of the medial meniscus secondary to severance of the cranial cruciate ligament. Vet Surg 9:121, 1980.
47. Flo G, DeYoung D, Tvedten H, et al: Classification of meniscal injuries in the canine stifle based upon gross pathological appearance. J Am Anim Hosp Assoc 19:325, 1983.
48. Flo GL: Meniscal injuries. Vet Clin North Am 23:832–843, 1993.
49. Flo GL, DeYoung D: Meniscal injuries and medial meniscectomy in the canine stifle. J Am Anim Hosp Assoc 14:683, 1978.
50. Cox JS, Nye CE, Schaefer WW, et al: Degenerative effects of partial and total resection of the medial meniscus in dogs' knees. Clin Orthop 109:178, 1975.
51. DeYoung D, Flo GL, Tvedten HW: Total medial meniscectomy in the dog. Abstract Vet Ortho Soc Annual Meeting, 1980.
52. DeYoung D, Flo GL, Tvedten H: Experimental medial meniscectomy in dogs undergoing cranial cruciate ligament repair. J Am Anim Hosp Assoc 16:639, 1980.
53. Hannan N, Ghosh P, Bellenger C, Taylor T: Systemic administration of glycosaminoglycan polysulfate (Arteparon) provides partial protection of articular cartilage from damage produced by meniscectomy in the canine. J Orthop Res 5:47, 1987.
54. Farrow CS: Sprain, strain, and contusion. Vet Clin North Am 8:169, 1978.
55. Vasseur PB, Arnoczky SP: Collateral ligaments of the canine stifle joint: Anatomic and functional analysis. Am J Vet Res 42:1133, 1981.
56. Hulse DA, Shires P: Multiple ligament injury of the stifle joint in the dog. J Am Anim Hosp Assoc 22:105, 1986.
57. Welches CD, Scavelli TD: Transarticular pinning to repair luxation of the stifle joint in dogs and cats: A retrospective study in 10 cases. J Am Anim Hosp Assoc 26:207, 1990.
58. Aron D: Traumatic dislocation of the stifle joint: Treatment of 12 dogs and one cat. J Am Anim Hosp Assoc 24:333, 1988.
59. Pond MJ: Avulsion of the extensor digitorum longus muscle in the dog: A report of four cases. J Small Anim Pract 14:785, 1973.
60. Bennett D, Campbell JR: Unusual soft tissue orthopaedic problems in the dog. J Small Anim Pract 20:27, 1979.

18

Fractures of the Tibia and Fibula

Fractures of the tibia are relatively common in dogs and cats, comprising 21 percent of long-bone fractures,[1] and 11.7 percent of appendicular fractures.[2] The entire spectrum of internal and external fixation devices are applicable to these fractures. The AO Vet fracture classification scheme (see Table 2–1) will be used for nomenclature,[1] and treatment recommendations are keyed to the Fracture Patient Scoring System detailed in Table 2–6 when applicable.[3,4]

FIXATION TECHNIQUES

Coaptation

A variety of coaptation devices are applicable in tibial fractures, particularly in type A1 and A3 diaphyseal fractures in skeletally immature animals, where a relatively short healing time in 69 fractures of about 4 weeks has been reported.[5] Some distal fractures are amenable to external fixation, but very few proximal fractures can be adequately stabilized by this method, due to their inherent instability and the difficulty of securing good immobilization of the distal femur.

The long leg cylinder cast (see Fig. 2–21) is useful for the tibia if care is taken to carry the cast high enough to immobilize the distal femur. This is difficult in short-legged and muscular breeds. The same comments apply to the long lateral splint (see Fig. 2–24). Thomas splints (see Fig. 2–25) provide good fixation of the tibia, with the ability to cause either cranial or caudal pull on either segment of the bone by varying the application of the wrapping and padding. With all of these devices it is important to maintain at least normal standing angles of flexion in both the stifle and hock joints to both keep the device as short as possible and to minimize joint stiffness. The Robert-Jones dressing (see Fig. 2–33) is an excellent emergency splint for the tibia, and is particularly useful in type I open fracture to prevent protrusion of sharp bone fragments until definitive treatment is started.

Intramedullary Pins, Cerclage Wires, Lag Screws

The main shortcoming of an intramedullary (IM) pin as the sole method of fixation is that it permits rotation at the fracture site. This method of fixation is reserved for transverse, short oblique, and minimally fragmented fractures of the tibia in skeletally immature or smaller mature dogs and cats.

The pin is best inserted from the proximal end of the tibia. Results of one study indicate that even when the pin is directed in a craniomedial direction, retrograde pinning from the middiaphyseal region has the potential for a significantly more caudal exit point on the tibial plateau, invasion of the joint space, damage to the insertion of the cranial cruciate ligament, and interference with the femoral condyles.[6] In a similar study no significant differences were found between craniomedially directed retrograde pins and normograde pins, although nondirected retrograde pins did cause more interference with the cranial cruciate ligament and femoral condyles.[7] This study also found that if the pin was not seated less than 1.5 cm from the tibial plateau, interference with the femoral condyle was seen with all techniques. We continue to advocate normograde pinning, since, as in the femur, it eliminates some variables that can cause complications. Closed normograde pinning may be used for those fractures that can be reduced closed with a minimum of manipulation and trauma to the soft tissue in the area.

NORMOGRADE IM PIN TECHNIQUE ■ Figure 18–1A shows a short oblique fracture of the tibia. The proximal aspect of the left tibia shows the menisci and limits of the articular surface (Fig. 18–1B). It is usually advanta-

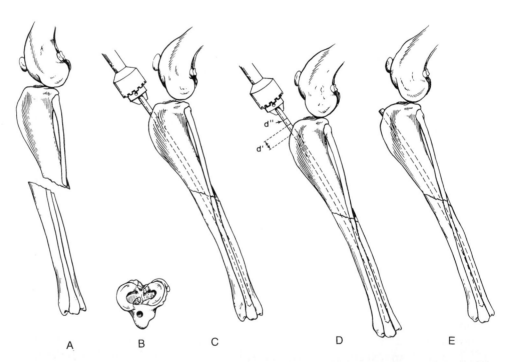

FIGURE 18–1. Intramedullary pinning technique for the tibia. (A) Serrated short oblique fracture of the tibia. (B) Proximal aspect of the left tibia showing menisci and limits of articular surface. Circle depicts the approximate location for insertion of an intramedullary pin. The stifle should be flexed at a right angle. The pin is inserted through the skin along the medial border of the patellar ligament, entering the proximal end of the tibia approximately ¼ inch caudal to the tibial tubercle. (C) Reduced fracture and intramedullary pin, lateral view. The pin should be inserted well into the distal end. (D) Pin retracted about ¼ inch (d'); pin cut (d''). (E) With a countersink and mallet, the pin is returned to the original depth. Sufficient pin is left protruding for removal at the time of clinical union.

geous to have the stifle flexed at a right angle and the animal in dorsal recumbency. The pin is then inserted through the skin and along the medial border of the patellar ligament, entering the proximal end of the tibia approximately one third to one half the distance from the cranial surface of the tibial tubercle to the medial condyle of the tibia (Fig. 18–1B, C). Entering the pin too far caudally will not allow full extension of the stifle joint due to interference of the pin with the femoral condyle. The pin is started close to the medial border of the tibial plateau and angled slightly medially and caudally. After entering the marrow cavity increased resistance and a coarse grating will be felt as the pin strikes the medial cortex. Drilling motion should stop and the pin simply pushed until it bends slightly and then glides along the medial cortical surface. Because of the bending of the pin, a slightly smaller than normal diameter pin is necessary, typically about 50 percent of the medullary canal diameter. This bending causes the Steinmann pin to function more as a Rush pin than as a static intramedullary pin, giving increased stability. If the pin is too large to bend it will straighten the normal S-curve of the tibia and cause valgus angulation of the distal tibia and hindpaw. Drilling back-and-forth quarter turns must be resumed as the pin is seated in the trabecular bone of the distal metaphysis (Fig. 18–1D), just short of the articular cartilage of the tibial trochlea. Palpation of the medial malleolus is used as a guide as to depth of penetration, using the radiograph to estimate how far the malleolus overhangs the surface of the tibial trochlea. The pin is retracted about 1/4 in (6 mm), then cut. With a countersink and mallet, the pin is returned to the original depth. This seats the pin so that the proximal end does not interfere with movement of the stifle joint and still keeps the pin protruding sufficiently for removal (Fig. 18–1E). The fracture site should be compressed by counterpressure from the distal end of the bone while the pin is redriven with the countersink and mallet. If the pin is of small enough diameter to allow bending, the pin can be driven to the desired depth, bent craniomedially, and cut short with a pin cutter. The bend will ensure that the pin does not interfere with the femoral condyle.

A second method is to use a true Rush pin placed through the insertion of the patellar ligament on the tibial tuberosity (Fig. 18–2). The pilot hole is drilled caudally and slightly medially from the tuberosity at an angle of 20 degrees to the long axis of the bone. The hook end of the Rush pin is driven close to the bone and produces no soft tissue reaction and therefore rarely needs to be removed. Rush pins can also be driven from the same point on the tibial plateau as described for Steinmann pins (Fig. 18–2).

INTRAMEDULLARY PIN AND CERCLAGE WIRES ■ The use of cerclage wires in addition to an intramedullary pin works well on long oblique or spiral fractures and certain reducible wedge fractures. Guidelines for cerclage application are given in Chapter 2, and Figure 18–2D presents an example of this method. Note that it is usually necessary to place the cerclage wires around the fibula from the midshaft distally due to the interosseous ligament. The intramedullary pin is usually removed after clinical union and the cerclage wires left in place.

INTRAMEDULLARY PIN AND LAG SCREWS ■ Figure 18–2E shows the same fracture, immobilized with the use of an intramedullary pin and lag screws inserted off center to avoid the intramedullary pin. This procedure is most amenable to larger dogs. Lag screws and intramedullary pins of relatively small diameter are used. The intramedullary pin is usually removed after clinical union and the lag screws left in situ.

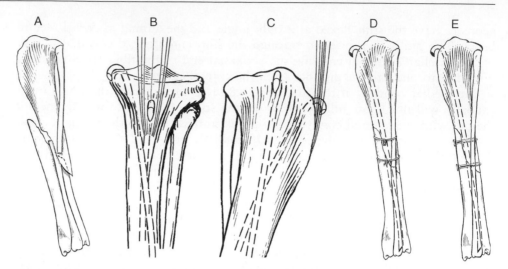

FIGURE 18–2. (*A*) Long oblique fracture of the tibia. (*B, C*) Insertion points in the proximal tibia for Rush pins. Either site can be used for a single pin, and both are used for double pinning. The cranial pin is placed through the tibial tuberosity at the insertion of the patellar ligament. The axial alignment of the pilot hole relative to the tibial shaft is approximately 20 degrees caudal and 5 degrees medial. The medial pin is positioned similarly to the Steinmann pin (see Fig. 18–1), but can be angled more laterally to provide for bending of the Rush pin. (*D, E*) Fracture immobilized by Rush pin through the tibial tuberosity and cerclage wires, or, in large breeds with lag screws inserted off center to avoid the pin.

External Fixators

This splint may be used on practically all fractures of the tibial shaft, including delayed unions and nonunions. Choosing between bone plates and external fixators in many cases is merely a matter of personal choice by the surgeon. All type of fixators are applicable to the tibia because both the medial and lateral aspects of the bone are available. Type I splints are placed on the medial surface of the leg. In this position, they are less subject to being bumped or becoming hooked on objects and do not interfere with walking. Type IA one-plane splints, with the fixation pins placed in the same plane and connected by a common connecting bar are used when there is load sharing between the bone and the fixator, as in simple, wedge, and segmental fractures (Fig. 18–14), as well as in most fractures of skeletally immature patients. Type IIA and B bilateral one-plane fixators (Fig. 18–12*B, C*) are indicated when no load sharing is possible, as in nonreducible complex wedge fractures. Type IB two-plane (see Fig. 18–16) and type III bilateral two-plane splints are used when there is a very short proximal or distal segment.

A very important advantage of the external fixator in tibial fractures is the ability to employ the *biological osteosynthesis* concept by applying the splint with the fracture closed, or with a very limited open approach and reduction. Because of the limited musculature of the crus, closed reduction is more feasible than in the humerus or femur. The animal is prepped and draped for surgery with the limb suspended as shown in Figure 2–12. Sterile towels or bandage material are wrapped around the suspending material a sufficient distance to prevent the chance of accidental contamination of the surgeon during reduction.

Although any type fixator can be used, the type II has special application during closed reduction. If the most proximal and distal fixation pins are in-

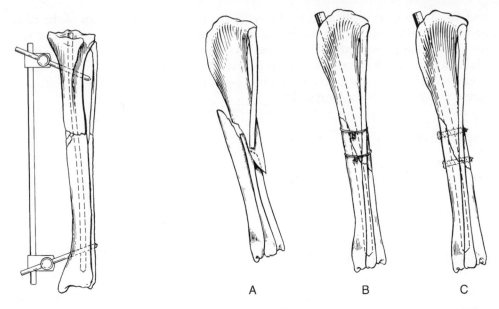

A   B   C

FIGURE 18–3. Intramedullary pin and external fixator, 1/1 pin (half Kirschner) splint, for unstable fractures. If this does not accomplish stability, use a 2/2 pin external fixator.

serted first, at 90 degrees to the bone, they become a visual indicator of the adequacy of reduction in the frontal plane, since they will be parallel to each other when angular deformity in this plane is reduced. Additionally, they can be employed to anchor a fracture distractor to aid in the reduction if desired. If difficulty is encountered in reducing the fracture closed, a limited open approach to the tibia will allow reduction under direct vision, but with minimal disruption of the fracture site, thus maintaining maximal vascularity of the fracture segments. The open approach also allows the use of auxiliary fixation such as K-wires, or lag screws, both of which can be inserted with minimal disruption of soft tissues.

The external fixator is particularly adaptable to open fractures because the segments can be immobilized without invading or placing metallic fixation in the contaminated open area. On the other hand, the external fixator can also be used in combination with other supplemental fixation (e.g., cerclage wires, lag screws, and intramedullary pins [Fig. 18–3]), although there seems little reason for the latter. The main reason for combining IM pinning with the external fixator in the humerus and femur is to allow early removal of the fixator and subsequently better limb function. Function with the fixator on the tibia is not a problem, however, as dogs walk well even with bilateral fixators. It would seem to make better sense to simply employ the appropriate fixator for the fracture and not use the IM pin.

Bone Plates

Plates can be used on most fractures of the tibial shaft, including nonunions, or corrective osteotomies.[8,9] Choosing between bone plates and external fixators in many cases is merely a matter of personal choice by the surgeon. Plates are usually placed on the medial or craniomedial surface of the bone. Contouring of the plate to fit closely the curvature of the medial cortex (see Figs. 18–13 and 18–15) is critical. Failure to do so results in marked deformity of the tibia and lower limb. Most commonly the distal end of the plate is underbent and the distal tibia moved laterally (valgus deviation), as in the case of the too large Steinmann pin. Whenever possible, it is best to apply plates so that compression is exerted at the fracture site. See Figure 2–74 for proper selection of plate and screw size relative to body weight.

Lag Screws

Bone screws applied in lag fashion to produce interfragmentary compression are applicable in many tibial fractures (see Figs. 18–2, 18–5, 18–13, and 18–20). See Figure 2–74 for proper selection of screw size relative to body weight.

PROXIMAL FRACTURES

Fractures of the proximal segment are not common, comprising only about 7 percent of tibial fractures.[1] Most clinical fractures are the simple types, with multifragmentary types being extremely rare. These types are included here mainly to make the classification system complete.

OPEN APPROACHES ■ Exposing the medial side is done by simple skin incision over the area of interest, an extension of the approach to the diaphysis shown below. Exposing the lateral aspect will involve elevating a variable portion of the origin of the tibialis cranialis muscle from the tibial tuberosity and the lateral border of the tibial plateau.

Fracture Type 41-A; Proximal, Extra-articular (Fig. 18–4A)

Type A1, Avulsion

Avulsion of the tibial tuberosity occurs infrequently and is limited to younger animals, usually between 4 and 8 months of age. The tuberosity is a separate growth center and becomes fused to the proximal epiphysis and then to the metaphysis of the tibia as the animal reaches skeletal maturity. In large dogs, the endochondral ossification process of the physis may be irregular as seen radiographically. Frequently, this is mistaken for a pathological process. The

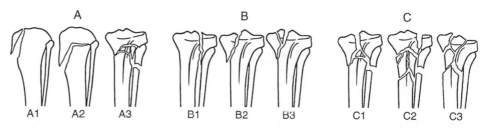

FIGURE 18–4. Proximal fractures of the tibia. (*A1*) Avulsion, (*A2*) simple, and (*A3*) multifragmentary. (*B1*) Lateral simple, (*B2*) medial simple, and (*B3*) unicondylar multifragmentary. (*C1*) Simple, metaphyseal simple, (*C2*) simple, metaphyseal multifragmentary, and (*C3*) multifragmentary. (From Unger M, Montavon PM, Heim UFA: Classification of fractures of the long bones in the dog and cat: Introduction and clinical application. Vet Comp Orthop Trauma 3:41–50, 1990, with permission.)

tibial tuberosity serves as the insertion point of the quadriceps muscles through the patellar ligament and avulsions occur due to contraction of the muscle while the stifle is flexed and the foot firmly on the ground. Such a mechanism could easily occur during jumping, running, or perhaps in a fall.

Clinically, the detached tuberosity (Fig. 18–5A) can usually be palpated, and is dislocated proximally and the distal end is rotated cranially. The patella also

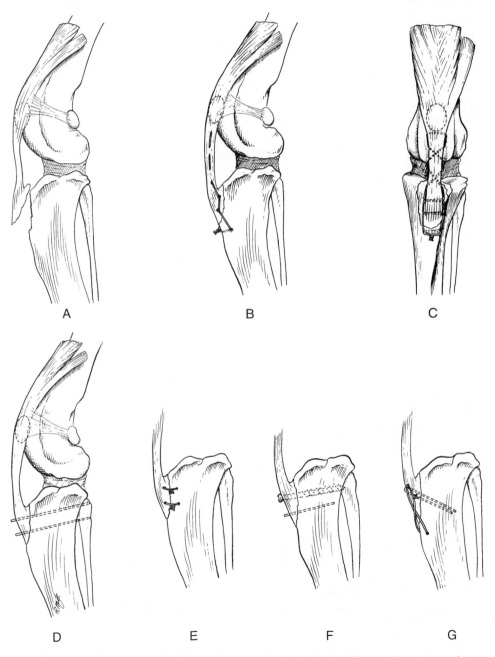

FIGURE 18–5. Operative treatment for the avulsed tibial tubercle. (A) Type A1 avulsion. (B, C) Ligament-bone suture technique using nonabsorbable suture material. (D) Two Kirschner wires. (E) Two stainless steel wire sutures. (F) Cancellous bone screw and pin. (G) Tension band wire.

rides higher in the trochlear groove of the femur and may be noted in radiographs, but not by palpation. Considerable joint effusion, soft tissue swelling, ecchymosis, and lameness characterize the first 3 to 4 postinjury days. There are varying degrees of avulsion, from just a few millimeters to complete detachment as seen in Figure 18–5A. If in doubt about the displacement, the radiograph should be compared with one of the contralateral stifle.

Closed Reduction and Fixation

Conservative management can be considered when the displacement is only partial—that is, 2 to 3 mm—with only a slight angulation of the tuberosity. If the breed is small, and optimal athletic function is not of paramount interest to the owner, then external fixation will be adequate. It is less likely to be successful in the large, active breeds, due in some part to the difficulties maintaining external fixation on these vigorous young dogs. Any of the splints/casts mentioned above in the section Fixation Techniques are applicable, and should be maintained 2 to 3 weeks.

Open Reduction and Internal Fixation

When avulsion is complete, failure to return the tibial tubercle to its original position results in loss of power to the quadriceps muscles and in extension of the stifle joint. Loss of function can be significant in large, athletic breeds, and especially in racing greyhounds. Reduction and internal fixation should be accomplished early in these cases.

A longitudinal incision is made just medial or lateral to the patella, the patellar ligament, and the tibial tuberosity. The blood and fibrin clot is removed from the original location of the tuberosity (Fig. 18–5A). With the hip flexed and the stifle extended and a hook or small pointed reduction forceps attached to the ligament at its insertion on the tuberosity, the tuberosity is slowly and gently pulled back into its original position. A pull is necessary to fatigue and overcome the spastic contraction of the quadriceps muscles. At this stage, the tuberosity can be rather friable, and care must be taken to avoid fragmentation. The tuberosity is then anchored in place using one of the methods shown in Figure 18–5.

1.   Ligament-bone suture technique using nonabsorbable suture material (Fig. 18–5B, C).
2.   Two Kirschner wires (Fig. 18–5D). Recommended only for small breeds and in less than total avulsion.
3.   Two stainless steel wire sutures (Fig. 18–5E). In very young animals the bone may not be well ossified and the wire could tear out. Recommended only for small breeds and in less than total avulsion.
4.   Cancellous bone screw and pin (Fig. 18–5F). There is some danger of implant loosening or breakage due to being loaded in bending rather than tension.
5.   Pins and tension band wire (Fig.15–5G). This is the preferred technique, because it is biomechanically sound and is universally applicable in both large and small breeds.

Aftercare

Additional support such as an off-weight-bearing sling (see Fig. 2–32) may be indicated for the first 2 weeks in poorly controlled or unruly patients. Exercise should be restricted for an additional 2 to 3 weeks. If the animal has a considerable amount of growth potential remaining (large and medium breeds under 6 months and small breeds under 3.5 to 4 months), the fixation should be removed as early as possible to help avoid premature fusion of the tuberosity to the shaft and eventual distal translocation of the tuberosity.

Complications

Fixation complications include avulsion of the tuberosity from the implant, wire breakage, bending of a pin, patellar luxation, and a pin through the proximal tibial growth plate.[10] These can be eliminated in the main part by close attention to good reduction and proper placement and size of implants (see discussion in Chapter 2). An additional problem reported by Goldsmid and Johnson was deformity of the tibial plateau thought to be due to injury to the germinal cells of the proximal tibial epiphysis (Salter type V injury), premature fusion of the tuberosity to the epiphysis, or a combination of both. Although they recognized distal translocation of the tuberosity, they did not attribute any interference with function to this, unlike our experience, where late lameness has been associated with this complication.

Type A2, Simple, Physeal

These are usually Salter type I (Fig. 18–6A) or II (Fig. 18–6B) injuries; for further discussion see Chapter 21. After skeletal maturity, fractures in this region are slightly more distal (Fig. 18–7). The entire epiphysis and tibial tuberosity is usually involved, and the tendency is for dislocation in a caudolateral direction in relation to the tibial shaft. Very occasionally the epiphysis will separate from the tuberosity. This injury may be accompanied by damage to the ligamentous structures (collateral ligaments in particular), which may vary from a sprain to a complete rupture. If the fracture is not reduced and maintained in position, both function and appearance are affected.[9]

Closed Reduction and Fixation

In some cases, further reduction is not essential, or it can be accomplished by closed means. Immobilization is accomplished by the use of a modified Thomas splint (see Fig. 2–25) or long lateral splint (see Fig. 2–24) for 2 to 3 weeks. The splints are usually applied with the stifle in the angulation of the standing position. In addition, the Thomas splint can be attached so that some outward force is exerted on the medial surface of the proximal tibia, which aids in maintaining reduction. If this technique is used, the modified Thomas splint must remain firmly attached and kept in good repair. Loosening invariably results in a crooked leg.

Open Reduction and Internal Fixation

In most cases, an open approach is necessary for returning the epiphysis to its proper position. A longitudinal skin incision is made on the craniomedial surface of the proximal tibia and stifle. In some instances, it is advantageous to make the skin incision on the craniolateral surface of the proximal tibia and stifle. Reflection of the proximal belly of the tibialis cranialis muscle may aid in exposing the fracture to best advantage for reduction and fixation, particularly if a portion of the metaphysis remains attached to the epiphyseal end laterally. By gentle elevation of the epiphysis with an osteotome or similar instrument, the dislocated part can usually be levered back into position. It may be necessary to dislocate the proximal end farther, remove the blood and fibrin

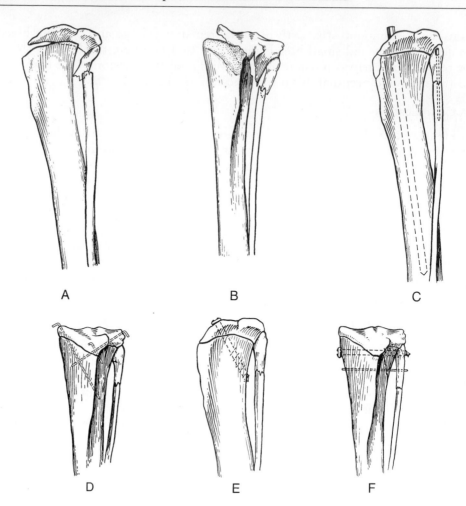

FIGURE 18–6. Fixation methods for type A2 simple fractures. (*A*) Epiphyseal separation of the proximal tibia and fracture of the fibula. (*B*) Fracture-separation of proximal tibia and fibular fracture. (*C, D*) Insertion of pins through the epiphysis distally into the tibia. If it is unstable, the fibula may also be pinned. (*E*) Insertion of a cancellous bone screw. (*F*) Insertion of bone screws in a transverse direction, indicated in some impacted fractures.

clot, and then reduce by levering. If the fibula is fractured and overriding, reduction of the fibula may be helpful in supporting and restoring length to the lateral surface. If the fibula cannot be reduced and is interfering with reduction of the epiphysis it can be shortened to eliminate the interference. The method of fixation varies. Usually, one of the techniques shown in Figure 18–6 will accomplish the objective.[8,9]

1. Insertion of a Steinmann pin in the usual manner through the epiphysis and distally into the tibia (Fig. 18–5C, D). There may not be good rotational stability in some cases. The fibula may also be pinned in large breeds or an angled transfixation added, as described below, to provide rotational stability.

2. Transfixation by multiple Kirschner wires or small Steinmann pins (Fig. 18–6D). This is probably the easiest and most versatile fixation method. The medial and lateral pins are started near the periphery of the tibial plateau, where they do not interfere with the femoral condyles. These pins should penetrate

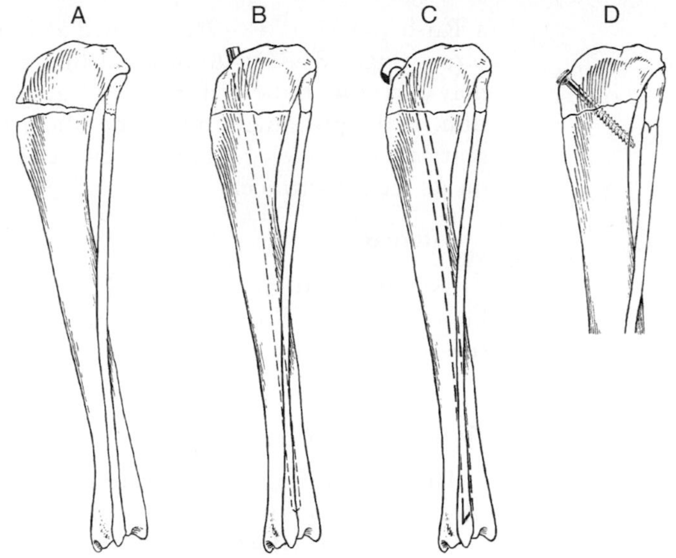

FIGURE 18–7. (*A*) Type A2 simple fracture of the proximal metaphyseal area of the tibia and fibula. (*B*) Fracture reduced and Steinmann intramedullary pin inserted. (*C*) Fixation with Rush pin. (*D*) Fixation with a cancellous lag screw.

the opposite cortex for best stability, and the proximal ends are bent away from the bone to further protect the femoral condyles. One pin medially and one laterally are often adequate, but a third in the tibial tuberosity adds even better three-point stability. This pin need not penetrate the opposite cortex.

3. Insertion of a cancellous bone screw (Fig. 18–6E). This method is restricted to those patients that are close to skeletal maturity so that there is no interference with growth.

4. Insertion of one or more cancellous bone screws in a transverse direction, indicated in some Salter type II fractures (Fig. 18–6F).

Aftercare

Additional support such as an off-weight-bearing sling (see Fig. 2–32) may be indicated for the first 2 weeks in poorly controlled or unruly patients. Exercise should be restricted for an additional 2 to 3 weeks. If the animal has a considerable amount of growth potential remaining (large and medium breeds under 6 months and small breeds under 3.5 to 4 months), screw fixation should be removed as early as possible to help avoid interference with the growth plate. Pin fixation need not be removed unless it loosens and migrates.

Type A2, Simple, Nonphyseal

Fractures occurring in the proximal metaphysis of the tibia and fibula are usually transverse, impacted, or short oblique in nature.[8,9] If the proximal segment is dislocated, it will usually be tilted caudally (Fig. 18–7A).

Closed Reduction and Fixation

In some instances, reduction can be accomplished by closed manipulation and fixation may be accomplished by use of a modified Thomas splint (see Fig. 2–25), long lateral splint (see Fig. 2–24), or a Steinmann or Rush intramedullary pin that is inserted normograde.

Open Reduction and Fixation

Most often, an open approach is indicated for reduction. In these cases, fixation is usually accomplished by the insertion of a Steinmann pin (Fig. 18–7B), a Rush pin (Fig. 18–7C), a medial bone plate, or, rarely, a cancellous bone screw (Fig. 18–7D). Additional filling with autogenous cancellous bone graft may rarely be indicated in some fractures in which deficit remains after reduction. If the proximal end of the fibula is fractured and detached, it should be reattached by use of a bone screw because the lateral collateral ligament inserts on its lateral surface.

Aftercare

Usually, no auxiliary immobilization is needed with intramedullary pinning, bone screw fixation, or bone plating with fractures of this type. Exercise is severely restricted until clinical union, with a gradual return to full activity 1 month later.

Type A3, Multifragmentary

This is an infrequent fracture in the dog and cat. There is no real possibility of closed reduction and external fixation due to the instability of the fracture pattern. Open reduction and internal fixation are the norm, and the fracture is approached as described above. Buttress plate fixation by means of a T-plate is the most practical method of fixation (Fig. 18–8). The plate must be applied on the side of the comminution in order to function as a buttress. Contouring of the plate is complicated on the lateral side by the extreme curvature of the metaphysis in this region. The two proximal screws must be carefully directed to avoid entrance into the joint surface. If it is possible a third screw is directed into the proximal fragment. Aftercare is as described above for type A2 nonphyseal fracture.

Use of an external fixator may be possible if plate fixation is not an option. A hybrid type II/III splint can be applied as illustrated for distal radial fractures (see Fig. 12–23). If the proximal segment is long enough for three fixation pins the type IB two-plane fixator shown below will be applicable (see Fig. 18–16A).

Fracture Type 41-B; Proximal, Partial Articular
(Fig. 18–4B)

Unlike the case in man, these fractures (Fig. 18–9A) are uncommon in quadrupeds; however, when they occur they are potentially devastating injuries inasmuch as severe degenerative joint disease follows when untreated or inappropriately treated. Fractures involving the medial condyle of the tibia are more demanding, since there are more weight-bearing forces on the medial side than

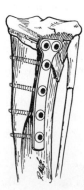

FIGURE 18–8. Fixation of some type B3 partial articular, and most type C complete articular fractures will require a buttress plate. The T-plate is usually the most adaptable to this situation.

FIGURE 18–9. (*A*) Type B1 lateral simple fracture of the proximal tibia. (*B*) Fixation by two cancellous lag screws. The proximal screw is inserted parallel, and as close as possible, to the tibial plateau articular surface. The second screw ideally should be perpendicular to the fracture line, but the acute curvature of the lateral cortex here makes it difficult to insert the screw at that angle.

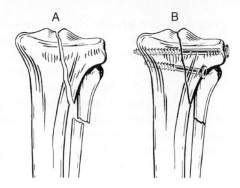

the lateral. As with all intra-articular fractures, precise anatomical reduction and rigid internal fixation are essential.

Reduction and Internal Fixation

Open approach to the area is via a medial or lateral parapatellar approach to the stifle,[11] with extension of the skin incision distally to expose the metaphyseal region as for extra-articular fractures. The reduction must be viewed from within the joint to ensure the accuracy of reduction.

Fixation by lag screw is imperative in order to obtain good fixation (Fig. 18–9B). The interfragmentary compression obtained by screw fixation is the only method that will resist the shear forces present at the fracture line. Simple pin fixation is not appropriate here. Two lag screws are advisable if the fragment is large enough. The screws are paired either horizontally or vertically, depending on the shape of the fragment.

Aftercare

Additional support such as an off-weight-bearing sling (see Fig. 2–32) may be indicated for the first 2 weeks in poorly controlled or unruly patients. Exercise should be severely restricted for an additional 4 to 6 weeks, then slowly returned to normal at about 12 weeks postoperatively. The implants are rarely removed.

Fracture Type 41-C; Proximal, Complete Articular
(Fig. 18–4C)

Even less common than type B partial articular fractures, these fractures are treated by a combination of methods described above in this section. Reconstruction of the articular surface and fixation by lag screws is the first consideration.

Plate fixation of the metaphyseal part of the fracture is the most common and easiest method, and is similar to that shown in Figure 18–8 for type A3 fractures. Because of the necessity for at least two, and preferably three screws in the proximal fragment, T-plates are the usual choice. If the animal is small enough that 2.7-mm screws are appropriate (see Fig. 2–74), two cuttable plates (Synthes Ltd. [USA], Paoli, PA) side-by-side can provide several screws in the proximal fragment. The proximal screws are usually put in in lag fashion to secure fragments. If the fragments are entirely reducible and can be compressed by lag screws (type C1), the plate will function as a neutralization plate. If the fragments are irreducible, as in type C2 and C3 fractures, the plate must function as a buttress. Aftercare is as described for type B fractures above.

Use of an external fixator for metaphyseal fixation may be possible if plate fixation is not an option. The intra-articular portion of the fracture must be reduced and stabilized by lag screws. Depending on the position and planes of the fracture lines it may be possible to apply a hybrid type II/III splint as illustrated for distal radial fractures (see Fig. 12–23). The fixation pins can be applied across, but not within, fracture lines. If the proximal segment is long enough for three fixation pins the type IB two-plane fixator shown below may be applicable (see Fig. 18–16A).

DIAPHYSEAL FRACTURES

The tibia is the third most common long bone fractured, following the femur and radius/ulna,[2] and diaphyseal fractures account for 75 to 81 percent of all tibial fractures.[1,5] Oblique and spiral fracture patterns are the most common in all ages, while multifragmentary fractures are seen most often in adults, as are open fractures.[5] Although it is commonly held by clinicians that tibial fractures, especially of the distal diaphysis, heal more slowly and less predictably than with other long bones, this is not supported by facts; in a series of 195 fractures of canine and feline tibial diaphyseal fractures the nonunion rate was only 4.1 percent.[5] Treatment recommendations are keyed to the Fracture Patient Scoring System detailed in Table 2–6.[3,4]

OPEN APPROACH ■ Shaft fractures are invariably approached from a medial or craniomedial skin incision, since there are no significant muscles on the medial side of the crus (Fig. 18–10). If access is required to the lateral cortex it is easily attained by elevating the tibialis cranialis muscle.

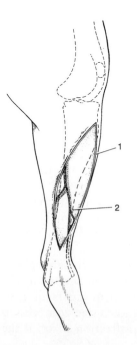

FIGURE 18–10. Approach to the shaft of the tibia.[11] (*1*) Craniomedial skin incision showing approximate location of medial saphenous vessels and nerve. (*2*) With care, the saphenous vessels and nerve, which cross the field obliquely in the middle third of the tibia, can be avoided. This approach can expose the entire length of the tibia.

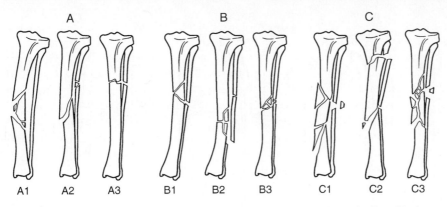

FIGURE 18–11. Diaphyseal fractures of the tibia. (*A1*) Incomplete tibial or fibula intact, (*A2*) simple oblique tibial, and (*A3*) simple transverse tibial. (*B1*) One reducible wedge, (*B2*) reducible wedges, and (*B3*) nonreducible wedges. (*C1*) Reducible wedges, (*C2*) segmental, and (*C3*) nonreducible wedges. (From Unger M, Montavon PM, Heim UFA: Classification of fractures of the long bones in the dog and cat: Introduction and clinical application. Vet Comp Orthop Trauma 3:41–50, 1990, with permission.)

Fracture Type 41-A; Diaphyseal, Simple or Incomplete (Fig. 18–11*A*)

Type A1, Incomplete Tibial or Fibula Intact

Fracture Patient scores of 9 to 10 are typical for these fractures, which are seen primarily in immature animals. Because an intact fibula in the immature animal will maintain length, these fractures can be handled either with a long leg cylinder cast (see Fig. 2–21) or Thomas splint (see Fig. 2–25). In a young animal, less than 6 months old, a long lateral splint (Fig. 2–24) will usually suffice. See the discussion above in Fixation Techniques relative to cast fixation.

Type A2, Simple Oblique Tibial

Because of their instability relative to shortening, these fractures are not suitable to external fixation.

Open Reduction and Fixation

A variety of fixation choices are available, depending on Fracture Patient score and available equipment.

INTRAMEDULLARY PIN ■ In immature animals, typically with a Fracture Patient score of 9 to 10, simple Steinmann pinning will suffice (Fig. 18–2), since early callus formation would be expected to aid in providing rotational stability.

INTRAMEDULLARY PIN AND AUXILIARY FIXATION ■ With the long oblique fracture shown in Figure 18–2*A* the Fracture Patient score typically would be 8 to 9. If the fracture line length is at least twice the bone diameter, cerclage wires are placed at about 1-cm intervals (Fig. 18–2*D*). In large patients there may be an option to replace the cerclage wires with lag screws (Fig. 18–2*E*). If the length of the fracture line is less than twice the bone diameter the fracture is treated as a transverse type A3 fracture.

EXTERNAL FIXATOR ■ Type IA or IIA and B (Fig. 18–12) external skeletal fixators are easily applied here, often by closed, or minimal open, reduction as

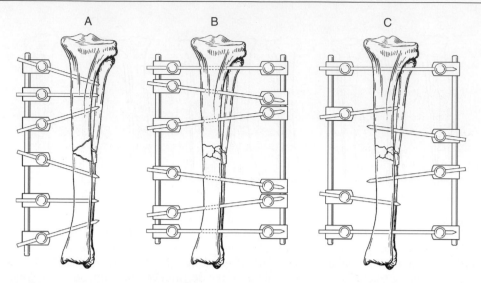

FIGURE 18–12. External skeletal fixation of diaphyseal fractures of the tibia. (*A*) Type IA fixator on a wedge fracture. (*B*) Type IIA full pin fixator on fracture with several wedges. (*C*) Type IIB fixator with half pins in the middle positions is simpler to apply than the type IIA, at a cost of some loss of stiffness.

explained above in Fixation Techniques. Auxiliary fixation in the form of interfragmentary K-wires or lag screws can be used in oblique fractures.

BONE PLATE ■ Neutralization plating of these fractures is an elegant method in the sense that it is applicable to all size animals, the results are quite predictable, and minimal aftercare is required. The technique is identical to the medial neutralization plate shown applied to a type B1 wedge fracture in Figure 18–13 below. Six to eight cortices should be captured by the plate screws; see Figure 2–74 for choice of plate size.

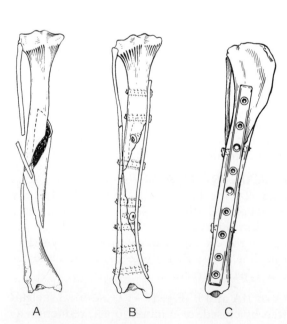

FIGURE 18–13. (*A*) Multiple fracture of the tibia. (*B, C*) Shaft has been anatomically reconstructed using two lag screws. Neutralization plate applied on medial surface of tibia.

Type A3, Simple Transverse Tibial

In skeletally immature dogs, a Fracture Patient score of 9 to 10 is usual, while in older animals and larger breeds it may go down to 8.

Closed Reduction and Fixation

In theory these fractures are treatable by closed reduction and external fixation by cast or splint. This method should be reserved for fractures at or below midshaft, as it is difficult to get good stability of the proximal fragment by cast or splint if the fragment is short. Short-legged or heavily muscled breeds also present a problem in this regard. See the discussion above in Fixation Techniques relative to cast fixation.

Reduction and Internal Fixation

Providing rotational stability is the primary concern in these fractures. Age and size of the patient are important determinants as to type of fixation.

STEINMANN PIN ■ If the patient is less than approximately 6 months, the exuberant callus expected will compensate to a considerable degree for lack of rotational stability, and simple Steinmann pin fixation would be adequate. In mature dogs however, some additional auxiliary fixation is needed. If the patient is less than 15 to 20 pounds (7 to 9.5 kg), interfragmentary wire fixation is often adequate. These patterns are described in Chapter 2 (Fig. 2–62). They must be properly oriented on the bone to counteract the external rotation of the distal fragment that characterizes tibial fractures. Such wire fixation must be very carefully applied in order to ensure that the wire is truly tight, and this author is very conservative in recommending it.

EXTERNAL FIXATOR ■ Fixators are applicable as described above for type A2 fractures, and are usually applied in a closed manner (Fig. 18–12).

BONE PLATE ■ Compression bone plate fixation is a very simple and highly effective method of treatment in all size animals, and especially in large and giant breeds. Six to eight cortices should be captured by the plate screws (see Fig. 2–74 for choice of plate size).

Aftercare

See aftercare suggestions at the end of this Diaphyseal Fracture section.

Fracture Type 42-B; Diaphyseal, Tibial Wedge
(Fig. 18–11B)

None of these fractures are amenable to coaptation fixation due to their instability. Fracture Patient scores will usually be in the 4 to 7 range, and occasionally as low as 3. If the wedges are reducible a reconstructive approach can be taken with several fixation methods. If the wedges are not reducible, the choice of fixation is limited to either bone plating or external skeletal fixators.

Type B1; One Reducible Wedge

If there is only one reducible wedge, and the fracture lines are long enough for cerclage wire fixation, then an intramedullary pin is possible, especially in small- and medium-size breeds with a Fracture Patient score of 6 to 7. Lag screw and neutralization plate fixation is a better option in larger animals (Fig.

18–13), where the Fracture Patient score could be 5 to 6. A minimum of six cortices must be captured by plate screws in each of the proximal and distal segments. Cerclage wire fixation can be substituted for lag screws in some cases. An external fixator of either type I or II could be substituted for the bone plate (Fig. 18–12).

Type B2; Several Reducible Wedges

Increasing instability and complexity drive Fracture Patient scores to 4 to 6. Intramedullary pinning and cerclage wire fixation is not reliable, especially in large breeds. Neutralization plating or external fixators are the primary choices for fixation. Although the wedges are reducible, there is also the option of bridging fixation as described below for type C3 fractures.

Type B3; Nonreducible Wedges

Although not all the fragments can be reduced and stabilized, nevertheless, the bone is able to assume some buttress function, and shortening of the bone is not the major problem as long as the major diaphyseal sections are held in alignment. It is best to take a biological osteosynthesis approach to these fractures, since total reduction is not possible; on the other hand a bridging or buttress fixation isn't needed. Fracture Patient scores of 3 to 5 are routine.

Reduction and Internal Fixation

BONE PLATE ■   The principles of biological osteosynthesis can be respected during plate fixation only if the temptation to attempt reduction of the fragments is resisted. The fracture hematoma and fragments should be disturbed as little as possible consistent with reduction of the major diaphyseal fragments. If it is possible to place the fracture under compression with the plate, and this will add stability. Six to eight cortices must be captured by plate screws in each major segment.

The *major problem with plate fixation* occurs when the nonreducible fragments are on the lateral cortex, which is the natural buttress cortex. Failure to bone graft this area (see Chapter 3) can lead to plate failure due to repetitive bending stresses applied to the plate over a very short segment of the plate. If the fragmented area of the lateral cortex is relatively small, or in other areas of the cortex, autogenous cancellous bone graft will stimulate early callus formation and relieve the bone plate of bending stress. Larger nonreduced areas on the lateral cortex can be physically reinforced by onlay or inlay grafts supplemented with autogenous cancellous graft (see Fig. 3–3E).

EXTERNAL FIXATOR ■   Bending stresses due to loss of the lateral cortex are less critical with type II fixators than with plates. A minimum of six fixation pins are advisable (Fig. 18–12). Closed reduction or limited open reduction (biological osteosynthesis) is the best choice for application, as this will result in the least disruption of the vascular supply to the fragments. See the discussion above in the section Fixation Techniques. Proximal or distal fractures with a very short segment may require a type IB biplanar splint (Fig. 18–16A) with three pins in the short fragment.

Aftercare

See aftercare suggestions at the end of this Diaphyseal Fracture section.

Type 41-C; Diaphyseal, Tibial Complex (Fig. 18–11C)

As stated above for wedge fractures, none of these injuries are amenable to coaptation. Fracture Patient scores will be 1 to 3 or 4.

Type C1, Reducible Wedges

These fractures are similar to type B2 fractures, differing mainly in the amount of the diaphysis involved with the wedges, and their fixation is similar. Although the wedges are reducible, there is also the option of bridging fixation as described below for type C3 fractures.

Type C2, Segmental

Segmental fractures are treatable by either plates or external fixators (Fig. 18–14). With dynamic compression plates both fracture lines can be compressed, as shown in Figure 2–71. A minimum of four cortices must be captured by plate screws in each of the bone segments. The disadvantage with plate fixation can be the need for a very long plate if the middle bone fragment is long. External fixators of type I or II are both applicable to this type fracture. A minimum of two fixation pins are required in each fragment, or three pins in each end segment.

Type C3, Nonreducible Wedges

Plate fixation in the bridging or buttress mode is applicable to these fractures (Fig. 18–15), and is supplemented with autogenous cancellous bone graft in the fragmented area.

Although bone plate fixation is feasible, these fractures heal more certainly and faster when a more biological approach is taken, with closed or limited open reduction and external skeletal fixation. Closed reduction or limited open reduction (biological osteosynthesis) is the best choice for application, as this will result in the least disruption of the vascular supply to the fragments. See the discussion above in the section Fixation Techniques. Type II external fixators (Fig. 18–12B, C) are sufficient for those patients with the highest Fracture Patient scores for this type fracture. A short proximal or distal segment is an

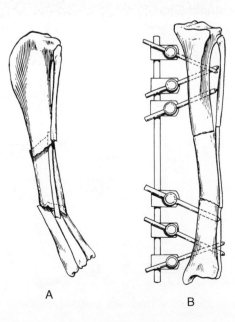

FIGURE 18–14. Unilateral external fixator, 3/3 pins. (A) Open multiple fracture of the tibia. (B) Splinting offers rigid uninterrupted fixation of fracture segments without invading the contaminated area. The use of 3/3 pins helps to further distribute the forces to which the pins are subjected, thus reducing the possibility of pin loosening before clinical union.

A

B

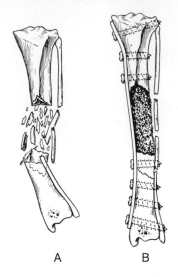

FIGURE 18–15. Multiple fracture of the tibia in a 10-year-old dog. (A) Entire center portion markedly comminuted. (B) Following application of a buttress plate, the small fracture fragments were left in place and the imperfections were filled in with autogenous cancellous bone. Fracture of this type may also be treated by use of frozen cylindrical allograft and a DCP plate.

A   B

indication for the type IB biplanar splint (Fig. 18–16), or a type III splint in the largest breeds (see Fig. 2–46).

Aftercare

Ideally the animal would be allowed early limited active use of the limb. This requires totally stable internal fixation, good owner compliance with confinement and exercise restrictions, and a patient that will not overstress the repair due to hyperactivity. If any of these elements are less than optimal, an off-weight-bearing sling (see Fig. 2–32) is advisable for 2 to 3 weeks, although this will not be possible if an external fixator has been placed. Exercise should be severely restricted for 6 weeks, with a gradual return to unrestricted activity 3 to 4 weeks after clinical union. Radiographs should be taken at 6 to 8 weeks to confirm clinical union before any increase in exercise is allowed.

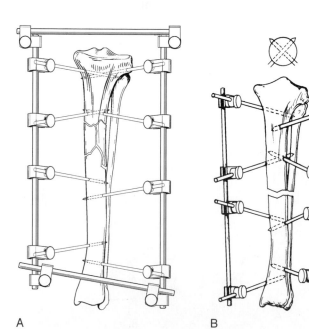

FIGURE 18–16. (A) Type IB two-plane external fixator is useful when there is one short metaphyseal segment. (B) The type III bilateral two-plane external fixator is used when there is a large area of bone loss or fragmentation, especially in gunshot fractures, when there is need for maximum stiffness and long term stability.

A   B

DISTAL FRACTURES

Fractures of the distal tibia account for about 21 percent of all tibial fractures.[1] The predominant fracture patterns were physeal and malleolar, 41 percent were in animals less than 1 year of age, and 37 percent were open fractures, primarily shearing injuries of the malleoli in a series of 43 fractures.[12] Despite the percentage of physeal fractures, growth disturbance of the distal epiphysis is rare. Pin and wire fixation is the predominant method, as complex fractures are uncommon.

OPEN APPROACHES ■ Since the region has no muscular covering, the bone is virtually subcutaneous. Proximal extension of the approaches to the malleoli shown in Figure 18–17 allow exposure of the metaphysis.

Fracture Type 43-A; Distal Tibia, Extra-articular
(Fig. 18–18A)

This fracture is observed primarily in the immature animal as a physeal fracture of Salter type I or II (see Chapter 21). In mature animals it is a metaphyseal fracture with a very short distal segment (Fig. 18–19).

Closed Reduction and Fixation

Reduction and fixation vary with the individual case. Sometimes reduction may be accomplished closed by a combination of traction, countertraction, and manipulation. If any degree of stability is obtained following reduction, fixation may be accomplished by use of a long leg fiberglass cast or a modified Thomas splint (see Figs. 2–21 and 2–25). Flexing the hock joint slightly beyond the normal standing angle increases the stability. In very young patients a short lateral splint may suffice (see Fig. 2–26). Clinical union is usually achieved by 3 to 4 weeks.

Reduction and Internal Fixation

An open approach may be mandatory for satisfactory reduction in most cases. In this situation, the approach is usually made on the medial side.

TRANSFIXATION PINS ■ The insertion of two small diagonally placed pins starting at the medial and lateral malleoli is often the only practical method of fixation because of the shortness of the fragment (Fig. 18–19C). Supplemental fixation using a short lateral splint (see Fig. 2–26) is indicated, since rotational stability from the pins alone can be marginal. Additional rotational stability can also be gained by a tension wire placed between the protruding pins on one or both sides.

RUSH PIN ■ A small Rush pin can often be started on the medial malleolus and driven proximally into the shaft (Fig. 18–19D). Because it is difficult to insert this pin from the lateral malleolus, a small transfixation pin is used on the lateral side to ensure rotational stability. A short lateral splint (Fig. 2–26) can be added if there is any doubt about rotational stability.

STEINMANN PIN ■ Another method of internal fixation is use of a Steinmann intramedullary pin. The pin inserted from the proximal end traverses the entire length of the tibial shaft and is anchored into the distal tibial epiphysis. The amount of anchorage gained is small but adequate if well supported by

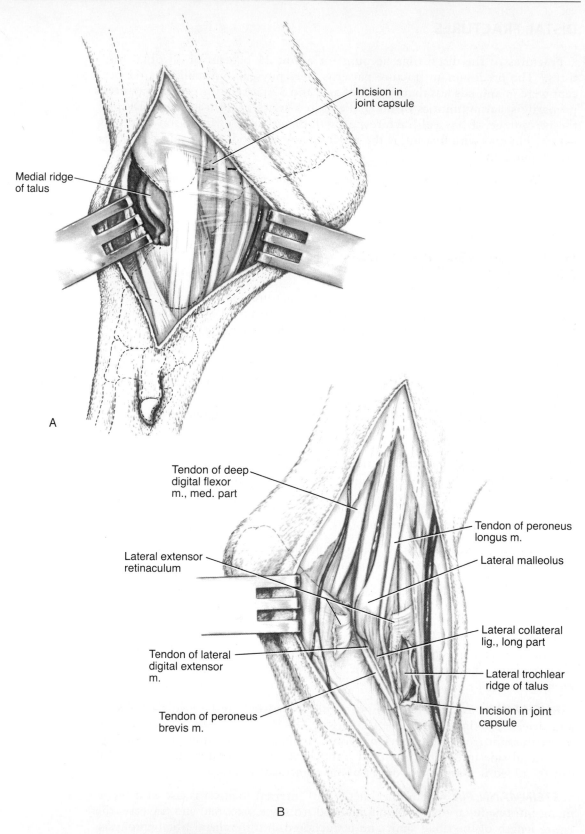

Incision in joint capsule

Medial ridge of talus

A

Tendon of deep digital flexor m., med. part

Lateral extensor retinaculum

Tendon of lateral digital extensor m.

Tendon of peroneus brevis m.

Tendon of peroneus longus m.

Lateral malleolus

Lateral collateral lig., long part

Lateral trochlear ridge of talus

Incision in joint capsule

B

FIGURE 18–17. *See legend on opposite page*

external fixation, usually a fiberglass cast or short lateral splint (see Figs. 2–21 and 2–26). A transfixation pin from the medial malleolus can also be used for additional rotational stability.

Aftercare

Whichever form of immobilization is used, activity is restricted during the healing period. The external fixation can be removed when adequate primary callus has formed (within approximately 3 weeks). The intramedullary pin or transfixation pins are usually removed after clinical union has been reached.

Type A2, Wedge

These fractures can be handled basically as were type A1 fractures, with the addition of some form of interfragmentary fixation of the wedge. Ideally this would take the form of lag screw fixation, but cerclage wires may be possible in some cases. Some fractures can be adequately fixed entirely by lag screws. Transfixation by K-wires is not as stable, but is often adequate; supplementary external support is often essential.

Type A3, Complex

Fortunately, these are very rare injuries in the dog and cat because they are rarely injured while skiing, unlike their human masters. Buttress fixation is essential.

BONE PLATE ■ Plate fixation is the best method of accomplishing the required buttress fixation. As many of the fragments as possible are stabilized by lag screws, either directly in the fragments or through the plate holes. The type of plate used is variable, depending on the size of the dog and the fracture pattern. Straight plates may be applicable in some cases, especially in large dogs. T-plates are useful if the length of the fracture area is not too long. Multiple cuttable plates spaced around the tibia may provide a method of getting sufficient screws in the distal end to provide good buttressing. The drawback of this method is that the largest screws that can be used are 2.7 mm. Any cortical defects should receive autogenous bone grafting. External support, as described above for type A1 and A2 fractures, is probably required in most cases.

EXTERNAL FIXATOR ■ There are at least two methods of utilizing external fixators in this situation. The first is the use of a hybrid type II/III splint as illustrated for distal radial fractures (see Fig. 12–23), placing fixation pins across but not within fracture lines. The second method is a splint that bridges the joint and places it under tension (ligmentotaxis). Tension is applied to the distal tibial articular fragment via the collateral ligaments to maintain the bone in position. Some transarticular fixator patterns are illustrated in Chapter 19. The fragments can be reconstructed as best possible by interfragmentary compression or transfixation pinning, or simply left unreduced to maximize their blood supply; a biological osteosynthesis approach. This is definitely a last-ditch effort when nothing else is possible.

FIGURE 18–17. (A) Approach to the medial malleolus and talocrural joint. (B) Approach to the lateral malleolus and talocrural joint. (From Piermattei DL: An Atlas of Surgical Approaches to the Bones and Joints of the Dog and Cat, 3rd ed. Philadelphia, WB Saunders Co, 1993, pp 303, 305, with permission.)

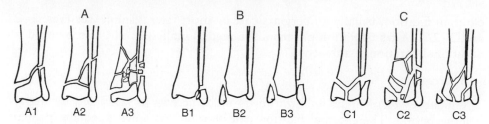

FIGURE 18–18. Distal fractures of the tibia. (*A1*) Simple, (*A2*) wedge, and (*A3*) complex. (*B1*) Lateral malleolar, (*B2*) medial malleolar, and (*B3*) multimalleolar. (*C1*) Simple, metaphyseal simple, (*C2*) simple, metaphyseal multifragmentary, and (*C3*) multifragmentary. (From Unger M, Montavon PM, Heim UFA: Classification of fractures of the long bones in the dog and cat: Introduction and clinical application. Vet Comp Orthop Trauma 3:41–50, 1990, with permission.)

Fracture Type 43-B; Distal, Partial Articular (Fig. 18–18*B*)

Fractures of either or both malleoli give rise to instability of the tarsocrural joint, resulting in subluxation or dislocation. Many of these malleolar fractures are a result of shearing injury, and are discussed in Chapter 19. The two most important factors in the treatment of articular fractures of the tarsocrural joint are:

1. Maintenance of integrity of the joint "mortise" created by the malleoli.
2. Complete re-establishment of the weight-bearing surfaces of the tibia and tibial tarsal bone.

The hock is functionally a hinge with motion in one plane, flexion and extension. The bony structure is designed as a mortise and tenon with considerable inherent stability. The mortise is formed by the lateral malleolus (the distal end of the fibula), the distal articular surface of the tibia, and the medial malleolus.

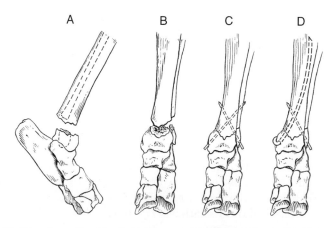

FIGURE 18–19. Fixation of a distal tibial type A1 physeal fracture. (*A, B*) Salter-Harris I fracture of the distal tibia and fibula. (*C*) Diagonally placed transfixation pins or Kirschner wires are started at the medial and lateral malleoli and driven into the opposite cortices. Supplemental coaptation fixation is also needed. (*D*) Slightly more stability can be provided by placing a Rush pin from the medial malleolar region. Coaptation splintage may not be necessary if good stability is achieved. It is not usually possible to similarly place a Rush pin from the lateral side, as the fibular malleolus interferes. A transfixation K-wire can be used for additional rotational stability.

The tenon is the trochlea and body of the tibial tarsal bone, which is shaped to fit snugly into the mortise. The tibia and fibula and tibial tarsal bone are bound together by numerous ligaments.

Complete malleolar fractures create ligamentous instability of the tarsocrural joint, and treatment by external fixation always results in malunion, continued instability, and eventual degenerative joint disease. Intraperiosteal fractures of the malleolus without displacement may be seen in immature animals, and these usually respond to casting or splinting.

Reduction and Internal Fixation

Rigid fixation can be best instituted by the use of bone screws, transfixation pins, or tension band wire and pins.

LATER AL MALLEOLUS ■ The lateral malleolus is part of the fibula and usually fractures some distance from the end, particularly in the cat (Fig. 18–20A). Fixation of the fracture is indirect; the fragment is fixed to the tibia. Screws are usually used in medium- and large-size dogs, and threaded Kirschner pins are used in small dogs and cats, although miniscrews in the 1.5- and 2.0-mm sizes are applicable in small breeds. The screws or pins should pass in a proximal direction and anchor completely through the cortex on the opposite side of the tibia (Fig. 18–20B, C). Stability of the joint should be tested after fracture fixation, and ligaments that have been ruptured should be repaired by suturing (see Chapter 19). Supplemental fixation may be indicated in the form of a short lateral splint (see Fig. 2–26) for 3 to 4 weeks postoperatively.

MEDIAL MALLEOLUS ■ Immobilization may be accomplished by use of a cancellous bone screw in large breeds (Fig. 18–20E, F). More widely applicable

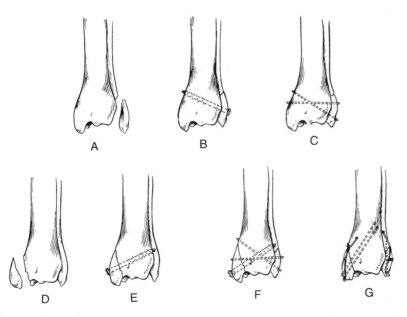

FIGURE 18–20. Malleolar fractures. (*A*) Fracture of the lateral malleolus (distal end of fibula). (*B*) Immobilization using a cancellous screw or (*C*) two threaded Kirschner wires. (*D*) Fracture of the medial malleolus. (*E*) Immobilization using a cancellous bone screw. (*F*) Fractures of both malleoli with fixation. (*G*) Fixation with two Kirschner wires and a figure-of-8 tension band wire.

is the Kirschner wires and figure-of-8 tension band wire method (Fig. 18–20*G*). In small breeds the fixation can be accomplished with one K-wire. With this fixation and restricted activity, no additional external fixation is usually needed. Bilateral malleolar fractures are treated in a similar manner (Figs. 18–20*F, G*).

Fracture Type 43-C; Distal, Complex Articular (Fig. 18–18C)

The least common of tibial fractures, these injuries are treated by a combination of methods illustrated above for type A and B fractures. Type C2 and C3 fractures are often a result of gunshot injury. As is typical for all complex fractures, the first order is to reconstruct the articular surface with lag screws parallel to the joint surface. The remaining extra-articular metaphyseal fracture is handled by the methods detailed above for type A fractures. In some multifragmentary fractures there is no hope of preserving a functional joint and these should receive arthrodesis as primary treatment. See Chapter 19 for a discussion of tarsocrural arthrodesis.

References

1. Unger M, Montavon PM, Heim UFA: Classification of fractures of the long bones in the dog and cat: Introduction and clinical application. Vet Comp Orthop Trauma 3:41–50, 1990.
2. Johnson JA, Austin C, Bruer GJ: Incidence of canine appendicular musculoskeletal disorders in 16 veterinary teaching hospitals from 1980 through 1989. Vet Comp Orthop Trauma 7: 56–69, 1994.
3. Palmer RH, Hulse DA, Aron DN: A proposed fracture patient score system used to develop fracture treatment plans (abstract). Proc 20th Ann Conf Vet Orthop Soc, 1993.
4. Palmer RH: Decision making in fracture treatment: The fracture patient scoring system. Proc (Sm Anim) ACVS Vet Symposium, 1994, pp 388–390.
5. Boone EG, Johnson AL, et al: Fractures of the tibial diaphysis in dogs and cats. J Am Vet Med Assoc 188:41–45, 1986.
6. Pardo AD: Relationship of tibial intramedullary pins to canine stifle joint structures: A comparison of normograde and retrograde insertion. J Am Anim Hosp Assoc 30:369–374, 1994.
7. Dixon BC, Tomlinson JL, Wagner-Mann CC: Effects of three intramedullary pinning techniques on proximal pin location and articular damage in the canine tibia. Vet Surg 23: 448–455, 1994.
8. Brinker WO: Fractures. *In* Canine Surgery, 2nd Archibald ed. Santa Barbara, American Veterinary Publications, Inc, 1974, pp 949–1048.
9. Butler HC: Fractures of the tibia. *In* Brinker WO, Hohn RB, Prieur WD: Manual of Internal Fixation in Small Animals. New York, Springer-Verlag, 1984, pp 180–190.
10. Goldsmid S, Johnson KA: Complications of canine tibial tuberosity avulsion fractures. Vet Comp Orthop Trauma 4:54–58, 1991.
11. Piermattei DL: Atlas of Surgical Approaches to the Bones and Joints of the Dog and Cat, 3rd ed. Philadelphia, WB Saunders Co, 1993.
12. Boone EG, Johnson AL, Hohn RB: Distal tibial fractures in dogs and cats. J Am Vet Med Assoc 188:36–40, 1986.

19

Fractures and Other Orthopedic Injuries of the Tarsus, Metatarsus, and Phalanges

Injuries to the tarsus generally involve fracture of one or more bones, impairment of ligaments, or, occasionally, a combination of these. Ligamentous injuries are most commonly seen in athletic animals, whereas fractures are common in a variety of animals. Ligamentous injuries of the tarsus resulting in varying degrees of instability are relatively common in athletic breeds because of the propulsive force supplied by the hindlegs. Unlike those of the carpus, tarsal injuries are more apt to be caused by spontaneous overstress rather than by outside traumatic forces. Conservative treatment of second- and third degree ligamentous injuries (see Chapter 7 for further discussion) by cast immobilization is not recommended because permanent instability is the usual result. Aggressive surgical treatment is much more rewarding, but it does require a good working knowledge of the anatomy of the region. Unfortunately, the official terminology of the tarsus differs markedly from that in current popular use.

ANATOMY OF THE HINDPAW ■ The bony anatomy of the hindfoot is complicated and must be well understood before any repairs are attempted. Figure 19–1 reviews these bones and provides a comprehensive resource for interpreting radiographs. Ligaments of the hock and tarsus are shown in Figure 19–2. Beginning at the tarsocrural joint and continuing distally, the terms *cranial* and *caudal* are replaced by the terms *dorsal* and *plantar*.

The bones of the tarsus are arranged in several levels, with a complex arrangement of ligaments. The joint between the tibia and fibula and the talus and calcaneus is the *tarsocrural* joint, often called the tibiotarsal, talocrural, or hock joint. It consists of both the talocrural and talocalcaneal joints, which are continuous with each other. *Intertarsal* joints include all articulations between tarsal bones, with four of them named specifically:

1. *Talocalcaneal joint*. The joint between the talus and calcaneus.
2. *Talocalcaneocentral joint*. This joint is primarily an articulation between the talus and central tarsal bone, but the joint capsule is continuous with the calcaneus.

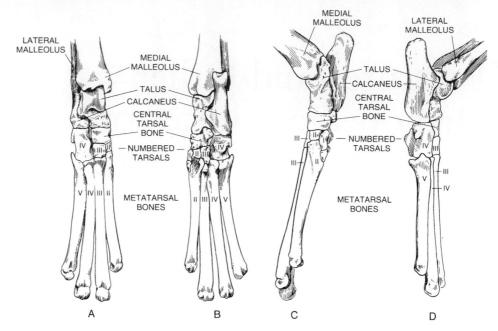

FIGURE 19–1. Bones of the tarsus, metatarsus, and phalanges. (*A*) Dorsal view. (*B*) Plantar view. (*C*) Medial view. (*D*) Lateral view.

3.   *Calcaneoquartal joint.* The joint between the calcaneus and the fourth tarsal. This joint and the talocalcaneocentral joint collectively are popularly known as the proximal intertarsal joint. This name is useful to the surgeon because of the awkwardness of the official names.

4.   *Centrodistal joint.* The joint between the central tarsal bone and the distal numbered tarsal bones. The popular name is the distal intertarsal joint.

The remainder of the joints of the hindpaw include;

1.   *Tarsometatarsal joints.* The joints between the distal tarsal and metatarsal bones.

2.   *Metatarsophalangeal joints.* The joints between the metatarsal bones and the first phalanges.

3.   *Interphalangeal joints.* The joints between the first and second and second and third phalanges.

The most common ligamentous injuries of this region involve the collateral ligaments of the tarsocrural joint (Fig. 19–2) and the plantar ligaments and tarsal fibrocartilage. Both collateral ligaments have long and short parts. The long parts serve to limit extension, and the short parts prevent hyperflexion. The plantar ligaments and tarsal fibrocartilage are tension bands that limit extension of the intertarsal and tarsometatarsal joints. The remaining ligaments are much smaller and shorter, connecting individual bones.

SURGICAL APPROACHES AND TECHNIQUE ■   Several approaches to the bones and joints of the tarsus have been described[1]; generally, approaches to the various bones are made directly over the injured bone or ligament because there are no muscles of any size covering them. Nerves, vessels, and tendons are retracted as necessary to allow exposure.

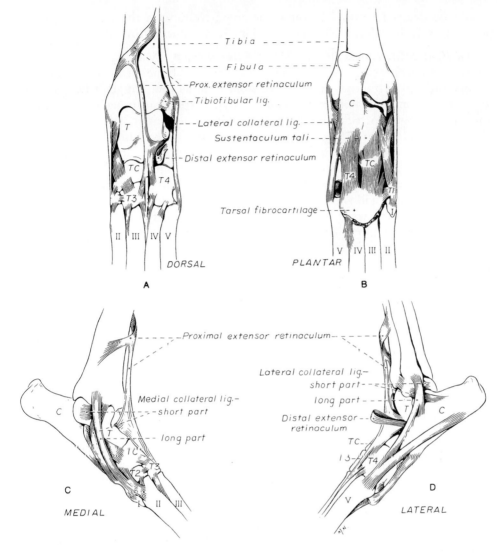

FIGURE 19-2. Ligaments of the left tarsus (*A*) Dorsal aspect. (*B*) Plantar aspect. (*C*) Medial aspect. (*D*) Lateral aspect. C = calcaneus; T1, T3, T4 = first, third, fourth tarsals; T = talus; I through V = metatarsals; TC = central tarsal. (From Evans HE: Miller's Anatomy of the Dog, 3rd ed. Philadelphia, WB Saunders Co, 1993, pp 253, 254, with permission.)

Surgery of the lower limbs can be done with a tourniquet, which is invaluable for decreasing oozing hemorrhage and so increasing visibility and decreasing operating time. Although pneumatic cuffs are the best way of creating the tourniquet more proximally in the limbs, distal tourniquets can be made more simply. Vetrap (3M Animal Care Products, St. Paul, MN) elastic bandage material has proven very satisfactory for this purpose, as illustrated in Figure 13–4. Although the bandage is best sterilized in ethylene oxide, it can be steam sterilized at minimal time and temperature, similar to the method of sterilizing rubber gloves (250°F for 12 minutes). Use of the tourniquet has the disadvantage of producing more postoperative swelling. Application of casts or splints should be delayed 48 to 72 hours postoperatively, with the lower limb supported in a Robert-Jones bandage (see Fig. 2–33) during this time.

CLINICAL SIGNS AND DIAGNOSIS OF INJURIES ■ Many tarsal injuries are a result of overstress of ligamentous structures and bone and occur without a history of known trauma. Sudden exertion, such as jumping, can be sufficient to damage plantar ligaments and cause a hyperextension injury or fracture of a metatarsal bone. Affected animals are usually non–weight-bearing, have varible swelling in the tarsal region, and show varying degrees of instability of the tarsus or metatarsus. The limb is commonly carried in flexion. Palpation will usually be sufficient to localize the area of probable injury.

Radiographs are necessary to verify the diagnosis and to localize the damage. Stress radiographs will show the area of instability. Standard dorsoplantar and lateral or medial views, plus obliques, will also identify avulsions and other fractures. Nonscreen film or fine-detail screens are essential.

THE TARSUS

Tarsocrural Luxation and Subluxation

Many complete luxations of this joint are accompanied by fracture of one or both malleoli, and internal fixation of the fractures results in stability of the joint. Treatment of such injuries is described in Chapter 18.

Clinical Signs

Rupture or avulsion of the collateral ligaments—grade 3 sprains—produces subluxation (Fig. 19–3A, B). Medial injuries allow valgus (lateral) deviation of the foot, and lateral injuries allow varus (medial) angulation. These deviations are easily palpated and confirmed radiographically. Rupture of just the long or short part of the ligament produces only moderate instability and may be difficult to diagnose preoperatively.

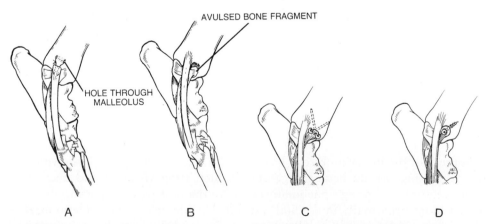

FIGURE 19–3. Collateral ligament injuries of the tarsocrural joint. (*A*) The long part of the medial collateral ligament is torn near its origin on the malleolus. A hole is drilled through the malleolus, and a locking loop suture is passed through this hole to pull the ligament against the bone. (*B*) An avulsion of the origin of the short part of the medial collateral ligament. (*C*) Diverging Kirschner wires used to stabilize the avulsed fragment. (*D*) Lag screw fixation is ideal if the fragment is large enough to allow screw placement.

Treatment

Principles of treatment are similar to those described in Chapter 7, such as imbricating, suturing, reattaching, or replacing ligaments as indicated. It is important to repair both the long and short part of the ligament in order to achieve good function. Reattachment of the long part of the ligament is illustrated in Figure 19–3A. A bone tunnel is used in the malleolus to anchor the suture. An avulsion of the short part is depicted in Figure 19–3B, fixed with two diverging Kirschner wires passed through the fragment into the tibia or a small lag screw (Fig. 19–3C, D). If good repair or reattachment of the ligament is not possible, the repair can be augmented by synthetic ligaments (Fig. 19–4C, D).

AFTERCARE ▪ Ligamentous repairs are protected with a short lateral splint for 4 to 6 weeks followed by an elastic bandage for an additional 2 weeks (see Chapter 7). Exercise is restricted to leash walking until 8 weeks, then gradually increased to normal at 10 to 12 weeks.

Shearing Injury of the Tarsus

This abrasion injury occurs when the dog's lower limb is run over by the tire of an automobile with its brakes locked attempting to avoid the animal. Soft tissues in contact with the pavement are simply ground away, often eroding skin, muscle, ligaments, and even bone. The medial tarsal and metatarsal region is most commonly affected, with the medial malleolus and collateral ligaments

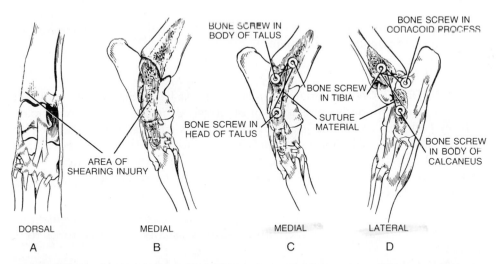

FIGURE 19–4. Shearing injury of the tarsus. (A, B) The medial malleolus and medial aspects of the proximal tarsal bones have been ground away, resulting in instability and valgus deformity. (C) Placement of medial synthetic ligaments.[2] The proximal screw is placed as distally as possible while the tibial cochlea is avoided. One screw is placed in the body of the talus to simulate the short part of the ligament, and another screw is placed in the head of the talus to simulate the long ligament. Two strands of size 0–2 braided polyester suture are placed between each of the screws and tied with the short portion taut in flexion and the long portion taut in extension. (D) Placement of lateral synthetic ligaments.[2] Placement is similar to that of the medial side, with the screws placed in the coracoid process and base of the calcaneus.

often completely destroyed (Fig. 19–4*A*, *B*). One or more tarsal or metatarsal joints may be open and various amounts of debris are ground into all the tissues. The lateral side is less commonly involved and represents a less serious injury than a comparable injury on the medial side. Owing to the fact that the dog normally stands with a few degrees of valgus (lateral) deviation of the hindpaw, ligamentous stability of the medial side of the tarsus and metatarsus is much more critical than on the lateral aspect.

Best results are obtained by treating these wounds in an open manner, with early stabilization of the joints and any accompanying fractures. Skin grafting is delayed and indicated only where granulation tissue does not adequately close the skin, which is a rare occurrence. Early or delayed arthrodesis is indicated in those cases for which it is not possible to restore reasonable joint function. Variables to be considered in choosing a plan of action are:

1. Assuming that the joint(s) can be stabilized, is there enough articular surface to allow good function? Loss of bone in the tarsocrural articulation is critical. If the answer is no, arthrodesis is indicated.

2. What will the owner accept as reasonable function? A large, active breed presents different problems from a small and sedentary animal. In the former, aggressive ligamentous repair, augmentation, or replacement is necessary, while in the latter case it may be possible to obtain good results by very conservative methods. Stabilization of joints by scar tissue may well provide adequate support in the smaller and less active animals, but it rarely will support the tension loads of the medial side in large, athletic individuals.

3. How will support for the joints or fractured bones be provided? Regardless which approach is taken to the ligamentous instability, the involved joints must be stabilized during the healing period. Because of the necessity for daily bandage changes for 2 to 3 weeks when treating these large open wounds, the use of conventional casts or splints is difficult. External skeletal fixators have greatly aided in solving this problem.

Treatment

RECONSTRUCTION ■   Initial debridement must be meticulous but not too aggressive, with emphasis on removal of obviously dead tissue and foreign matter from both soft tissue and joint spaces. Copious irrigation with Ringer's or saline solution is very important at this time. Addition of 10 percent povidone-iodine or 0.2 percent chlorhexidine is favored by some. After adequate debridement, it may be possible to partially close the wound by suturing skin. This can be helpful, but care must be taken to:

1. Leave adequate open area for unimpeded wound drainage. Placement of Penrose or tube drains under the sutured skin is usually advisable for 2 to 5 days.

2. Avoid closing skin under tension. Serious circulatory stasis develops owing to the tourniquet-like effect of excessive skin tension in the lower limbs.

3. When in doubt about tissue viability, *do not suture skin*. Delayed primary closure can be done in a few days with no loss of healing time.

Several debridements over a number of days may be necessary to adequately remove all devitalized tissue owing to the difficulty in determining viability of badly traumatized tissue. If there are portions of ligaments, joint capsule, or other tissues that can be sutured to support the joint and to close the synovial membrane, this should be done. Monofilament or synthetic absorbable suture is most trouble free. Re-establishment of the tibiotarsal collateral ligament complex is usually hampered by loss of bone, and small bone screws may have to be used to anchor the synthetic ligament. There is a tendency to use monofilament wire in this contaminated area, but heavy braided polyester or monofilament nylon suture is a much more functional ligament and has resulted in very few problems related to suture sinus drainage tracts.

Three bone screws are positioned to mimic the normal ligaments as closely as possible (Fig. 19–4C, D). Precise placement of these bone screws for attachment of heavy braided polyester suture and adequate soft tissue debridement are necessary for successful treatment.[2] The proximal screw is placed as distally in the tibia as possible, bearing in mind that the tibial cochlea is recessed a considerable distance into the distal tibia and can be seen by stressing the tarsus to open the joint. The screw must not enter the joint. The distal screws are placed to simulate the insertion points of the long and short parts of the collateral ligaments. Medially (Fig. 19–4C), both screws are placed in the talus, the proximal one in the body. This screw should be angled slightly distad to avoid the trochlear sulcus of the talus. The distal screw is placed in the head of the talus, approximately halfway between the base of the medial trochlear ridge and the distal articular surface. Laterally (Fig. 19–4D) the screws are similarly placed in the calcaneus. The proximal screw goes into the base of the coracoid process, and the distal screw is placed halfway between the distal base of the coracoid process and the distal articular surface. Double strands of heavy braided polyester suture (size 0–2) or a single strand of 40- to 60-pound test monofilament nylon fishing line are placed between the screws. The short ligament should be moderately taut in flexion and the long portion taut in extension. The sutures are tied tightly enough to stabilize the joint, but motion without binding should still be possible. The long ligament is tied with the joint in extension, and the short with the joint flexed. Steel washers can be used on the screws to prevent the suture from slipping over the head of the screw.

Treatment of the open wound is simplified by use of transarticular external skeletal fixator to stabilize the joint (Fig. 19–5). Fixation is maintained until granulation tissue has covered the defect, usually 3 to 4 weeks. A recently introduced external fixator hinge joint has potential for application in this situation (Jorgensen Laboratories, Inc., Loveland CO). This device allows for joint motion in one plane and would stabilize the joint during healing while allowing motion, which should have a beneficial effect in organizing collagen to form a pseudoligament. In either case, sterile laparotomy sponges soaked in saline or saline solutions of povidone-iodine or chlorhexidine are loosely bandaged to the limb for several days, and debridement is repeated daily or every other day until all dead tissue is removed. The wound must be kept moist and provision made for adequate drainage of exudate.[3] Moist gauze with copious absorbent padding covered by a moisture barrier such as polyvinyl sheet and dressing changes are used daily until healthy granulation covers the wound. (Hydrocolloid, hydrogel, and polyethylene semiocclusive dressings have received considerable attention for treatment of full-thickness skin wounds. Hydrogel and polyethylene dressings were significantly better in all parameters tested in one study.[4]) At this point, nonadherent dressings, either dry or with antibacterial ointments, and minimal absorbent padding are used in place of the moist dressings. Intervals between dressing changes can gradually be spread out as discharge lessens. The wound must be kept protected until it is well epithelialized, which may take up to 10 to 12 weeks.

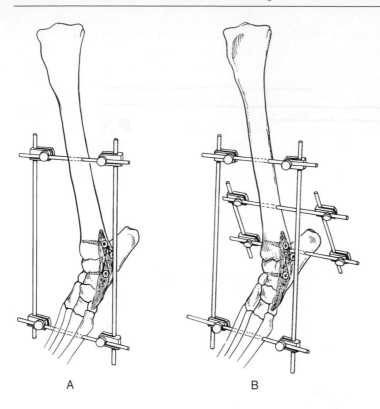

FIGURE 19–5. (*A*) A simple external skeletal fixation splint used to support and protect a medial tarsocrural ligament repair in small breeds. (*B*) A stiffer external fixator frame for support of ligamentous repair in large breeds.

A

B

Prognosis ■   A retrospective study of 98 shearing injuries by Beardsley and Schrader revealed some previously unknown facts regarding the outcome of these cases.[5] All were treated essentially as described above except that none received joint stabilization by means of external fixators; all were supported in some form of external coaptation. Healing time ranged from 2 to 9 weeks, depending on the size and depth of the wound and the amount of the wound that was able to be closed by suture. A mean of 1.7 surgical procedures were performed on each patient, and a mean of 5.5 rechecks were required after hospital discharge. Good to excellent outcome was attained in 91 percent of the dogs, defined as clinically normal or with only minimal functional abnormalities after healing of the injury. Only one case required skin grafting. As can be seen, these are expensive injuries due to the amount of care required, and those owners not prepared for this type care would be well advised to consider amputation as a primary treatment. It is our subjective opinion that support with external fixators simplifies treatment because owners can do more of it at home due to the absence of the coaptation splint, but we do not have data to suggest that it shortens the healing period or affects the final outcome.

Aftercare ■   When granulation tissue completely covers the wound, but not before 3 weeks postoperatively, the external fixator is removed. An elastic support bandage should be maintained for another 3 weeks with very restricted activity. Normal exercise is not allowed until weeks 8 to 12, depending on the stability achieved. Loosening of the bone screws and skin irritation from screw heads are both indications for removing the screws. This should not be done before 3 to 4 months postoperatively if possible. Failure to stabilize the joint adequately will result in degenerative joint disease and poor function. In such a situation arthrodesis offers the best chance of restoring function. See the discussion below regarding arthrodesis.

ARTHRODESIS ■ Some injuries are too extensive to be successfully reconstructed. These are invariably those with extensive bone loss of the medial malleolus, tibial trochlea, and less commonly the condyle of the talus. If the bone loss extends into the articular surface of the tibia there may not be sufficient articular support for the talus. Additionally, the ability to provide sufficient medial ligamentous support is questionable. In this situation, arthrodesis of the talocrural or tarsocrural joint is the best method of maintaining limb function. Although it is possible to attempt reconstruction and then follow with arthrodesis if reconstruction fails, a great deal of time and expense can be wasted.

By the use of external skeletal fixation (see Figs. 19–23 and 19–24A), the arthrodesis can be performed very early, before the wound is healed, with a high probability of successful fusion and a low chance of bone infection. The procedure can be delayed for a few days, until the debridement phase is complete and hopefully some granulation tissue has begun to appear. The tarsus is supported during this phase entirely by the bandage, sometimes augmented by thermomoldable plastic splints or wire frames. If it seems necessary to use the external fixator immediately to support the joint, the fusion is done at the same time. The technique is performed basically as described below in the section Tarsocrural Arthrodesis. The major difference is in the manner of applying the autogenous cancellous bone graft, since there must be sufficient soft tissue available to cover the graft and allow its early vascularization. Exudation is another contraindication to early grafting, as the exudate may physically carry the graft fragments away. In this situation the joint debridement and fixation is completed as usual, but grafting is delayed until there is a healthy granulation tissue bed, without exudation. At that point the granulation tissue is carefully elevated from the joint surfaces sufficiently to allow the graft to be packed into the joint spaces. The area is kept covered by petrolatum-impregnated gauze sponges for several days, until granulation tissue again covers the area. Aftercare from this point onwards is as described above.

Fractures of the Calcaneus

A calcaneal fracture is a very disabling injury because it destroys the ability of the gastrocnemius muscle and the rest of the common calcanean tendon apparatus to prevent hyperflexion of the hock joint, resulting in a plantigrade stance. As a result of muscle tension on the tendons, there is considerable pull on the free fragment and, therefore, marked displacement of the fragment.

Fractures occur most commonly at the tuber or in the shaft (see Figs. 19–7A and 19–8A) and less commonly near the base (see Fig. 19–9A). Because the plantar ligament of the calcaneoquartal part of the proximal intertarsal joint originates at the base of the calcaneus, fractures in this region cause subluxation and hyperextension of this joint (see below for further discussion of tarsal hyperextension). Calcaneal fractures are not uncommon injuries of the racing greyhound and are usually associated with central tarsal (Tc) bone fractures. When there is no accompanying Tc bone fracture there is invariably a plantar proximal intertarsal subluxation.[6]

OPEN APPROACH ■ The calcaneus is exposed by a lateral approach, with medial displacement of the tendon of the superficial digital extensor muscle when tension band wire fixation is employed (Fig. 19–6).

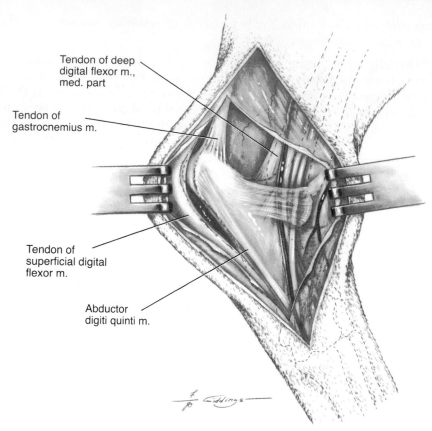

Tendon of deep
digital flexor m.,
med. part

Tendon of
gastrocnemius m.

Tendon of
superficial digital
flexor m.

Abductor
digiti quinti m.

FIGURE 19–6. Approach to the calcaneus from the lateral aspect. The superficial digital flexor tendon has been elevated by incising the retinaculum attaching it to the bone. (From Piermattei DL: An Atlas of Surgical Approaches to the Bones and Joints of the Dog and Cat, 3rd ed. Philadelphia, WB Saunders Co, 1993, p 309, with permission.)

Treatment

The bending loads on the free fragment make conservative treatment with an external cast impossible. Fixation by a Steinmann pin or a screw is very questionable as well because both will usually bend, even with the limb in a splint. Tension band wiring with Kirschner wires is an ideal fixation method in most cases because it allows the bending loads to be converted to compression forces, is applicable to any size animal, is inexpensive, and requires no special equipment. To be successful, however, the cortex opposite the tension band wire must be intact to act as a buttress. For further explanation of the tension band technique, see Figure 2–63.

TENSION BAND WIRE FIXATION ■ Surgical approach by means of a lateral incision to the calcaneus is not complicated. Reduction of the fracture and application of fixation are simplified if the tendon of the superficial digital flexor is freed from the tuber by incision of the lateral retinaculum and retracted medially. The tension band wires must be applied between the tendon and the bone, not superficial to the tendon (Fig. 19–7B, C).

Two methods of application of the tension band are shown. The method shown in Figure 19–7 is the conventional one and is used for fractures of the tuber. It has the disadvantage of creating some irritation of the tendon of the

FIGURE 19-7. (*A*) Fracture of the tuber calcanei. (*B, C*) Two Kirschner wires, 0.045 or 0.062 inch in diameter, placed side by side, as far medially and laterally as possible. Note that the tendon of the superficial digital flexor has been retracted medially. The exact position of the transverse hole for the wire is not critical and is usually at midshaft or slightly distal as shown here.

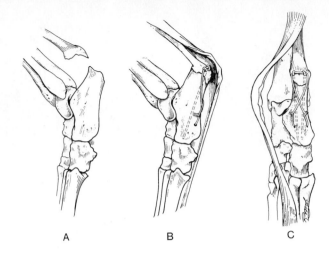

superficial digital flexor as it glides over the tuber. This is minimized by placing the pins as plantarolateral and medial as possible and seating the bent end of the pin close to the bone. Following bone healing, these pins and the wire occasionally must be removed because of soft tissue irritation. The method shown in Figure 19–8 eliminates these problems by countersinking the pin, but it is applicable only to fractures of the shaft or base. Note the option of placing the pins in the sagittal plane shown in Figure 19–8D; this is helpful in small breeds. The stainless steel tension wire must be adequate in size. The following sizes are recommended: up to 15 to 20 pounds, 22 gauge (0.635 mm); 20 to 40 pounds, 20 gauge (0.812 mm); and over 40 pounds, 18 gauge (1.02 mm).

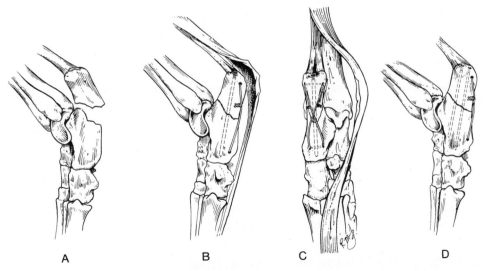

FIGURE 19-8. (*A*) Fracture of the shaft of the calcaneus. (*B, C*) A single Steinmann pin, 5/64 to 1/8 inch in diameter, has been countersunk in the tuber. This pin position allows the wire to be placed through a drill hole in the tuber, which minimizes irritation of the tendon of the superficial digital flexor. A single pin is used when the fracture reduces well and is stable relative to rotation in the reduced position. (*D*) If the fracture line is smooth or slightly comminuted, two smaller countersunk pins or Kirschner wires in the sagittal plane are used because they provide more rotational stability.

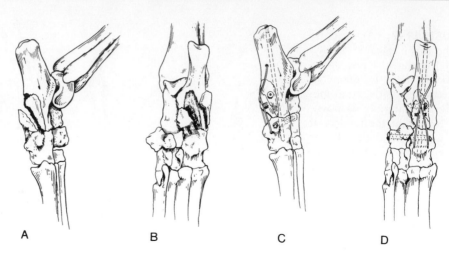

FIGURE 19–9. (*A, B*) Comminuted fracture of the base of the calcaneus. The tarsus hyperextends at this level. Further instability is created by a dorsomedial luxation of the central tarsal bone, a fairly common complication of this type of calcaneal fracture. (*C, D*) The central tarsal bone is reduced first to establish some stability at the proximal intertarsal joint. Fixation is done with a 3.5-mm bone screw through the central tarsal bone into the fourth tarsal bone. This screw is not lagged, but threaded into both bones with the central tarsal held in a reduced position with vulsellum forceps. (For more details, see Figure 19–29). The slab fracture on the lateral side of the calcaneus is lag screwed with a 2.0- or 2.7-mm screw. A ⁵⁄₆₄-inch Steinmann pin is placed in the calcaneus and seated in the fourth tarsal bone. The tension band wire is placed from midshaft in the calcaneus to the plantar tubercle of the fourth tarsal bone, dorsal to the tendon of the superficial digital flexor tendon. The tension band wire holds the second fragment in place. An additional lag screw may be useful in some cases.

TENSION BAND WIRE AND LAG SCREW FIXATION ■   Comminuted fractures involving the base of the calcaneus (Fig. 19–9*A, B*) usually require small lag screws for fixation of the slab-like bone fragments from the distolateral region of the bone, as illustrated in Figure 19–9*C, D*.

BONE PLATE ■   Occasionally, a comminuted fracture requires application of a bone plate, which is best placed laterally. When possible the plate should be supplemented with a tension band wire, placed as shown in Figure 19–8.

Aftercare ■   Generally, external casts are not necessary postoperatively except for severely comminuted fractures. In such cases, a short lateral splint (see Fig. 2–26) is applied for approximately 4 weeks or until some radiographic signs of bone healing are seen. A Robert-Jones bandage may be useful for a few days to minimize soft tissue swelling. Exercise is restricted until clinical union occurs. Prognosis is generally good.

Luxation of the Tendon of the Superficial Digital Flexor Muscle

This muscle and tendon form the most superficial part of the calcanean tendon group, and cross the tuber calcanei as a flat tendon, with a bursa between tendon and bone. The tendon continues distally to split into branches to each toe. Spontaneous rupture of the medial or lateral retinacular insertion of this tendon on the tuber calcanei allows the tendon to luxate medially (Fig. 19–

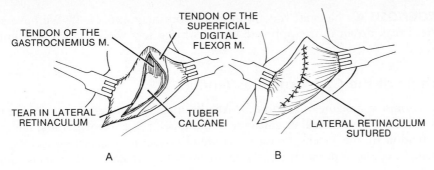

FIGURE 19–10. (A) Medial luxation of the tendon of the superficial digital flexor muscle follows tearing of the lateral retinaculum at the calcaneus. (B) Surgical repair consists of suturing the retinaculum with nonabsorbable suture material.

10A), or more commonly, laterally. The injury is usually associated with vigorous activity and may be caused by rotational force applied to the tendon's insertion on the calcaneus.[7] The medial insertion and retinaculum seems to be less well defined than the lateral and may rupture more easily.[7] Dysplasia of the tuber calcanei has been proposed as either the cause, or contributing to the luxation.[8] The groove of the calcaneus was observed to be shallow or absent, with a distolateral slant in some patients, both of which could lead to instability of the tendon. The sheltie and collie breeds seem overrepresented in our cases. Surgical repair that is made before extensive fibrosis develops is very successful. Chronic tendinitis and bursitis can cause marked changes in the tendon and decrease chances for success.

Clinical Signs

Lameness is not dramatic and may be intermittent. Moderate swelling on either side of the calcaneus can be noted, and a distinct popping sensation will be felt as the hock is flexed and extended. Accompanying bursitis may result in somewhat fluctuant swelling over the tuber calcanei. The tendon can sometimes be palpated in the luxated position and then reduced as the hock is extended. Flexion then results in reluxation.

Surgical Repair

An incision is made along the calcaneus on the side opposite the direction of the luxation, curving from the distal calcanean tendon toward the calcaneus. This approach is similar to that described above for the calcaneus. The bursa is opened and any fibrinous debris removed, and the tendon is reduced. Interrupted nonabsorbable sutures are placed from the edge of the tendon to adjoining retinacular insertion tissue to maintain the tendon in the reduced position (Fig. 19–10B). There may be redundant retinacular tissue due to stretching that can either be imbricated or excised. Because the medial soft tissue available for attachment is often scant, it may be necessary to create another method of attachment of the tendon to the calcaneus. One or two 1.5- to 2.0-mm screws can be inserted in the calcaneus near the tendon edge and sutures from the tendon attached to the screw heads. Alternatively, holes can be drilled through the calcaneus to allow a horizontal mattress pattern placement of sutures through the bone and tendon.[7]

AFTERCARE ■ The lower limb is supported in a short lateral splint (see Fig. 2–26) for 2 weeks, and exercise restricted for 2 to 3 more weeks.

PROGNOSIS ■ Normal function can be routinely expected.[7] We have seen shelties break down in the opposite limb within a few weeks of the first injury.

Avulsion of the Gastrocnemius Tendon

The common calcanean tendon, or Achilles mechanism, consists of three tendons that insert on the tuber calcanei of the talus: the gastrocnemius; the common tendon of the biceps femoris, semitendinosus, and gracilis muscles; and the tendon of the superficial digital flexor muscle. The gastrocnemius tendon is the largest of this group and the most powerful extensor of the tarsocrural joint. It can be avulsed from the tuber by normal activity, without outside trauma.[9] Most injuries develop during running and presumably occur as the animal pushes off the limb with the foot firmly planted. Affected dogs are primarily from the large sporting and working breeds and are usually 5 years of age and up. The Doberman pinscher and labrador retriever breeds seem to be over represented. These facts suggest that degenerative changes in the tendon may play a part in the pathogenesis of this injury, but this is only speculative at this time. Owing to contracture of the muscle, any attempt at nonsurgical treatment will invariably result in permanent deformity. It is necessary to surgically reattach the tendon to the bone to restore function.

Diagnosis

CLINICAL SIGNS ■ The lameness seen with this injury is severe and non–weight-bearing for several days, but within 1 to 2 weeks the animal starts using the leg again. During weight bearing at this time the stifle will be seen to be slightly extended, the tarsocrural (hock) joint moderately flexed, and the digits are flexed. The position of the digits results in a crab-like stance, with the foot resting on the distal ends of the digital pads. Because the superficial digital flexor tendon is intact, it is forced to take a longer course to reach the digits when the hock joint is flexed beyond the normal standing angle. The result is as if the digital flexor muscle was contracted, and so the digits stay flexed during weight bearing. They can easily be manually extended if the tarsocrural joint is extended with the stifle flexed. This is a type 2C injury in the Achilles tendon lesion classification system proposed by Muetstege.[10]

Shortly after the injury, regional edema and pain predominate the physical findings. Later the region becomes engulfed in fibroplasia and the gastrocnemius muscle contracts, pulling the distal end of the tendon proximally. Often, careful palpation will reveal the end of the tendon 2 to 3 cm proximal to the tuber and deep to the superficial digital flexor tendon. The distal end of the tendon mushrooms and becomes very firm on palpation owing to the fibroplasia. Eventually the gap between the tuber and the tendon becomes filled with fibrous tissue and gives the impression during palpation that the tendon is intact. Radiographs are useful at this time in establishing the diagnosis.

RADIOGRAPHIC SIGNS ■ During the acute phase, edema of the soft tissues will be appreciated, and it may be possible to visualize the retracted tendon if soft tissue radiographic technique is used. Small avulsed bone fragments near the tuber calcanei are diagnostic (Fig. 19–11). More chronic cases have visible roughening of the tuber and increased soft tissue density in the region between the tuber and the retracted tendon. Very rarely a large fragment from the tuber calcanei may be seen attached to the retracted tendon.

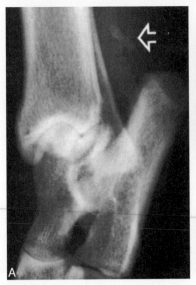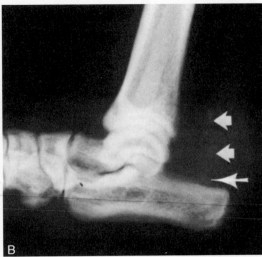

FIGURE 19–11. Avulsion of the tendon of the gastrocnemius muscle at the tuber calcanei. (*A*) A large bone fragment is visible here. The position of the fragment is an indication of how far the tendon has retracted. (*B*) Two avulsed bone fragments are seen with the retracted tendon (*broad arrows*). A roughened area on the tuber calcanei (*narrow arrow*) indicates the area of avulsion. Marked soft tissue density in the area suggests a chronic course.

Surgical Repair

A lateral paramedian approach is made over the distal tendon and tuber calcanei. Proximally the superficial digital flexor tendon is separated from the gastrocnemius tendon and its lateral retinacular insertion on the calcaneus is incised to allow medial retraction of the tendon (see the discussion above regarding reluxation of the tendon of the superficial digital flexor muscle). In acute injuries the avulsed end of the gastrocnemius tendon will be immediately evident (Fig. 19–12*A*). The tendon is debrided to create a smooth end for suturing. In chronic cases considerable debridement is necessary to free the tendon and tuber from the fibroplasia. The tuber should be cleared of all tissue prior to suturing and the tendinous end should be resected proximally until normal tendinous tissue is identified. With moderate tension it should be possible to bring the cut end into apposition with the tuber when the stifle and hock joints are at normal standing angles. Medial and lateral bone tunnels are drilled from the center of the tuber toward the medial and lateral cortices (Fig. 19–12*B, C*). These holes should emerge in an area where they will not interfere with gliding of the superficial digital flexor tendon. Alternatively, these tunnels can be drilled transversely through the calcaneus. Locking-loop sutures are placed medially and laterally in the tendon. Suture material should be large, size 0–2, and preferably monofilament nylon, polybutester, or polypropylene for ease of handling in the tendon. Braided polyester is also acceptable, but monofilament stainless steel wire should be avoided, as it will quickly fracture owing to movement in this area. One end of each suture is then passed through a bone tunnel, the hock is extended and the stifle flexed to relax the gastrocnemius, and each suture is tied over the bone to its opposite end. The lateral retinaculum of the superficial digital flexor tendon is sutured and the remaining tissues are closed in layers.

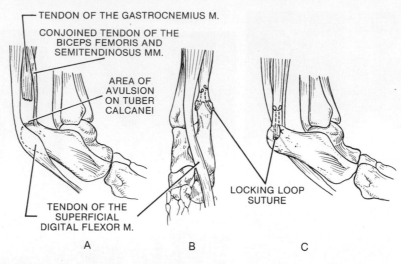

FIGURE 19–12. (*A*) Avulsion of the tendon of the gastrocnemius muscle from the tuber calcanei. Note that the tendon of the superficial digital flexor muscle and the conjoined tendons of the biceps femoris and semitendinosus muscles are intact and partially support the tarsocrural joint. (*B, C*) The tendon of the gastrocnemius muscle is reattached to the tuber calcanei with locking-loop sutures (see Fig. 7–1) of size 0–2 nonabsorbable suture secured through bone tunnels in the calcaneus.

In the event of a large bone fragment from the tuber being attached to the tendon, it may be possible to reattach this by the pins and tension band wire technique shown in Figure 19–7.[11]

AFTERCARE ■   A short leg cylinder cast (see Fig. 2–22) or lateral splint (see Fig. 2–26) is applied for 6 weeks. Alternatively, an external fixator, such as in Figure 19–5, could be used if there was difficulty in maintaining a coaptation device. It is not necessary to immobilize the stifle joint. The splint is followed by a Robert-Jones bandage for 7 to 10 days. Exercise is severely restricted until 8 weeks postoperatively, then slowly increased to normal at 12 weeks.

PROGNOSIS ■   Very good function has been obtained in our cases and has been reported by others.[9,11] Considerable periosteal bony proliferation of the tuber has been seen in some animals, but this abates and remodels with time and does not cause permanent changes.

Chronic Calcanean/Achilles Tendinitis

Chronic swelling of the common calcanean tendon just proximal to the tuber calcanei is seen occasionally in large-breed dogs. There is increased flexion of the digits, as described above for avulsion of the gastrocnemius tendon, and there may be pain with forced extension of the toes, but there is no increase in tarsocrural flexion. Lameness is variable but is usually slight to none. This may represent chronic tendinitis of the superficial digital flexor tendon, or perhaps a grade II strain injury (see Chapter 7) of the gastrocnemius tendon.

Treatment consists of resting the tendon by immobilizing the tarsocrural joint. This can be accomplished by coaptation such as a short-leg cylinder cast (see Fig. 2–22), or a lateral splint (see Fig. 2–26). Alternatively, an external fixator, such as in Figure 19–5, could be used if there was difficulty in maintaining a coaptation device. Immobilization is maintained for 6 to 8 weeks.

Osteochondritis Dissecans of the Talus

Osteochondritis dissecans (OCD) occurs in the same canine population as do the other manifestations of osteochondrosis, although the Rottweiler, labrador retriever, and bull mastiff are overrepresented (see Chapter 6). The disease may be bilateral and may affect either the medial (most common) or lateral ridge of the talus, where it is most commonly seen in the Rottweiler.[12] The cartilage flap usually contains bone since, unlike OCD of the shoulder, elbow, and stifle, the flap usually remains connected to and vascularized by the synovial membrane, allowing endochondral ossification to progress.

Surgical treatment of OCD of the talus is controversial, with conflicting results reported in the literature. In one study, surgical treatment resulted in a worse score for function and radiographic changes 16 to 79 months postoperatively (blinded assessments) than did nonsurgical treatment in another series of cases (11 dogs, 17 joints: 11 surgical, 6 nonsurgical).[13] All dogs had significant degenerative joint disease clinically and radiographically. Another study, involving 12 cases with a mean follow-up of 52 months, found that only 25 percent had attained full function postsurgically, and that osteoarthritic changes had progressed in all joints.[14] Despite these apparently discouraging figures for surgical treatment, Montgomery and co-workers[15] pointed out that of 98 treated joints (74 surgical, 24 nonsurgical) with treatment response reported in the literature, 39 percent of the surgically treated were free of lameness versus 8 percent of the nonsurgical. Some degree of lameness persisted in 57 percent of surgical cases, and in 79 percent of nonsurgical, while severe lameness was reported in 4 percent of surgical and 13 percent of nonsurgical cases. They concluded that surgical treatment was preferable to conservative treatment.

Early surgical removal (4 to 6 months of age) of the semidetached cartilage flap is essential for best results.[13] Each month that goes by decreases the chances of good results because of the progress of degenerative joint disease. Dogs older than 1 year at surgery have a poor prognosis and should probably be treated conservatively. Animals with severe lameness of short duration may have a poorer prognosis than those with less severe and slower development of lameness.[13] Degenerative joint disease may progress after surgery because of instability or incongruity of the joint following removal of a large flap. If the flap is large enough to be reattached, every effort should be made to do so in order to minimize postoperative instability. Early surgery increases the probability of being able to do this.

Diagnosis

Diagnosis of OCD is based on finding caudomedial and/or caudolateral tarsocrural joint swelling and effusion in appropriate breeds with a history of lameness beginning after 4.5 months of age, and appropriate radiographic signs.

CLINICAL SIGNS ■ Hindlimb lameness is characterized by a shortened stride. Often there is hyperextension at the tarsocrural joint. Caudomedial or caudolateral (less common) joint effusion is seen early, and thickening of the tarsus on the medial aspect of the joint develops later as degenerative changes progress within the joint; these are consistent signs. Less effusion and soft tissue changes are appreciated when the lateral ridge of the talus is involved. Pain may be manifested on flexion and extension of the joint, which may also show a decreased range of motion in flexion. Crepitus is occasionally present.

RADIOGRAPHIC SIGNS ■ Radiographs in the extended dorsoplantar and flexed lateral position will reveal a defect in the medial ridge of the trochlea

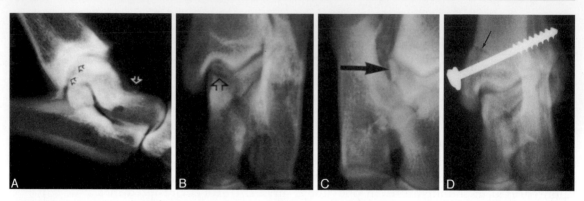

FIGURE 19–13. Osteochondritis dissecans of the talus. (A) In this chronic case many signs of degenerative joint disease are present, such as osteophytes and subchondral sclerosis. Note the flattening of the ridge of the talus (*black arrows*) and the free osteochondral fragment within the joint (*white arrow*); lateromedial view. (B) A large fragment can be seen on the medial ridge of the talus in this craniocaudal-lateromedial oblique view. (C) A displaced fragment of the lateral ridge of the talus is visualized in this caudocranial-mediolateral oblique view. (D) Postsurgical view after removal of a fragment from the medial ridge. Note the precise reduction of the malleolar osteotomy due to predrilling the lag screw hole before performing the osteotomy.

(Figs. 19–13A, B and 19–14). A dorsolateral-plantaromedial 45 degree oblique view in full extension further outlines the medial ridge of the talus. Increased joint space is often seen, and free ossicles may also be seen occasionally. Mediolateral views may show flattening of the dome of the talus. Lateral lesions are much more difficult to demonstrate owing to the superimposition of the calcaneus in conventional craniocaudal views. The dorsal 45 degree lateral-plantaromedial view (Fig. 19–13C) is usually helpful in outlining the lateral trochlear ridge.[12] A flexed dorsoplantar view has also been proposed for outlining the trochlear ridges without summation from the calcaneus.[16] With the dog in dorsal recumbency, the calcaneus is elevated from the table to allow the x-ray beam to be parallel to the metatarsus and capture a skyline view of the talar ridges. Changes are often subtle in lateral lesions, and arthrography or computed tomography (CT) scanning may be needed for a definitive diagnosis.

SURGICAL TECHNIQUE ■   For lesions of the medial ridge a medial approach to the joint is made with arthrotomies proximal and distal to the collateral ligament.[1] Synovial incision lateral to the deep digital flexor tendon allows medial retraction of the tendon to permit visualization of the caudomedial part of the joint.[17] If exposure is inadequate owing to lesion size or position, the medial

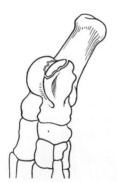

FIGURE 19–14. Osteochondritis dissecans lesion on the medial ridge of the talus. The lesion can be located anywhere on the ridge but is most likely to be centrally placed, as here, or more proximally.

malleolus can be osteotomized. Accurate reduction of the malleolar fragment is essential to minimizing postoperative degenerative joint disease due simply to this intra-articular osteotomy. Predrilling and tapping a screw hole before osteotomy helps ensure accurate reduction and fixation of the malleolus (Fig. 19–13D). The exposure provided by osteotomy allows inspection and removal of dislodged cartilage fragments that become adherent to the fibrotic synovial membrane in the medial collateral ligament area. An approach distal to the collateral ligament can be made to the lateral ridge, where lesions are more commonly located on the distal part, near the body of the talus. If the lesion cannot be fixed in place, the loose cartilage fragment is removed and minimal curettage is performed, in order to minimize the amount of instability produced. There is evidence that some lateral lesions may actually be traumatic osteochondral fractures.[18] If large enough, these lesions may lend themselves to fixation as explained below; small fragments are excised.

Because the tendon sheath of the deep digital flexor is confluent with the tarsocrural joint, free cartilage fragments can escape proximally into the sheath. In this situation they can in some cases be "milked" distally into the joint. Failing this the tendon sheath must be opened proximally.

AFTERCARE ■ A padded bandage is maintained for 2 weeks, and normal exercise is not allowed until 4 to 6 weeks postoperatively.

PROGNOSIS ■ Although the argument over surgical versus conservative treatment remains open, the message is clear: Surgical treatment must be done early, and the lesion must be small for surgical treatment to be worthwhile. In any case the prognosis is not encouraging, and the owner should be forewarned regarding long-term function of the dog.

Fractures of the Talus

Fractures of this bone may be intra-articular, involving either the medial or the lateral ridge of the trochlea (Figs. 19–15 and 19–16), or may be extra-articular in the neck (Fig. 19–17), the body, or the base (Fig. 19–18). Fractures of the ridges, especially the lateral, are difficult to visualize radiographically. Dorsolateral oblique views in both flexion and extension are most useful. See the discussion above for diagnosis of OCD of the talus for further discussion of radiographic views. Lameness is severe, and there is generally some effusion

FIGURE 19–15. (A) Fracture of the medial ridge of the talus. (B) Medial malleolus osteotomized and reflected to allow placement of two Kirschner wires, which are countersunk beneath the surface of the articular cartilage. Alternatively, 1.5- or 2-mm screws could be used. The malleolus is replaced by the pin and tension band wire technique (see Fig. 2–63).

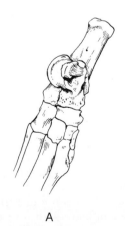
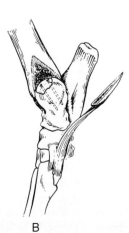

A   B

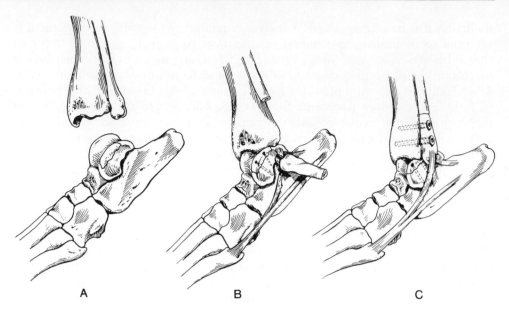

FIGURE 19–16. (*A*) Fracture of the lateral ridge of the talus. (*B*) The fibula is osteotomized 1.5 to 2 cm from the tip of the malleolus, dissected free from the tibia, and rotated caudally or distally on the intact short part of the collateral ligament. (See Fig. 19–3 for more detail.) It is necessary to cut a short ligament between the tibia and fibula to reflect the fibula. When the foot is supinated (rolled inward), the fracture can be visualized. It is fixed by two or three Kirschner wires countersunk beneath the articular cartilage. Alternatively, 1.5- or 2-mm screws could be used. (*C*) The fibula is attached by two lag screws, small pins, or Kirschner wires. The small cut ligament is not sutured. *Note*: If exposure of the caudal portion of the condyle is essential, the short collateral ligament is cut close to the fibula. It is reattached with a suture that engages the ligament and is then passed medial to lateral through two drill holes in the malleolus and tied on the lateral side.

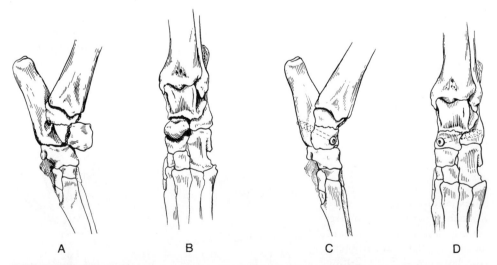

FIGURE 19–17. (*A, B*) Fracture of neck of talus with typical luxation of body and base. (*C, D*) Reduction is obtained by flexion and lateral bending at the proximal intertarsal joint and is maintained with vulsellum forceps. A 3.5- or 4.0-mm screw (shown here) is used in average- to large-size breeds. It is not essential that this screw be lagged if the bone is properly reduced and held in place with forceps.

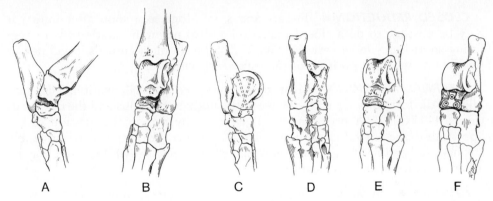

A   B   C   D   E   F

FIGURE 19–18. (*A, B*) Fracture through the body of the talus. (*C–E*) Kirschner wires are crossed in the bone. The proximal pin must be cut close to the bone to avoid irritation of the deep digital flexor tendon. (*F*) T-plates of the 1.5-, 2-, and 2.7-mm series can be used in some cases. Here, a 2.7-mm plate has been cut to fit the bone. Because only one screw is placed in the proximal fragment, external support is essential.

in the joint. Severely comminuted fractures may require arthrodesis (see below). The etiology is usually obscure but may involve a fall or jump. Prognosis for intra-articular fractures is variable, depending on the accuracy of reduction of the fracture. Moderate to severe degenerative joint disease is common following these injuries. The prognosis is good for neck and body fractures.

Fracture of the Trochlear Ridges

INTERNAL FIXATION ■ These fractures are generally stabilized by 0.035- or 0.045-inch (0.9 to 1.2-mm) Kirschner wires that are countersunk beneath the articular surface. Lag screw fixation is preferable, but the fragments are often too small; when fragment size permits, 1.5- and 2.0-mm screws can be used. The screw heads may be countersunk beneath the cartilage surface when used in an articulating area. Fractures of the medial ridge (see Fig. 19–15) are approached by incision of the joint capsule proximal and distal to the collateral ligament (see discussion above regarding OCD of the talus) when possible. Osteotomy of the medial malleolus of the tibia gives much better visualization, but is a second choice due to the morbidity (degenerative joint disease) that accompanies this procedure. Nevertheless, it is often the only way of accessing the joint for fixation. In the same way, the lateral ridge is approached by osteotomy of the distal fibula (see Fig. 19–16) to allow maximum exposure of the lateral side if simple arthrotomy is not sufficient.

Aftercare ■ A lateral splint (see Fig. 2–26) is placed on the lower limb for 4 weeks, followed by a support bandage for 2 weeks. Exercise is restricted for 8 to 12 weeks.

Prognosis ■ The outlook ranges from poor to good, depending on the exactness of reduction and stability achieved. Degenerative joint disease is the sequela when this joint fracture does not heal perfectly, but may ensue regardless of exact reduction and good stability.

Fracture of the Talar Neck

A fracture of the talar neck (Fig. 19–17A, B) is usually accompanied by luxation of the body of the bone, the fracture surface rotating dorsally and distally.

CLOSED REDUCTION ■ In cats and small dogs seen soon after injury, it may be possible to do a closed reduction and to maintain fixation by a snug-fitting short-leg cylinder cast (see Fig. 2–22), but in most animals it will not be possible to maintain position of the fragments with a cast.

INTERNAL FIXATION ■ Most animals require internal fixation, best supplied in the form of a lag screw between the body of the talus and the calcaneus (Fig. 19–17C, D). A neck fracture is exposed by proximal extension of the approach to the central tarsal bone.[1] The 3.5-mm cortical screw is considerably stronger in bending than the 4.0-mm cancellous screw shown here and may be a better choice in this application.

Aftercare ■ Because the lag screw crosses the tarsal sinus (a gap between the calcaneus and talus), it is somewhat subject to bending with early weight bearing; the screw is thus best protected by a short lateral splint (see Fig. 2–26) for 4 weeks. Exercise is restricted for 8 to 12 weeks.

Prognosis ■ Good long-term function is expected in this injury.

Fracture of the Talar Body

In these cases (Fig. 19–18A, B), the base of the talus does not luxate, but there is a slight subluxation of the talocalcaneal joint.

INTERNAL FIXATION ■ Fixation is usually by means of multiple Kirschner wires because the neck of the bone is often too small to accommodate a lag screw. Ideally, two wires are crossed in the bone (Fig. 19–18C, D, E). In some cases, bone plates can be used for fixation. T-plates of the 1.5-, 2.0-, and 2.7-mm series can be adapted to this fracture and provide relatively good stability (Fig. 19–18F). The bone is approached by a combination of the approaches to the medial malleolus and the central tarsal bone.[1]

Aftercare ■ Neither fixation is very rigid and both should be protected for 4 to 6 weeks postoperatively by a short lateral splint (see Fig. 2–26). Exercise is restricted for 8 to 12 weeks.

Prognosis ■ Good long-term function is expected in this injury.

Luxation of the Base of the Talus

This is an infrequent but very disabling injury (Fig. 19–19A) that is difficult to repair if it is not diagnosed early. Surgical stabilization is quite successful and is indicated in most animals, but closed reduction and casting have been satisfactory in cats and small dogs.

Diagnosis

Considerable swelling and deformity of the proximodorsal tarsus is evident, with lameness typified by the animal's carrying the leg. Because of possible concurrent damage of the insertion of the medial collateral ligament, the tarsus should be evaluated for medial instability. Radiographs are necessary to confirm the diagnosis.

Internal Fixation

The bone is exposed by a proximal extension of the approach to the central tarsal bone.[1] The base of the talus can be reduced after the proximal intertarsal joint is opened by flexion and lateral (varus) stress on the metatarsus. A posi-

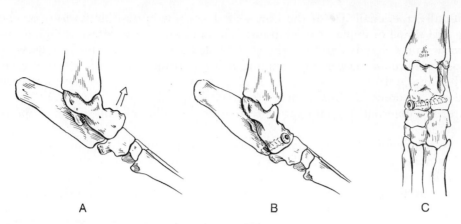

FIGURE 19–19. Luxation of the talus. (*A*) The base of the talus luxates dorsally. There may also be injury to the insertion of the medial collateral ligament. (*B*, *C*) A positional screw is placed distally in the talus to avoid the tarsal sinus. The screw is driven into the calcaneus.

tional screw is placed between the talus and calcaneus and is placed as distally as possible in the talus to avoid crossing the tarsal sinus (Fig. 19–19*B*, *C*). If medial instability remains at the talocentral joint, joint cartilage of the calcaneocentral joint is debrided, and a second bone screw is placed in the medial side of the central tarsal bone. Stainless steel wire is placed around the head of both screws and tightened, similar to the procedure illustrated for distal intertarsal instability in Figure 19–34*D* and *E*.

AFTERCARE ■ A short lateral splint (see Fig. 2–26) is applied and maintained for 4 weeks. Exercise is limited through the eighth postoperative week.

Talocrural Arthrodesis

Indications for arthrodesis of the hock joint are not uncommon in small animal practice under these circumstances:

1. Severe shearing injury.
2. Degenerative joint disease (most commonly due to OCD).
3. Chronic instability or hyperextension.
4. Comminuted intra-articular fractures.
5. Irreparable injury of the calcanean tendon apparatus.
6. Sciatic nerve palsy when combined with transposition of the long digital extensor tendon.[19]

Assuming there are no disease conditions of the hip or stifle, function of the fused limb is satisfactory. These joints must flex more than normal to compensate for fusion at the hock level, and if they do not function normally, the leg will be circumducted markedly during the forward swing phase of gait. As with all arthrodeses, additional strain is placed on adjacent joints and may lead to degenerative joint disease, particularly in the more distal tarsal joints. For this reason, pantarsal arthrodesis is receiving increased attention as a substitute for talocrural arthrodesis.[20,21]

Surgical fusion of the talocrural joint is a severe challenge to the surgeon because of the magnitude and orientation of the forces of weight bearing. Additionally, the small size of the bones of the tarsus impose limitations on the size and shape of implants used in internal fixation. Failure rates, as high as 50 percent in our hands[22] and in others[20] have led us to be much more aggressive in using more and larger implants and in supporting them with external casts and splints until fusion is certain. It also seems useful to cross the joint with one of the screws or pins in order to neutralize shear forces. Lag screw, bone plate, and external skeletal fixation techniques are all applicable when properly executed.

The talar and tibial articular surfaces can be prepared either by osteotomy with a bone saw (Fig. 19–20A), or by curettage manually or with a high-speed bur (Fig. 19–20B). Osteotomy by saw provides a flat surface that is more stable relative to bending shear forces, but makes rotational alignment more difficult.

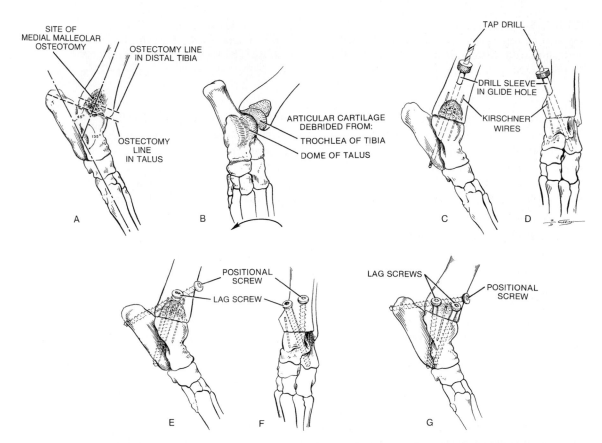

FIGURE 19–20. Arthrodesis of the tarsocrural joint by screw fixation. (A) The angle chosen here for the fusion is 135 degrees. The complementary angle of 45 degrees also describes the angle to be cut through the talus, since the tibia is best cut 90 degrees to its axis. The joint is exposed medially by a malleolar osteotomy.[1] (B) An alternative method of removing articular cartilage involves debridement with a power bur or curettes, following the normal contour of the articular surface. (C, D) Temporary fixation is obtained by two Kirschner wires placed across the joint at an angle. A 4.5-mm (or 3.5-mm) glide hole has been drilled, and the 3.2-mm (or 2.0-mm) tap drill is inserted through a drill sleeve. The drill penetrates the plantarolateral cortex of the calcaneus near its base. (E, F) The hole is tapped and a screw of appropriate length and diameter is inserted. A second hole is drilled from the cranial aspect of the distal tibia into the tuber calcanei with a tap drill sized for the screw diameter selected. Soft tissue in the space between the distal tibia and calcaneus must be protected. *Both* bones are tapped and the screw inserted. (G) In dogs over 10 kg body weight it is preferable to insert two screws across the joint. In this situation a single Kirschner wire is placed between the screws.

Reference K-wires can be placed in the tibia and tarsus to help realign the parts before fixation is applied.

Screw Fixation

Single lag screw fixation is suitable only for cats and dogs under 8 to 10 kg body weight. All others should receive two or three screws. The joint is approached medially by malleolar osteotomy.[1] The malleolus and medial collateral ligaments are detached, and the bone is cut into very small chips with a rongeur to be used as bone graft to supplement autogenous cancellous bone from the proximal tibia. The functional angle for dogs is typically between 135 and 145 degrees; in cats it is 115 to 125 degrees. This angle should be carefully checked in the opposite limb preoperatively. In Figure 19–20A, the angle chosen is 135 degrees; the complementary angle is 45 degrees. Since it is most convenient to cut the distal tibia at 90 degrees to its long axis, the talus is cut at a 45-degree angle to the axis of the tarsus-metatarsus. Considerable bone must be removed from the tibia because of the depth of the cochlea. The cartilage can also be removed with power burs, curettes, or rongeurs by following the bony contours (Fig. 19–20B). In some cases the fibula will prevent apposition of the tibia and talus after bone and cartilage removal and it may be necessary to resect the lateral malleolus or perform a short supramalleolar ostectomy of the fibula through a separate short lateral incision.

Initial fixation and rotational alignment is obtained by two Kirschner wires driven across the contact surfaces in a plantarolateral direction (Fig. 19–20C). Drilling for the lag screw can then proceed without motion of the contact surfaces. Screws of 4.5 mm are appropriate for animals of 15 to 18 kg or larger, and 3.5-mm screws are ideal for smaller animals. Full-threaded screws are preferred because of their ease of removal and greater strength. The glide hole is drilled in the tibia first (Fig. 19–20C, D). The tap hole is then drilled through the talus and calcaneus. Placement of 4.5-mm screws is illustrated in Figure 19–20. The glide hole is started at a point on the tibia 2 to 2.5 cm from the end of the bone and at an angle of 15 to 20 degrees from the tibial sagittal plane. The hole is measured with the depth gauge and is tapped, and a screw of appropriate length is inserted and tightened (Fig. 19–20E, F). An alternate technique consists of drilling the 3.2-mm tap hole first, then enlarging the tibial hole with the 4.5-mm glide drill. A second hole is drilled from the cranial aspect of the distal tibia into the tuber calcanei with a tap drill sized for the screw diameter selected. Soft tissue in the space between the distal tibia and calcaneus must be protected. *Both* bones are tapped and the screw is inserted. This positional screw protects the lag screw from bending loads. In dogs over 10 kg body weight it is preferable to insert two screws across the joint (Fig. 19–20G). In this situation a single Kirschner wire is placed between the two screws. Autogenous cancellous bone graft (Chapter 3) is packed into and around the contact surfaces. The Kirschner wires are left in place.

Aftercare ■ External support is *imperative* to prevent bending loads on the screws. A short lateral splint or cylinder cast (see Figs. 2–26 and 2–22) is maintained for 6 to 8 weeks, or until radiographic signs of fusion are evident. Exercise is severely restricted until radiographic fusion is complete, then slowly increased to return to normal 6 weeks later. Implants should be removed routinely about 6 months postoperatively. Because of bending loads exerted on the fusion site, micromotion eventually results in screw loosening or breakage, which causes irritation and pain. Fully threaded screws are more easily removed than are partially threaded cancellous screws.

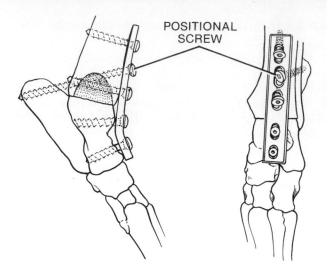

FIGURE 19–21. Talocrural arthrodesis with a cranially placed bone plate is possible if one screw is placed through the plate and into the calcaneus to act as a positional screw. All four cortices are tapped. Care must be taken to avoid extending the plate beyond the proximal intertarsal joint.

Bone Plate Fixation

Talocrural arthrodesis with a *cranially* placed bone plate is possible if one screw is placed through the plate and into the calcaneus to act as a positional screw (Fig. 19–21). All four cortices are tapped, as the purpose of this screw is to prevent bending loads on the plate. Care must be taken to avoid extending the plate beyond the proximal intertarsal joint. Autogenous cancellous bone graft (Chapter 3) is packed around the arthrodesis site before closing the soft tissues.

Talocrural arthrodesis with a *laterally* placed straight plate (Fig. 19–22) is possible with a plate that allows a large number of screws per unit of length, such as the Veterinary Cuttable Plate (VCP) (Synthes Ltd. [USA], Paoli, PA). Because the plate is loaded on edge, it is very resistant to the bending loads of

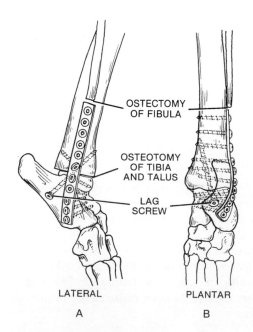

OSTECTOMY
OF FIBULA

OSTEOTOMY
OF TIBIA
AND TALUS

LAG
SCREW

LATERAL

A

PLANTAR

B

FIGURE 19–22. Talocrural arthrodesis with a laterally placed plate is possible only with a plate that allows a large number of screws per unit of length, such as the AO/ASIF Veterinary Cuttable Plate (Synthes Ltd. [USA], Paoli, PA). Here, a 1.5-mm thick plate and 2.7-mm screws are used, following the method of Sumner-Smith and Kuzma.[23] At least one screw must cross the joint as a lag screw, to provide compression at the arthrodesis site. The distal one third of the fibula is resected to allow lateral placement of the plate, which is molded around the calcaneus distally.

this joint. Despite this mechanical advantage, such techniques have not been satisfactory in the past owing to inability to place a sufficient number of screws distal to the arthrodesis site. The VCP solves this difficulty by the number of screw holes available. Additionally, the plates are available in both 1- and 1.5-mm thickness and can be stacked to increase their thickness and stiffness. In Figure 19–22 a 1.5-mm thick plate and 2.7-mm screws are used, following the method of Sumner-Smith and Kuzma.[23] The distal one third of the fibula is resected, and the joint surfaces are prepared as in Figure 19–20. A lag screw (3.5- to 4.5-mm diameter) is placed across the joint to provide compression at the arthrodesis site, from the calcaneus distally, through the talus, and into the tibia proximally (Fig. 19–22A). Drilling the glide hole from the talus to the calcaneus before reduction ensures accurate placement of this hole. In small breeds, the lag screw may be passed from the distal plate hole.

The plate is molded to the tibia and around the calcaneus distally, where a sharp bend and slight twist are necessary to fit the bone closely. Screw placement starts distally with two screws in the calcaneus. The next screw is placed in the distal tibia and is positioned eccentrically in the plate hole to provide compression. Two more screws are similarly placed in the tibia, taking care to avoid the lag screw. The rest of the screws are placed in the center of the plate holes, and the lag screw is retightened. Autogenous cancellous bone graft (Chapter 3) is packed around the arthrodesis site before closing the tissues.

A second method of lateral plating involves the use of a reconstruction plate (Synthes Ltd. [USA], Paoli, PA). These plates can be curved on the flat dimension to follow the curvature from the tibia to the tarsus (see Fig. 19–24B). The illustration shows application for pantarsal arthrodesis; for talocrural arthrodesis the plate would be shortened to extend only to the distal end of the calcaneus. Lag screw fixation across the talocrural joint is accomplished as described above for the cuttable plate.

Aftercare ■ External support is *imperative* to prevent bending loads on the screws. A short lateral splint or cylinder cast (see Figs. 2–26 and 2–22) is maintained for 6 to 8 weeks, or until radiographic signs of fusion are evident. Exercise is severely restricted until radiographic fusion is complete, then slowly increased to return to normal 6 weeks later. Implants should be removed routinely about 6 months postoperatively. Because of bending loads exerted on the fusion site, micromotion eventually results in screw loosening or breakage, which causes irritation and pain. Fully threaded screws are more easily removed than are partially threaded cancellous screws.

External Skeletal Fixator

Fixation by means of the external fixator (Fig. 19–23) is particularly applicable to open or shearing injuries of the hock. Open luxation with comminuted fractures of the tibial trochlea or condyles of the talus is also a relatively common injury best treated by arthrodesis. Minimal metal at the area of contamination lessens infection problems, and all the metal can easily be removed. Because of the morbidity associated with the prolonged casting/splinting needed for the procedures described above, the external fixator has become the method of choice in our hands. A variety of configurations are useful, depending on patient size. Mechanical studies of transarticular fixators are lacking, so their application is more art than science. In all methods the contact surfaces are prepared as already described after adequate soft tissue debridement (see Fig. 19–20A).

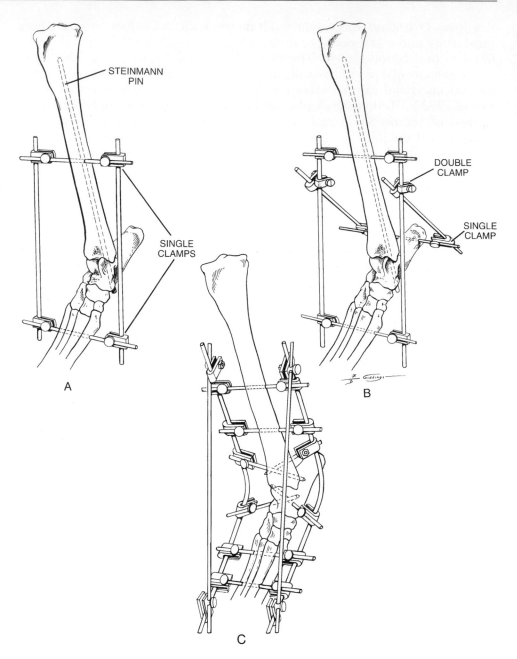

FIGURE 19–23. Arthrodesis of the talocrural joint by external skeletal fixation. (*A*) The joint surfaces are prepared as in Figure 19–20*A* or *B*. A Steinmann pin is driven from the calcaneus into the proximal tibia with the joint at the selected angle. Transfixation pins are driven through the tibia and metatarsal bones. These pins are connected with bilateral rods secured by single clamps. (*B*) Additional stability in large dogs is provided by a second transfixation pin in the calcaneus. This pin is connected to the first set of connecting rods with single clamps distally and double clamps proximally. (*C*) When no intramedullary pin is used, a more rigid frame is used to prevent bending loads at the arthrodesis site. One of the easier methods is shown here, using a curved connecting rod to eliminate the need for double clamps. Using half pins for the middle sets of fixation pins simplifies the problem of fitting the pins to the connecting rods on both sides when drill guides are not available. At least one of the fixation pins should cross the tarsocrural joint to neutralize shear forces.

TYPE II FIXATOR AND STEINMANN PIN ▪ A Steinmann pin is driven through the calcaneus and talus into the distal tibia with the joint at the desired angle (Fig. 19–23A). If the pin follows the medullary canal, it is driven into the proximal metaphyseal region. If the pin penetrates the tibial cortex, it is driven completely through the cortex. The pin is cut about 1 cm from the calcaneus and left protruding through the skin. An alternative method consists of driving the pin from the proximal tibia as described for fracture repair in Chapter 18. After penetrating the calcaneus, the pin is pulled from the distal end until the proximal end is below the proximal articular surface of the tibia and cut distally. Centrally threaded positive-thread-profile transfixation pins are driven through the tibia and through the bases of the metatarsals. These pins are connected by single clamps and connecting rods in small dogs and cats (Fig. 19–23A). A large autogenous cancellous bone graft taken from the proximal tibia will significantly speed healing and can be used in a contaminated site. Fixation can be made even more rigid in larger breeds (10 to 20 kg) by placing a transfixation pin through the calcaneus, and connecting it with double clamps to the proximal ends of the other connecting rods (Fig. 19–23B). Double clamps can be avoided by using single clamps outboard of the tibial fixation pin clamps.

TYPE IIB FIXATOR ▪ In larger breeds over 20 kg, a more rigid frame is used to neutralize bending loads at the arthrodesis site. One of the easier methods is shown in Figure 19–23C, using curved connecting rods, which are prepared to the desired angle of the joint as described above. Using half pins for the middle sets of fixation pins simplifies the problem of fitting the pins to the connecting rods on both sides. At least one of the fixation half pins should cross the talocrural joint to control shearing motion at the arthrodesis site. Three half pins each side of the joint can be substituted for the second full pin as illustrated in Figure 19–24A, which simplifies application. The use of double clamps can be avoided by using single clamps attached outboard of the proximal and distal pin clamps.

Aftercare ▪ Healing of the arthrodesis will be slow in the case of open injuries and fixation may need to be maintained for 10 to 12 weeks or until

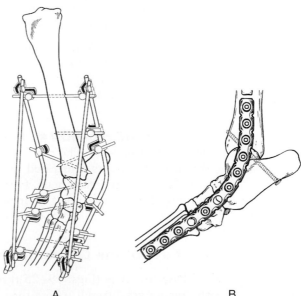

FIGURE 19–24. Pantarsal arthrodesis. (A) The type IIB external fixator used for tarsocrural arthrodesis (Fig. 19–23C) has been extended to place fixation pins in the central and fourth tarsal bones. Also note that all the fixation pins except the proximal and distal are half pins, which simplifies construction of the frame. (B) The reconstruction plate can be contoured on edge to follow the curvature of the lateral aspect of the tibia and tarsus. The distal fibula is ostectomized as in Figure 19–22 to allow good contact of the plate with the tibia.

A

B

radiographic signs of fusion are present. Closed cases generally show radiographic fusion by 8 to 10 weeks. Exercise should be restricted to the house, a small pen, or a leash until the apparatus is removed. The transfixation pins are removed when good fusion is present, but Steinmann pins can be left in place for several months to absorb some of the bending stress on the arthrodesis during the remodeling phase of bone healing.

Pantarsal Arthrodesis

We have noted that some dogs with apparently successful talocrural fusion do not return to full function. In many of these, no specific reason for the decreased function has been found, but in some cases progressive degenerative joint disease of the more distal tarsal joints has been documented.[20,21] Because the talocrural joint is the site of most motion in the tarsus, when it is fused the other joints are subjected to increased functional loads that they are not designed to accommodate. Chronic sprain injury to the ligaments as well as degenerative joint disease may well account for the functional problems observed. For this reason pantarsal arthrodesis may well be a better solution to talocrural problems, just as carpal panarthrodesis has yielded better function than antebrachiocarpal arthrodesis. Gorse and co-workers found a tendency for better function with panarthrodesis than with lag screw fixation of the talocrural joint.[21]

Surgical Techniques

The basic preparation of the talocrural joint and establishing the angle of the joint are carried out as described above. The additional consideration is curettage of articular cartilage in the other joints involved and the additional fixation required to immobilize them. Although the small joints of the tarsus do not require as thorough debridement as do the large joints, nonetheless bony bridging will progress more surely if most cartilage is removed. It is difficult to get curettes into the small joints, and if high-speed power burs are not available, several passes with a powered twist drill will suffice. The intertarsal joints often fuse spontaneously when they are bridged by a screw or pin, but the transverse joints require more preparation. The curettage is done primarily from the dorsal, medial, and lateral aspects, leaving the large plantar ligaments intact. Multiple incisions may be necessary to approach all the joints.[1]

EXTERNAL FIXATOR ■   Perhaps the simplest method of fixation is the type IIB fixator (Fig. 19–24A). This is essentially the same device shown in Figure 19–23C for talocrural arthrodesis, modified to place fixation pins in the central and fourth tarsal bones. Aftercare is as described above for talocrural arthrodesis with the external fixator.

BONE PLATE FIXATION ■   Reconstruction plates can be used for panarthrodesis (Fig. 19–24B). The plate is applied laterally to the tibia after resection of the distal fibula, as illustrated in Figure 19–22, and then contoured to allow attachment to the calcaneus, fourth tarsal, and proximal metatarsus. A minimum of three screws must be anchored in the tibia and in the metatarsal bones. Aftercare is as described above for plate fixation of talocrural arthrodesis.

Fractures of the Central Tarsal Bone

These fractures (Figs. 19–25 through 19–28) are seen infrequently except in the racing greyhound, where they are usually seen in the right foot.[24,25] When

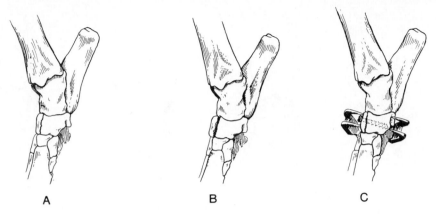

FIGURE 19–25. (A) Dorsal slab fracture of the central tarsal bone with minimal displacement (type 1). (B) Dorsal slab fracture of the central tarsal bone, slightly displaced (type 2). (C) A 2.7-mm lag screw is placed in the center of the fragment. The fragment is held in the reduced position with vulsellum forceps and the screw is placed between the teeth of the forceps.

they occur in other breeds, there is no predeliction for right or left. In the racing Greyhound the right foot is the "off" foot—toward the outside of the track— and the bone is subject to tremendous compression forces during turns. These forces literally explode the bone out of its position in the midst of the other six tarsal bones, producing a variety of fractures and subluxations of the bone. The fracture types are explained in detail below. In nonracing animals, the simpler fracture types are seen; more commonly, however, the bone is luxated intact except for a portion of the plantar process. Fixation is by one or two lag screws, followed by coaptation in a lateral splint or short cast; closed reduction and

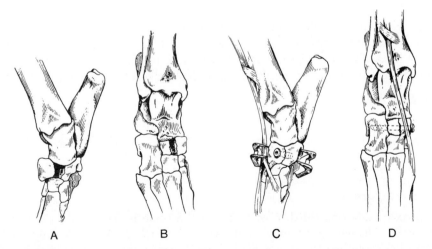

FIGURE 19–26. (A, B) Dorsomedial displacement of the medial portion of the central tarsal bone (type 3). (C, D) The 3.5- or 4.0-mm lag screw has been inserted in a mediolateral direction. The tendon of insertion of the tibialis cranialis muscle and the ligament between the central and third tarsal bones are shown for orientation. Reduction is accomplished by laterally displacing and flexing the metatarsus to allow the fragment to be wedged back into the joint space. It is held by vulsellum forceps while the screw is inserted.

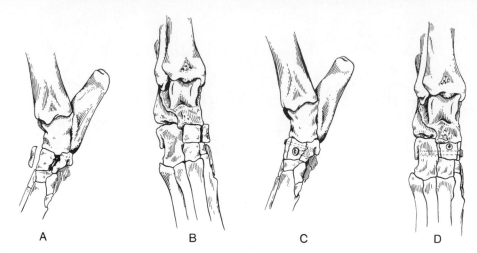

FIGURE 19–27. (*A, B*) Dorsal and medial displacement of two fracture fragments of the central tarsal bone (type 4). There may be comminution of the central part of the bone with slight varus deformity of the foot. (*C, D*) The medial fragment is reduced first and the 4.0-mm lag screw is placed mediolaterally as far distally in the bone as possible. The 2.7-mm lag screw is placed next in a dorsoplantar direction. Because this screw must not enter the proximal intertarsal joint, the exact angle of the drill hole is critical. Using partially threaded 4.0-mm screws for the mediolateral lag screw gives an extra millimeter of clearance between the two screws over the fully threaded 3.5-mm screw.

simple coaptation is not effective. The bone is approached by a dorsomedial incision.[1] The details of fixation for each fracture type follow.

Type 1 Fracture

A small slab is seen on the dorsal surface of the bone, with minimal displacement (Fig. 19–25A). In the past, these fractures have been treated primarily with a short lateral splint. Generally, they heal well with 4 to 6 weeks of immobilization, but occasionally they displace a little more during healing and thus create a slight incongruity at the proximal intertarsal joint space. For this reason, type 1 fractures are best treated with a lag screw, as are type 2 fractures.

Type 2 Fracture

Slightly more displacement of the dorsal slab differentiates a type 2 fracture from a type 1 fracture (Fig. 19–25B). A single 2.7- or 3.5-mm lag screw centered in the middle of the fragment is placed in a dorsoplantar direction (Fig. 19–25C).

Type 3 Fracture

Approximately one third to one half of the bone is fractured in the median plane and is displaced medially or dorsally (Fig. 19–26A, B). A single 3.5- or 4.0-mm lag screw is placed in a mediolateral and slightly plantar direction and seats in the fourth tarsal bone. The screw is placed just proximal to the origin of the ligament between the central and third tarsal bones (Fig. 19–26C, D).

Type 4 Fracture

Type 4 fractures are most common (68 percent) and are usually accompanied by associated fractures of the fourth tarsal bone (T4), the calcaneus, or T4 and

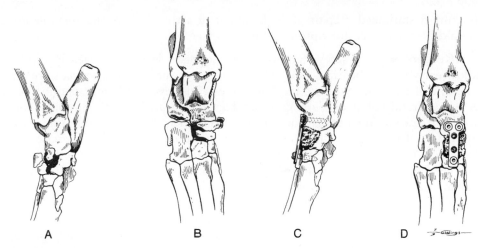

A   B   C   D

FIGURE 19-28. (A, B) Comminuted fracture of the central tarsal bone (type 5). Note the varus deformity of the tarsus and metatarsus. (C, D) A finger plate (2.7-mm screws) has been used as a buttress plate to restore the joint space occupied by the tarsal bone. No fixation of the fragments is possible because of their small size. The fragments are placed loosely back into the space, and the entire area is packed with autogenous cancellous bone graft obtained from the proximal tibia.

the lateral aspect of the base of metatarsal V.[26] This injury is a combination of fracture types 2 and 3 (Fig. 19-27A, B). The distance between the talus and T1-3 may be narrowed if the lateral undisplaced half of the bone is comminuted. This will lead to slight hyperextension and varus deformity of the foot. Because of the severe instability of the tarsus induced by this injury, fractures of other tarsal bones, especially the base of the calcaneus and T3 and T4, should be suspected.

Fixation is a combination of the two lag screws used for type 2 and 3 fractures. Exact placement of the screws is critical to ensure that both of them will be able to be placed in this small bone (Fig. 19-27C, D). The mediolateral screw must be placed first at the junction of the middle and distal third of the bone. The dorsoplantar screw is placed at the junction of the proximal and middle third of the bone. The angle of the drill bit is important because it must pass proximal to the first screw and also avoid entering the proximal intertarsal joint. If other fractures are present, they are often reduced spontaneously during reduction of the central tarsal bone. Fixation of these fractures is illustrated in Figures 19-9, 19-30, and 19-31.

Type 5 Fracture

Severely comminuted and displaced (Fig. 19-28A, B), these injuries carry the poorest prognosis for racing. If soundness of the animal for kennel activity is the only consideration, closed reduction and immobilization in a short cylinder cast for 6 weeks are sufficient. These animals will have slight hyperextension and varus deformity of the foot. If optimal results are desired, a buttress plate and cancellous bone graft (see Chapter 3) are utilized (Fig. 19-28C, D). The objective is to restore and maintain the normal joint space and thereby prevent deformity of the foot. Fragments of the bone are left in place, and cancellous graft is packed into the spaces. Ligamentous injury on the lateral side of the joint may accompany these fractures and may be difficult to evaluate until the fracture is stabilized. Repair of the ligament or arthrodesis of the unstable joint should be performed for optimum function (see below).

Aftercare ■   Lag screw fixation in these cases is not sufficiently rigid to allow early weight bearing, especially in the greyhound. These animals are very tolerant of pain and will use the limb excessively, even in kennel confinement. A short lateral splint or short cast (see Figs. 2–26 and 2–22) is applied for 4 weeks. Close confinement is maintained for 8 weeks, at which point radiographs are made. If fracture healing is satisfactory, gradually increasing exercise is allowed; at 12 weeks postoperatively, regular training is allowed. Bone screws do not need to be removed unless the screw enters the proximal intertarsal joint, as may happen with the dorsoplantar screw in type 4 fractures (Fig. 19–27C, D). These animals remain slightly lame until the screw is removed. A screw in the joint may also loosen and back out, again requiring removal. The plate used in type 5 injuries should be removed in most cases at 3 to 6 months postoperatively, especially if any attempt will be made to race the dog. Motion in the tarsus will cause the screws to loosen, which causes pain and prevents return to racing form.

Prognosis ■   With anatomical reduction and rigid fixation, good healing and return to competitive racing can be anticipated in 71 percent of dogs with fracture types 1 through 4.[27] Type 5 injuries carry a more guarded prognosis for racing, although most patients will become sound for breeding or pet purposes. Some type 4 and 5 injuries also have fractures of the base of the calcaneus (see Fig. 19–9) or proximal intertarsal plantar ligament injuries with subluxation and hyperextension of that joint (see below). Again, the prognosis for racing is poor, but soundness of condition for kennel activity can be expected. Treatment is a combination of the methods described above with the methods for a fracture of the calcaneus and for hyperextension at the proximal intertarsal joint.

Fracture-Luxation of the Central Tarsal Bone

Unlike most fractures of the central tarsal bone, which are almost exclusively a fracture of the racing greyhound, fracture-luxation of this bone (Fig. 19–29A,

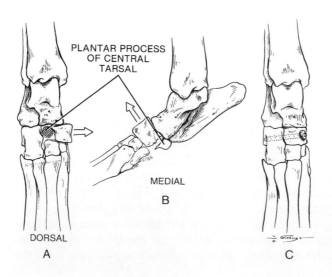

FIGURE 19–29. Fracture-luxation of the central tarsal bone. (A) The central tarsal luxates dorsomedially. (B, C) Fixation is by means of a positional screw through the central tarsal into the fourth tarsal bone. A threaded Kirschner wire or small pin may be substituted in small dogs.

PLANTAR PROCESS OF CENTRAL TARSAL

MEDIAL

B

DORSAL

A

C

B) is seen sporadically in all breeds. Fracture of the bone occurs at the plantar tubercle, which remains attached to the plantar ligaments, while the rest of the bone displaces dorsomedially. Closed reduction and cast fixation are rarely successful, and surgical stabilization is always advisable. Good function can be anticipated.

Diagnosis

Protrusion of the bone is readily palpable because there is minimal soft tissue swelling. If the bone is luxated completely out of contact with the talus and distal tarsal bones, mild varus deformity and hyperextension may be noted. Radiographs confirm this diagnosis.

Internal Fixation

The bone is approached by an incision directly dorsal to it.[1] The bone is reduced by flexing and lateral bending at the joint. A positional screw is directed laterally into the fourth tarsal bone (Fig. 19–29C). A further illustration of placement of this screw is found in Figure 19–26. Threaded Kirschner wire has been successfully substituted for the bone screw in toy breeds.

Aftercare ■ A short lateral splint (see Fig. 2–26) is applied and maintained for four weeks. Exercise is limited through the eighth postoperative week.

Fractures of Numbered Tarsal Bones

In our experience, we have not seen fractures of the first and second tarsal bones. Occasionally, the third tarsal bone may be fractured on the dorsal surface in racing greyhounds (Fig. 19–30A). A slab fracture similar to the central tarsal type 1 and 2 fractures, it may be treated either by a closed reduction and casting or, preferably, by lag screw fixation (Fig. 19–30B, C). Fractures of the fourth tarsal bone seen in nonracing animals are usually nondisplaced and respond well to casting. More serious injuries are seen in greyhounds, usually in conjunction with fractures of the central tarsal bone (Fig. 19–31A). Some of these require internal fixation, whereas others heal well with a cast following internal fixation of the central tarsal bone. The decision is based primarily on the amount of displacement, always bearing in mind that the fracture will probably displace farther while in the cast. If internal fixation of the central tarsal bone is indicated, it is very little additional work to place a screw or Kirschner wire

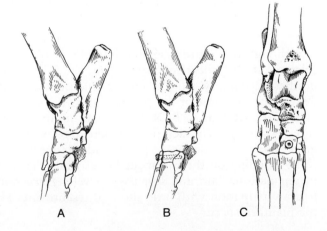

FIGURE 19–30. (*A*) Dorsal slab fracture of the third tarsal bone. (*B, C*) Lag screw fixation with 2.7-mm screw placed in the center of the fragment.

A   B   C

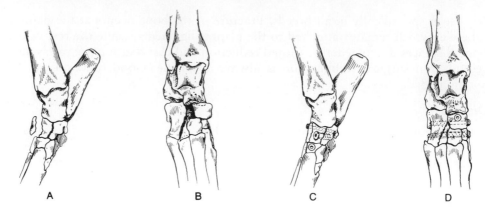

FIGURE 19–31. (*A, B*) Type 4 fracture of the central tarsal bone with fracture of the head of the fourth tarsal bone. (*C, D*) Double lag screw (4.0 and 2.7 mm) fixation of the central tarsal bone is accomplished first, followed by placement of a 3.5-mm lag screw that is started in the second tarsal bone and passes through the third and into the fourth tarsal bone.

in the fourth tarsal bone (Fig. 19–31*C, D*). The third and fourth tarsal bones are exposed by incision directly over the bones. The third tarsal incision is simply a distal continuation of the approach to the central tarsal bone.

Aftercare ■   A short lateral splint or short cast (see Figs. 2–26 and 2–22) is applied for 4 weeks. Exercise restrictions for racing animals are the same as for animals with central tarsal fractures. For nonracing animals, close confinement is maintained for 6 weeks, followed by 4 weeks of gradual return to normal activity.

Hyperextension with Subluxation of the Proximal Intertarsal Joint

This is a common injury of the tarsus in small animals (Fig. 19–32*A*). The majority of affected animals have no history of known trauma. Although hyperextension (dorsiflexion) is seen in all breeds of dogs, the Shetland sheep dog and collie seem to be predisposed, while the injury is apparently unrecorded in the cat. Affected animals fall into two groups: highly athletic animals such as racing greyhounds or coursing dogs, and obese, poorly conditioned dogs.

Diagnosis

Although the entire proximal intertarsal joint is affected, the primary instability is at the calcaneoquartal joint. Stability of the talocentral joint distinguishes this injury from complete luxation, described below (Fig. 19–33*A*). Tearing or avulsion of the plantar ligament between the fourth tarsal and calcaneus (Fig. 19–32*A, B*) is the primary injury. Loss of this tension band structure results in a characteristic hyperextension and variable degrees of plantigrade stance. The degree of plantigrade stance varies, the worst cases appearing to be standing on the calcaneus bone, while many have only 30 to 40 degrees of angulation. Pain and soft tissue swelling are not severe, and most animals tolerate palpation with little show of resentment. The joint is unstable only on the plantar aspect.

FIGURE 19–32. Arthrodesis of the calcaneoquartal joint for hyperextension with subluxation of the proximal intertarsal joint. (*A, B*) Tearing or avulsion of the plantar ligament of the calcaneoquartal joint allows hyperextension (dorsiflexion) at the proximal intertarsal joint. (*C, D*) The joint is exposed by a plantarolateral approach with medial retraction of the superficial digital flexor tendon.[1] The calcaneoquartal joint cartilage is debrided, and an autogenous cancellous bone graft is inserted. A tension band wire (18 to 20 gauge) is placed between the calcaneus and plantar tubercle of the fourth tarsal but not tightened. A small Steinmann pin ($5/64$ to $1/8$ inch in diameter) is driven through the calcaneus into the fourth tarsal and then countersunk beneath the cartilage of the tuber calcanei. The tension band wire is now tightened. (*E*) Plantarolateral view of the completed fixation. The superficial digital extensor tendon is retracted medially.

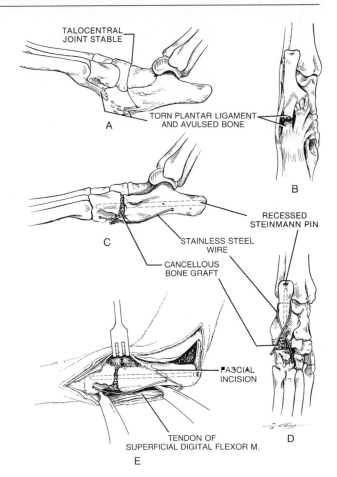

A mediolateral radiograph, with the joint stressed in extension, will confirm the site of instability and may demonstrate avulsed fragments of bone from either the fourth tarsal bone or the base of the calcaneus (Fig. 19–32*A*). Note that the talocentral joint remains unaffected by the instability of the calcaneoquartal joint.

Arthrodesis

Primary repair of the soft tissue injury or cast fixation is rarely successful and arthrodesis of the calcaneoquartal joint is recommended. Arthrodesis of this joint causes little functional disability, although racing animals rarely return to the track. The tension band wire fixation described here is applicable to any size animal and is relatively simple to perform.

The joint is exposed by a plantarolateral approach, with medial retraction of the tendon of the superficial digital flexor.[1] Fragments of the torn or avulsed ligament are excised to allow access to the joint. Articular cartilage is debrided on the joint surfaces with a high-speed bur or by curettage. A hole is drilled transversely through the midportion of the calcaneus and the plantar tubercle of the fourth tarsal bone (Fig. 19–32*C, D*). An 18 to 20 gauge (1.0- to 0.8-mm) stainless steel wire is threaded through both holes in a figure-of-8 manner. A pilot hole for the intramedullary pin is drilled through the shaft of the calcaneus, favoring the dorsal aspect of the medullary canal. This hole is best made with a slightly undersize bone drill rather than a pin because of the extreme

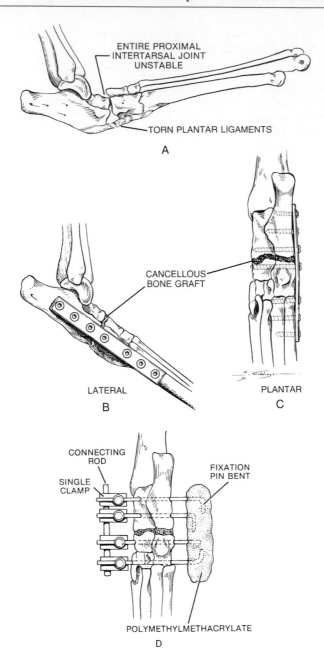

ENTIRE PROXIMAL INTERTARSAL JOINT UNSTABLE

TORN PLANTAR LIGAMENTS

A

CANCELLOUS BONE GRAFT

LATERAL

B

PLANTAR

C

CONNECTING ROD

SINGLE CLAMP

FIXATION PIN BENT

POLYMETHYLMETHACRYLATE

D

FIGURE 19–33. Arthrodesis for hyperextension with luxation of the proximal intertarsal joint. (*A*) Complete luxation is differentiated from subluxation by marked dorsal displacement of the distal tarsus at the proximal intertarsal joint. (*B, C*) Following curettage of the proximal intertarsal joint. Bone plate fixation requires smoothing of the lateral surface of the calcaneus and base of the fifth metatarsal. Plates are usually of the 3.5- or 2.7-mm screw size. At least three screws are placed in the calcaneus. The No. 3 screw is angled to engage the head of the talus, and number 4 screw spans the tarsus. The distal screws are placed in metatarsals 4 and 5. (*D*) External skeletal fixation is applicable to this surgery. Illustrated are both the use of conventional clamp fixation (*left*), and the use of polymethylmethacrylate dental tray cement as a connecting rod (*right*). Fixation pins are bent for more stability in the cement. See text for details.

hardness of this bone. Autogenous cancellous bone graft from the proximal tibia is placed into the joint space with the joint extended to open it. A single pin (from $\frac{5}{64}$ to $\frac{1}{8}$ inch; 1.9 to 3.2 mm in diameter) is started at the proximal calcaneus and driven to the distal end of the fourth tarsal bone. The pin is retracted 1 cm, cut, and countersunk beneath the surface of the tuber calcanei to protect the superficial digital flexor tendon. The tension band wire is now tightened by twisting in both halves of the figure-of-8 (Fig. 19–32D, E). The twists are cut and bent flat against the bone. The lateral retinaculum of the superficial digital flexor tendon is sutured as in Figure 19–10B to prevent its luxation and the skin is closed routinely.

Aftercare ■ Although external casts or splints are not required, a padded bandage is useful during the first postoperative week. Exercise is restricted to the house, a small pen, or a leash until radiographic signs of fusion are noted, usually 6 to 8 weeks postoperatively. At this time, activity can be slowly increased to normal at 12 weeks.

Hyperextension with Luxation of the Proximal Intertarsal Joint

A much less common injury than subluxation, this luxation (Fig. 19–33A) is usually a result of severe trauma and may be complicated by fractures of the tarsal bones. Arthrodesis of the joint is the preferred method of fixation, since primary repair of the ligaments is fruitless. Function is excellent with this fusion. Because the entire proximal intertarsal joint is involved, bone plate fixation results in more stable fixation of the talocalcaneal portion of the joint than does tension band wire fixation as shown in Figure 19–32. The tension band wire method can be used if modified to provide additional stability of the talocalcaneal joint by adding the medial wire fixation shown in Figure 19–34C, D, and E. External skeletal fixators are also adaptable to this procedure.

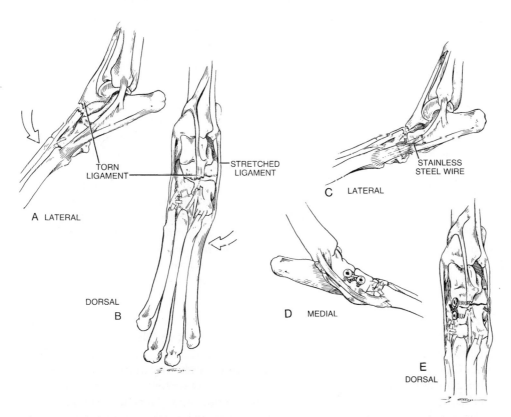

FIGURE 19–34. Surgical repair of proximal intertarsal subluxation with dorsal instability. (A, B) Excessive flexion and often varus deformity occur when the dorsal ligaments are ruptured. (C) Lateral instability is stabilized with stainless steel wire (20 to 22 gauge) placed through drill holes in the bony prominences of the distolateral calcaneus and proximolateral fourth tarsal bones. (D, E) Dorsomedial instability is stabilized by placing stainless steel wire (20 to 22 gauge) between screws placed in the base of the talus and central tarsal bones.

Diagnosis

This condition is differentiated from subluxation by instability of the joint in all planes and is confirmed radiographically by marked dorsal displacement of the distal segment rather than hinging at the dorsal aspect of the proximal intertarsal joint. This shows clearly in stressed mediolateral radiographs.

Arthrodesis

BONE PLATE FIXATION ■   The joint is exposed by a lateral incision from the tuber calcanei to the base of the metatarsals. Articular cartilage is removed from the entire joint by high-speed bur or curettage. The lateral side of the base of the calcaneus must be flattened to allow firm seating of the bone plate. This may involve sacrifice of a portion of the insertion of the long part of the lateral collateral ligament, which can be reattached by a suture running beneath the plate. A seven-hole plate of a 3.5- or 2.7-mm screw size is typically used (see Fig. 19–33B, C), although the VCP (Synthes Ltd. [USA], Paoli, PA) is particularly useful here to ensure an adequate number of plate holes to match the bones. A minimum of three screws are placed proximally, one penetrating the calcaneus and talus and the rest attached only to the calcaneus. One screw spans the tarsus distal to the proximal intertarsal joint, and at least three screws are placed in metatarsals 4 and 5. Autogenous cancellous bone graft (Chapter 3) is used in the joint space.

In larger breeds it may be possible to place three screws in the fourth tarsal bone by using the cuttable plate. If so, the plate does not have to be extended distally to the metacarpal bones; this saves some complications explained below.

Aftercare ■   External support is advisable because the plate is not in the tension band position. A short lateral splint or cylinder cast (see Figs. 2–26 and 2–22) is maintained until radiographic signs of fusion are present, usually 6 to 8 weeks. If the plate crosses the tarsometatarsal joint, it will always loosen as a result of joint motion, which causes the metatarsal screws to loosen. The plate should be left in place at least 4 months, preferably 6 months. If the distal metatarsal screws loosen before this, it is advisable to remove them, but the tarsal screws should be left in until 4 to 6 months have passed. Loss of blood supply to the skin as a result of the original or surgical trauma may lead to skin necrosis over the plate. This should be treated as an open granulating wound, with the plate left in place. The plate is removed about 4 months postoperatively if fusion is good, and if still present the skin defect is grafted or allowed to granulate.

EXTERNAL SKELETAL FIXATOR ■   Stabilization of this arthrodesis is also possible by means of a type II external skeletal fixator. This method is advantageous when there are open wounds associated with the injury and when bone plate fixation is not available. The fixation pins can be connected conventionally with clamps, as on the left side of Figure 19–33D or by means of polymethylmethacrylate cement (dental tray cement or hoof repair acrylic: see Chapter 2), as on the right side of Figure 19–33D. The joint is approached from a dorsal incision centered over the joint, and articular cartilage is removed by high-speed bur or curettage. Autogenous cancellous bone from the proximal tibia is placed in the joint space (see Chapter 3). Two fixation pins are placed transversely in the calcaneus and talus. If the fixation will use connecting clamps, care must be taken to ensure that the pins are spaced widely enough to allow placement of the clamps. Two more pins are placed distally in the tarsal bones. If there is not sufficient room to place both pins in the tarsus, the distal pin is driven through the bases of the metatarsal bones. The pins are then connected by clamps or cement. If cement is to be used, the fixation pins can be bent at a right angle at the protruding end in order to give more surface contact for the cement. The latter is mixed until reaching a dough–like consistency, then molded into a rod approximately $\frac{3}{4}$ inch (2 cm) diameter and hand packed onto the fixation pins. The arthrodesis site must be stabilized until the cement has hardened, typically 8 to 10 minutes from the start of mixing.

Aftercare ■ The animal is closely confined and the fixator maintained until radiographic signs of bony fusion are well defined. This will typically take 8 to 10 weeks. Exercise is slowly returned to normal 4 weeks after fixator removal.

Proximal Intertarsal Subluxation with Dorsal Instability

This injury is much less common than hyperextension at the proximal intertarsal joint. Although the primary damage is to the dorsal ligaments (Fig. 19–34A, B), there is often a medial or lateral instability, with varus deformity resulting from lateral instability being most common. The condition is evidently caused by overstress (i.e., self-induced), because outside trauma is rarely reported by the owner, although some animals have sustained this injury while climbing woven wire fences.

Diagnosis

Diagnosis of the condition can be difficult because the subluxation can be demonstrated only by palpation. There are few clinical signs with this condition other than a mild hindlimb lameness. The dog stands normally because the plantar ligaments are intact, but instability creates inflammation and pain in the joint and causes a mild lameness, which is worse if there is medial or lateral instability superimposed. Physical examination will reveal abnormal flexion at the proximal intertarsal joints. Medial and lateral stability should be tested, and stress-position radiographs should be made to confirm the physical findings. Figure 19–34A and B illustrates the dorsolateral instability.

Treatment

Because the dorsal ligaments do not function as tension bands, conservative treatment by casting for 3 to 4 weeks is often effective if there is no medial or lateral laxity. The smaller the patient, the more likely is conservative treatment to succeed. In larger breeds and in athletic animals, surgical treatment is more commonly indicated.

ARTHRODESIS ■ Surgical repair is indicated when dorsal ligamentous instability is complicated by medial or lateral instability. Surgery becomes even more important in a large athletic dog. Stabilization from both the medial and lateral sides is usually indicated. Because primary repair of such small ligaments is usually not possible, arthrodesis is preferred. The areas are approached by incisions directly over the bones. Medial and dorsal instability can be eliminated by placing stainless steel wire of 20 to 22 gauge (0.8 to 0.6 mm) between screws placed in the talus and central tarsal bones (Fig. 19–34D, E). Articular cartilage of the proximal intertarsal joint is debrided before screw placement, and suturing of any available ligament fragments is useful. Bone grafting is not routinely needed. If there is significant lateral instability, a tension band wire can be added laterally (Fig. 19–34C). Bony projections are available on both the distal calcaneus and proximal fourth tarsal to allow bone tunnels to be drilled for wire placement. Stainless steel wire of 20 to 22 gauge (0.8 to 0.6 mm) is used for the tension band.

Aftercare ■ A short lateral splint (see Fig. 2–26) is applied for 4 weeks, with activity restricted through 8 weeks postoperatively. If the joint does not completely fuse, the screw may loosen and back out, thus requiring removal.

Distal Intertarsal Subluxation with Dorsomedial Instability

This injury (Fig. 19–35A) can be seen in isolation or combined with hyperextension at the proximal intertarsal joint or tarsometatarsal luxation with dorsal instability. Cast fixation has been disappointing in our experience, and we advise surgical stabilization.

Diagnosis

Valgus deformity resulting from dorsomedial ligamentous instability can be appreciated on palpation. Soft tissue swelling is minimal. Radiographs in the stressed position confirm the site of instability and should be studied carefully for fractures of the fourth tarsal bone, a frequent complication.

Treatment

Because primary repair of such small ligaments is usually not possible, arthrodesis is preferred. The technique shown here is combined with proximal intertarsal arthrodesis when this condition is concurrent with hyperextension.

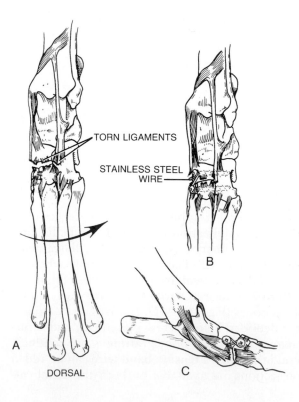

TORN LIGAMENTS

STAINLESS STEEL WIRE

A

DORSAL

B

C

FIGURE 19–35. Distal intertarsal subluxation with dorsomedial instability. (*A*) Valgus deformity is evident following rupture of the medial and dorsal ligaments of the centrodistal joint. (*B, C*) Bone screws are placed through the central and distal tarsals into the fourth tarsal. Articular cartilage of the centrodistal joint is debrided, and stainless steel wire (20 to 22 gauge) is looped around the screw heads and tightened.

ARTHRODESIS ■ The area is exposed by a distomedial extension of the approach to the central tarsal bone.[1] Articular cartilage is removed from the centrodistal joint by high-speed bur or curettage. Bone screws are placed from the central and second tarsal bones laterally into the fourth tarsal bone. Stainless steel wire, 20 to 22 gauge (0.8 to 0.6 mm), is looped around the screw heads and twisted tightly (Fig. 19–35B, C).

Aftercare ■ A short, lateral splint (see Fig. 2–26) is applied and maintained for 4 weeks. Exercise is limited through the eighth postoperative week.

THE METATARSUS, PHALANGES, AND SESAMOIDS

Fractures of these bones are virtually identical to fractures of the corresponding bones of the metacarpus and forefoot and are covered in Chapter 13.

Hyperextension with Subluxation of the Tarsometatarsal Joints

This injury (Fig. 19–36A) is not as common as proximal intertarsal hyperextension. The plantar tarsal fibrocartilage is torn in this situation.

Diagnosis

This condition seems to be more often related to known trauma than does proximal intertarsal hyperextension; thus, more soft tissue swelling is seen. The injury often happens when an animal becomes tangled in a wire mesh fence while attempting to climb it. Pain is not marked, and most animals will attempt weight bearing within a few days, with a typically plantigrade stance. Radiographs taken with hyperextension stress readily confirm the injury (Fig. 16–36A). In some cases, more complete luxation with plantar displacement of the bases of one or more metatarsal bones will be seen. Rarely are all four metatarsals completely luxated.

Treatment

As with other hyperextension injuries, conservative treatment by cast fixation is virtually never successful. Arthrodesis of the tarsometatarsal joints is the best treatment and yields good results and virtually normal function is anticipated.

ARTHRODESIS ■ The joints are exposed by means of a dorsal or plantar approach.[1] The digital flexor or extensor tendons are alternately retracted medially and laterally to allow debridement of articular cartilage of the joints. These joints do not form a straight line across the tarsus; therefore, each one must be curetted independently. Several fixation techniques are adaptable to this condition.

Intramedullary (IM) Pin and Tension Band Wire ■ This method works well and requires minimal equipment (Fig. 19–36C, D). Transverse holes for the wire (18 to 20 gauge) are drilled in the bases of the calcaneus and the metatarsal bones. Placing the proximal end of the wire in the base of the calcaneus shortens the wire compared to placing it over the pin at the tuber calcanei, and causes the wire to cross closer to the tarsometatarsal joint. The wire must be placed deep to the superficial digital flexor tendon. Because of the collective "quarter-moon" cross-sectional shape of the proximal metatarsal

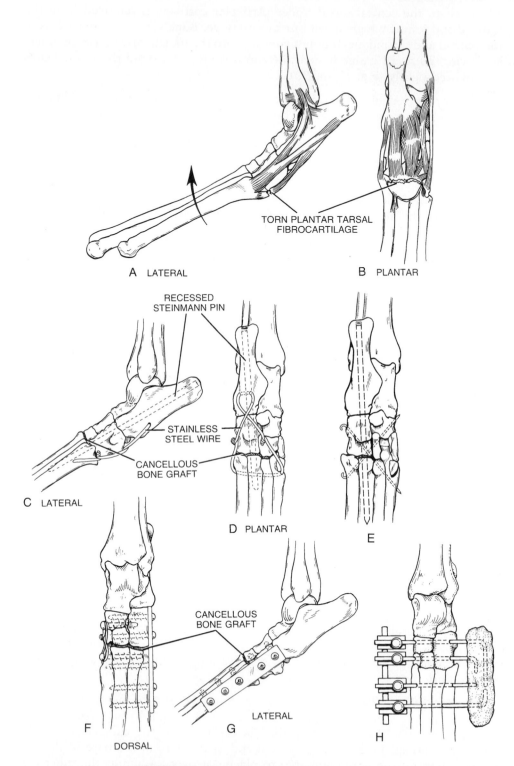

TORN PLANTAR TARSAL
FIBROCARTILAGE

A LATERAL

B PLANTAR

RECESSED
STEINMANN PIN

STAINLESS
STEEL WIRE

CANCELLOUS
BONE GRAFT

C LATERAL

D PLANTAR

E

CANCELLOUS
BONE GRAFT

F

DORSAL

G

LATERAL

H

FIGURE 19–36. *See legend on opposite page*

bones, it is unlikely that the drill will go through more than three of the four bones. A small Steinmann pin, $\frac{5}{64}$ to $\frac{1}{8}$ inch (2.0 to 3.2 mm) in diameter, is driven through the calcaneus, across the fourth tarsal bone, and into the base of metatarsal IV. It is then retracted 1 cm, cut short, and countersunk beneath the cartilage of the tuber calcanei. It is worthwhile to predrill a hole in the calcaneus for the pin with a slightly undersize bone drill. Autogenous cancellous bone graft (Chapter 3) is packed into the joint space before the wire is tightened. Because the pin crosses the calcaneoquartal joint, spontaneous fusion of the joint often follows. If the joint doesn't fuse, the IM pin will usually migrate proximally and irritate the superficial digital flexor tendon, necessitating removal of the pin.

Intramedullary Pin and Transfixation Pins ■ A simplified method of tarsometatarsal arthrodesis has been reported by Penwick and Clark.[28] The tension band wire is replaced by transfixation pins that cross the joint in an X pattern (Fig. 19–36E). The advantage of being able to do the procedure from a dorsolateral approach and so avoid the more complicated plantar area for wire implantation is offset by the need for coaptation splintage until fusion. The Steinmann pin can be placed in a retrograde manner from the distal surface of the fourth tarsal proximally through the calcaneus, where it is retracted and then driven distally into metatarsal IV. The Steinmann pin can either be countersunk in the calcaneus, or left protruding for later removal.

Bone Plate ■ Lateral plate fixation (Fig. 19–36F, G) also provides excellent stabilization. A five-hole plate of appropriate size is attached to the fourth, central, and distal tarsal bones proximally and to the metatarsals distally. Ideally, three screws should be placed in the fourth tarsal bone, but this is rarely possible with normal plates. The VCP (Synthes Ltd. [USA], Paoli, PA) is particularly adaptable to the small and medium size breeds, for it will ensure an adequate number of screws in each bone. Rarely will more than three of the metatarsals be engaged by any drill hole. A lateral bony projection of the base of metatarsal V will have to be removed to allow seating of the plate. Addition

---

FIGURE 19–36. Hyperextension of the tarsometatarsal joints. (*A, B*) Rupture of plantar tarsal fibrocartilage removes the tension band support for the joint and allows hyperextension to develop. (*C, D*) Arthrodesis by pin and tension band wire. A plantar approach is used to expose the joint for cartilage debridement.[1] Stainless steel wire (18 to 20 gauge) is placed through bone tunnels in the distal calcaneus and proximal metatarsals. The Steinmann pin ($\frac{5}{64}$ to $\frac{1}{8}$ inch; 2.0 to 3.2 mm in diameter) is driven into the fourth metatarsal and recessed into the calcaneus to prevent damage to the superficial digital flexor tendon. (*E*) A technically simpler method than the tension band wire involves replacing the wire with two transfixation pins placed to penetrate tarsal and metatarsal bones. The cost of this simpler procedure is the use of coaptation splintage until fusion is present. (*F, G*) Lateral bone plate fixation for arthrodesis. Two screws in the fourth tarsal bone and three screws in the metatarsals are minimum for this situation. The cuttable plate (Synthes Ltd. [USA], Paoli, PA) will simplify placing an adequate number of screws in each segment. In large breeds, bending loads on the medial side are neutralized with screw and wire fixation. External support in a cast or splint is necessary. (*H*) External skeletal fixation is applicable to this surgery. Illustrated are both the use of conventional clamp fixation (*left*), and the use of polymethylmethacrylate dental tray cement as a connecting rod (*right*). Fixation pins are bent for more stability in the cement. See text for details.

of wire and screw fixation medially is indicated in large breeds because of the difficulty of extending the plate screws to metacarpal II. Autogenous cancellous bone grafting (Chapter 3) of the joint spaces is advisable.

External Fixator ■   Stabilization of this arthrodesis is also possible by means of a type II external skeletal fixator. This method is advantageous when there are open wounds associated with the injury and when bone plate fixation is not available. The fixation pins can be connected conventionally with clamps as on the left side of Figure 19–36H or by means of polymethylmethacrylate cement (dental tray cement or hoof repair acrylic; see Chapter 2), as on the right side of Figure 19–36H. The joint is approached and articular cartilage is removed by power bur or curettage as described above. Autogenous cancellous bone from the proximal tibia is placed in the joint space (see Chapter 3). Two fixation pins are placed transversely in the distal tarsal bones. If the fixation will use connecting clamps, care must be taken to ensure that the pins are spaced widely enough to allow placement of the clamps. Two or more pins are placed distally in the metatarsal bones. The pins are then connected by clamps or cement. If cement is to be used, the fixation pins can be bent at a right angle at the protruding end in order to give more surface contact for the cement. The latter is mixed until reaching a dough-like consistency, then molded into a rod approximately ¾ inch (2 cm) in diameter and hand packed onto the fixation pins. The arthrodesis site must be stabilized until the cement has hardened, typically 8 to 10 minutes from the start of mixing.

Aftercare ■   External casting is not needed with the tension band wire or external fixator technique, but it is advised with bone plating because the plate is not in a tension band position, and for the pin and transfixation pin method. A short lateral splint or cast (see Figs. 2–26 and 2–22) or the external fixator is maintained until radiographic signs of fusion are noted, usually 8 to 10 weeks postoperatively. Exercise should be severely limited through this period and is slowly returned to normal 4 weeks after splint or fixator removal. If the calcaneoquartal joint does not fuse spontaneously with IM pin and tension band wire or transfixation pin fixation, the pin may migrate due to motion at the joint. This will create considerable soft tissue irritation and require removal of the pin after fusion is complete.

Tarsometatarsal Subluxation with Dorsomedial Instability

Although angular displacement may not appear severe with this injury (Fig. 19–37A), it is nonetheless a disabling problem. This is because the medial tarsus is the tension side, and attempted weight bearing further aggravates valgus deviation.

Diagnosis

This injury is rarely spontaneous, most of the time being directly attributable to trauma; thus, it may be associated with other local or remote injuries. The instability can be appreciated on palpation but probably cannot be differentiated from distal intertarsal subluxation. Radiographs of the animal in the stressed position are necessary to confirm the diagnosis.

Treatment

Cast fixation generally yields poor results, primary repair of these small ligaments is rarely possible, but simple arthrodesis carries a good prognosis.

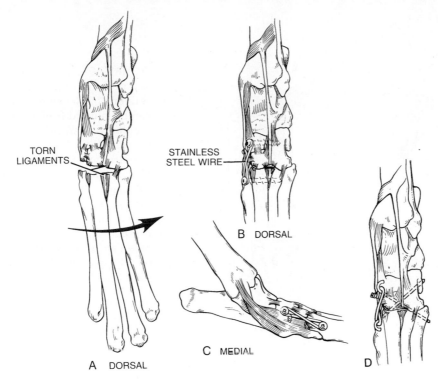

FIGURE 19–37. Tarsometatarsal subluxation with dorsomedial instability. (*A*) Valgus deformity develops as a result of disruption of the dorsomedial tarsometatarsal ligaments. (*B, C*) A direct medial approach exposes the affected joints, and articular cartilage is removed. Bone screws are placed in the central and fourth tarsal and metatarsals 2, 3, and 4. Stainless steel wire (20 to 22 gauge) is placed around the screw heads and tightened. (*D*) Support can also be provided with Kirschner wires and a tension band wire placed between the pins.

ARTHRODESIS ■ A medial incision is made directly over the affected joints. Articular cartilage is debrided in the second and third tarsometatarsal joints by high-speed bur or curette. Bone screws are placed in the central and fourth tarsal bones and in the bases of metatarsals II, III, and IV. Stainless steel wire (20 to 22 gauge; 0.8 to 0.6 mm) is looped around the screw heads and tightened (Fig. 19–37B, C). A second technique applicable here is cross pinning of the tarsometatarsal joint with Kirschner wires (Fig. 19–37D). A tension band wire placed between the pins provides good stability.

Aftercare ■ A short lateral splint or cast (see Figs. 2–26 and 2–22) is applied and maintained for three weeks. Exercise is limited throughout the eighth postoperative week. The pins may migrate after active weight–bearing starts and should be removed in this circumstance.

Tarsometatarsal Subluxation with Dorsal Instability

As with dorsal instability at the proximal intertarsal level, this injury (Fig. 19–38A) is apparently self-induced in most cases; it is rarely associated with known trauma.

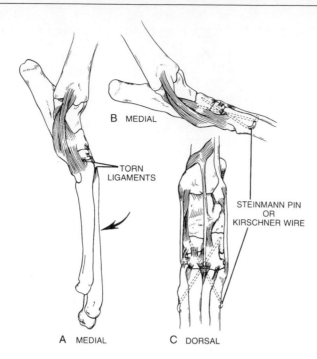

B MEDIAL

TORN
LIGAMENTS

STEINMANN PIN
OR
KIRSCHNER WIRE

A MEDIAL   C DORSAL

FIGURE 19–38. Tarsometatarsal subluxation with dorsal instability. (*A*) Flexion deformity can be induced from tearing of the dorsal ligaments of the tarsometatarsal joints. (*B, C*) Cross pinning through paired medial and lateral incisions is sufficient to stabilize this condition. The pins should be seated close to the bones to prevent skin irritation. These pins can also be driven from the tarsus in the opposite direction.

Diagnosis

History and clinical signs are similar to those of proximal intertarsal dorsal instability; that is, a rather vague and intermittent lameness. Because the deformity is not seen when the dog is standing, palpation to exert flexion stress is important in diagnosis. Radiographs showing the stress position will confirm the site of instability.

Treatment

This is perhaps one of the lesser tarsal injuries, often responding to cast fixation for 3 to 4 weeks. The larger the dog and the more instability present, the greater the need for surgical treatment. All chronic cases should undergo surgical treatment. Primary repair of these small ligaments is rarely possible, but simple arthrodesis carries a good prognosis. Because the plantar ligaments and fibrocartilage are intact only minimal fixation is required.

ARTHRODESIS ■ Paired medial and lateral incisions expose the joints. Small pins or Kirschner wires are driven from the proximal metatarsals into the tarsal bones in an X fashion (Fig. 19–38B, C). It is best not to cross the proximal intertarsal joint with the pins. Each pin is driven to the desired depth, retracted 1 cm, and cut 1 cm from the bone. A hook is bent in the pin and is then tapped back against the bone. Pins can also be driven in the opposite direction, from the tarsus into the metatarsals.

Alternatively, combined medial and lateral screw and wire fixation similar to Figure 19–37B and C can be used.

Aftercare ■ A short-leg lateral splint or cast (see Figs. 2–26 and 2–22) is maintained for 4 weeks. Exercise is restricted through 8 weeks postoperatively. The pins will almost certainly migrate when active weight bearing starts; they should then be removed.

Luxation and Subluxation of the Metatarsophalangeal and Interphalangeal Joints

These injuries are identical to those of the forefoot (see Chapter 13, Figs. 13–39 through 13–43).

References

1. Piermattei DL: An Atlas of Surgical Approaches to the Bones and Joints of the Dog and Cat, 3rd ed. Philadelphia, WB Saunders Co, 1993.
2. Aron DN: Prosthetic ligament replacement for severe tarsocrural joint instability. J Am Anim Hosp Assoc 23:41, 1987.
3. Swaim SF: Management and bandaging of soft tissue injuries of dog and cat feet. J Am Anim Hosp Assoc 21:329, 1985.
4. Morgan PW, Binnington AG, et al: The effect of occlusive and semi-occlusive dressings on the healing of acute full-thickness skin wounds on the forelimbs of dogs. Vet Surg 23:494–502, 1994.
5. Beardsley SL, Schrader SC: Treatment of dogs with wounds of the limbs caused by shearing forces: 98 cases (1975–1993). J Am Vet Med Assoc 207:1071–1075, 1995.
6. Ost PC, Dee JF, Dee LG: Fractures of the calcaneus in racing Greyhounds. Vet Surg 16:53, 1987.
7. Mauterer JV, Prata RG, et al: Displacement of the tendon of the superficial digital flexor muscle in dogs: 10 cases (1983–1991). J Am Vet Med Assoc 203:1162–1165, 1993.
8. Reinke JD, Mughannam AF, Owens JM: lateral luxation of the superficial digital flexor tendon in 12 dogs. J Am Anim Hosp Assoc 29:303–309, 1993.
9. Bonneau NH, Olivieri M, Breton L: Avulsion of the gastrocnemius tendon in the dog causing flexion of the hock and digits. J Am Anim Hosp Assoc 19:717, 1983.
10. Muetstege FJ: The classification of canine achilles tendon lesions. Vet Comp Orthop Trauma 6:53–55, 1993.
11. Reinke JD, Mughannam AF, Owens JM: Avulsion of the gastrocnemius tendon in 11 dogs. J Am Anim Hosp Assoc 29:410–418, 1993.
12. Weisner RE, Berry CR, et al: Osteochondrosis of the lateral trochlear ridge of the talus in seven Rottweiler dogs. Vet Surg 19:435–439, 1990.
13. Smith MM, Vasseur PB, Morgan JP: Clinical evaluation of dogs after surgical and nonsurgical management of osteochondritis dissecans of the talus. J Am Vet Med Assoc 187:31, 1985.
14. Breur GJ, Spaulding KA, Braden TD: Osteochondritis dissecans of the medial trochlear ridge of the talus in the dog. Vet Comp Orthop Trauma 4:168–176, 1989.
15. Montgomery RD, Hathcock JT, et al: Osteochondritis dissecans of the canine tarsal joint. Comp Cont Ed 16:835–845, 1994.
16. Miyabayashi T, Biller DS, et al: Use of a flexed dorsoplantar radiographic view of the talo-crural joint to evaluate lameness in two dogs. J Am Vet Med Assoc 199:598–600, 1991.
17. Dew TL, Martin RA: A caudal approach to the tibiotarsal joint. J Am Anim Hosp Assoc 29:117–121, 1993.
18. Aron DN, Mahaffey MB, Rowland GN: Free chondral fragment involving the lateral trochlear ridge of the talus in a dog. J Am Vet Med Assoc 186:1095–1096, 1985.
19. Lesser A, Solimen SS: Experimental evaluation of tendon transfer for the treatment of sciatic nerve paralysis in the dog. Vet Surg 9:72, 1980.
20. Doverspike M, Vasseur PB: Clinical findings and complications after talocrural arthrodesis in dogs: Experience with six cases. J Am Anim Hosp Assoc 27:553–559, 1991.
21. Gorse MJ, Earley TD, Aron DN: Tarsocrural arthrodesis: Long-term functional results. J Am Anim Hosp Assoc 27:231–235, 1991.
22. Klause SE, Piermattei DL, Schwarz PD: Tarsocrural arthrodesis: Complications and recommendations. Vet Comp Orthop Trauma 12:119, 1989.
23. Sumner-Smith G, Kuzma A: A technique for arthrodesis of the canine tarsocrural joint. J Small Anim Pract 30:65, 1989.
24. Dee JF, Dee J, Piermattei DL: Classification, management, and repair of central tarsal fractures in the racing greyhound. J Am Anim Hosp Assoc 12:398–405, 1976.
25. Taylor RA, Dee JF: Tarsus and metatarsus. In Slatter D (ed): Textbook of Small Animal Surgery, 2nd ed. Philadelphia, WB Saunders Co, 1993, p 1885.
26. Boudrieau RJ, Dee JF, Dee LG: Central tarsal bone fractures in racing greyhounds: A review of 114 cases. J Am Vet Med Assoc 184:1486, 1984.
27. Boudrieau RJ, Dee JF, Dee LG: Treatment of central tarsal bone fractures in the racing greyhound. J Am Vet Med Assoc 184:1492, 1984.
28. Penwick RC, Clark DM: A simple technique for tarsometatarsal arthrodesis in small animals. J Am Anim Hosp Assoc 24:183–188, 1988.

PART IV

OTHER FRACTURES AND RECONSTRUCTION OF BONE DEFORMITY

20

Fractures and Luxations of the Mandible and Maxilla

Fractures of the jaws are usually caused by automobile or other forms of trauma and are characterized by swelling, deviation of the segments, malocclusion of the teeth, and blood-stained saliva.[1] With few exceptions, all jaw fractures are open and contaminated or infected. These fractures may be unilateral or bilateral with single or multiple fracture lines. Mandibular fractures accounted for 3 percent of all canine and 15 percent of all feline fractures in two studies.[2,3] Symphyseal fractures were the most common injury in cats (73 percent), and fracture in the premolar region of the mandibular body the most common site in the dog in these same studies. Fractures of the maxilla are relatively rare compared to mandibular fractures. Vehicular trauma is the most common cause of fractures in the head; therefore, associated life-threatening trauma of other regions is often present.

In general, healing is rapid (3 to 5 weeks) in the rostral mandible, but more delayed (4 to 17 weeks) in the caudal region.[2] The exception to this general statement on healing is fractures through infected sockets and symphyseal fractures in the elderly toy breeds where considerable osteoporosis precedes the fracture. Complications are fairly common, 34 percent in dogs, with malocclusion being the most common, followed by infection and delayed union.[2]

DIAGNOSIS AND GENERAL TREATMENT

Diagnosis is usually based on a history of trauma, sudden onset, appearance, and a palpable fracture. Radiography is also helpful in discerning fracture lines and displacement but is supplemental to a thorough physical examination under anesthesia or sedation because fracture lines can be difficult to see and to orient radiographically.

The objective of treatment should be restoration of functional occlusion by fixation that allows the animal to have sufficient use of the mouth to eat and drink following reduction and fixation. With few exceptions, this goal can be achieved.

Treatment varies considerably, and in many cases, some type of internal fixation is indicated. The tension band side of both jaws is the alveolar border, and fixation should be applied as close to this side as possible (Fig. 20–1). With a few exceptions, bone fragments are replaced in the reduction process and are not discarded. Realignment is usually best checked with the jaw closed and the teeth occluded. Following reduction and fixation, the torn gingiva is sutured to

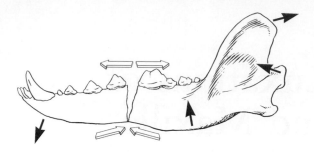

FIGURE 20–1. Masticatory forces exerted by muscles (*closed arrows*) cause ventral bending of the mandible, with tension forces on the lingual border and compressive forces on the ventral border (*open arrows*). (From Sumner-Smith G: Fractures of the mandible and maxilla. In Brinker WO, in Small Animals. New York, Springer-Verlag, 1984, pp 210–218, with permission.)

keep food and contaminants out of the wound. Suturing also aids in stabilizing the fracture segments and in converting the area to a closed fracture. Even though the tissues in the mouth are very effective in eliminating infection, systemic antibiotics are advisable.[3] Chronic osteomyelitis in connection with primary jaw fractures is rare when treated with antibiotics at the time of fixation.

In performing the fixation procedure in many cases, particularly the more complicated ones, a tracheostomy—or, preferably, a pharyngostomy—is done to maintain anesthesia. This technique ensures an open airway while the animal's mouth is closed and the teeth can be occluded during the procedure, ensuring adequate reduction during application of fixation. After the animal is stabilized on gas anesthesia, the tracheal tube is changed to pass through the pharyngostomy opening (Fig. 20–2). After the surgery is completed, the tracheal tube is removed, and the pharyngostomy opening is allowed to heal by granulation. In some cases a stomach tube is implanted through the pharyngostomy for postoperative feeding, although direct gastrostomy intubation is preferred.

FRACTURES OF THE MANDIBLE

Mandibular Symphysis

The method of immobilization depends on the presence or absence of incisor teeth, the stability of the reduced fragments, presence of infection or osteoporosis, and to some extent on the size of the patient.[1,4]

Fixation Methods

INTERDENTAL WIRING ■ If the incisor teeth are present and the fracture-separation is stable, a simple, stainless steel interdental wire may be adequate,

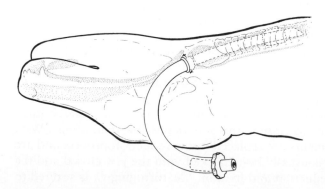

FIGURE 20–2. Pharyngostomy tube. After the animal is stabilized on gas anesthesia, the tracheal tube is changed to pass through a pharyngostomy opening and down the trachea. This allows fixation to be applied with the mouth closed and the teeth occluding.

especially in smaller patients (Fig. 20–3A). If the bases of the third incisor and canine teeth fit too close together to permit passage of the wire, a hand chuck may be used to force a Kirschner wire between them, allowing easy placement of the wire (Fig. 20–3B). Wire gauge size 20 to 22 (0.8 to 0.6 mm) is usually applicable.

CERCLAGE WIRE ■ The most often used method in smaller dogs and cats consists of using an encircling wire (Fig. 20–3C, D). The wire is inserted through the skin via an 18-gauge hypodermic needle from the ventral midline

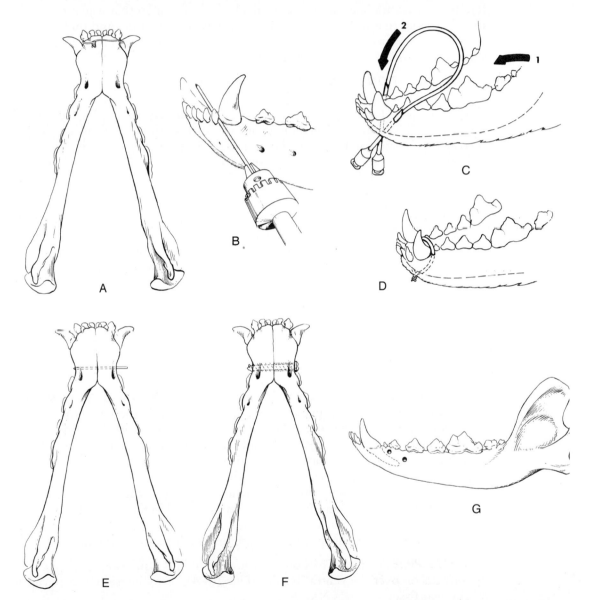

FIGURE 20–3. Fixation of the mandibular symphysis. (A) Simple, interrupted stainless steel wire suture. (B) A hand chuck forces a Kirschner drill wire between the base of the third incisor and canine teeth, allowing easy placement of wire sutures. (C, D) Immobilization by use of an encircling wire. The wire (usually 20 gauge) is inserted by using two 16-gauge needles and twisted outside the skin on the ventral surface. The mouth is closed with the teeth occluding when the final twisting is done. (E) Insertion of a transmandibular pin, smooth or threaded, or a bone screw (F) to improve stability. (G) Suggested location from the lateral surface for insertion, which is usually just rostral to the mental foramen.

at a point that will cause the wire to be placed at the caudal gingival margin of the incisor teeth. The needle is directed along the bone on one side to follow the bone under the skin and gums, and the wire is inserted through the needle. The needle is withdrawn so the wire protrudes ventrally, after which the needle is redirected through the same skin hole to the opposite side of the mandible. The free oral end of the wire is inserted into the needle and the needle and wire withdrawn ventrally. The wire is *tightened until no vertical shearing motion can be induced* between the mandibles. It is important that this motion be tested for, as the fracture line cannot be seen. The twist is cut so that it just protrudes from the skin; removal is done by cutting the wire intraorally and pulling it out ventrally by means of the twist. Wire of 20 gauge (0.8 mm) is used in cats and small dogs, with 18 gauge (1.0 mm) for larger breeds.

TRANSFIXATION PIN OR LAG SCREW ■   Stability may be improved by the insertion of a transmandibular pin (smooth or threaded) or a bone screw to neutralize shear forces at the fracture site (Fig. 20–3E, F, G). Figure 20–3G suggests the location from the lateral surface for insertion, which is usually just rostral to the mental foramen. These methods, especially the lag screw, are indicated when gross instability is present, as is often the case when this fracture is associated with other mandibular fractures. Combining cerclage wiring and transfixation pinning is also a simple way of providing excellent stability.

AFTERCARE ■   Good stability is usually achieved by these fixation methods, and postoperative care is not complicated. Food should be fairly soft and no chew-toys or bones should be allowed. Fractures in this area usually heal rapidly, but there is little that can be done to evaluate healing, as no callus is usually seen radiographically. Inasmuch as the implants cause little irritation, there should be no urgency to remove them. Eight weeks is adequate for healing in most cases, and allows for the delay seen in older osteoporotic patients or where delay due to infection is present.

Mandibular Body

A wide variety of fractures may be encountered here, as it is the most common location in the dog[2]; ingenuity is required to devise the best type of fixation. No single technique is applicable to all fractures, and the choice often must be made between several applicable methods. A method or combination of methods must be used that gives stability at the fracture site, and critical to understanding the mechanics of fixation in the mandible is to appreciate that normal masticatory muscle forces will bend the rostral fragment ventrally (Fig. 20–1). Thus the gingival margin of the bone is loaded in tension and the ventral cortex is loaded in compression, and the effects of both these forces must be evaluated relative to each specific fracture and each fixation technique.

OPEN APPROACH ■   The body of the mandible is quite simply approached by an incision over the ventral border (Fig. 20–4), or by incision and elevation of gingival tissue.

Fixation

TAPE MUZZLE COAPTATION ■   Simple tape muzzles are commonly used on many shaft fractures. Muzzling the upper and lower jaws together provides mediolateral stability to the mandible by the interdigitation of the canine teeth, and stability in the vertical plane by simply limiting motion. Muzzles are used

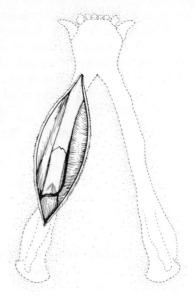

FIGURE 20–4. Ventral approach to the body of the mandible showing the digastricus muscle (caudal), platysma muscle (lateral), and mylohyoid muscle (medial). A branch of the facial vein crosses the digastricus muscle.

for both primary fixation and for support and protection of internal fixation. Primary fixation muzzles are most useful for stable body fractures in the mid- and caudal regions, and are not suitable for rostral fractures. Neither are they suitable for cats and brachycephalic breeds, and soft tissue injuries of the facial or mandibular regions can complicate muzzle application.

Muzzles are best applied to the sedated or anesthetized patient. Typically they are not applied tightly enough to totally shut the mouth; rather, an opening large enough for the tongue is left rostrally so that liquids can be consumed. A 1- to 3-ml syringe casing works well as a bite block during muzzle application as shown in Figure 20–5. Feeding consists of slurried dog food. The small

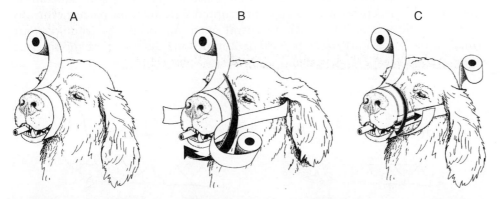

FIGURE 20–5. Tape muzzle application. (*A*) A bite block, such as a syringe case, is placed between the incisor teeth. The block should be just thick enough to allow passage of the tongue for drinking. Adhesive tape is placed around the jaws with moderate pressure. (*B*) A headstall, to prevent slippage of the muzzle, is fashioned by a second piece of tape applied with the adhesive side out. (*C*) Additional circular wraps of tape anchor the headstall, which is then folded back on itself to cover the exposed adhesive side. A ventral chinstrap can be added at the caudal end of the mandible to prevent the headstall from coming over the top of the head. Test to be certain that there is room for the tongue to protrude.

amount of motion of the mandible permitted by this opening does not create a problem if the fracture is reasonably stable. However, if the muzzle is used for unstable fractures it must be applied tightly, and feeding by stomach, pharyngostomy, or jejunostomy tube is necessary. This results in considerable nursing care, and is a good reason to consider internal fixation for unstable fractures. Fixation for 3 to 4 weeks is adequate in many midbody fractures, especially in immature patients.

INTERARCADE WIRE ■ Wiring the mandible to the maxilla can be substituted for muzzle application when the muzzle can't be used for the reasons stated above. The basic method shown in Figure 20–6 can be applied at many levels of the mandible, taking care to avoid teeth roots. As with the muzzle, the mouth can be left slightly open to allow liquids to be consumed, or closed tightly for maximum stability. Maximum stability is provided by the method shown in Figure 20–16.

INTERDENTAL WIRE ■ Wiring around the crowns of the teeth near the gingival margin works best when there is a solid tooth on each side of the fracture line and when the fracture is simple in nature (Fig. 20–7A, C). The wire functions as a tension band, and the ventral cortex must be intact to buttress the compression forces. Occasionally, wire placement is modified so that the wire is passed between the roots of the adjacent teeth when the shape of the crown prevents secure wire anchorage (Fig. 20–7B). The guide hole is made with a small Kirschner wire and a pin chuck. The wire is passed through gingival tissue, with no attempt made to elevate the soft tissue. The twisted ends should be kept on the labial side of the gum, and must be carefully bent flat with the gum to ensure no soft tissue irritation. Pressure necrosis of gingiva will result in eventual complete or partial covering of the wire by gum tissue and little irritation as long as the wire remains tight and stable. See aftercare instructions below.

INTERFRAGMENTARY WIRE ■ Additional stability can be added to interdental wiring by supplementing it in some oblique, multiple, and noncomminuted unstable fractures with simple interrupted wire fixation placed ventrally on the mandible (Fig. 20–8). After ventral open approach, the fragments are drilled, usually with a Kirschner wire or 2-mm bone drill, so that the inserted

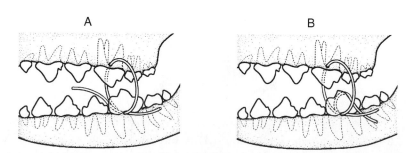

FIGURE 20–6. Interarcade wiring is useful when the tape muzzle is not applicable due to soft tissue injuries, in brachycephalic dogs, and in cats. (*A*) A Kirschner wire is used to develop a hole at the margin of the alveolar bone between the roots of the fourth premolar teeth, and a loop of 20- to 22-gauge (0.9- to 0.7-mm) wire is placed through the holes. (*B*) With a bite block in place as in Figure 20–5, one end of the wire is brought over or around the crown of the lower premolar and twisted. Test to be certain that there is room for the tongue to protrude.

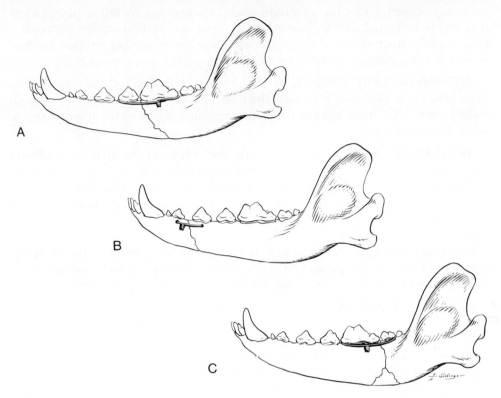

FIGURE 20–7. Fixation of a fracture of the body of the mandible. (*A*) Interdental wire around the bases of the fourth premolar and the first molar. (*C*) Interdental wire around the bases of the first and second molars. (*B*) Modified method, with wire through drill holes between the roots of the adjacent teeth.

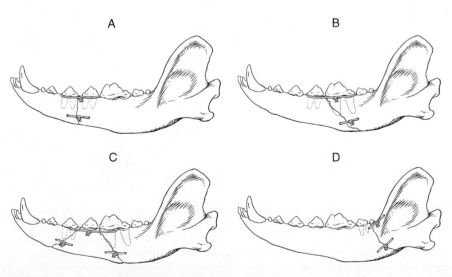

FIGURE 20–8. (*A–D*) Examples of combined interdental and interfragmentary wiring of stable mandibular body fractures.

wire crosses the fracture line at a right angle. These wires are left in place unless removal is indicated due to loosening or infection. Stability must be accomplished at the fracture site; if not, some modification or another fixation method is in order. See aftercare instructions below.

INTRAMEDULLARY PINNING ■ Although intramedullary pin fixation has been used for mandibular fractures, the difficulty of pin insertion and marginal stability provided argue against their continued use when so many other methods are available.

INTRA-ORAL SPLINT ■ A simple intraoral splint can be used for midbody and rostral fractures (Fig. 20–9). A Steinmann pin of $\frac{5}{64}$ to $\frac{1}{8}$ inch diameter (2.0 to 3.2 mm) is bent to fit on the lingual side of the mandible along the gingival margins. It is then secured to the mandible by wire that is looped around the pin and then passed through the bone to the labial side, where the wire ends are twisted and bent flat.

Intraoral splinting with dental acrylic molded to the crowns of the teeth has been used by some, but results have not been encouraging, with accumulation of food particles and exudate complicating postoperative treatment.[6]

EXTERNAL FIXATOR ■ This device[1,4-6] is useful for:

1. Nonunion fractures; bone grafting is indicated in many cases (see Chapter 3).
2. Multiple fractures (Fig. 20–10A, B).
3. Bilateral fractures (Fig. 20–10C).
4. Unstable or gunshot fractures where bone is missing (Fig. 20–10D). The gums are sutured following reduction and fixation. In the healing process, the

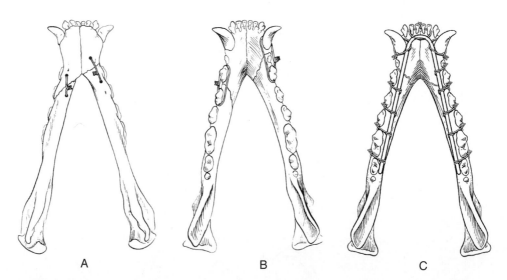

A   B   C

FIGURE 20–9. (A, B) Dorsal and ventral views of a rostral stable bilateral body fracture treated with both interfragmentary and interdental wires. (C) Dorsal view of bilateral rostral body fracture stabilized with an intraoral splint fashioned from a Steinmann pin. The splint is bent to shape and wired to the mandible through holes in the mandibular body placed between teeth or between tooth roots. Rostrally the wiring incorporates the canine and incisor teeth. The most rostral wire may also be placed through a drill hole if good wire security cannot be obtained on the teeth.

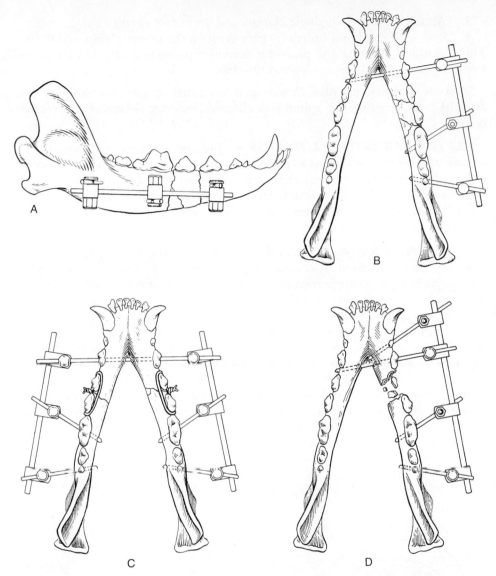

FIGURE 20–10. External fixator. (*A*, *B*) Multiple fractures. (*C*) Bilateral fractures. (*D*) Unstable fracture with bone missing. In most cases, the splint can be applied so that it does not extend beyond the length of the mandible, thus it does not interfere with eating or drinking. If the bone chips are left in place and the gums closed, in most cases the bone deficit will bridge over without the addition of a bone graft.

missing segment may fill in if bone chips and periosteum are still present. In others, a bone graft is indicated.

Surgical Procedure ■   Two pins are usually inserted in each fragment, but one pin in the rostral fragment may be sufficient if it passes transversely through both halves of the mandible (Fig. 20–10*A*, *B*, *C*). The procedure is usually as follows:

1. Close the animal's mouth with the fracture reduced and the teeth occluding.

2. Insert the rostral and caudal pins through the skin and soft tissues into the bone as ventrally as possible to avoid tooth roots, nerves, and vessels.

3.   Attach the bar with single clamps and an empty center clamp.

4.   Insert the third and fourth (?) pins through the center clamp and tighten. This essentially lines up the pins in a common plane and attaches them with single clamps and a common connecting bar.

In some patients, interdental wiring is indicated to improve stability (Fig. 20–10C). In general, the splint is well tolerated. See aftercare instructions below.

ACRYLIC BAR EXTERNAL FIXATOR ■ Because the external fixator splint has some inherent limitations in pin placement and connecting bar attachment, polymethylmethacrylate (nonsterile dental acrylic) may be substituted as the connecting bar and is often simpler to apply than the splint with clamps (Fig. 20–11).[6] See Chapter 2 for more complete description of the application of this type connecting bar.

Surgical Procedure ■ A tracheal tube is inserted through a pharyngostomy or tracheostomy incision to ensure an open airway. The mouth is closed, and functional reduction of the fracture occurs as a result of occlusion of the teeth. At least two or more pins should be placed in each major bone segment. Small fragments may be skewered with divergent Kirschner wires. A major advantage of this technique is the ability to stabilize multiple fragments from a variety of angles, usually using more and smaller diameter pins than with clamp fixation. The protruding pins are bent to better hold the molded acrylic connecting bar (Fig. 20–11). The acrylic usually takes about 8 to 10 minutes to set, and the teeth are maintained in occlusion until hardening is well advanced. Although a bilateral technique is illustrated, the splint can be substituted for clamp splints on unilateral fractures as well. See aftercare instructions below. Following healing, the pins can be cut between the acrylic and jaw and removed with a hand chuck. Alternatively the acrylic bar can be cut with a saw between each pin to allow pin removal. Because bilateral fixation extends rostrally beyond the lower jaw, it may interfere with eating, and hand feeding of semisolid food may be necessary.

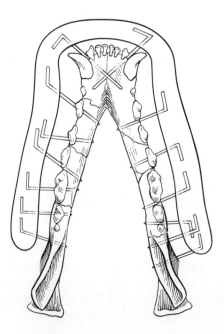

FIGURE 20–11. Modified acrylic external fixator. With the mouth closed, the fracture reduced, and the teeth occluding, two or more Kirschner wires are inserted into each major segment. The wires are bent and included in an acrylic mold. This apparatus has the disadvantage of protruding beyond the length of the jaw, thus making it more vulnerable to bumping and cumbersome when eating. In many cases, the same configuration can be applied by first bending the connecting bar of the external fixator, then inserting the Kirschner pins through the holes in the clamps and through the skin and soft tissue and into the bone.

BONE PLATES ■ These are particularly useful for the more complex fractures and bilateral fractures.[5,6] They afford good rigidity and almost unrestricted use of the jaws immediately after surgery.

Surgical Procedure ■ A pharyngostomy or tracheostomy incision is made, with insertion of a tracheal tube to ensure an open airway. The jaw is exposed with a ventral incision. Compression forceps are applied to compress the fracture segments and hold them in the reduced position while the bone plate is contoured to fit the surface perfectly (Figs. 20–12A, B). The plate is then attached with bone screws. Contouring the plate is a most important step in ensuring proper occlusion of the teeth. Reduction and occlusion will be lost as the screws are tightened unless the contouring is almost perfect. The plate is usually placed laterally near the ventral border to avoid placing the screws in the mandibular canal and injuring tooth roots. The reconstruction plate (Synthes Ltd. [USA], Paoli, PA) is particularly useful to allow bending to follow the curve of the ventral cortex of the mandible (Fig. 20–12C). See Figure 2–74 for suitable plate and screw sizes. In some cases, it is advisable to add interdental wiring for additional tension band stability.

AFTERCARE ■ Postoperative treatment in all cases of internal fixation consists primarily of restricting the animal's jaw activity by feeding soft, small pieces of food. Chew bones, toys, or play that would stress the jaws should be eliminated until healing is evident. Wire fixation requires the most protection, and plates or fixators the least. Some care must be exercised with fixators to keep food particles cleaned from between the lips and the splint, particularly when the splint is bilateral.

Vertical Ramus

Because of the extensive musculature covering this region, there is often little displacement of the fragments, and most ramus fractures can be treated conservatively by muzzling or interarcade wiring. Various methods of internal fixation may be used when conservative treatment is not practical, including Kirschner wires, interfragmentary wire, and mini bone plates. External fixators are not applicable because of the mediolateral thinness of the ramus.

Figure 20–13 illustrates a lateral approach to the ramus and temporomandibular joint. Fixation methods for fractures of the ramus are shown in Figure 20–14. Fractures of the condyles are usually not amenable to fixation due to the small size of the bone fragments. Initial conservative treatment is indicated; if good function does not return after removal of the muzzle/interarcade wires, then excision arthroplasty will permit adequate function. The condyle is excised to remove bony contact between the mandible and temporal bone and to allow fibrous tissue invasion and a subsequent false joint.

Luxation of the Temporomandibular Joint

The temporomandibular (TM) joint can luxate either cranially or caudally as a result of trauma, and may occur as an isolated injury (especially in the cat), or associated with fractures of the mandible.

DIAGNOSIS ■ The mandible and lower canine teeth are visibly displaced to either side of the upper canines. Palpation will establish mediolateral laxity of the mandible, but it is usually not possible to be sure of the direction of luxa-

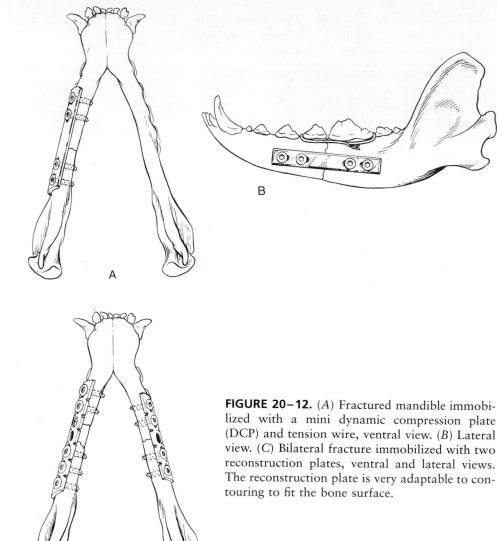

FIGURE 20–12. (A) Fractured mandible immobilized with a mini dynamic compression plate (DCP) and tension wire, ventral view. (B) Lateral view. (C) Bilateral fracture immobilized with two reconstruction plates, ventral and lateral views. The reconstruction plate is very adaptable to contouring to fit the bone surface.

tion. Standard position radiographs adequately outline the canine TM joint, but in the cat, slight rotation of the head in the lateral view gives better visualization. The mandibular condyle can be seen either cranial or caudal to the mandibular fossa. When the luxation is cranial the rostral mandible will be displaced to the contralateral side, and with a caudal luxation displacement will be ipsilateral.

REDUCTION ■   Closed reduction is usually possible. A fulcrum is introduced at the level of the last molar teeth on the affected side. This is usually a plastic tuberculin syringe for a cat, to a 3- or 5-ml syringe for a large dog. The syringe is placed transversely between the upper and lower last molars, and the rostral end of the mandible is squeezed dorsally towards the maxilla and so levering the caudal end ventrally and "unlocking" the luxation. While holding the mandible in this position the rostral end is levered in the appropriate direction to

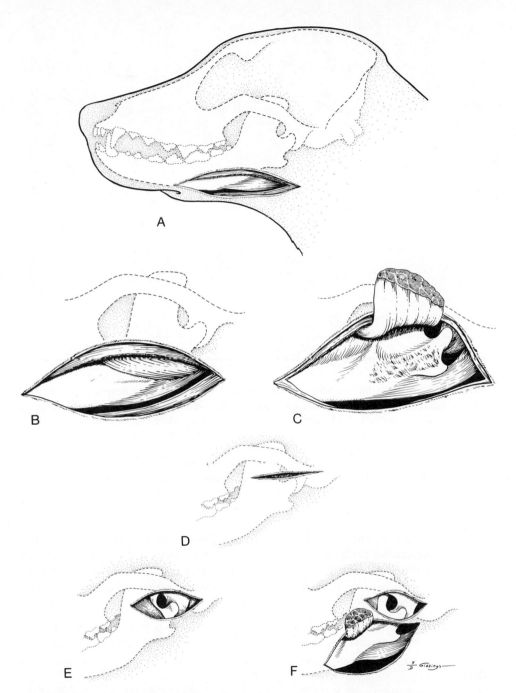

FIGURE 20–13. Surgical approach to the ramus and temporomandibular joint. (*A*) Ventrolateral approach to the caudal angular portion of the ramus. Skin incision along the ventrolateral border; separation of the platysma muscle exposes the digastricus muscle. (*B*) Further separation of the soft tissue exposes portion of the mandible, masseter muscle, and digastric muscle. (*C*) Subperiosteal reflection of the masseter muscle exposes angular and condyloid processes and masseteric fossa. (*D*) Longitudinal skin incision along ventral border of zygomatic arch and temporomandibular joint. (*E*) Platysma muscle and fascia incised along same line. This tissue is reflected ventrally, exposing the lateral surface of the joint and the upper portion of the condyloid process. (*F*) The tissue between the two incisions is tunneled beneath the visualization, reduction, and fixation.

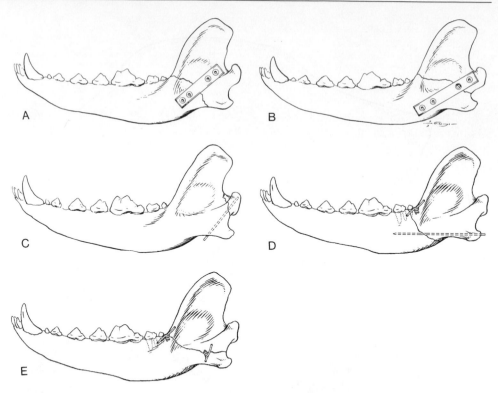

FIGURE 20–14. Fixation methods for fractures of the ramus. (*A*) Fracture just rostral to the angular process immobilized by a bone plate. (*B*) Fracture between the angular and condyloid processes immobilized by use of a bone plate. (*C*) Condyloid process fracture immobilized by an intramedullary pin placed from the ventral border of the mandible. (*D*) Fracture rostral to the angular process immobilized with an intramedullary pin placed through the angular process and an intraoral wire at the angle of the mandible. (*E*) Fracture between the angular and condyloid processes immobilized by an interfragmentary wire and an intraoral wire at the angle of the mandible.

reduce the luxation, and then slowly released. Reduction is verified by interdigitation of the canine teeth, as several attempts may have to be made to obtain reduction. Failure to reduce may lead to open reduction, but there is little in the way of joint capsule to imbricate, and excision arthroplasty as described above for condylar fractures may be indicated.

Aftercare ■   In the rare instance where the luxation is stable after reduction, no stabilization is necessary, only soft food as described above for fractures. In most cases 1 to 2 weeks of support with a tape muzzle or interarcade wiring is indicated.

FRACTURES OF THE MAXILLA

Fractures of the incisive and maxillary bones are usually readily diagnosed by observation and palpation.[4-6] They are accompanied by bleeding from the nose and mouth, swelling, and varying degrees of malocclusion. The primary objective is re-establishment of dental occlusion and closing any communication between nasal passages and the mouth. Accomplishing this goal usually returns approximately normal appearance to the nose, upper jaw, and face.

Maxillary Fractures of the Facial Region

Many undisplaced fractures require no fixation at all. Closed reduction and taping or wiring the jaws together represents the next level of stabilization. Wiring of fragments is easily accomplished and useful especially when fragments are depressed into the nasal cavity. Open approach and reduction of these non-oral fractures is done by incision directly over the affected areas. Fractures in this thin bone area frequently collapse inward and are reduced with a small hook-shaped probe that can be used to lever the fragments outward from below. Occasionally, a flat spatula or probe can be inserted from the nares to aid in reduction. Most of these fractures do not need fixation, and those that do can be handled by interfragmentary wire or Kirschner wire stabilization. Little stability is required once the fragments are reasonably reduced. In the case of multiple fractures with marked displacement, the acrylic bridge external fixator is valuable. The fragments are "speared" on K-wires, reduced, and then connected by acrylic. This technique is applicable to a variety of situations.

Intraoral Maxillary Fractures

Midsagittal fracture of the hard palate in the cat is the most common injury of this area. Most of these are a result of hitting the nose on the ground after a fall or an automobile strike. A wire suture(s) inserted underneath the mucosal covering of the hard palate and anchored to a tooth on each side is the simplest method of stabilization (as in Fig. 20–15). The torn gingiva of palate can be

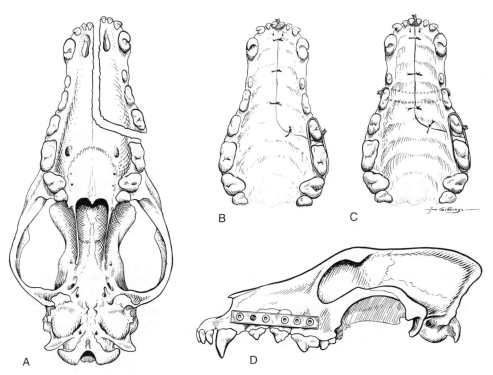

FIGURE 20–15. Fixation of fractures of the upper jaw. (*A, B*) Suturing of a torn gingiva and palate with interdental wiring of adjacent teeth. (*C*) Insertion of wire suture underneath mucosal covering of hard palate and anchored to a tooth on either side, in addition to the above. (*D*) Bone plate fixation.

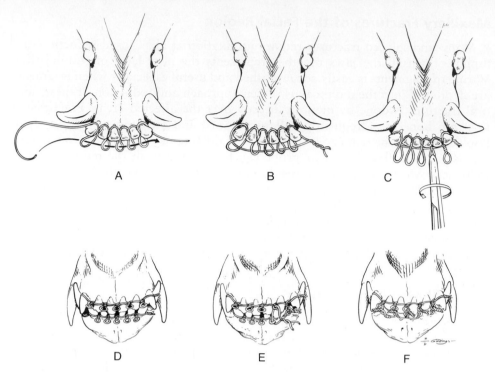

FIGURE 20–16. Surgical procedure for bilateral fractures of both upper and lower jaws if they cannot be stabilized separately. (A–F) Procedure for wiring the jaws together using the eyelet method.

sutured, although this is not necessary if the fracture is well reduced and stabilized.

Various other fracture patterns are seen. Fixation can usually be accomplished by placing a stainless steel wire around the base of the teeth on each side of the fracture line (Fig. 20–15A, B, C). Some fractures of the incisive bone or maxilla are amenable to bone plate fixation (Fig. 20–15D). Exposure is gained by incising the gums along the base of the teeth and reflecting the soft tissue dorsally to expose the fracture area. The intraoral pin splint (Fig. 20–9) is adaptable to the maxilla and is useful for fractures of the incisive bone that leave the entire rostral end of the jaw loose.

Occasionally, massive bilateral fractures of the nasal and maxillary bones and mandible are encountered. Reconstruction and immobilization may include using an acrylic pin external fixator[6] or wiring the jaws together using the eyelet method of wiring to maintain occlusion during the healing period (Fig. 20–16). Food and liquids may have to be given by use of an implanted pharyngostomy, jejunostomy, or gastrostomy tube. Healing is usually rapid, and the jaws are wired together for 3 to 6 weeks. *Note:* Occasionally, this style of wiring can be used to advantage on certain fractures of the mandible to provide immobilization of the entire lower jaw.

References

1. Brinker WO: Fractures. In Canine Surgery, 2nd Archibald ed. Santa Barbara, American Veterinary Publications, Inc, 1974, pp 949–1048.

2. Umphlet RC, Johnson AL: Mandibular fractures in the dog: A retrospective study of 157 cases. Vet Surg 19:272–275, 1990.
3. Umphlet RC, Johnson AL: Mandibular fractures in the cat: A retrospective study. Vet Surg 17: 333–337, 1988.
4. Rudy RL: Internal fixation of jaw fractures. 19th Annual AO/ASIF Course on Surgical Fixation of Fractures. Ohio State University, Columbus, OH, 1988.
5. Sumner-Smith G: Fractures of the mandible and maxilla. In Brinker WO, Hohn RB, Prieur WD (eds): Manual of Internal Fixation in Small Animals. New York, Springer-Verlag, 1984, pp 210–218.
6. Egger EL: Skull and mandibular fractures: In Slatter D (ed): Textbook of Small Animal Surgery, 2nd ed. Philadephia, WB Saunders Co, 1993, pp 1910–1921.

21

Fractures in Growing Animals

This chapter describes separations and fractures involving the physis before closure and diaphyseal fractures in animals up to 4 or 5 months of age. Beyond this period of time, treatment of shaft fractures is basically the same as for the adult animal. A variety of fractures involve the growth plate and all have the potential to retard or arrest bone growth and create limb deformities due to shortening or angular changes.[1] Correction of these deformities is discussed in Chapter 22.

Although the growth plate of long bones is often referred to as the epiphyseal plate, in truth, it is the metaphyseal growth plate. The term *physis*, referring to the zone of growth in a long bone, is more convenient and is used throughout this text. The epiphysis is a separate center of ossification found at the ends of long bones, is initially entirely cartilaginous, grows by endochondral ossification, and forms the articular surface in many bones. Fractures involving the physis may, but do not necessarily, involve the epiphysis.

The shafts of long bones are more resilient and elastic than older bones and thus withstand greater deflection before incomplete or complete fracture. Incomplete, or "greenstick," fractures are common in puppies and kittens. The periosteum is attached loosely to the diaphysis and strips easily when subjected to trauma. Blood collects beneath it, and the resulting subperiosteal hematoma is soon converted to callus. The periosteum is thick and may act as a restraining and stabilizing sleeve, helping to prevent displacement of bone fragments and generally adding stability.

Healing is rapid (2 to 4 weeks, depending on age), and most animals produce an abundant callus regardless of the method of stabilization. Remodeling is very active and is completed quickly, with all evidence of the fracture obliterated within a few weeks. Nonunion is very unusual. Physeal fractures are accompanied by considerable hemorrhage, rapid organization of callus, and often considerable displacement due to muscle forces. Because these changes occur so quickly following trauma, it is fundamental that reduction and fixation of physeal fractures be carried out as soon as possible. In articular fractures, anatomical reduction and rigid fixation are necessary to restore a functional joint.

DIAPHYSEAL FRACTURES

External Fixation

Some fractures may be treated by closed reduction and supported by coaptation (Fig. 21–1) as described in Chapter 2. If limb splintage is used, it must

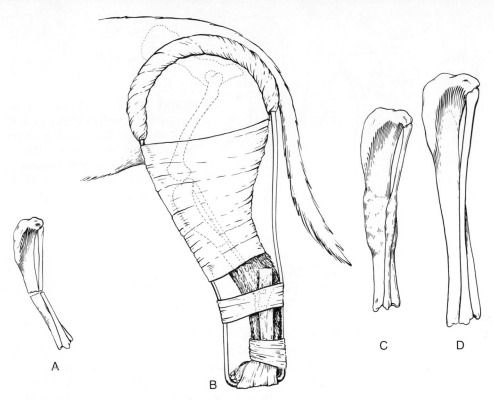

FIGURE 21–1. (*A*) Transverse fracture of the tibia in a toy poodle 8 weeks of age. (*B*) After reduction, a modified Thomas splint was applied. (*C*) Splint removed 2 weeks after treatment. (*D*) Fracture remodeled 4 weeks after treatment.

be properly applied and kept in good repair; otherwise hazards may be encountered, including valgus deformity, rotation, ligamentous laxity, joint stiffness, and others. Immobilization of the hindlimb so that the hip joint is deprived of weight-bearing forces causes coxa valga and increased anteversion, and the result is identical to the pathology of congenital hip dysplasia, as described in Chapter 15. This effect is most pronounced in the large breeds, but can affect all size dogs. Hindlimb immobilization also can result in quadriceps tie-down and fibrosis of the stifle joint. Immobilization of the forelimb commonly causes laxity and hyperextension to develop in the carpus. Fortunately this is usually reversible, whereas the hip and stifle problems are not. Coaptation should be left in place for the absolute minimal amount of time necessary for clinical union.

Internal Fixation

Internal fixation is used primarily for these types of acute fractures:

1. Fractures causing rotational deformity or excessive shortening.
2. Fractures resulting in incongruency of an articular surface.
3. Fractures affecting the physeal plate and thus future bone growth.
4. Fractures of the femur, especially in large breeds.

The following types of fixation are applicable:

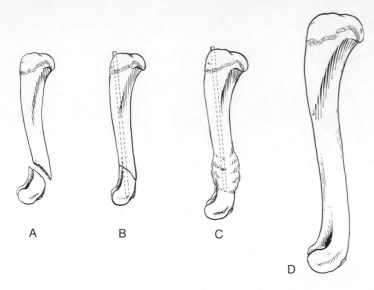

FIGURE 21–2. (*A*) Oblique fracture of the distal humerus in a 7-week-old animal. (*B*) Postoperative Steinmann pin fixation. (*C*) Pin removed 2 weeks postoperatively. (*D*) Fracture remodeled 4 months postoperatively.

INTRAMEDULLARY PIN ■   In proportion, pins used in the young are relatively smaller in diameter than those used in the adult.[2] Because cancellous bone is present in a high percentage of the medullary cavity, the pin stabilizes the fracture better in young animals. Auxiliary fixation is rarely used, as the rapid development of periosteal callus stabilizes rotational and shortening forces (Fig. 21–2).

EXTERNAL FIXATOR ■   The fundamentals of using the splint are the same in the young as in adult animals; however, healing is rapid, less fixator stiffness is required, and 2/2 pins are usually sufficient (Fig. 21–3). The fixation pins should not traverse the physis or penetrate paired bones such as the radius and ulna. The splint must not bridge the physis; keep all fixation pins in the diaphysis and metaphysis. Because fissure fractures of the shaft commonly accompany

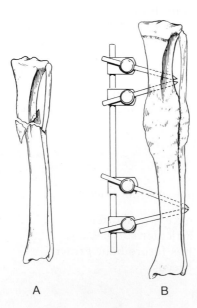

FIGURE 21–3. (*A*) Comminuted open fracture of the tibia in a 9-week-old animal. (*B*) Clinical union at 2½ weeks; external fixator removed at this time.

complete fractures, care must be taken to not place fixation pins into these fissures. It is acceptable to cross the fissure lines with pins.

BONE PLATE ■ Although commonly disregarded, bone plates offer many advantages in juvenile patients, especially in femoral fractures of the large breeds. Highly unstable and multiple fragment fractures of this bone are difficult to handle by any other means (Fig. 21–4). Latte has devised a unique approach to plate application in growing animals, specifically in femoral fracture stabilization.[2] The femoral cortex in growing animals is quite thin, more so than in other long bones. This, combined with the rigidity of bone plates relative to the bone, causes screw loosening in many cases, especially when contact of the main fragments cannot be re-established. He proposes using relatively small and flexible plates, 2.7-mm size, combined with 3.5-mm screws, and placing the screws only in the end holes of the plate, where the bone is metaphyseal in nature; that is, containing much trabecular bone within the medullary canal. This allows avoiding the thin cortex in the middiaphyseal area. There will be some motion of the fracture, but since callus formation is rapid and quickly stabilizes the fracture, this motion is not important. Latte's recommendations for biological osteosynthesis of femoral fractures include:

1.   Wait 36 hours following injury before fixation to allow for some attachment to fragments and organization of the hematoma.

2.   Do not attempt to reduce fragments. Correct angular and rotational malalignment and restore length only to the extent possible without disruption of the hematoma. Use only pointed reduction forceps on the major fragments to avoid damage to periosteum.

3.   Use radiographs of the normal limb to measure and contour the plate. Do not cross growth plates with the plate.

4.   Do not use any lag screws, and do not place screws close to the fracture line. Three screws on each major fragment are needed. No tapping is done in metaphyseal areas.

5.   Do not use any limb splintage postoperatively.

Good results have been reported using conventional plating technique in fractures of the radius in growing animals.[3] The cortex of the radius, humerus, and

FIGURE 21–4. (*A*) Type C complex diaphyseal fracture with nonreducible wedges in an 11-week-old large-breed dog. (*B*) Postoperative view showing plate fixation in the manner of Latte.[2] A 2.7-mm plate is attached in the metaphyseal regions with 3.5-mm screws. No screws are used in the diaphysis, and the fragments are not reduced. (*C*) At 6 weeks the femur is completely healed and remodeled. The bone has continued to increase in length distally, which is the normal pattern. The plate is removed at this time.

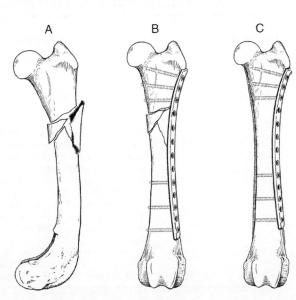

tibia in the young animal is much thicker than the femur, and screw loosening is not an issue. When used, bone plates should be removed early, after approximately 3 to 5 weeks, depending on age and circumstances. Early removal is necessary to prevent entrapment of the plate by appositional bone growth.

PHYSEAL FRACTURES

Longitudinal growth of bone is the result of enchondral ossification occurring in the epiphyseal and metaphyseal areas. The process is a sequence of coordinated events: multiplication, growth, and degeneration of the cartilage cell; followed by calcification and vascularization of the cartilage matrix; then production of primary spongiosa; which is followed by bony trabeculae of the metaphysis. Excess load applied to the immature bone may result in dislocation, fracture, or a crushing type injury. Because the strength of the fibrous joint capsule and ligaments is two to five times greater than that of the metaphyseal-physeal junction, the latter is more prone to injury (e.g., separation, dislocation, fracture).

Growth plates can be classified on the basis of their locations. There are two types: pressure and traction growth plates. *Pressure growth plates* are located at the ends of the long bones and transmit forces through the adjacent joint. Pressure growth plates produce the majority of the longitudinal growth. *Traction growth plates* are located where muscles originate or insert. A traction growth plate contributes little to bone length (e.g., the tibial tuberosity).

Salter and Harris (Table 21–1 and Fig. 21–5) have anatomically classified physeal injuries into five types.[4] Although the original intent was to give prognostic information based on fracture type, this has not proven to be a valid concept. In a histological study of 13 physeal fractures, 10 were shown to have damage to the physeal proliferative zone cartilage.[5] Most physeal fractures occur in the proliferative zone because it is the weakest area of the physis. It

TABLE 21–1. SALTER-HARRIS CLASSIFICATION OF SEPARATIONS OR FRACTURE-SEPARATIONS INVOLVING A GROWTH PLATE AND THE ADJACENT METAPHYSIS AND EPIPHYSIS

TYPE OF FRACTURE	RADIOGRAPHIC FINDINGS	PRINCIPAL ANATOMIC REGION INVOLVED
Type 1 (Fig. 21–5A)	Physeal separation; displacement of the epiphysis from the metaphysis at the growth plate	Proximal humerus and femur, distal femur
Type 2 (Fig. 21–5B)	Small corner of the metaphyseal bone fractured, with displacement of the epiphysis from the metaphysis at the growth plate	Distal femur and humerus, proximal humerus, proximal tibia
Type 3 (Fig. 21–5C)	Fracture through the epiphysis and part of the growth plate, but the metaphysis unaffected	Distal humerus
Type 4 (Fig. 21–5D)	Fracture through the epiphysis, growth plate, and metaphysis; several fracture lines may be seen	Distal femur, distal humerus
Type 5 (Fig. 21–5E)	Soft tissue swelling, but no bony abnormalities seen following the injury	Distal ulna, distal radius, distal femur
Type 5 (Fig. 21–5F)	Two months after trauma, shortening of ulna and partial closure with angular deformity of radius	

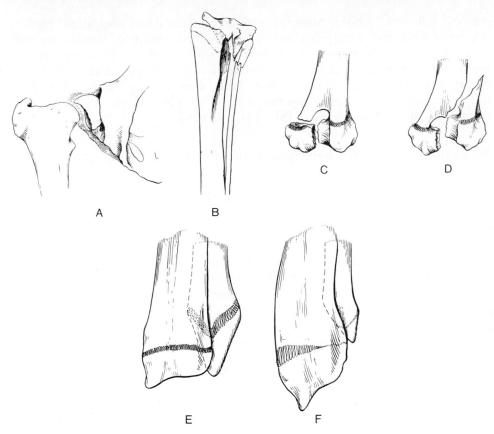

FIGURE 21–5. Salter-Harris classification of epiphyseal fractures involving the growth plate, adjacent metaphysis, and epiphysis. (*A*) Type 1 physeal fracture; displacement of the epiphysis from the metaphysis at the growth plate. (*B*) Type 2 small corner of the metaphyseal bone fractured with displacement of the epiphysis from the metaphysis at the growth plate. (*C*) Type 3 fracture through the epiphysis and part of the growth plate. Metaphysis unaffected. (*D*) Type 4 fracture through the epiphysis, growth plate, and metaphysis. (*E*) Type 5 soft tissue swelling but no bony abnormalities seen immediately following the injury. (*F*) Type 5 2 months after the trauma; closure and shortening of the ulna and partial closure with an angular deformity of the radius are evident.

would appear that growth disturbance is not only related to the type of fracture, but that other factors are important, such as the age of the patient, extent of displacement, degree of reduction, time since injury, and type of fixation. The various types of injuries are the result of different types of forces being applied to various areas of the leg at different stages of maturity of the growth plate. The younger the animal, the greater the chance for growth deformity even with early reduction and fixation. Despite failure to fulfill the original expectations, the Salter-Harris classification remains as a standard system for nomenclature.

Incidence[6]

About one fourth to one third of long-bone fractures involve the physes, and Salter II injuries predominate. The physis most important to the length of the bone is most often involved, except in the humerus, where the distal physis is more commonly injured than the proximal. The distal femoral physis is most injured, followed by distal humerus, proximal femur, distal ulna, distal radius, proximal tibia, and distal tibia. Between 5 and 10 percent of these cases will develop growth deformities, of which the majority will require corrective osteotomy to restore normal function. The tendency to develop a growth abnormality is most likely in medium- to large-breed dogs that are less than 5 months old at time of injury. Salter V injuries of the distal ulnar physis are more likely to produce significant deformity than any other injury.

Treatment of Salter-Harris Type I–IV Injuries

Open reduction and internal fixation of fractures involving joints are indicated if congruent articular surfaces cannot be obtained and maintained by conservative means. The majority of fractures in small animals need open reduction and rigid internal fixation.[1] Kirschner wire fixation of bone fragments is an excellent method; healing is rapid, and the wires can be removed in 2 to 4 weeks. With meticulous surgery, early reduction, and rigid fixation, the response to type I–IV injuries is very encouraging for healing and return to normal or at least satisfactory function. The surgical approach and fixation methods are similar to those described for the corresponding areas in the adult animal and have been covered in Chapters 10, 12, 16, and 18. Figures 21–6 and 21–7 depict most fracture-separations that occur in the region of the physes and suggest methods of stabilization.

Principles of Treatment

1. Do the least reduction and fixation that is compatible with good function and rapid healing. The younger the animal, the less reduction and fixation needed.

2. Closed reduction and fixation is preferable when possible, as in the distal tibia, distal radius, and occasionally the distal humerus. The ability to successfully perform a closed reduction is limited to cases that are seen early and have minimal displacement. Be aware of the problems associated with coaptation splintage in growing animals as mentioned above in the section regarding diaphyseal fracture treatment. Splints can usually be removed in 2 weeks for physeal fractures in animals under 5 months of age.

3. Reduce physeal fractures as early as possible. Within 72 hours many are virtually impossible to reduce due to rapid organization of the copious fracture hematoma, along with severe muscular contracture.

4. During open reduction:
    - Be aware of the epiphyseal blood supply and spare it during all manipulations
    - Do not grind germinal cartilage off the epiphyseal fragment in type I–III injuries during the reduction process.
    - Be careful with bone clamps, as they can easily crush the epiphysis or damage articular cartilage. Pointed reduction clamps will minimize these injuries, but reduction should be accomplished by traction and leverage of the epiphysis via the ligaments attached to the adjoining long bone.

5. Regarding internal fixation:
    - Do not bridge the physis with any fixation that prevents increase in bone length (e.g., lag screws, bone plates, tension band wires, threaded pins, external fixators). The younger the animal, the more important this is to prevent growth disturbance.

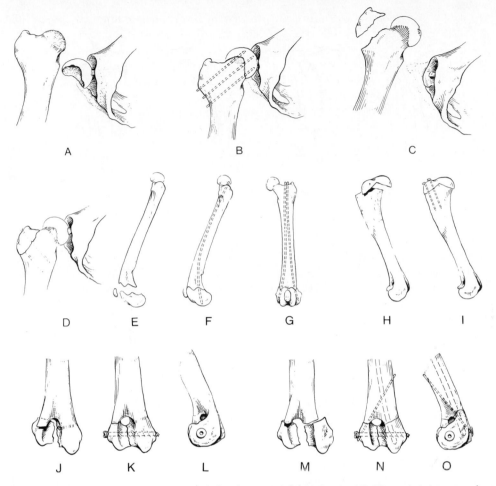

FIGURE 21–6. Physeal fractures of the femur and humerus. (*A*) Type 1 injury to the pressure physis; separation of the proximal femoral physis. (*B*) Fixation with three smooth Kirschner wires. (*C, D*) Type 1 injury to the traction physis; avulsion or fracture of the trochanter major and dislocation of the coxofemoral joint. After reduction of the femoral head, the trochanter is relocated and fixed in place with two Kirschner wires. (*E–G*) Type 1 injury to the pressure physis; separation of the distal femoral physis. Reduction and fixation using two small intramedullary pins. (*H, I*) Type 1 injury to the pressure physis; fracture of proximal humeral epiphysis. Fixation by insertion of two Kirschner wires entering on the ridge of the greater tuberosity. (*J–L*) Type 3 injury to the pressure physis; fracture between the medial and lateral aspects of the humeral condyle with separation at the lateral part of the epiphyseal line. Fixation with a transcondylar lag screw. (*M–O*) Type 3 bicondylar fracture of the humeral condyles with separation along the entire epiphyseal line. Fixation with a transcondylar screw and two pins.

- Small-diameter, smooth Steinmann pins or Kirschner wires are adequate fixation in most cases. Diameters typically range from 0.035 to $^5/_{64}$ inch (1 to 2 mm). With smooth pins, the epiphysis is free to grow in length and glide along the pin, which often becomes completely buried within the epiphysis. Bone will quickly grow into threads, locking it to the implant and preventing growth unless the pin slides backwards with epiphyseal growth. Lag screws are needed in type III

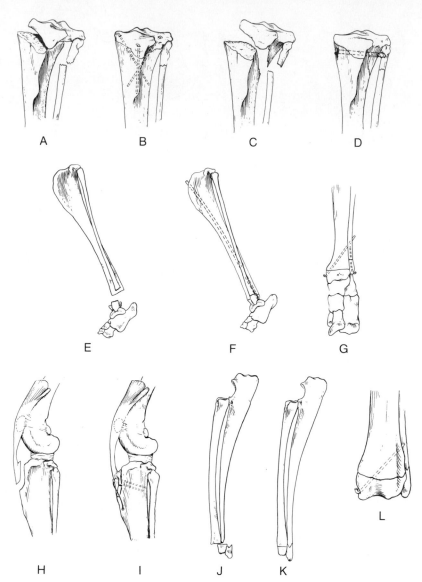

FIGURE 21–7. Physeal fractures of the tibia and radius and ulna. (*A, B*) Type 1 injury to the pressure physis. Fracture of the proximal tibial physis with a fracture of the fibula. Fixation with three obliquely inserted Kirschner wires. (*C, D*) Type 2 injury to the pressure physis; fracture of the proximal tibial physis and a small portion of the metaphysis. Fixation with a cancellous screw under the physis. (*E–G*) Type 1 injury to the pressure physis. Fracture of the distal tibial and fibular physis. If the parts are stable on reduction, the hock is flexed to a right angle and fixed in this position for 2 to 3 weeks with a cast. The right angle places the bone segments in the most stable position. If this fracture is unstable on reduction, a small intramedullary pin is inserted from the proximal end of the tibia down into the epiphysis, or two small pins are inserted through the malleoli. A cast is applied for additional stabilization. (*H, I*) Type 1 injury to the traction physis. Avulsion of the tibial tubercle. Fixation by a tension band wire. (*J, L*) Type 1 separation of the distal physis of the radius and fracture of ulna. The segments are usually stable on reduction (*K*) but require external stabilization with a coaptation splint. If segments appear unstable after reduction, a Kirschner wire (*L*) should be inserted diagonally through the radial styloid process into the diaphysis.

and IV injuries, but these run parallel to the physis and do not cross it.

- Pins should cross the physeal plate at an angle as perpendicular as possible to minimize any effect on the plate. Angles of more than 45 degrees will cause some locking effect and predispose to epiphysiodesis. Rush pins will produce a locking effect due to the hook end, preventing movement of the epiphysis along the pin. These hooks should be cut off after the pin is seated.
- If a form of fixation that does bridge the physis is unavoidable in order to secure fixation, it should be used. The first priority is to obtain fracture healing with a functional reduction. In this situation the fixation is removed as soon as possible, usually within 3 to 4 weeks, and as early as 2 weeks in very young animals.
- Strive for stable internal fixation that will allow early, limited, active weight bearing on the limb to minimize secondary bony deformity due to disturbed stress/strain patterns on other bones.

References

1. Brinker WO, Braden TD: Fractures in immature animals. In Brinker WO, Hohn RB, Prieur WD (eds): Manual of Internal Fixation in Small Animals. New York, Springer-Verlag, 1984, pp 225–238.
2. Latte Y: Semi-rigid internal fixation for the treatment of diaphyseal fractures of the femur in growing dogs. European Society of Veterinary Traumatology, Frankfort, Germany, 1987.
3. McLain DL, Brown SG: Fixation of radius and ulna fractures in the immature dog and cat: A review of popular techniques and a report of eight cases using plate fixation. Vet Surg 11: 140–145, 1982.
4. Salter RB, Harris WR: Injuries involving the epiphyseal plate. J Bone Joint Surg 45-A:587, 1953.
5. Johnson JM, Johnson AL, Eurall J: Histological appearance of naturally occurring canine physeal fractures. Vet Surg 23:81–86, 1994.
6. Maretta SM, Schrader SC: Physeal injuries in the dog: A review of 135 cases. J Am Vet Med Assoc 182:708–710, 1983.

22

Correction of Abnormal Bone Growth and Healing

Angular and rotational deformities of long bones induce considerable functional problems in cases when the deformity is beyond the ability of the animal to compensate. Angular deformities have the effect of shortening the limb, and although dogs and cats have remarkable ability to compensate for this, there is a point beyond which the gait is markedly altered. Both rotational and angular deformity cause abnormal stress and strain on adjacent joints and this will induce degenerative joint disease with time. These deformities are most commonly caused by premature arrest of long-bone growth plates, or by healing of a long-bone fracture in a position of incomplete reduction. Many deformities can be corrected by division and repositioning of the bone, which is the subject of this chapter.

OSTEOTOMY

An osteotomy is the surgical division of the bone and is usually indicated to correct bony deformities that may include length, angular, or rotational changes. These changes may occur in one plane; however, most involve two or more planes.

Angular deformities are most common and include varus, valgus, hyperextension, and hyperflexion. Length can be shortened or (rarely) lengthened, and rotation can be internal or external. Malunion can include the above plus over-riding of diaphyseal segments in all planes and directions. These deformities are treated by corrective osteotomy; simple osteotomies are commonly performed as part of a surgical approach or as part of another procedure such as arthrodesis.

Common Indications for Corrective Osteotomy

- Angular deformity of the radius and ulna due to premature physeal arrest of the radius and/or ulna.
- Angular deformity of the distal tibia due to premature physeal arrest of the distal tibia and/or the distal fibula.
- Correction or prevention of hip dysplasia.
- Malunion of all long bones and pelvis.

Osteotomy Types

TRANSVERSE ■ This technique is used for correction of rotational deformity (Fig. 22–1*A*, *B*, *C*). Kirschner wires may be inserted in each section of bone (*dashed lines*) before the osteotomy is done so that the amount of derotation can be determined.

OPENING WEDGE ■ This is a transverse osteotomy used to correct an angular deformity (Fig. 22–1*D*, *E*). Rotational correction is also possible and length is maintained.

CUNEIFORM ■ This is a closing wedge procedure, with a predetermined size wedge of bone removed from the point of maximal deformity (Fig. 22–2*A*, *B*). Some limb length is lost. Figure 22–17 is a case illustration of its use.

OBLIQUE ■ An oblique cut is usually made parallel with the articular surface to be realigned. The point of the long segment is inserted into the medullary cavity of the articular fragment (see Fig. 22–7). This procedure maintains or increases length slightly and can be used to correct rotation and varus or valgus deformity. It is most frequently used in corrective surgery for radius curvus. It is less suitable to diaphyseal osteotomies because of the large gaps that it creates.

STAIR-STEP LENGTHENING ■ A simple method for lengthening is the stair-step method illustrated in Figure 22–2*C* and *D*.

Surgical Principles of Corrective Osteotomy

- Because this is an elective procedure, there is no urgency. The animal must be in optimal condition to undergo anesthesia and surgery, the procedure should be well planned, and all equipment and implants necessary should be available.

- Plan the procedure by radiographing the bone in two planes, 90 degrees apart; commonly craniocaudal and mediolateral. Tracings made of these films allow the osteotomy to be preplanned to some degree (see Fig. 22–17). Because rotational changes cannot be ad-

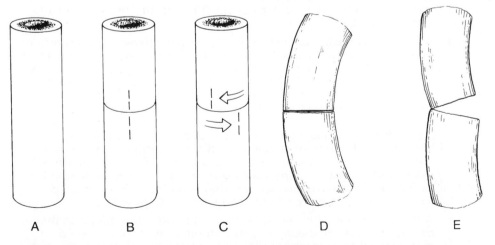

A	B	C	D	E

FIGURE 22–1. Transverse osteotomy. (*A–C*) Correction of a predetermined rotational deformity. (*D–E*) Open wedge type. A single transverse cut is made, rotational and angular deformities are corrected, stabilization is applied, and the deficit is filled with a bone graft.

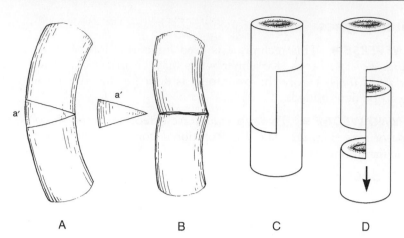

FIGURE 22–2. (*A, B*) Cuneiform osteotomy, closing wedge type. A predetermined size wedge of bone (*a'*) is removed from the point of maximal deformity. (*C, D*) Lengthening osteotomy. The sagittal osteotomy is twice as long as the desired lengthening in order to provide good bone contact for healing.

equately appreciated radiographically, a certain amount of error is introduced that must be compensated for at the surgery table. Nevertheless, it is useful to have a plan preoperatively, even if it is not reduced to paper.

- For angular deformity, the osteotomy must be done as close as possible to the point of maximum angular change (see Fig. 22–17). This will minimize the overall cosmetic deformity induced by the osteotomy. Make the osteotomy parallel to the joint surface to be realigned.

- When practical, make the osteotomy so the cut surfaces will fit together. Although this is useful to minimize the amount of bridging callus necessary, it is often not possible, as in the oblique osteotomy (see Fig. 22–7). It is more important to minimize the osteotomy gap in diaphyseal locations than in metaphyseal areas.

- Axially align the proximal and distal joints relative to the shaft. The animal should be draped in a manner that will allow good visualization of the distal limb because, in the end, the final alignment is done visually.

- An open approach is carried out to expose the operative bone area. In skeletally immature dogs, a longitudinal incision is made through the periosteum, which is peeled back as a layer using the osteotome or periosteal elevator. The bone is osteotomized using a powered bone saw, Gigli wire, or osteotome. With the power saw, constant irrigation is necessary to dissipate the heat generated in the cutting process. The osteotome should not be used as the primary cutting instrument in the diaphysis, as there is undue risk of splintering the bone. Instead, a row of closely spaced holes is drilled on the osteotomy line with a K-wire or 1.5- to 2.0-mm drill, and a narrow osteotome is used to connect the holes. This is a very good method, as it produces an irregular surface that tends to lock together, unlike the smooth surface of the power saw or Gigli wire cut.

- Autogenous cancellous bone graft (see Chapter 3) is added at the osteotomy site in diaphyseal osteotomies. It is not needed in metaphyseal osteotomies in skeletally immature patients.

- Fixation appropriate to a similar fracture pattern in the same bone is applied, and the surgical area is closed in layers.

- Aftercare is as for a similar fracture pattern in the same bone.

TREATMENT OF PREMATURE PHYSEAL GROWTH ARREST

Salter-Harris type V injury to the growth plate can result in temporary delay in growth, altered growth, or premature closure and cessation of growth.[1] The entire growth plate or a localized eccentric region within the growth plate may close prematurely. This is recognized radiographically by replacement of the radiolucent growth plate with uniform bone density, known as bone bridging. In paired bones, the premature closure may involve one or both bones, resulting in partial or complete growth impairment. The degree of alteration of growth is proportional to the growth potential remaining at the time of injury. Frequently, the immediate resultant pathology may be too insignificant for clinical observation, but with time (1 to several weeks) angular and/or rotational deformities begin to appear. The most common of these injuries involve the distal radial and ulnar physes in medium to large canine breeds.

Clinical characteristics of premature partial or complete closure of the physes include lameness, shortened limb, angular deformity, valgus or varus (Fig. 22–3), rotation, discomfort, crepitation, and restricted range of movement. Radiography should include both limbs, with special attention to the physis, the adjacent metaphysis, and the joints above and below the growth arrest. This study should determine (1) length of bone or bones, (2) width of the joint space at either end of the shortened bone, (3) direction of diaphyseal bowing, (4) angulation of the foot, (5) range of movement, and (6) extent of pathological changes in the joints above and below the physeal injury. An excellent description of the radiological changes of forelimb growth disturbances is the publication by O'Brien, Morgan, and Suter.[2]

The treatment of pathological changes in Salter-Harris Type V injury presents more complex problems when paired bones (e.g., radius and ulna or tibia and fibula) are involved. The most common problems involve the radius and ulna, where each bone must grow in a synchronous manner to promote normal growth and maintain congruency of their common articular surfaces. The ulna grows from two growth plates. The proximal physis, which closes between approximately 187 and 222 days, contributes only to olecranon length and is usually not significant relative to premature physeal closure anomalies. The distal ulnar physis is responsible for 100 percent of the longitudinal growth distal to the elbow joint and must equal the combined growth of the proximal and distal radial physis. The radius grows from both the proximal physis (40 percent) and distal physis (60 percent) and provides the major weight-bearing surface of the elbow joint (75 to 80 percent). Closure of these physes ranges

FIGURE 22–3. (A) Eccentric injury to the physeal growth plate (*) can result in complete cessation or reduction in rate of bone formation in that part of the physis. (B, C) Diaphyseal angular deformity and varying degrees of subluxation of the adjacent joint follow due to a greater amount of bone growth on the uninjured side. (From O'Brien T, Morgan JP, Suter PF: A radiographic study of growth disturbances in the forelimb. J Small Anim Pract 12:19–35, 1971, with permission.)

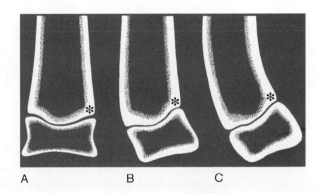

A   B   C

from about 220 to 250 days.[3] Abnormal development from asynchronous growth between the radius and ulna can result from retarded growth of the distal ulnar physis, distal radial physis, or proximal radial physis. Resultant dysplasias are common orthopedic problems and vary depending on the physis or physes involved, the age of the animal at time of involvement, and the span of time since injury.

Two cardinal considerations in planning corrective surgery are (1) the operative procedure should increase or at least maintain length because closure of the physis always results in a shorter bone (limb), and (2) corrective surgery should be carried out early to avoid or to at least minimize irreversible pathological changes in the adjacent joints. In the discussion below concerning surgical treatment, the following criteria will be used:

SKELETALLY IMMATURE ■   Two to 3 months of growth potential remaining: giant breeds—not over 7 to 8 months; large breeds—not over 5 to 6 months; small breeds—not over 3 months.

SKELETALLY MATURE ■   Growth plates not necessarily totally closed, but little lengthening remaining: giant breeds—over 8 months; large breeds—over 7 months; small breeds—over 4 months.

Distal Ulnar Physis Closure

Premature closure of the distal ulnar physis and subsequent deformities are the most common complications of forelimb physeal injuries, comprising 83 percent of forelimb growth disturbances in 39 dogs.[2] The conical shape of the distal ulnar physis is unique to the dog. In all other animals, the radial and ulnar physes are flat and predisposed to shearing fractures, and after reduction, the prognosis for uninterrupted growth is usually good. The canine distal ulnar physis is unable to shear because of the conical configuration, and thus shear forces are transformed to compressive forces and injury to germinal cartilage.[4] Significant retardation in growth of the distal ulnar physis results in a shortened ulna, which, because of the interosseous ligamentous connections between the bones, acts as a bowstring to restrict longitudinal growth of the radius.

Clinical and Radiographic Signs

Retardation of ulnar growth produces varying degrees of cranial and/or lateral bowing of the distal radius, radial shortening, valgus deformation and external rotation (supination) of the foot, elbow subluxation, and degenerative joint disease in the carpal and elbow joints (Figs. 22–4 and 22–5). Measurement of carpal valgus and cranial bowing can be done from the radiograph as shown in Figure 22–6. With cessation of growth of the ulnar diaphysis and continued growth of the radius, the humeral condyle is forced proximally relative to the ulna. In normal straight-limbed dogs this usually results in subluxation of the humeral condyle and damage to the anconeal process. The most severe lesion occurs in the distal half of the trochlear notch, resulting in degenerative cartilage changes, fracture of trabeculae in the subchondral bone, and alteration in joint morphology. Another effect is seen at the distal radial physis, where the compression of the physis laterally can cause eccentric slowing or complete cessation of growth and further carpal valgus and cranial bowing deformities. In brachycephalic breeds, the radial head usually subluxates laterally and rests on the lateral edge of the humeral condyle articular surface, where it causes mechanical damage to both the radial head and humeral condyle.

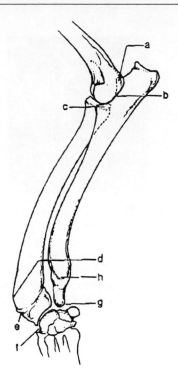

FIGURE 22–4. Radiographic changes characteristic of premature closure of the distal ulnar physis. With a cessation of growth of the ulna and continued growth of the radius, there is remodeling of the anconeal process with sclerosis (*a*), elbow subluxation with flattening of the trochlear notch (*b*) and distal displacement of the styloid process (*c*), anterior bowing of the radius (*d*), opening of distal radial physis (*e*) with increased angulation of the radiocarpal joint (*f*), and secondary arthritic changes. There is proximal relocation of the ulnar styloid (*g*) because of the shortened ulna. The distal ulnar physis is closed (*h*).

Because the radius is released from some of the compression force there may be less carpal valgus and cranial bowing.

Lameness is usually the first clinical sign of premature closure of the distal ulnar growth plate. Elbow subluxation may be accompanied by regional pain. Beginning radiographic changes are usually visible at this time. If radiographs are taken at the time of injury, they will often reveal a fracture line in the region of the growth plate.

Surgical Correction

Skeletally Immature

Early corrective surgery is indicated to avoid or to at least minimize subsequent changes. It is important to decide if the distal radial physis has bridged laterally or caudolaterally; if this is seen radiographically, see the description below for combined ulnar and distal radial physeal closure.

CARPAL VALGUS LESS THAN 25 DEGREES ■ *Partial ulnar ostectomy* of the distal ulna is required to remove the bowstring effect and to allow radial remodeling. The distal ulna is approached laterally and the lateral digital extensor muscle is retracted.[5] The easiest section to excise is just proximal to the physis. The length of the excised ulnar segment should be about 1.5 times the bone diameter, and it is critical that it be exposed extraperiosteally so that no periosteum is left to cause rapid bony bridging. Cutting of the bone is done with a power saw, Gigli wire saw, or osteotome, which can be used here because the bone is still quite soft at this age. Care must be exercised to avoid severing the radial artery on the caudal side of the radius. A fat graft placed in the defect will discourage bone bridging.[6] The fat can be collected from the falciform ligament or the subcutaneous gluteal region. It should be collected in a single

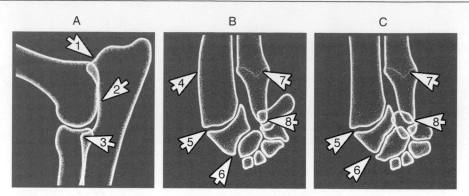

FIGURE 22-5. Common bony changes seen radiographically following premature closure of the distal ulnar physis. (*A*) Elbow region. (1) sclerotic and remodeled anconeal process with decrease of the distance between the process and the radial head; (2) trochlear notch shallow and subluxation of the humeroulnar joint; (3) distal displacement of the coronoid processes. (*B, C*) Region of the distal radius and ulna. Lateral view (*B*), and dorsopalmar view (*C*): (4) cranial bowing of the radial diaphysis and metaphysis; (5) open distal radial growth plate; (6) cranial and medial subluxation of the distal radius with increased angulation of the antebrachiocarpal joint and secondary degenerative joint disease; (7) closed distal ulnar growth plate; (8) proximal location of ulnar styloid process due to shortened ulna. (From O'Brien T, Morgan JP, Suter PF: A radiographic study of growth disturbances in the forelimb. J Small Anim Pract 12:19–35, 1971, with permission.)

block and handled gently to avoid necrosis. The fat should be large enough to fit tightly in the available space and soft tissues closed to secure it. A firm padded bandage is maintained for 7 to 10 days postoperatively. If bilateral procedures are done, the limbs should be lightly splinted for 2 weeks to avoid motion at the graft site which interferes with incorporation of the graft.[6] Moderate malalignment of the elbow will correct following distal ostectomy as the ulna is pulled proximally by triceps brachii muscle forces. More severe malalignment accompanied by elbow pain requires proximal dynamic proximal ulnar osteotomy and is described below (see Fig. 22–9).

The original report on partial ulnar ostectomy concluded that partial correction of the radial deformity was obtained.[6] No mention was made of the exact

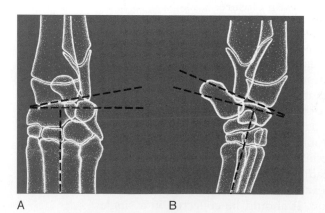

FIGURE 22-6. (*A*) Lining method for determination of angulation of the carpus from dorsopalmar radiographs. Zero to 10° is normal. (*B*) Lining method for determination of angulation of the carpus from lateromedial radiographs. Zero to 8° is normal. (From O'Brien T, Morgan JP, Suter PF: A radiographic study of growth disturbances in the forelimb. J Small Anim Pract 12:19–35, 1971, with permission.)

amount of carpal valgus preoperatively. A later report found the procedure to be effective only in young dogs (median age 5 months) with less than 25 degrees of carpal valgus or in older animals (median age 6.5 months) with less than 13 degrees of valgus.[7] This further reinforces the urgency of early surgical treatment.

CARPAL VALGUS GREATER THAN 25 DEGREES ■ Corrective osteotomy of the radius to realign the foot should be performed at the same time as the partial ulnar ostectomy.

Use of the external fixator is usually the preferred method of fixation. Type I external fixators can be used (Fig. 22–7E), or type II (Fig. 22–7C, D). Because the osteotomy is in the metaphyseal area in an immature animal, healing is rapid; the fixator can usually be removed by 6 weeks postoperatively.

The type II fixator is preferred by the author because of the ease of final alignment. The proximal full pin is placed in the frontal plane of the proximal radius; this will be perpendicular to the humerus when the elbow is flexed 90 degrees. The distal full pin is placed as close to the joint as is practical. A small

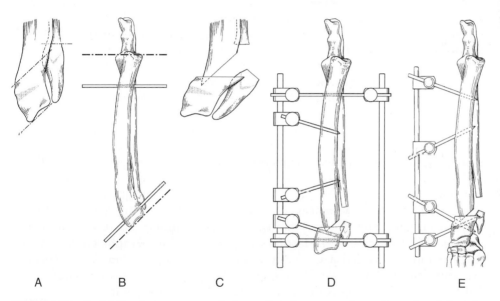

A   B   C   D   E

FIGURE 22–7. Oblique osteotomy of the radius for correction of angular deformity caused by premature arrest of the distal ulnar growth plate. (*A, B*) The osteotomy line is drawn parallel with the antebrachiocarpal joint surface at the area of greatest radial curvature. A transverse osteotomy of the ulna is planned at or slightly proximal to the radial osteotomy. Center-threaded fixation pins are placed proximally and distally in the radius, parallel to the adjacent joint surfaces. The distal pin is also positioned to keep it in the frontal plane of the rotated carpus/metacarpus. These pins are placed before the osteotomy is done. (*C, D*) The pointed proximal segment of the radius is reduced into the center of the distal segment. Connecting bars and clamps are loosely positioned on the fixation pins, and the foot is derotated and held so that it is in a straight line with the proximal portion of the radius and ulna and its frontal plane is continuous with the plane of the proximal segment. The two full pins should be approximately parallel to each other and in the same frontal plane at this point. The connecting bar clamps are tightened and the half pins are driven through the empty clamps to complete the type IIB fixator. (*E*) The type IA fixator can also be applied. As above, the proximal and distal fixation pins are placed before the osteotomy is done.

hypodermic needle is used to probe for the joint space and is left in place to mark the distal end of the radius. This pin is placed in the frontal plane of the distal radius, carpus, and metacarpus. It will be perpendicular to the paw when the carpus is flexed 90 degrees. Because of possible supination of the distal radius the pins will be in different planes as viewed from the distal end of the limb.

The ulnar osteotomy is performed first from a lateral approach, as described above. The osteotomy is done at or distal to the proposed radial site; if cut too proximally the cut end will protrude laterally after angular correction. The radial osteotomy site is approached cranially with separation and retraction of the carpal and digital extensor tendons.[5] Periosteum is incised longitudinally and elevated from the bone and the osteotomy performed as described above. Connecting bars and clamps are positioned loosely, with three empty clamps on the medial bar.

The distal segment is aligned first by placing the pointed end of the radius within the medullary canal and then by rotating the full pins until they are in the same plane, and then by angulating the distal bone until the pins are parallel to each other in the frontal plane. The foot should be in axial alignment with the proximal radius. Rotational alignment is checked by flexing the elbow and the carpus; the paw should be aligned with the humerus. It is often difficult to completely reduce the cranial bowing due to contracture of the flexor apparatus. At this point the four clamps on the full pins are tightened, and a half pin is driven through the distal empty clamp into the distal fragment and the clamp tightened. Two more half pins are then driven into the proximal segment to complete the fixation. Bone grafting is not necessary, and closure is routine.

Type I fixators (Fig. 22–7E) are applied in a similar fashion, with the proximal and distal pins inserted first and the remaining pins driven after realignment. Prognosis for satisfactory function is good, regardless of degree of deformity, when performed at this age.[7] Some limb shortening can be expected in most animals.

Figure 22–8A, B shows a healed fracture of the radius with premature closure of the distal ulnar physis in a 5-month-old Afghan hound. Treatment originally consisted of application of a Mason metasplint. The radiographs taken 3 weeks after the injury revealed a clinically healed radius, leg shortening of 10 mm, premature closure of the distal ulnar growth plate, moderate valgus deformity of the foot, and early signs of incongruency of the elbow joint.

The primary objectives were to restore congruency of the elbow joint and to correct the cranial bowing of the radius and valgus deformity of the foot. Removal of a 1½-inch section of the ulna (including periosteum) corrected the bowstring effect, and, in most instances (with minor deformity), the proximal ulna will readjust in position and make the correction needed for congruency at the elbow joint. An oblique osteotomy of the radius at the fracture site was used to derotate the foot and straighten the radius. In Figure 22–8C the type I external fixator is in place, following partial ulnar ostectomy and corrective osteotomy of the radius. At 4 weeks postoperatively, the radius was healed and the elbow joint was congruent and had a full range of movement (Fig. 22–8D). The external fixator was removed at this time.

DYNAMIC PROXIMAL ULNAR OSTEOTOMY ■ If there is marked incongruency of the elbow, with or without distal changes, a proximal ulnar osteotomy (Fig. 22–9) allows the proximal end to shift proximally and re-establish

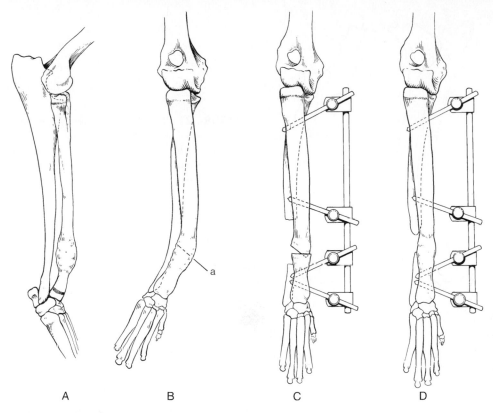

A   B   C   D

FIGURE 22–8. (*A, B*) Healed fracture of the radius with premature closure of the distal ulnar physis in 5-month-old Afghan hound. Preoperative lateral and craniocaudal views. (*C*) A 1½-inch section of the ulna (including periosteum) was removed, the oblique cut (*a*) in the radius was made at the point of greatest curvature, the point of the radius was inserted into the medullary cavity of the distal radial segment, the foot and distal section of radius was held so that it was in line with the proximal end of the leg, and the external fixator was applied on the medial surface. (*D*) At 4½ weeks postoperatively, healing of the radius has occurred and the elbow joint is congruent with a good range of motion; the external fixator was removed at this point.

congruency as well as possible with the deformed articulating surfaces.[8] A caudal approach to the proximal ulna exposes the ulna and the humeroulnar joint,[5] which can be inspected for fibrous tissue invasion and osteophytes; these are removed as indicated. The osteotomy is made slightly distal to the coronoid process. In most cases the bone will spring apart after cutting, but in some cases a periosteal elevator is needed to break down the interosseus and annular ligaments. A small smooth Steinmann pin driven normograde is used for stabilization. In immature dogs, a fat graft, as described above, is used to prevent premature osseous bridging.

Skeletally Mature

After cessation of most long-bone growth there is no hope of meaningful correction of carpal valgus by eliminating the bowstring effect of the short ulna, and all attention should be directed toward correcting angular and rotational deformities and in re-establishing elbow congruity. Angular and rotational de-

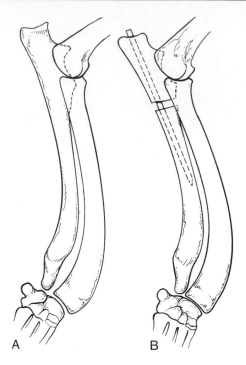

FIGURE 22–9. (*A*) Incongruency and subluxation of the elbow joint due to shortening of the ulna. (*B*) Dynamic proximal ulnar osteotomy of the ulna just distal to the coronoid processes allows the ulna to move into physiological reduction due to muscle and weight-bearing forces. A smooth Steinmann pin or Kirschner wire is used for stabilization.

formities are eliminated by corrective radial osteotomy, as described above. Bone plate fixation is possible only with moderate angular deformity and little or no rotational component. A closing wedge osteotomy is advisable when using plate fixation, which further shortens the limb. If the elbow incongruity is minor it will correct itself after the distal ulnar osteotomy, but if the incongruity is marked and accompanied by pain in the elbow region the dynamic proximal osteotomy described above will provide more rapid and complete realignment.

Distal Ulna and Eccentric Distal Radial Closure

It seems probable that the primary injury in this situation is distal ulnar physis closure. The bowstring effect of the short ulna can create a compression of the lateral or caudolateral region of the distal radial physis that can cause complete shutdown of the growth plate in this region and replacement by a bone bridge. As the medial side of the physis continues to grow, the valgus angulation of the distal radius continues, even after the ulna is sectioned, and probably accounts for some of the failures of ulnar ostectomy alone to correct radial deformities. If the bridging involves primarily the caudolateral aspect of the physis, increased cranial bowing accompanies the lateral deviation. Careful inspection of fine-detail screen or nonscreen radiographs is necessary to verify the bone bridge, which has the same density as surrounding bone, compared to the radiolucent active physis.

Surgical Correction

Skeletally Immature

In this situation simple partial ulnar ostectomy will fail because the radial bone bridge will prevent radial correction. Ulnar ostectomy should be accom-

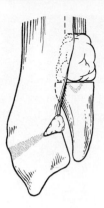

FIGURE 22–10. Premature closure of the distal ulnar growth plate accompanied by lateral closure and bone bridge of the radial growth plate (see also Fig. 22–7A). A partial ulnar ostectomy of the distal ulna is accompanied by resection of the lateral bone bridge in the radius. Both bone defects are packed with fat grafts to discourage bone healing.

panied by resecting the bone bridge to free its restriction to radial remodeling (Fig. 22–10).[9]

A skin incision is made over the craniolateral region of the radial physis and fascia is incised to expose the epiphysis. A small-gauge hypodermic needle is used to probe for the growth plate beginning medially and working laterally. The needle easily penetrates the cartilage of the active physis and is used to locate the medial limits of the bone bridge. A curette, fine-nose rongeur, osteotome, or power saw is then used to create a generous V-shaped bone defect corresponding to the location of the original growth plate and extending medially into the active physeal cartilage. The point of the V should be in the active growth cartilage. It is important to be sure that the bone bridge be completely removed. A fat graft (see discussion above regarding partial ulnar ostectomy) is collected from the gluteal region and placed into the defect and soft tissue sutured over it. The partial ulnar ostectomy is then completed as described above.

There seems to be little published regarding the outcome of this surgery. One case available for follow-up by Vandewater and Olmstead returned to normal,[9] and the author's experience has been encouraging. As with the other techniques that depend on bone remodeling, the earlier they are done, the better the prognosis.

Skeletally Mature

Correction at this age is corrective osteotomy as described above for distal ulnar physis closure.

Retained Cartilaginous Cores in the Distal Ulnar Physis

This condition is seen in growing large and giant breeds of dogs and is caused by delayed endochondral ossification of a zone of distal ulnar metaphysis, resulting in cores or "candlesticks" of hypertrophied cartilage cells rather than bony trabecula (Fig. 22–11A).[10] This cartilage core slows distal ulnar lengthening, and the ulnar styloid is seen to not extend distally to the ulnar carpal bone. This results in some loss of lateral support for the carpus, and mild carpal valgus deformity ensues. The distal radius may also respond to the ulnar shortening by cranial bowing (Fig. 22–11B), although lateral deviation or elbow incongruity have not been seen.

The cause of retained cartilage cores is unknown, although some think it is a form of osteochondrosis.[11] Although the role of hypernutrition and acceler-

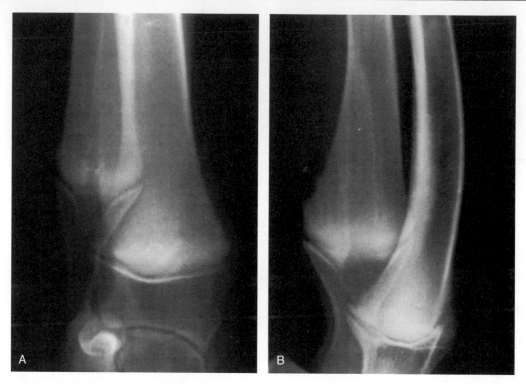

FIGURE 22–11. (*A*) Four-month-old female Great Dane with painful forelegs. Note the "candlestick" core of cartilage extending from the ulnar epiphysis into the metaphysis. (*B*) Five-month-old male St. Bernard with increased valgus angulation of the carpus and pain elicited upon palpation of the carpus. Note the "candlestick" formation in the ulna and cranial bowing of the radius with secondary thickening of the caudal cortex (Wolff's law).

ated growth remains to be proven, we advise decreasing the plane of nutrition to slow growth when presented with a 3 to 4-month-old puppy with these changes. Corrective osteotomy is occasionally indicated in a mature dog with functional problems due to deformity.

Proximal or Distal Radial Physis Closure

Less common than premature closure of the distal ulnar physis is premature closure of either the proximal or distal radial physis. Of all forelimb growth arrests there was an 11 percent incidence of distal closure, and a 6 percent incidence of proximal closure.[2] Premature closure of either physis results in shortening of the radius, although the leg may remain straight if the distal closure is symmetrical. Asymmetrical distal closure usually results in some degree of angular deformity, either varus or valgus.

Clinical and Radiographic Signs

PROXIMAL CLOSURE ■ As the ulna grows, the shortened radius is pulled distally by the radioulnar ligament, bringing about an increase in joint space between the radial head and humeral condyle (Figs. 22–12 and 22–13*A*).[2] As discrepancy of growth between the radius and ulna continues, the medial and lateral collateral ligaments of the elbow impinge the humeral condyle on the coronoid processes with subsequent displacement and an increase of humer-

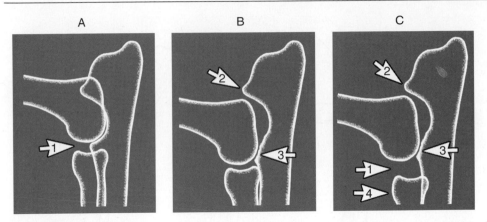

FIGURE 22–12. Common bony changes seen radiographically following premature closure of the proximal or distal radial physis. (*1*) Increased space at the humeroradial joint, resulting in subluxation of the entire elbow joint. (*2*) As a result of the increased distance between the anconeal process and radial head the anconeal process appears displaced proximally. (*3*) Sclerosis and remodeling of the coronoid processes, accompanied by varying degrees of degenerative joint disease. (*4*) Displacement of the radial head caudally and laterally. (From O'Brien T, Morgan JP, Suter PF: A radiographic study of growth disturbances in the forelimb. J Small Anim Pract 12:19–35, 1971, with permission.)

oulnar joint space, elongation of the articular notch, and sometimes fragmentation of either coronoid process[2,12,13] and degenerative joint disease. There is usually shortening of the limb.

DISTAL CLOSURE ■ Several variables determine the types of abnormalities seen.[14] Because ulnar growth usually continues, elbow malarticulation develops as described for proximal closure. With complete *symmetrical* closure the limb usually remains straight and shortened, but carpal varus has been reported.[15] There are also changes in the antebrachiocarpal joint, which may include an increase in joint space and later degenerative joint disease. A caudal bowing of the radius and ulna may occur in some cases. *Asymmetrical* distal closure is more common and *lateral* closure results in valgus deformity and external rotation (supination) of the paw similar to that seen with distal ulnar closure. Indeed, some degree of closure of the distal ulnar physis may be concurrent. *Medial* closure of the radius is less often seen and causes varus angular deformity and inward rotation (pronation) of the paw. In some cases, particularly with lateral closure, caudal closure is more pronounced than cranial, resulting in caudal angulation of the antebrachiocarpal joint.

The first clinical sign of closure is a gradual onset of lameness and pain in the elbow region. Radiographic changes are present at this time, and early surgery is indicated to check or minimize joint changes.

Surgical Correction

Skeletally Immature

The most pressing problem is restoration of congruency of the elbow joint because degenerative changes occur rapidly. A choice must be made regarding the existing radial shortening: the ulna can be shortened by partial ostectomy or the radius lengthened by osteotomy to achieve contact of the radial head

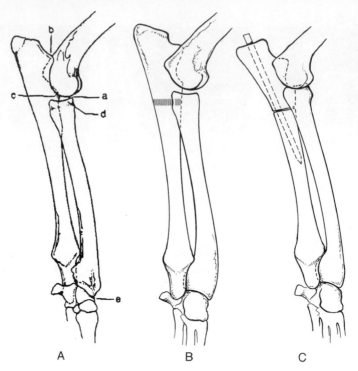

A   B   C

FIGURE 22–13. (A) Bony changes characteristic of premature closure of the distal or proximal radial physis (also see Fig. 22–12). With a cessation of growth of the radius, there is increased width of the humeroradial joint space (a), proximal displacement of the anconeal process (b), remodeling of the trochlear notch and coronoid process (c), and development of secondary degenerative joint disease. There is caudal and lateral displacement of the radial head (d). Angular deformity may or may not be present; however, there is usually some increase in radiocarpal joint space (e) and evidence of radial physis closure. (B) If lengthening of the radius is not possible, the ulna is shortened by dynamic proximal ulnar ostectomy, removing a section of ulna (*shaded area*) slightly longer than the distance between the humeral condyle and radial head. The ostectomy is immediately distal to the coronoid processes. (C) Shortening of the ulna due to weight-bearing and muscular forces results in physiological reduction of the humeroradial joint. A smooth Steinmann pin or Kirschner wire is used for stabilization.

with the humeral condyle. The ideal choice would always be radial lengthening, but technical and economic considerations often prevent employing this method. Shortening the ulna is technically much easier and good results can be anticipated.[15] If limb length is sufficient for reasonably good function, it is probably the preferred method. If distal angular and rotational deformity is present, it generally must be corrected by osteotomy. There is also the possibility with eccentric distal closure for resection of the bone bridge and achieving correction in younger animals.[14] Corrective ostectomy could be done later if the deformities persist.

DYNAMIC PARTIAL ULNAR OSTECTOMY ■ For cases in which the radial shortening is minimal and the animal is nearly mature, one can remove a short section (ostectomy) of the ulna to restore congruency of the radial head with the humeral condyle (Fig. 22–13B, C).[8] The proximal ulna and elbow joint are approached from a caudal incision.[5] The ulnar segment removed should be slightly longer than the observed gap between the humeral condyle and radial head. A small Steinmann pin is used for stabilization. Muscular forces and weight bearing will cause the ulna to shorten by sliding on the smooth pin until the radial head contacts the condyle. Fragments of the lateral coronoid process can be removed from the same caudal approach to the proximal ulna, but those of the medial coronoid will probably require a separate medial approach.[5] Analgesic and anti-inflammatory agents are given to encourage early postoperative weight bearing.

The advantage of this approach over a static shortening ostectomy with rigid fixation is that the radial head will find its own position relative to the humeral condyle and so form a more physiological joint. This procedure is often combined with a distal corrective osteotomy of the radius and ulna to correct angular and rotational defects,[15] or with resection of the bone bridge of the distal physis.

BONE BRIDGE RESECTION ■ When the distal radial physis closure is eccentric, resection of the bone bridge can allow varying degrees of angular and rotational correction due to continuing growth of the remaining growth plate.[14,15] This is most applicable to younger patients with considerable bone growth remaining and is usually combined with partial ulnar ostectomy. The technique has been explained above in the section Distal Ulnar and Eccentric Distal Radial Closure (Fig. 22–10).

DYNAMIC LENGTHENING OSTEOTOMY OF THE RADIUS ■ Progressive spreading of a radial osteotomy has the potential for elongating the radius to match the ulna and so reduce the elbow incongruity. Although the conventional external fixator applied with threaded connecting rods or the Charnley apparatus have been employed to lengthen the radius, correction of angular deformity is restricted to one plane. The advent of the Ilizarov type ring fixator (see Fig. 2–35E) gives the possibility of simultaneous lengthening with angular and rotational correction.[14,16,17] Such apparatus is now commercially available for veterinary use in North America (Jorgensen Laboratories, Inc., Loveland, CO) and in Europe.

After placement of the fixation wires and reflection of periosteum, transverse radial osteotomy is performed as has been explained above. If the ulna is seriously deformed, it is also osteotomized. The wires are attached to rings and the rings connected by threaded rods and nuts. Angular and rotational deformities are reduced to the extent possible and the bones distracted to the limits of soft tissue. One-millimeter daily spreading of the osteotomy divided into two to four increments is continued until the elbow is reduced, typically 4 to 6 weeks. Frequent radiographic evaluation is necessary to monitor the progress (Fig. 22–14). After the distraction phase is complete the fixator is left in place for another 4 to 6 weeks to allow solidification of the distracted callus.

If only the proximal physis is closed, or if there is no angular deformity with distal closure, simple axial lengthening is all that is required. This can be accomplished with the Charnley apparatus (Synthes Ltd. [USA], Paoli, PA), or with slightly modified conventional Kirschner style apparatus applied in type IIA configuration. Threaded $^3/_{16}$-inch (3.2-mm) rods are substituted for normal connecting rods. These threaded rods are available commercially at hardware outlets. There are two methods for providing the sliding motion necessary for distraction. In the first, conventional medium clamps are attached to the two distal fixation pins, and these are tightened to the rod in the normal manner. The proximal pin clamps are modified by drilling or filing the connecting rod

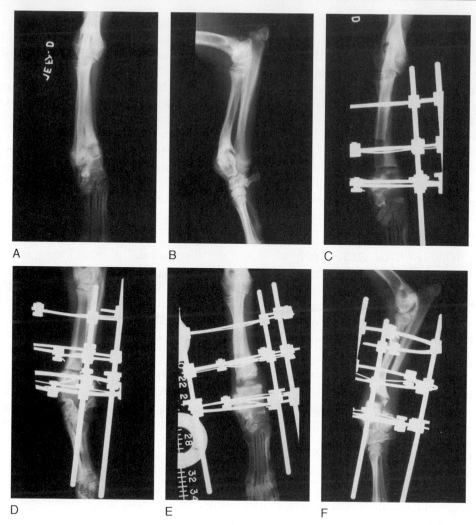

FIGURE 22–14. Limb lengthening with a ring (Ilizarov) fixator. The patient was a 4-month-old greyhound with a deformed left antebrachium. (*A, B*) Premature closure of the distal radial physis and malunion of a distal radial metaphyseal fracture. Varus deviation of the distal limb and cranial bowing of the radius. The elbow joint is stable and congruent. (*C, D*) Postoperatively after transverse radial osteotomy and segmental ulnar ostectomy. The angular deformity and cranial bowing have been corrected with the ring fixator. Distraction was started 10 days later at the rate of 0.25 mm four times daily. (*E, F*) At 20 days postoperatively, and after 10 days of distraction, new bone formation is evident in the osteotomy gap. The elbow joint has become incongruent. *Figure continued on opposite page*

hole to ³/₁₆-inch diameter with a fixation pin in the bolt and the nut tightened (modified clamps are available from Imex Veterinary, Inc., Longview, TX). This allows the clamps to slide on the threaded rod, and they are secured to the rod by a normal nut on each side of each clamp. Distraction is accomplished by loosening the nuts on the proximal side of the clamps and tightening the distal clamps. The second method is to divide the connecting rods in the middle area and connect each pair of rods by a threaded turnbuckle. Rotation of the turnbuckle causes the rod to lengthen. The distraction procedure is managed as explained above.

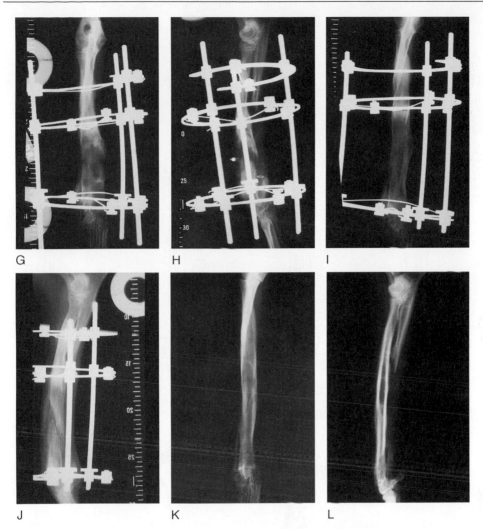

FIGURE 22–14. *Continued* (G, H) Approximately 5 cm of lengthening has occurred at 8 weeks postoperatively. Regenerate new bone appears as axially oriented striations, and the elbow has realigned. (I, J) Distraction has been discontinued at 4 months postoperatively and approximately 8 cm of length has been gained. The fixator was left in place an additional 6 weeks to allow maturation of new bone formation. (K, L) Eleven months postoperatively and 5.5 months after removal of the fixator. The limb is 5 mm longer than the opposite, and function is normal. There is good axial alignment and the elbow appears normal. The quality of the regenerate bone is excellent. (Photos and case material courtesy of Dr. Erick Egger.)

STATIC LENGTHENING OSTEOTOMY OF THE RADIUS ■ Bone lengthening with plate fixation or conventional external fixators is also possible. For animals over 5 to 6 months of age, one lengthening will usually be sufficient. For those under this age, the procedure may need to be repeated in 6 to 8 weeks to restore length and congruency. If the closure is accompanied by angular deformity, corrective osteotomy for this defect may be delayed until the lengthening osteotomy is about healed.

Figure 22–15 shows premature closure of the distal growth plate of the radius, with shortening and early secondary incongruency of the articular surfaces

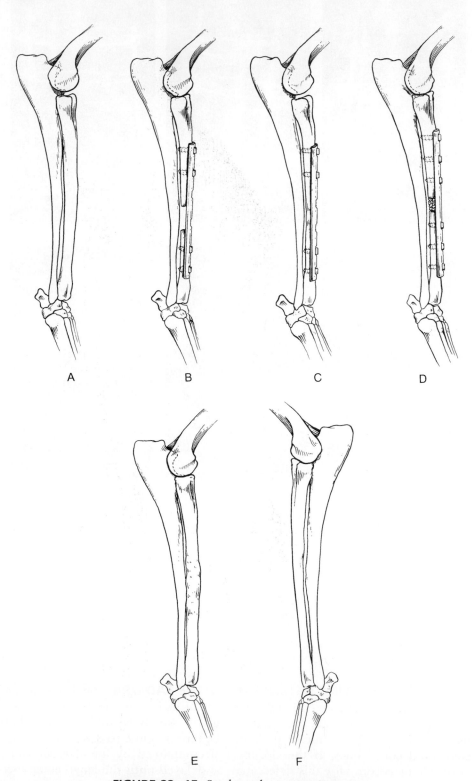

A   B   C   D

E   F

FIGURE 22–15. *See legend on opposite page*

in the elbow joint in a 4-month-old large-breed dog. The animal had started to favor the leg 2 weeks before presentation. The leg appeared to be straight from both lateral and cranial views. The objective was to restore approximately normal length to the radius and thus restore congruency to the articular surfaces of the elbow joint. Because the animal had approximately 4 months of growth left, the operative procedure was expected to be repeated to maintain a good elbow joint.

A transverse midshaft osteotomy of the radius was performed (Fig. 22–15B). The bone segments were wedged apart 15 mm with a bone spreader, and a semitubular plate was inserted for fixation. Congruency of the elbow joint was restored. At the 3-month re-examination, the osteotomy area was filled with bone. Shortening of the radius and incongruency of the elbow were again evident. Lameness returned about 3 weeks prior to this re-examination. Discrepancy between the coronoid process of the ulna and the articular surface of the radius was evident (Fig. 22–15C). The bone plate was removed, and the radius was again osteotomized and lengthened by 10 mm. A semitubular plate was applied for fixation (Fig. 22–15D). At the 2-month follow-up, the leg was straight, the elbow joint range of motion appeared normal, and function was good (Fig. 22–15E). The overall length in comparison to the opposite leg was 16 mm shorter; however, this was not evident on standing or moving. The normal opposite leg is shown in Figure 22–15F.

Partial or complete premature closure of the distal and proximal radial physes in the same limb is illustrated in Figure 22–16. For this condition, the objectives of corrective osteotomy were to restore congruency of the elbow joint and realign the foot. Because the leg was already shorter than the opposite leg, a lengthening procedure was planned. The 6½-month-old Doberman had suffered a foreleg injury approximately 8 weeks previous to being treated. Lameness was intermittent at first but became continuous and progressive during the preceding 3 weeks. Radiographs revealed premature closure of the proximal radial physis, shortening of the radius, and incongruency of the elbow joint (Fig. 22–16A, B). There was also evidence of damage to the distal radial physis with altered growth, resulting in some valgus deformity and outward rotation of the foot, which was becoming more pronounced. The first objective was to restore radial length and elbow congruency; the second objective was to correct the angular deformity and external rotation of the foot at a later date.

A transverse osteotomy was performed and the segments were wedged apart by 11 mm using a bone spreader; this restored length to the radius and con-

---

FIGURE 22–15. (A) Premature closure of the distal physis of the radius with shortening and early secondary incongruency of the articular surfaces in the elbow joint in a 4-month-old dog. (B) Transverse midshaft osteotomy of radius was performed. Bone segments wedged apart 15 mm and semitubular plate inserted for fixation. Congruency of elbow joint restored. (C) At the 3-month follow-up, osteotomy area is filled with bone. There is evidence of shortening of radius and incongruency of elbow; lameness has returned. Note the discrepancy between the coronoid process of the ulna and the articular surface of the radius. (D) The bone plate was removed, the radius again osteotomized and lengthened 10 mm, and another semitubular plate applied for fixation. The osteotomy area deficit was filled with autogenous cancellous bone. (E) At the 2-month follow-up, the leg is straight, the elbow joint's range of motion appears normal; overall length in comparison with opposite leg is 16 mm shorter, although this is not evident when the animal moves or stands. The plate was removed. (F) Normal opposite leg.

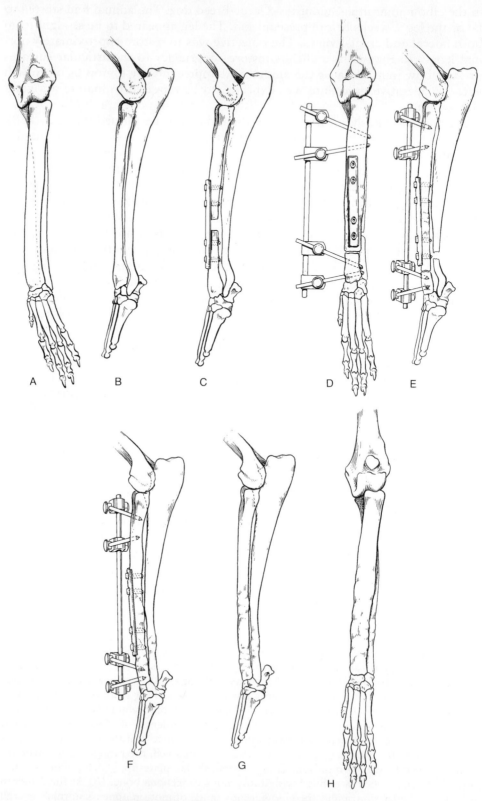

FIGURE 22–16. *See legend on opposite page*

gruency to the articulating surfaces of the elbow joint. A semitubular plate (buttress plate) was applied for fixation (Fig. 22–16C). In 1 month, healing at the osteotomy site was well underway, and the elbow appeared stable. Leg function had improved markedly. At this time, the ulna and radius were again osteotomized, angulation and rotation were corrected, and an external fixator was applied for fixation (Fig. 22–16D, E). In 7 weeks, the osteotomy sites were well healed. The bone plate and external fixator were removed. When the animal was rechecked at 1 year of age, good functional use of the leg was evident (Fig. 22–16G, H). The leg appeared straight from both lateral and cranial views. There was a 10-degree loss of flexion at the elbow joint; however, it was not discernible at the walk or running. The affected radius was slightly shorter than the opposite normal radius. The animal adjusted by slightly increasing extension at the shoulder and elbow joints; this was not evident on standing or moving.

Skeletally Mature

The objectives of treatment of mature animals are identical to those detailed above for immature animals, and the same procedures are applicable, with the exception of resection of physeal bone bridges. The elbow joint may need to be explored to resect fibrous tissue and osteophytes and to remodel bone deformity.[14] Partial ulnar ostectomy alone or combined with distal corrective osteotomy for angular and rotational deformity are the most common procedures. Static lengthening of the radius by stair-step osteotomy is simpler than in the growing animal because only one procedure will be needed. Because of the degenerative changes present due to elbow incongruity, the prognosis for function is not as good as in animals treated early in life.

Distal Tibial Deformity

Deformity as a result of disturbed growth of tibial physes is very rare. Trauma involving the proximal tibia totaled 3.7 percent of 135 cases and the distal physis 3 percent in one report, and none of these developed any deformity.[18] However, as in the radius/ulna, in a two-bone system there is a possibility of premature closure of the distal fibula with resulting valgus deformity of the

---

FIGURE 22–16. Growth plate injury with closure of the proximal radial physis and partial closure of the distal radial physis. (A, B) Eight-week-old foreleg injury in a 6-month-old Doberman with progressive lameness, shortening of the radius, and incongruency of the elbow joint. Damage to the distal radial physis with partial closure resulted in some progressive valgus deformity and outward rotation of the foot. (C) Lateral view following transverse osteotomy. The segments were slowly wedged apart 11 mm by exerting constant pressure with a bone spreader, restoring length to the radius and congruency to the elbow joint. A semitubular buttress plate was applied. In 1 month, healing at the osteotomy site was nearly complete, the elbow joint appeared congruent, leg function had markedly improved. (D, E) The ulna and radius were osteotomized, derotation and straightening of the foot were carried out, and an external fixator was applied to the medial surface of the radius. (F) After 7 weeks, both osteotomy sites were well healed and the plate and external fixator were removed. (G, H) At 1 year, the leg was straight when viewed laterally and cranially; there was a 10-degree loss of flexion at the elbow joint, the elbow joint appeared congruent, the affected leg was slightly shorter than the opposite normal leg, function was good.

tibia, as there is at least one such case reported.[19] Premature closure of the medial side of the distal tibial growth plate without traumatic injury may be an inherited condition in the dachshund, and was termed "pes varus" by Johnson and co-workers.[20] Lameness of the affected limbs before skeletal maturity was seen in both types of cases.

Surgical Correction

Valgus Deformity

Either an opening wedge or closing wedge[19] osteotomy can be performed according to the principles described above. A closing wedge method is illustrated in Figure 22–17. In addition to the fixation illustrated in Figure

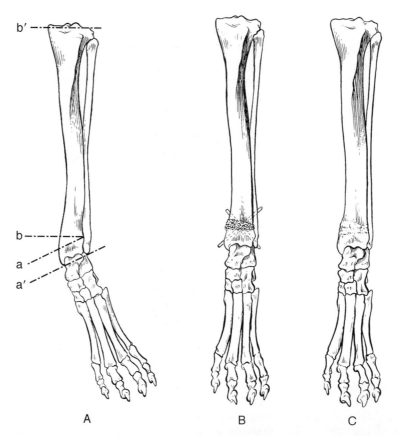

A   B   C

FIGURE 22–17. Cuneiform closing wedge osteotomy used for correction of an angular deformity caused by partial premature closure of the distal tibial physis. (*A*) Preoperative craniocaudal view. To plan the size wedge to remove, a paper tracing is made from the radiogram. *Line a* is drawn parallel to the distal joint surface, *line a'*, and intersects the medial cortex at the apex of the curvature. *Line b* is parallel to the proximal joint surface, *line b'*, and connects to *line a* at the lateral cortex. Because angular deformities and rotation encompass more than one plane, final adjustments will need to be made before application of fixation. (*B*) Because the distal segment was relatively short, cross pins were used for fixation at the osteotomy site. The removed wedge of bone was cut in small pieces and laid in the area as a bone graft. The fixation was further stabilized with a coaptation splint. (*C*) Clinical union was present at 7 weeks, and the splint and pins were removed.

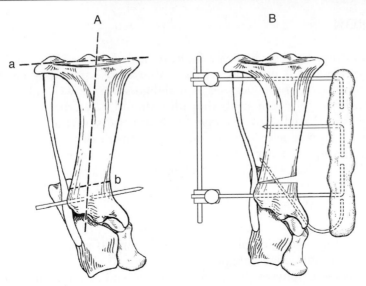

FIGURE 22-18. Opening wedge osteotomy for pes varus in the dachshund. (*A*) Preoperative planning is complicated by the fact that the plane of the proximal joint, *line a*, is not perpendicular to the sagittal plane of the tibia. Radiographs of the normal limb are essential to understanding the correction needed. The planned osteotomy, *line b*, is parallel to the distal joint surface at the point of maximum curvature of the tibia. The distal full fixation pin is parallel to *line b* and is placed before the osteotomy is completed. (*B*) The proximal fixation pin is placed perpendicular to the sagittal plane of the tibia. The wedge is opened by lateral angulation of the distal segment until the full pins are parallel to each other, at which point the lateral connecting bar is attached and clamps tightened. A 0.062-inch (1.5-mm) Kirschner wire is driven through the medial malleolus and across the osteotomy into the medial cortex and a second pin is placed in the proximal segment. A molded acrylic connecting bar simplifies connecting the fixation pins medially. (From Johnson SG, Hulse DA, et al: Corrective osteotomy for pes varus in the dachshund. Vet Surg 18:373–379, 1989, with permission.)

22–17C, an external fixator similar to that described for varus deformity below (Fig. 22–18) could be employed. Bone plate fixation could be applicable if the osteotomy can be made proximally enough to allow at least two plate screws in the distal fragment.[19] The Veterinary Cuttable Plate (VCP) (Synthes Ltd. [USA], Paoli, PA) is helpful in this situation if 2.7-mm screws are suitable for the size animal (see Fig. 2–74).

Varus Deformity

Opening wedge osteotomy and type II external fixators (Fig. 22–18) were used in a series of five cases for correction of pes varus in dachshunds.[20] As pointed out by these workers, the proximal and distal tibial articular surfaces are usually not parallel in the dachshund, so careful study of craniocaudal radiographs of the normal tibia is necessary to determine the angular correction needed. The method of application of the external fixator illustrated allowed the osteotomy to be made very distally, at the point of maximum curvature. Because the fixation pin in the medial malleolus was only 0.062 inch, methylmethacrylate acrylic bars were used instead of conventional clamps.

MALUNION

Malunion may be described as a fracture healed or healing in malalignment. Function of the part is disturbed to a variable degree depending on the type of deformity induced. Minor degrees of malalignment are well tolerated by animals, for which the veterinary orthopedist should be eternally grateful. When function is interrupted, however, corrective surgery is advisable.

Malunion can be due to lack of fracture treatment or to inappropriate treatment. Recognition of a developing malunion during fracture healing, while the callus is still plastic, provides an opportunity for treatment by augmenting the fixation after closed reduction of the deformity. Closed application of external skeletal fixation works well in most diaphyseal fractures. The following classification has been proposed by Kaderly[21]:

1. Overriding—long diaphyseal fragments pulled past each other by muscular forces but still axially aligned.
2. Angular—diaphyseal fragments in end-to-end contact with axial angular deformity.
3. Rotational—diaphyseal fragments in end-to-end contact with torsional deformity.
4. Intra-articular—malalignment of articular surfaces.

Most clinical cases exhibit a mixture of the types named above. A secondary effect of most malunions is that joints may become malaligned and subsequently suffer from degenerative joint disease. Ligamentous tissues are abnormally stressed and joint instability can follow. Soft tissues adjacent to involved bones may become impinged by the bone. Valgus and external rotation seem to be more poorly tolerated by the limb than do their opposites. Bowing in the craniocaudal direction causes limb shortening, but is relatively well tolerated because joint surfaces remain parallel to each other and to the ground plane.

Surgical correction by osteotomy is the preferred method of treatment when the malunion is well healed and is producing significant functional, as opposed to cosmetic, problems. Consideration must be given to the extent of the soft tissue shortening when the angular deformity is severe. It may not be possible to achieve significant straightening of the limb in a single procedure without endangering soft tissue vascularity. This situation requires either multiple procedures, or gradual lengthening such as described above for correction of bone growth abnormalities. The choice of an appropriate osteotomy technique will depend on the type and location of deformity and the age of the patient. Adequate internal fixation is imperative for uninterrupted healing, and generally is identical to that required for a type A fracture of the bone as described in previous chapters. It would be tragic to convert a malunion into a nonunion due to poor choice of fixation.

Clinical Considerations in Common Malunions

Femur

Malunion of the femoral shaft can be disastrous due to the complexity of the resulting changes. The proximal femur and neck undergo anteversion and valgus angulation, especially in immature animals. Both changes destabilize the hip joint and lead to dysplasia-like changes. Proximal femoral intertrochanteric varus and derotational osteotomy may be needed to correct the hip changes.

Severe degenerative changes in the hip probably warrant total hip replacement or excision arthroplasty.

Torsional and angular changes in the shaft also can predispose to patellar luxation, usually lateral. Conventional patellar stabilization techniques may suffice if the structural changes are minor, but diaphyseal osteotomy may be necessary in more severe cases. Closing wedge techniques are usually preferred due to their inherent stability and because loss of length is rarely a problem.

Marked overriding of fragments results in severe shortening of the quadriceps and hamstring muscles. Lengthening osteotomies may be difficult to perform due to these soft tissue changes. Sciatic nerve entrapment and hyperextension of the stifle are potential problems associated with femoral malunions and must be dealt with appropriately.

Other Long Bones

Malunion of the tibia and radius/ulna typically result in tarsal/carpal valgus and external rotation. Treatment of humeral malunion, as with fractures of this bone, requires identification and protection of the radial nerve.

Pelvis

Pelvic malunion may affect the rectum and/or the hip joint. Chronic constipation results from narrowing of the pelvic canal. Treatment is pubic osteotomy, followed by spreading to enlarge the canal (see Chapter 14) or by triple pelvic osteotomy (see Chapter 15). Malarticulation of the hip joint due to pelvic fracture can result in severe degenerative joint disease. If treated early, triple pelvic osteotomy may stabilize the joint. After severe degenerative joint disease is present, only excision arthroplasty or total hip replacement offers relief.

Mandible

Mandibular malunions may result in poor mastication and wear of the teeth. They are usually better handled by extraction of the involved teeth than by osteotomy of the mandible.

References

1. Salter RB, Harris WR: Injuries involving the epiphyseal plate. J Bone Joint Surg 45-A:587–622, 1953.
2. O'Brien T, Morgan JP, Suter PF: A radiographic study of growth disturbances in the forelimb. J Small Anim Pract 12:19–35, 1971.
3. Noser G, Carrig CB, Merkley D, et al: Asynchronous growth of the canine radius and ulna: Effects of cross-pinning the radius to the ulna. Am J Vet Res 38:601–610, 1977.
4. Skaggs S, DeAngelis MP, Rosen H: Deformities due to premature closure of the distal ulna in fourteen dogs: A radiographic evaluation. J Am Anim Hosp Assoc 9:496–500, 1973.
5. Piermattei DL: An Atlas of Surgical Approaches to the Bones and Joints of the Dog and Cat, 3rd ed. Philadelphia, WB Saunders Co, 1993.
6. Vandewater A, Olmstead ML, Stevenson S: Partial ulnar ostectomy with free autogenous fat grafting for treatment of radius curvus in the dog. Vet Surg 11:92–99, 1982.
7. Shields LH, Gambardella PC: Premature closure of the ulnar physis in the dog: A retrospective clinical study. J Am Anim Hosp Assoc 25:573–581, 1989.
8. Gilson SD, Piermattei DL, Schwarz AD: Treatment of humeroulnar ulnar subluxation using a dynamic ulnar osteotomy. A review of 13 cases. Vet Surg 18:114, 1989.
9. Vandewater A, Olmstead ML: Premature closure of the distal radial physis in the dog: A review of eleven cases. Vet Surg 12:7–12, 1983.
10. Riser WH, Shirer JF: Normal and abnormal growth of the distal foreleg in large and giant breed dogs. J Am Vet Radiol Soc VI:50–64, 1965.
11. Olsson SE: Osteochondrosis in the dog. In Kirk RW (ed): Current Veterinary Therapy VI. Philadelphia, WB Saunders Co, 1980.
12. Macpherson GC, Lewis DD, et al: Fragmented coronoid process associated with premature distal radial physeal closure in four dogs. Vet Comp Orthop Comp Trauma 5:93–99, 1992.

13. Olson NC, Brinker WO, Carrig CB, et al: Asynchronous growth of the canine radius and ulna: Surgical correction following experimental premature closure of the distal radial physis. J Vet Surg 10:3, 1981.
14. Egger EL: Premature radial physeal closure. In Slatter D (ed): Textbook of Small Animal Surgery, 2nd ed. Philadephia, WB Saunders Co, 1993, pp 1754–1756.
15. Shields LH, Gambardella PC: Partial ulnar ostectomy for treatment of premature closure of the proximal and distal radial physes in the dog. J Am Anim Hosp Assoc 26:183–188, 1990.
16. Elkins AD, Morandi M, Zembo M: Distraction osteogenesis in the dog using the Ilizarov external ring fixator. J Am Anim Hosp Assoc 29:419–426, 1993.
17. Latte Y: Treatment of radius curvus by Ilizarov apparatus. Proc Vet Orthop Soc 16:1989.
18. Manfretta SM, Schrader SC: Physeal injuries in the dog: A review of 135 cases. J Am Vet Med Assoc 182:708–710, 1983.
19. Jevens DJ, DeCamp CE: Bilateral distal fibular growth abnormalities in a dog. J Am Vet Med Assoc 202:421–422, 1993.
20. Johnson SG, Hulse DA, et al: Corrective osteotomy for pes varus in the dachshund. Vet Surg 18:373–379, 1989.
21. Kaderly RE: Delayed union, nonunion, and malunion. In Slatter D (ed): Textbook of Small Animal Surgery, 2nd ed. Philadelphia, WB Saunders Co, 1993, pp 1682–1684.

PART V

MISCELLANEOUS CONDITIONS OF THE MUSCULOSKELETAL SYSTEM

23

Disease Conditions in Small Animals

Panosteitis

Panosteitis is a very common condition of long bones in large breeds of young dogs, especially the German shepherd and bassett hound. The condition is also called eosinophilic panosteitis, osteomyelitis, enostosis, fibrous osteodystrophy, juvenile osteomyelitis,[1] and "eo pan" or "long-bone disease" by breeders.

Although this disease causes severe lameness, it is self-limiting, and there is no permanent impairment. Therefore, because the condition gets better "by itself," intensive investigations of the various stages of this disease have been lacking. Many contradictions exist as to its clinical features.

The etiology of panosteitis is unknown, although infection, metabolic disease, endocrine dysfunction, allergy, autoimmune mechanisms, parasitism, and hereditary factors have been postulated.[1] Viral infection appears the most probable cause of panosteitis.[2] In a recent review of this condition,[3] there is no new information as to its cause.

Clinical Signs

The clinical picture is that of a healthy dog with lameness of acute onset but no history of trauma. Males are affected four times more often than females.[4] The lameness may be marked, and often the dog will "carry" or favor the limb. This lameness may last a few days to several weeks.[4] In about 53 percent of cases, other limbs have become involved, thereby characterizing the condition as causing a "shifting leg lameness."[5] These recurring bouts usually subside by the time the animal reaches 2 years of age.[1] However, dogs up to 5 years of age have incurred panosteitis.[5,6]

Examination

Gentle palpation along the distal, middle, and proximal areas of long bones may elicit exquisite pain when the involved area is reached, even in stoic animals. This reaction may consist of crying out, wincing, pulling the leg away, or, occasionally, snapping at the examiner. When palpating, the clinician's fingers should push aside muscle bundles (especially of the humerus and femur) so that bone is reached prior to squeezing. This avoids misinterpretation arising from hurting normal muscle tissue trapped in the palpation.

Depending on when thorough veterinary attention is sought and how elaborate the workup completed, other factors may be present, such as fever,[1,4] muscle atrophy,[4] eosinophilia,[1,4] decreased activity, and inappetence. Others have disclaimed the occurrence of fever, muscle atrophy,[6] and eosinophilia.[6] Eosinophilia has been reported to be seen only in the first 2 days of clinical signs.[1]

Radiographic Signs

Radiographically, the disease may be separated into three stages.[6] Often, the clinician sees the case in the middle phase and the other stages only during extensive studies of this condition.

EARLY PHASE ■ Although the limb may be asymptomatic, radiographic changes may be detected during a survey of all the long bones. These consist of blurring and accentuation of trabecular patterns, best seen at the proximal and distal ends of the diaphysis (Figure 23–1). The contrast between the cortex and medullary canals is diminished. In some cases, a few granular densities are seen.

MIDDLE PHASE ■ Patchy, mottled, sclerotic-looking densities appear, especially around the nutrient foramen in the early stages (Fig. 23–2). In some cases, the entire diaphysis is involved; in others, there may be only pea-sized lesions (Fig. 23–3). In a third of panosteitis cases, the periosteum becomes involved. Initially, a subtle roughening appears that becomes more dense within 1 or 2 weeks and eventually becomes as dense as the cortex (Figs. 23–2 and 23–3).

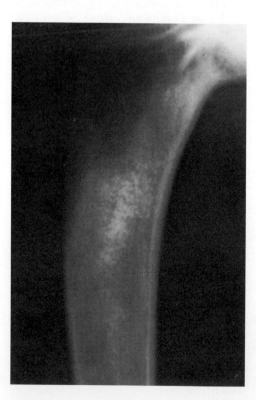

FIGURE 23–1. Early stage of eosinophilic panosteitis in the humerus of a 9-month-old male German shepherd. Granular densities are seen.

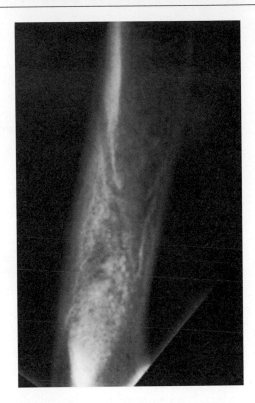

FIGURE 23-2. Middle stage of eosinophilic panosteitis with increased densities around the nutrient foramen in a 6-month-old male Great Pyrenees. Note the periosteal thickening caudal to the foramen.

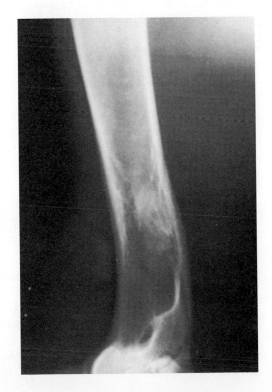

FIGURE 23-3. Middle stage of eosinophilic panosteitis showing a small sclerotic area in the distal humerus of a 6-month-old German shepherd. Note the thickened caudal cortex adjacent to the sclerotic patch.

LATE PHASE ■   In the process of recovery, the medullary canal attains normal density while the coarse trabecular pattern remains. In about a third of the cases, the cortex remains thicker than normal. A few granular densities may be present. It may require several months for these changes to disappear completely. In general, the lesions affect the central part of the radius, the proximal third of the ulna, the distal and central parts of the humerus, the proximal third of the tibia, and the central and proximal parts of the femur.

Histopathology

Histopathological findings[6] of the lesions consist of accentuation of osteoblastic and fibroblastic activity in the periosteum, endosteum, and marrow. Fibrosis occurs in the marrow. There is evidence of neither acute or chronic inflammation nor malignancy. In highly mature lesions, the cortical thickening consists of thickened lamellar bone with haversian systems, whereas in immature lesions, cellular fiber bone is present with many osteoblasts and osteoclasts.

Differential Diagnosis

Differential diagnosis includes osteochondritis dissecans, fragmented coronoid process, ununited anconeal process, hip dysplasia, cruciate disease, coxofemoral luxation, and fractures. When there is a shifting leg lameness, other conditions such as rheumatoid arthritis, systemic lupus erythematosus (SLE), or bacterial endocarditis must be considered. The diagnosis of panosteitis is determined by palpation and radiography.

Treatment

Treatment is symptomatic to relieve pain by using aspirin, corticosteroids, and other agents. None of these has been documented to hasten the resolution of the condition.[1,3]

NUTRITIONAL DISORDERS

Although nutritional problems affecting bone and muscle are beyond the scope of this text,[1,7–11] some clinical situations that may confront the orthopedist are considered.

Clinical Problems

There are three clinical problems we see: obesity, consequences of the all-meat diet, and oversupplementation in large and giant breeds of dogs.

Obesity

Although obesity has not been proved to cause osteoarthritis, at least in mice,[12] common sense tells us that excessive weight on injured or congenitally deformed joints or spinal conditions can affect musculoskeletal performance. Prevention of obesity is obviously accomplished more readily than treatment. Interesting clinical studies in people have shown that obesity precedes and increases the risk of osteoarthrosis of the knee (especially women)[13,14] and probably results from mechanical stresses.[15] In addition, other studies suggest that weight loss can both prevent the onset of symptomatic osteoarthrosis of the knee[16,17] and alleviate pain when present.[16] If the veterinary clinician observes patients gaining weight, or if an animal has a potential for arthritis or back problems or becomes neutered, the client should be warned to watch the animal's weight carefully and to cut back food intake before weight gain becomes unmanageable. In known periods of inactivity (e.g., the winter months, or cessation of the hunting season), food intake should be diminished.

If an animal is obese, the endocrine system, especially the thyroid, should be examined. For a "diet," we usually recommend cutting the total daily caloric intake by one third to one half in order to reduce the animal's weight. Canine vitamin supplementation may be administered to alleviate the owner's apprehension concerning dietary restriction. Often, if the owner is sincere and conscientious, decreasing the amount of presently fed food by one third to one half is all that is necessary. Owners (even those who are themselves overweight) seem to understand and accept "the more weight your pet carries, the more it abuses its bad joint, which could potentially hasten joint destruction, necessitating surgery or leading to a painful life." When this does not seem to be effective, prescribed reducing diets may be tried. Our usual goal is to achieve a conformation in which there is an observable indentation or "waist" along the flank region and the presence of individually palpable ribs. Some clients may need to be told, "Your dog needs to lose 4 pounds," instead of these guidelines. For a lighter weight breed, the owner may monitor progress using a bathroom scale at home.

The All-Meat Diet

Publicity concerning all-meat diets has been widespread enough that the syndrome is rarely seen today. Low in calcium and high in phosphorus, this diet has the tendency to cause secondary nutritional hyperparathyroidism (SNH), a condition in which the parathyroids are stimulated to secrete parathormone. This hormone increases the resorption of calcium from bone in order to maintain proper serum levels. In the young animal, the result may be loss of skeletal density and thinning of the bone cortex. Lameness or pathological fracture may result (Fig. 23–4). In an adult animal that is fed an all-meat diet, the process is slow and can result in osteopenia. Treatment involves feeding the animal a balanced commercial diet as well as supplementation with calcium.

Hypernutrition and Oversupplementation

The most perplexing nutritional problem facing the orthopedist is presented when a breeder asks the veterinary clinician to test serum calcium and phosphorus levels in a young dog of large or giant breed that has poor bony conformation. Although it may appear that improper nutrition is to blame, this may or may not be the answer. A few points are worth emphasizing in this regard. In giant breeds, the phosphorus may be twice as high in the dog 3 to 6 months old as in the adult (8.7 mg/100 ml versus 4.2 mg/100 ml). The calcium may be slightly higher in a younger animal (11.1 mg/100 ml versus 9.9 mg/100 ml for an adult).[7] In those dogs with known dietary excesses or imbalances of calcium and phosphorus, the serum calcium and phosphorus levels usually are in the normal range as a result of the dog's homeostatic mechanisms, if the parathyroid gland is working properly. More sensitive indicators of dietary imbalance are the quantities of calcium and phosphorus excreted in the urine over 24 hours and the creatinine clearance ratios.

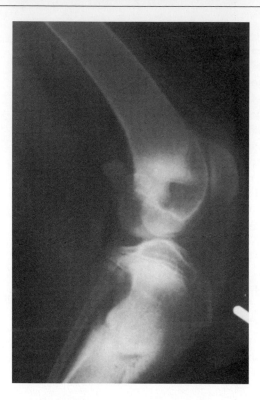

FIGURE 23–4. Five-month-old male Gordon setter with pathological fracture of the tibia from secondary nutritional hyperparathyroidism. Note the thin cortices of the femur. This dog was fed a balanced home diet by a breeder using egg shells (which are not absorbed in the canine intestine) for the calcium source.

Most commercial dry dog foods contain the proper quantities of and balance between calcium and phosphorus. People owning large breeds feel that this commercial diet may be good for the normal "run-of-the-mill" dog, but not for their dog, which is going to be large. Often the owner feeds a mixture of foods suggested by the breeder, for whom the diet produced champions. These mixtures include vitamins, dicalcium phosphate, bone meal, high-protein cereals, meat, milk, cottage cheese, eggs, wheat germ, and other nutrients. This highly palatable diet may lead to an ingestion of excessive quantities of nutrients that can lead to a nutritional imbalance. Young Great Danes fed a balanced diet ad libitum had accelerated bone growth, sinking of the metacarpophalangeal joints, lateral deviation of the forepaws (valgus deformity of the carpus), cow-hocked rear limbs, enlargement of the distal radial and ulnar metaphyses, enlargements of the costochondral junctions, pain, arched backs, and inactivity. Those dogs fed two thirds of the quantity of protein and calories of the other group had slower bone growth and better conformation, and they were more active and playful.[9] It is therefore wise for the veterinarian to discuss diet with the owners of these large breeds. The importance of slow bone growth should be stressed, and the owners should be warned not to push their dogs nutritionally.

Signs of overnutrition may be mistaken for "rickets" and therefore improper acceleration of the plane of nutrition prescribed. Rickets is extremely rare and has been seen usually only under starvation or research conditions.

The valgus deformity of the carpus may correct itself when the diet is changed while the dog is still growing. Severe deformities, however, may require corrective osteotomy after skeletal maturity is complete.

HYPERTROPHIC OSTEODYSTROPHY

Hypertrophic osteodystrophy (HO), vitamin C deficiency, metaphyseal osteodystrophy, or scurvy,[19] is a syndrome seen in young dogs of medium and giant breeds (Great Danes, Irish setters, boxers, Labrador retrievers). The condition is characterized by grossly observable swellings of the distal metaphyses of the radius, ulna, and tibia. This disorder has been misinterpreted by some clinicians as joint swellings. The etiology is unknown.

Clinical Signs

Often the dog appears to show systemic involvement with pyrexia, anorexia, pain, arched back, and reluctance to move,[1] and often has a history of diarrhea the preceding week.[19] Cranial bowing of the forelegs and a valgus deformity of the carpus may occur.[5] The acute phase may last 7 to 10 days[1]; however, recurrences have been seen.[19]

Radiographic Signs

Radiographically, the initial finding is a thin, radiolucent line in the metaphysis parallel to the epiphyseal plate especially of the radius. Secondarily, there is an extraperiosteal cuff of calcification along the metaphysis (Fig. 23–5). The lucent line disappears and is replaced by an increased radiodensity. If relapses occur, a new radiolucent line appears between the physis and the radiodense region.[20] As the dog matures, these extraperiosteal thickenings often regress (Figs. 23–6 and 23–7), but may leave a permanently thickened metaphysis.[21]

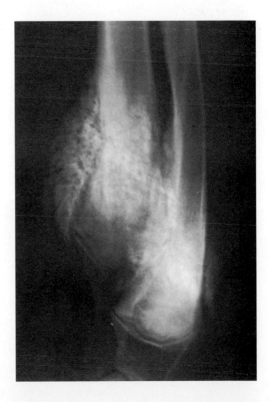

FIGURE 23–5. Six-month-old male Great Dane with extraperiosteal proliferation and calcification of the distal radius and ulna.

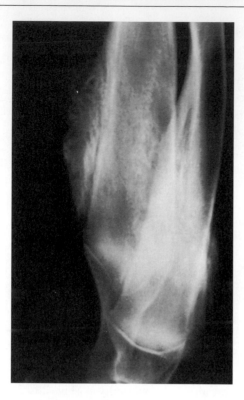

FIGURE 23–6. Same dog as shown in Figure 23–5, now 9 months old.

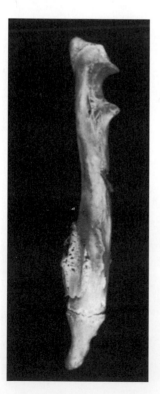

FIGURE 23–7. Gross specimen of the ulna shown in Figure 23–6.

Pathogenesis

The scurvy theory arises from the radiographic similarity to scorbutic changes seen in children.[1] Whether hypertrophic osteodystrophy and scurvy are the same disease or whether vitamin C deficiency is involved at all remains to be proved.[19] The mean value of serum ascorbic acid in 18 dogs with hypertrophic osteodystrophy was only slightly below the mean of serum ascorbic acid in 28 normal young large breeds of dogs.[19] Since serum ascorbic acid levels vary with exercise, food intake, and stress, these values may be meaningless, since dogs with hypertrophic osteodystrophy are under stress and anorexic. There is circumstantial evidence that the canine distemper virus may be involved with HO especially after vaccination. Virus has been detected in bones of some dogs with HO.[22]

Treatment

This disease appears to improve with whatever treatment is undertaken. In one study, 24 dogs were managed by one of these methods: no treatment; antibiotics; antibiotics and corticosteroids; or antibiotics, corticosteroids, and vitamin C. There was no statistical difference in the rates of recoveries between these treatments.[19] Most dogs recovered from systemic signs in 7 to 10 days,[1,19] whereas bony changes have required several months for resorption.[21] In severe cases, if bacteremia has been proven by blood cultures, broad-spectrum antibiotics are indicated.[20] Death has been reported in some instances.[19] Generally, analgesics and antidiarrheal medications are indicated.

RENAL OSTEODYSTROPHY

Although renal osteodystrophy, or "renal rickets," is infrequently seen by the orthopedist, it can occasionally produce pathological fractures or give appearance of generalized skeletal demineralization upon radiography. With renal disease, phosphorus is retained, which causes secondary hyperparathyroidism similar to that caused by nutritional imbalances or excesses of phosphorus.

When an adult dog spontaneously fractures a leg or jaw or experiences minimal trauma such as falling down two stairs, particular attention should be paid to the density of the bone on the radiograph. It is only with chronic severe kidney disease that the bone will show obvious demineralization, and usually the client would have sought veterinary attention because of the problems related to uremia.

HYPERTROPHIC PULMONARY OSTEOPATHY

Hypertrophic pulmonary osteopathy (HPO) has been known as hypertrophic pulmonary osteoarthropathy (HPOA)[23] and hypertrophic osteoarthropathy (HOA).[24] HPOA is a misnomer because the joints are not really involved, and some prefer HOA because the lung occasionally is not involved.[24]

Clinical Signs

This syndrome is characterized by lameness, reluctance to move, and firm swellings of the distal limbs. The lungs usually are involved. In a study of 60

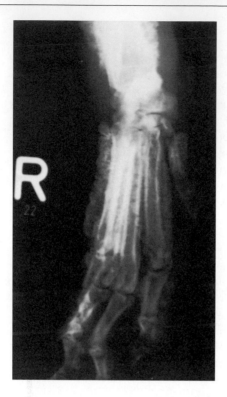

FIGURE 23–8. Phalanges, metacarpus, radius, and ulna affected with hypertrophic pulmonary osteopathy in a 5-year-old female collie mix with metastatic carcinoma to the lungs from the ovaries or uterus.

cases, 30 percent showed thoracic disease signs prior to musculoskeletal signs.[24] Lung disease was eventually seen in 95 percent of the cases. The cause of the thoracic disease was cancer in 91 percent. *Spirocerca lupi* infestation of the esophagus and dirofilariasis can also cause HPO.

Radiographic Signs

The classic radiographic signs of HPO consist of extensive, rough periosteal formation beginning in the distal phalanges, metacarpal bones, and metatarsal bones (Fig. 23–8). Other bones may become involved (Fig. 23–9). In peracute

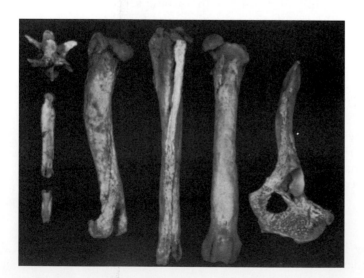

FIGURE 23–9. Gross appearance of an 8-year-old German shepherd with hypertrophic pulmonary osteopathy affecting the vertebrae, pelvis, long bones, and metacarpal and phalangeal bones.

cases with swollen limbs, the radiographs may not show the extensive periosteal changes, but such changes will be apparent within a few days.

Pathogenesis

The pathogenesis of these periosteal changes is speculative. Some theories include chronic anoxia, obscure toxins,[1] and autonomic neural vascular reflex mechanisms mediated by afferent branches of the vagus or intercostal nerves.[2,25] When HPO is diagnosed, a thorough diagnostic workup, especially of the thorax, is indicated. The probability of finding a nonlethal cause is low. Lung lobectomy may allow regression of bony lesions until death occurs or until additional lung cancer intercedes.[2,24,26] Bony changes may take 3 to 4 months to regress after lobectomy.[26] With possible nonlethal causes (i.e., *Spirocerca lupi* infestation, dirofilariasis), the removal of the inciting cause may or may not bring about regression of HPO signs.[23,24]

CRANIOMANDIBULAR OSTEOPATHY

An uncommon proliferative bone disease, craniomandibular osteopathy (CMO) ("lion jaw") usually involves the mandibular rami and the tympanic bullae in Scottish, cairn, and West Highland white terriers.[27] Other breeds that occasionally experience this condition include the Boston terrier, Labrador retriever, Great Dane, Doberman pinscher,[28] German shepherd, boxer, and a mongrel.[22] Other bones of the head and some long bones have occasionally been involved. In some animals, only the mandibles are involved, whereas in others only the tympanic bullae seem affected.

Occurrence

The occurrence of this disease is infrequently reported in the literature. At the small animal clinic at Michigan State University only seven cases were seen in 9 years (1970 to 1979), and during that time, a total of 130,000 admissions had been recorded. In a recent literature review,[22] collated data from 81 dogs was reported and information on an additional 13 cases was discussed.

Clinical Signs

The signs usually relate to persistent or intermittent pain around the mouth in growing male and female puppies 4 to 7 months of age. Mild cases may be asymptomatic and are discovered by palpation or radiography. If the angular processes of the mandible and tympanic bullae are involved, jaw movement is diminished, even under anesthesia. Temporal and masseter muscle atrophy is apparent. Nutrition may become inadequate if the condition is so severe that the dog cannot drink liquids. The mandibular thickening may be palpable and there may be intermittent fever. Exacerbations may recur every 2 to 3 weeks.[28] However, once skeletal maturation nears (11 to 12 months of age), the pain disappears and the exostoses may even regress.

Diagnosis

Diagnosis of craniomandibular osteopathy is made on the basis of breed, signs, physical findings, and radiography.

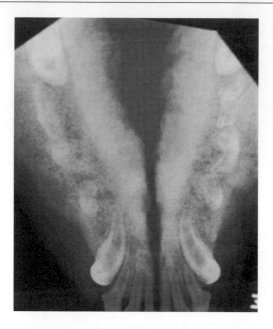

FIGURE 23–10. Open-mouth radiograph of a 6-month-old female West Highland white terrier with canine mandibular osteopathy. Note the bilateral roughened proliferations of the mandible.

Radiographic Signs

Radiography helps to document the condition. Changes consist of beadlike osseous proliferations of the mandible or tympanic bullae (Figs. 23–10 and 23–11). When the exostoses stop proliferating and eventually regress, the roughened borders become quite smooth. With early lesions, however, swellings may not be very radiopaque.

Histopathological Appearance

Histologically, normal lamellar bone is replaced by an enlarged coarse fiber (woven) bone. The bone marrow is replaced by a fibrous-type stroma and some inflammation.[27] Inflammatory cells at the periphery of the invading bone have

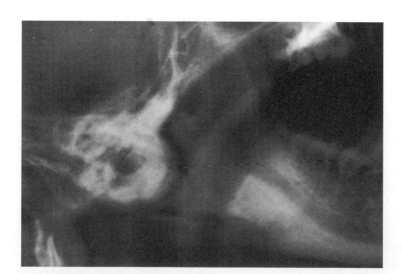

FIGURE 23–11. Proliferation of the tympanic bullae of a 7-month-old male Scottish terrier.

been documented and would seem to make this an inflammatory disease. However, others claim this to be a noninflammatory, nonclassifiable disease,[5,28,29] based upon earlier histopathological literature that may or may not have had sufficient case material to offer adequate study of the disease in various stages. Although the cause of CMO is unknown, one author has suggested possible infection (arising from the fever and histological inflammation at the periphery of the lesion), with a genetic influence, owing to its occurrence in the terrier breeds.[27] An autosomal recessive trait has been suggested.[30] A recent paper suggested that the canine distemper virus may be involved much like that suggested for hypertrophic osteodystrophy.[22]

Treatment

Treatment is usually aimed at decreasing pain and inflammation with medication such as aspirin, cortisone, and so forth. Signs may wax and wane spontaneously and the disease is self-limiting, which makes treatment responses in sporadic cases difficult to assess.[22] Surgical excision of the exostoses has resulted in regrowth within 3 weeks in one documented case.[29] Rostral hemimandibulectomy in one dog unable to move its jaws enabled better food intake resulting in weight gain.[22] Feeding highly nutritious fluids would be important in those dogs with minimal ability to open the mouth. Euthanasia may be necessary in a very few cases.

SYNOVIAL CHONDROMETAPLASIA

Synovial chondrometaplasia (SCM) is a condition in which nodules of sclerosis, fibrocartilage, and even bone form in the synovial layer of the joint capsule, causing chronic lameness in the dog.[31] Since that publication we have also seen SCM in a cat, as well as several more cases in the dog. SCM has been reported in the shoulder, stifle, and hock of dogs and in the tendon sheath and bursae of horses.[31-34] SCM affects the large joints in humans.[35]

The cause of the spontaneous nodular formation is unknown, but secondary SCM can be stimulated by traumatic, degenerative, or inflammatory conditions in humans.[35]

The diagnosis is made by radiography and histological examination of the joint capsule. Upon joint exploration, synovial biopsy should be performed when the synovial lining appears nodular. Differential diagnoses include synovial sarcoma, immune-mediated inflammatory joint disease, and infection. Multiple (10 to 100) joint mice seen radiographically, as well as nodular formation seen histologically, are diagnostic of the condition (Fig. 23–12). Surgical removal of loose bodies and partial synovectomy have resulted in marked improvement in most cases.[31]

SURGICAL ASPECTS OF LONG-BONE NEOPLASMS

Appendicular bone tumors may be separated into three categories:

1. Primary bone tumors (osteosarcoma, chondrosarcoma, or fibrosarcoma).

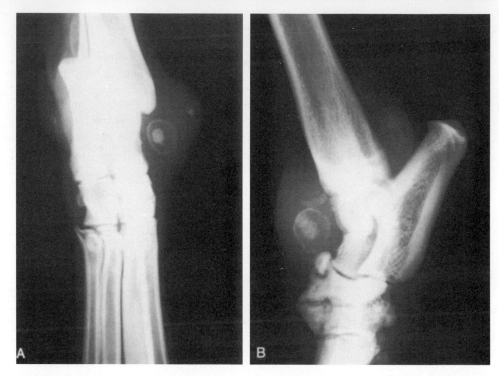

FIGURE 23–12. (A) Anteroposterior and (B) lateral radiographic views of a hock of a 1-year-old golden retriever with synovial chondrometaplasia (SCM). Note the severe soft tissue swelling and the multiple concentric loose bodies caudal to the distal tibia (in the flexor hallucis longus tendon sheath) and the talocrural joint.

    2.   Secondary metastatic tumors (rising most commonly from the mammary gland, lung, and prostate).

    3.   Local invasion from soft tissue tumors (such as synovial cell sarcoma).

All are malignant and carry a grave prognosis. Osteosarcoma is the most common tumor type seen in a dog's bone.

Often the presenting sign is lameness with or without systemic signs such as lethargy and anorexia. Neoplasia ought to be suspected and ruled out in the older dog with a rapidly progressive lameness (2 to 4 weeks) as well as swelling. Palpation may reveal muscle atrophy, swelling, and increased heat and sensitivity. Neoplasia should also be suspected in dogs sustaining fractures following minimal or no trauma. Careful scrutiny of good-quality radiographs is a must in such cases.

Fine-detail radiography is often the best diagnostic tool to use in finding bone neoplasia, but it may be inappropriate to predict histological type based upon radiographs.[36] However, often the radiograph is very characteristic and therefore diagnostic of osteosarcoma. Biopsy in such cases is sometimes misleading owing to the lack of tumor cells in small biopsy samples. Biopsy should be used, however, on uncharacteristic lesions, especially if potentially curable conditions exist (e.g., infection, cysts, undifferentiated carcinoma, lymphomas, transmissible venereal tumor, and plasma cell myeloma). Biopsy is also helpful when an owner wants a more knowledgeable answer as to the probable life expectancy of his pet. Chondrosarcoma and fibrosarcoma are slow growing, allowing slower progression until natural death.

Limb amputation is the most frequent surgical treatment in the dog and cat, with or without chemotherapy. It improves the quality of life, but 85 percent of dogs still die within 8 months after amputation.[37,38]

Recent advances in treatment of osteosarcoma in humans have increased overall survival rates to 60 to 70 percent in patients with nonmetastatic osteosarcoma.[39] However, 80 to 90 percent of humans do not have gross evidence of metastatic disease in the bone at the time of osteosarcoma diagnosis.[39] This is in contrast to our canine patients, in which 85 to 90 percent have metastatic disease when the primary tumor is removed.[38] Treatments in people include various chemotherapy regimens, pulmonary resection of metastases (often multiple surgeries), and limb salvage procedures. The goals of limb salvage procedures are to remove the tumor completely and to avoid local recurrence while reconstructing a functional extremity.[39] Endoprostheses (metal, allografts, or autoclaved autograft of resected tumor) may be inserted. However, the overall survival rates have not differed from those seen with amputation.[39] Ten percent of dogs undergoing amputation or limb sparing alone will survive 1 year.[40]

Limb salvage in dogs has been used in selected cases and includes tumor resection and stabilization using whole cortical allografts and bone plates.[38,41] The use of cisplatin is showing early improved survival rates with more than 50 percent of dogs living 1 year following treatment.[38] If limb sparing or amputation is combined with cisplatin, 35 to 50 percent will survive 1 year.[42] Newer immunotherapeutic regimens are being investigated,[4] but at this time the prognosis remains grave for long-term benefit.

References

1. McKeown S, Archibald J: The musculoskeletal system. In Cattcott ES (ed): Canine Medicine, 4th ed. Santa Barbara, American Veterinary Publications, Inc, 1979, pp 533–678.
2. Johnson KA, Watson ADH, Page RL: Skeletal diseases. In Ettinger SJ, Feldman EC (eds): Textbook of Veterinary Internal Medicine, 4th ed. Philadelphia, WB Saunders Co, 1995, pp 2077–2106.
3. Muir P, Dubielzig RR, Johnson KA: Panosteitis. Compend Cont Educ Pract Vet 18:29–34, 1996.
4. Barrett RB, Schall WD, Lewis RE: Clinical and radiographic features of canine eosinophilic panosteitis. J Am Anim Hosp Assoc 4:94–104, 1968.
5. Brown SG: Skeletal diseases. In Ettinger SJ (ed): Textbook of Veterinary Internal Medicine. Philadelphia, WB Saunders Co, 1975, pp 1715–1741.
6. Bohning R Jr, Suter P, Hohn RB, Marshall J: Clinical and radiographic survey of canine panosteitis. J Am Vet Med Assoc 156:870–884, 1970.
7. Fletch SM, Smart ME: Blood chemistry of the giant breeds—bone profile. Bull Am Soc Vet Clin Pathol 2:30, 1973.
8. Morris ML: Nutrition and disease. In Cattcott EJ (ed): Canine Medicine, 4th ed. Santa Barbara, American Veterinary Publications, Inc, 1979, pp 223–252.
9. Hedhammar A, Wu FM, Krook L, et al: Oversupplementation and skeletal disease: An experimental study in growing Great Dane dogs. Cornell Vet 64(Suppl 5):32–45, 1974.
10. Krook L: Nutritional hypercalcitoninism. In Kirk RW (ed): Current Veterinary Therapy. VI. Philadelphia, WB Saunders Co, 1977, pp 1048–1050.
11. Krook L: Metabolic bone disease in dogs and cats. Proc Am Anim Hosp Assoc, 38th Annual Meeting, 1971, pp 350–355.
12. Moskowitz RW: Symptoms and laboratory findings in osteoarthritis. In Hollander JL (ed): Arthritis and Allied Conditions. Philadelphia, Lea & Febiger, 1972, pp 1032–1053.
13. Felson DT: The epidemiology of knee osteoarthrosis: Results from the Framingham Osteoarthritis Study. Semin Arthritis Rheum 20:42–50, 1990.
14. Felson DT, Anderson JJ, Naimark A, et al: Obesity and knee osteoarthritis. The Framingham Study. Ann Intern Med 109:18–24, 1988.
15. Hartz AJ, Fischer ME, Bril G, et al: The association of obesity with joint pain and osteoarthritis in the HANES data. J Chronic Dis 39:311, 1986.

16. Felson DT: Weight and osteoarthritis. J Rheumatol Suppl 43:7–9, 1995.
17. Felson DT, Zhang Y, Anthony JM, et al: Weight loss reduces the risk for symptomatic knee osteoarthritis in women. The Framingham Study. Ann Intern Med 116:535–539, 1992.
18. Olsson SE: Osteochondrosis—a growing problem to dog breeders. Gaines Dog Research Progress, White Plains, NY, Gaines Dog Research Center, Summer 1976, pp 1–11.
19. Grondalen J: Metaphyseal osteodystrophy (hypertrophic osteodystrophy) in growing dogs. A clinical study. J Small Anim Pract 17:721, 1976.
20. Muir P, Dubielzig RR, Johnson KA: Hypertrophic osteodystrophy and calvarial hyperostosis. Compend Cont Educ Pract Vet 18:143–152, 1996.
21. Morgan JP: Radiology in Veterinary Orthopedics, 1st ed. Philadelphia, Lea & Febiger, 1972.
22. Watson ADJ, Adams WM, Thomas CB: Craniomandibular osteopathy in dogs. Compend Cont Educ Pract Vet 17:911–923, 1995.
23. Thrasher JP: Hypertrophic pulmonary osteoarthropathy. J Am Vet Med Assoc 39:441–448, 1961.
24. Brodey RS: Hypertrophic osteoarthropathy in the dog: A clinicopathologic survey of 60 cases. J Am Vet Med Assoc 159:1242–1255, 1971.
25. Holling HE, et al: Hypertrophic pulmonary osteoarthropathy. J Thorac Cardiovasc Surg 46:310–321, 1963.
26. Suter PF: Pulmonary neoplasia. In Ettinger SJ (ed): Textbook of Veterinary Internal Medicine. Philadelphia, WB Saunders Co, 1975, pp 754–766.
27. Riser WF, Parkes LJ, Shirer JF: Canine craniomandibular osteopathy. J Am Vet Radiol Soc 8:23–30, 1967.
28. Palmer N: Bones and joints. In Jubb KVF, Kennedy PC, Palmer N (eds): Pathology of Domestic Animals, 4th ed. San Diego, Academic Press, 1993, pp 1–181.
29. Pool RR, Leighton RL: Craniomandibular osteopathy in the dog. J Am Vet Med Assoc 154:657–660, 1969.
30. Padgett GA, Mostosky UV: Animal model: The mode of inheritance of craniomandibular osteopathy in the West Highland white terriers. Am J Genet 25:9–13, 1986.
31. Flo GL, Stickle RL, Dunstan RW: Synovial chondrometaplasia in five dogs. J Am Vet Med Assoc 191:1417–1422, 1987.
32. Schmidt E, Schneider J: Synovial chondromatosis in the horse. Monatsschr Vet 37:509, 1982.
33. Schawalder von P: Die synoviale osteochondromatose (synoviale chondrometaplasie) biem Hund. Schweiz Arch Tierheilk 122:673–678, 1980.
34. Kirk MD: Radiographic and histologic appearance of synovial osteochondromatosis of the femorotibial bursa in a horse. A case history report. Vet Radiol 23:167–170, 1982.
35. Schajowicz F: Tumor and Tumor-like Lesions of Bones and Joints. New York, Springer-Verlag, 1981.
36. Probst CW, Ackerman N: Malignant neoplasia of the canine appendicular skeleton. Compend Cont Educ Pract Vet 4(3):260–270, 1982.
37. Brodey RS, Abt DA: Results of surgical treatment in 65 dogs with osteosarcoma. J Am Vet Med Assoc 168:1032, 1976.
38. Withrow SJ, LaRue SM, Powers BE, et al: Osteosarcoma: New trends in treatment. In 10th Annual Kal Kan Symposium for the Treatment of Small Animal Disease, October, 1986.
39. Goorin Am, Abelson HT, Frei E: Osteosarcoma: Fifteen years later. N Engl J Med 313(26):1637–1642, 1985.
40. Spodnick GL, et al: Prognosis for dogs with appendicular osteosarcoma treated by amputation alone: 162 cases (1978–1988). J Am Vet Med Assoc 200:995, 1992.
41. Vasseur PB: Limb salvage in a dog with chondrosarcoma of the tibia. J Am Vet Med Assoc 187(6):620–623, 1985.
42. Withrow SJ, et al: Recent advances in surgical oncology. Compend Cont Educ Pract Vet 15:939, 1993.

INDEX

Note: Page numbers in *italics* refer to illustrations; page numbers followed by t refer to tables.

ISBN 0-7216-5689-7